Peripheral Nerve Injury

An Anatomical and Physiological Approach for Physical Therapy Intervention

Stephen J. Carp, PT, PhD, GCS
Doctor of Physical Therapy Program
Temple University
College of Public Health

F.A. Davis Company • Philadelphia

F. A. Davis Company
1915 Arch Street
Philadelphia, PA 19103
www.fadavis.com

Printed in the United States of America

Last digit indicates print number: 10 9 8 7 6 5 4 3 2 1

Senior Acquisitions Editor: Melissa Duffield
Developmental Editor: Andrea Edwards
Director of Content Development: George Lang
Design and Illustration Manager: Carolyn O'Brien

As new scientific information becomes available through basic and clinical research, recommended treatments and drug therapies undergo changes. The author(s) and publisher have done everything possible to make this book accurate, up to date, and in accord with accepted standards at the time of publication. The author(s), editors, and publisher are not responsible for errors or omissions or for consequences from application of the book, and make no warranty, expressed or implied, in regard to the contents of the book. Any practice described in this book should be applied by the reader in accordance with professional standards of care used in regard to the unique circumstances that may apply in each situation. The reader is advised always to check product information (package inserts) for changes and new information regarding dose and contraindications before administering any drug. Caution is especially urged when using new or infrequently ordered drugs.

Library of Congress Control Number: 2015935849

For Diane, Julia, Jennifer, and Emily. Thank you for a lifetime of love

I wish to thank all my teachers and mentors—especially Dick Williams, Carole Steinruck, Mark McCandless, Emily Keshner, and Mom and Dad. Your dedication to my education is as responsible for this publication as was my writing. A special thanks to all my students and especially to Dr. Michael O'Hara for his editorial assistance. Lastly, a thank you to Melissa Duffield who believed in my writing before I did.

PREFACE

Sadly, and for a multitude of reasons, the incidence and prevalence of peripheral neuropathy in the United States and around the world continue to increase. We are all well aware of the number of Americans affected by diabetes mellitus and one of its most common complications, peripheral neuropathy. Another complication of diabetes mellitus is chronic kidney disease. Kidney disease, separate from diabetes, is in itself an indirect cause of peripheral neuropathy. As the number of HIV infections continues to increase worldwide, we are seeing an increasing number of patients with HIV-related neuropathic complications. Peripheral neuropathy is a common side effect of scores of prescribed (and illegal) drugs. Cancers and their sequelae—paraneoplastic syndrome, complications of chemotherapy and surgeries, and space-occupying tumors—often lead to peripheral neuropathy. Nerve injuries may result from low-force, high-repetition activities such as keyboard typing, overhead work, and musical instrument playing. Exposure to environmental toxins such as lead, mercury, and arsenic, prevalent in some areas of the United States and the world, may cause nerve injury. A common risk factor for falls is lower extremity neuropathy. The list goes on and on. Peripheral neuropathy is becoming a very common presenting and comorbid diagnosis for rehabilitation professionals.

Peripheral neuropathy may affect motor neurons, sensory neurons, and regulatory (autonomic) neurons. The functional impact may range from minimal to severe. The spectrum of motor neuropathy may range from weakness of muscles within the myotomal distribution of one nerve (mononeuropathy) to weakness of many muscles innervated by many nerves (systemic polyneuropathy). The severity of weakness may range from subclinical to flaccid paralysis. The spectrum of sensory loss is even greater than that of motor neuropathy. There may be positive (additive) signs such as paresthesia, radicular pain, and multisegmental pain. There may be negative signs such as loss of tactile, temperature, pain, somatosensory (proprioception and kinesthesia), vestibular, and vibratory senses. Lastly, pathology of the regulatory neurons may lead to aberrant and inappropriate blood pressure and cardiac responses to positional change and exercise. There may be delayed healing, loss of toenails and fingernails, and trophic skin changes.

Peripheral Nerve Injury: An Anatomical and Physiological Approach to Pathology and Intervention is the first comprehensive textbook written for rehabilitation professionals—physical therapists, occupational therapists, physical therapy assistants, occupational therapy assistants, physician assistants, nurse practitioners, athletic trainers, and orthotists/prosthetists—with content related to the etiology and intervention of diagnoses of peripheral neuropathy. In addition, primary care physicians, nurses, vocational rehabilitation specialists, and insurance providers may find the text helpful with their practices.

The textbook is divided into five content areas:

1. Overview of the peripheral nervous system and biomechanics of peripheral nerve: This section includes chapters related to the anatomy and physiology of the peripheral nerve, the biomechanics of healthy and damaged nerve, and the pathophysiology of the peripheral nervous system. This section contains a focused blueprint of the impact of the inflammatory cascade on peripheral nerves associated with injury and illness.

2. Etiologies of peripheral nerve injury: This section examines common pathologies that either directly or indirectly injure peripheral nerves. Pathologies examined include vasculitic, connective tissue, and seronegative spondyloarthropathies; environmental toxins; critical illness myopathy/polyneuropathy; diabetes mellitus; infection; nutritional deficiencies; chronic kidney disease; and neuropathic complications of common medications.

3. Evaluation of a patient with suspected peripheral nerve injury: This section includes chapters on the physical examination of individuals with suspected peripheral neuropathy, the use of laboratory tests and

measures in the investigation of suspected neuropathy, and an overview of electroneurodiagnostic testing.

4. Evidenced-based interventions for individuals with peripheral nerve injury: These chapters provide a clear summary of the rehabilitative modalities and interventions that may be used to treat patients. In addition, chapters describe manual therapy techniques, the role of physical agents, and orthotic fabrication for use with these patients. This section ends with a chapter on behavioral modification techniques used by health care practitioners to address functional loss and chronic pain syndromes.

5. Current "hot topics" related to peripheral nerve injury: The topics addressed in this section include brachial plexus syndromes, Guillain-Barré syndrome, neuropathies associated with athletics, entrapment neuropathies in the upper and lower extremity, and neuropathic processes associated with HIV disease.

I authored half the chapters. The other half were authored by many who are national and international experts in their unique content areas.

Mary F. Barbe, PhD, Professor of Anatomy and Cell Biology at Temple University School of Medicine, Philadelphia, Pennsylvania, is one of the leading researchers in the growing field of repetitive strain injury. For the past 10 years, she has been involved in neurobiological, cell, and molecular biological studies examining the effects of repetition and force on musculoskeletal and neural systems and on sensorimotor function with a research colleague, Ann E. Barr, PT, PhD (now at Pacific University, Portland, Oregon). Drs. Barbe and Barr developed a unique voluntary rat model of work-related musculoskeletal disorders (also known as repetitive strain injury and overuse injury) with varying levels of repetition and force and have been working to characterize the short-term effects. They have now expanded to examining the long-term effects of repetitive and forceful tasks on musculoskeletal and nervous system pathophysiology, focusing on injury and inflammation and how these processes induce degenerative tissue changes and sensorimotor dysfunction. Dr. Barbe is currently exploring inflammation-induced catabolic tissue changes versus mechanical overload–induced tissue disruption using pharmaceutical methods to block inflammatory processes. This work is currently funded by the National Institute for Occupational Safety and Health and National Institute of Arthritis and Musculoskeletal and Skin Diseases.

Susan Bray, MD, Clinical and Associate Professor in the Division of Nephrology at Drexel University College of Medicine, Philadelphia, is a much honored clinical nephrologist, internist, author, and palliative care specialist. She currently maintains a clinical practice in Philadelphia.

Stephan Whitenack, MD, PhD, a graduate of Thomas Jefferson Medical College, Thomas Jefferson University, Philadelphia, is board certified in general surgery, thoracic surgery, and vascular surgery and is a preeminent researcher, writer, lecturer, diagnostician, and surgeon in the field of brachial plexopathies.

Emily A. Keshner, PT, EdD, received her Certificate in Physical Therapy at the College of Physicians and Surgeons, Columbia University, New York, New York. She received her doctoral degree in Movement Science at Teachers College, Columbia University. She then pursued postdoctoral fellowships at the University of Oregon, Eugene, Oregon, and the University Hospital in Basel, Switzerland, both in the area of postural control in healthy and vestibular-deficient adults. Subsequently she was a Research Associate in the Department of Physiology, Northwestern University, Chicago, Illinois, where she performed animal and human research. She then worked as a research scientist in the Sensory Motor Performance Program at the Rehabilitation Institute of Chicago with a faculty position in the Department of Physical Medicine and Rehabilitation at Northwestern University until she came to Temple University in 2006. Dr. Keshner has been continuously funded from the National Institutes of Health since 1989. She currently teaches in the PhD program in the Department of Physical Therapy. In addition to her appointment at Temple University, Dr. Keshner is Adjunct Professor, Department of Physical Medicine and Rehabilitation, Feinberg School of Medicine, Northwestern University and Director of the Virtual Environment and Postural Orientation Laboratory at Temple Univeristy. Dr. Keshner has authored more than 100 peer-reviewed publications. Jill Slaboda, PhD, at the time this article was written, was a post-doctoral research fellow in Dr. Keshner's laboratory. Currently, she is with the Geneva Foundation.

James W. Bellew, PT, PhD, is an associate professor at the Kranert School of Physical Therapy at the University of Indianapolis, Indianapolis, Indiana. Dr. Bellew has published more than 50 peer-reviewed scientific articles and abstracts in the areas of exercise training, balance, and muscle physiology and is the co-author of the textbook *Modalities for Therapeutic Intervention*, 5th ed., published by FA Davis Company. Edward Mahoney, PT, DPT, CWS, is currently Assistant Professor at Louisiana State University Health in Shreveport Louisiana. He obtained his Doctorate of Physical Therapy from Louisiana State University Health Sciences Center in Shreveport and his Master's in Science of Physical Therapy from Sacred Heart University. He has published extensively in the areas of wound healing and therapeutic modalities for tissue healing. He is a member of the American Board of

Wound Management as well as a site reviewer for the American Board of Physical Therapy Residency and Fellowship Education.

Roberta A. Newton, PT, PhD, FGSA, an internationally recognized expert in fall prevention programming for older adults and the author of 53 peer-reviewed publications, 5 books, and 16 book chapters. At the time of the authorship of this chapter, Dr. Newton was professor of Physical Therapy and Clinical Professor of Medicine at Temple University. Past posts at Temple have included director for the Institute on Aging, and regional coordinator and director of education of the Gerontology Education Center. Newton was also a tenured associate professor at the Department of Physical Therapy, School of Allied Health Professions, Medical College of Virginia of Virginia Commonwealth University. Newton earned a PhD in neurophysiology and a BS in physical therapy from the Medical College of Virginia, Virginia Commonwealth University, and a BS in biology from Mary Washington College. She is the recipient of the American Physical Therapy's Catherine Worthingham Fellow Award. Dr. Newton has written, along with Dennis W. Klima, PT, PhD, GCS, NCS, formerly Dr. Newton's doctoral student and now assistant professor in the Department of Physical Therapy at University of Maryland Eastern Shore, Princess Anne, Maryland, a wonderful chapter on fall risk identification, prevention, and management. Dennis Klima joined the faculty at University of Maryland, Eastern Shore, in the fall of 2002. Prior to his UMES appointment, Dennis served as Program Director of the Physical Therapist Assistant Program at the Baltimore City Community College for thirteen years. He received his Bachelor of Science degree in Physical Therapy from the Medical College of Virginia. He completed a PhD in Physical Therapy from Temple University where his dissertation focused on physical performance and fear of falling in older men. Dr. Klima received his geriatric and neurologic clinical specializations from the American Board of Physical Therapy Specialties. His APTA experience also includes serving as an on-site reviewer for both PT and PTA programs with the Department of Accreditation since 1990. He has presented geriatric and neurological continuing education courses both nationally and internationally. Areas of research include both management of adults with TBI and fall prevention in older adults.

Robert B. Raffa, PhD, is Professor of Pharmacology and Chair of the Department of Pharmaceutical Sciences at Temple University School of Pharmacy and Research Professor at Temple University School of Medicine. Dr. Raffa holds bachelor's degrees in Chemical Engineering and in Physiological Psychology, master's degrees in Biomedical Engineering and in Toxicology, and a doctorate in Pharmacology. Dr. Raffa was a Research Fellow and Team Leader for an analgesics discovery group at Johnson & Johnson and was involved in the elucidation of the mechanism of action of tramadol. He is co-holder of several patents, including the combination of tramadol with acetaminophen. Dr. Raffa is the co-author or editor of several books on pharmacology, including *Netter's Illustrated Pharmacology* and *Principles in General Pharmacology and Drug-Receptor Thermodynamics,* and has published more than 150 articles in refereed journals and more than 70 abstracts and symposia presentations. He is co-founder and editor of the journal *Reviews in Analgesia* and was an associate editor of the *Journal of Pharmacology and Experimental Therapeutics.* Dr. Raffa is active in several professional societies and is a past president of the Mid-Atlantic Pharmacology Society. He is the recipient of the Hofmann Research Award, Lindback Teaching Award, and other honors.

John P. Scanlon, DPM, is a graduate of the Temple University School of Podiatric Medicine and maintains a podiatric clinical practice in Philadelphia. Dr. Scanlon is also the Chief Medical Officer at Chestnut Hill Hospital in Philadelphia and directs the Chestnut Hill Hospital Podiatric Residency Program. Crystal N. Gonzalez, DPM, Benjamin R. Denenberg, DPM, and Krupa J. Triveda, DPM, were residents in Podiatry under Dr. John Scanlon at Chestnut Hill Hospital and are now all in private practice.

Joseph I. Boullata, PharmD, RPh, BCNSP, is a clinician-educator on the standing faculty of the University of Pennsylvania School of Nursing in Philadelphia. He received his Doctorate in Pharmacy from the University of Maryland in Baltimore after completing undergraduate degrees in Nutrition Science (Pennsylvania State University), State College, Pennsylvania, and in Pharmacy (Philadelphia College of Pharmacy & Science, Philadelphia). He completed a residency at the Johns Hopkins Hospital in Baltimore and a nutrition support fellowship at the University of Maryland Medical System. His teaching experiences have spanned well over a dozen years mostly in pharmacy education through didactic, small group, and bedside teaching. Outside the classroom, Dr. Boullata is involved with student mentoring and professional organizations as well as his clinical practice and scholarship. Dr. Boullata's research agenda generated from questions that arise during clinical practice and then developed further through interdisciplinary collaboration. His research areas have included pharmacotherapeutic issues within the intensive care unit setting, pharmacotherapeutic implications of nutrition regimens, and drug-nutrient interactions. The pharmacology and therapeutics of individual nutrients and natural health products in disease management as well as their interaction with medication require further exploration. Dr. Boullata has achieved and maintained board certification in nutrition support. He has also received recognition for his active membership in several multidisciplinary, national professional organizations including the American Society for Parenteral and Enteral Nutrition. He has also served on the editorial boards for *Nutrition in Clinical Practice* and *Current Topics in Nutraceutical Research*.

David M. Kietrys, PT, PhD, OCS, received his entry-level physical therapy degree from Hahnemann University in Philadelphia and his doctorate from Temple University. Dr. Kietrys is currently Associate Professor of Rehabilitation and Movement Sciences at the Rutgers School of Health Related Professions (formerly known as UMDNJ–School of Health Related Professions) in Stratford, New Jersey. Dr. Kietrys has published extensively in the field of HIV and exercise and repetitive strain injury. Mary Lou Galantino, PT, PhD, MS, MSCE, has a dual appointment: Adjunct Associate Professor of Family Medicine and Community Health at the Perelman School of Medicine, University of Pennsylvania, and Professor of Physical Therapy at Richard Stockton College. An accomplished funded researcher, Dr. Galantino has published extensively in the areas of HIV-related neuropathy, holistic medicine, and women's health.

Bill Egan, DPT, OCS, FAAOMPT, received a BA in psychology from Rutgers University, New Brunswick, New Jersey, in 1997, and an MPT from the US Army–Baylor University in San Antonio, Texas, in 1999. He served as an active duty Army physical therapist for 6 years. Dr. Egan completed the tDPT and Manual Therapy Fellowship program through Regis University in Denver, Colorado, in 2006, and he now serves as affiliate faculty for these programs. Currently, Dr. Egan is an associate professor in the Doctor of Physical Therapy program at Temple University. He is a board-certified Orthopedic Clinical Specialist and a Fellow of the American Academy of Orthopedic Manual Therapists. Dr. Egan serves as an adjunct instructor for various local physical therapy programs teaching manual therapy and thrust manipulation. He is also an instructor for Evidence In Motion. Dr. Egan maintains a part-time clinical practice at the Sports Physical Therapy Institute in Princeton, New Jersey. Scott Burns, PT, DPT, OCS, FAAOMPT, received his Master of Physical Therapy and transitional Doctor of Physical Therapy from the University of Colorado-Denver. He is currently Associate Professor and Assistant Chair in the Doctor of Physical Therapy Program at Temple University. Dr. Burns's teaching responsibilities include the Musculoskeletal Management course series, Orthopaedic Residency Coursework and Advanced Musculoskeletal Elective, and Clinical Decision Making. In addition to his teaching responsibilities, he maintains an active clinical schedule including research and patient care. His main research interests revolve around clinical decision making, clinical education strategies/models, patient outcomes, chronic pain management and manual physical therapy interventions for various musculoskeletal conditions. His work, entitled "Short-term response of hip mobilizations and exercise in individuals with chronic low back pain: a case series" was awarded the Dick Erhard Award for Best Platform Presentation at AAOMPT Conference in 2010. In 2014, Dr. Burns was selected as the recipient for the College of Public Health Excellence in Teaching Award.

Amy Heath, PT, PhD, OCS, is Chair and Assistant Professor of Physical Therapy at Simmons College. She received her BS in Health Studies and DPT from Simmons College, and her PhD in Educational Psychology from Temple University. Dr. Heath is credentialed by the American Physical Therapy Association as a Clinical Instructor.

Teri O'Hearn, DPT, CHT received a bachelor's degree in Health Science from the University of North Florida, Jacksonville, Florida, a master's of science degree in Physical Therapy from the University of North Florida, and a Doctor of Physical Therapy degree from Boston University, Boston. She became a Certified Hand Therapist in 2007. She is currently employed at Ministry Door County Medical Center in Sturgeon Bay, Wisconsin.

Megan Mulderig McAndrew, DPT, MS, is employed in the Drucker Brain Injury Center at Moss Rehabilitation Hospital in Elkins Park, Pennsylvania. Ms. McAndrew has presented and written extensively in the field of neurotrauma and neurorehabilitation. She is a graduate of the Moss Rehabilitation Neurological Physical Therapy Residency.

Elizabeth Spencer Steffa, OTR/L, CHT, is an occupational therapist, certified hand therapist, partner of Highline Hand Therapy, and a clinical faculty member at the University of Washington, Seattle, Washington, her alma mater. Ms. Steffa treats hand and upper extremity injuries, performs physical capacity evaluations, and participates in splinting/orthosis fabrication.

Each chapter begins with a title, germane quotation, objectives, key terms, and an introduction. The text is supplemented liberally with photographs, tables, and diagrams. Each chapter includes a case study and sample questions. A comprehensive list of references also is included with each chapter. At the end of the text is a comprehensive glossary of definitions of all key terms in the chapters. An index is also provided for ease of locating subject matter.

REVIEWERS

Kevin Ball, PhD
Assistant Professor
Physical Therapy
Director
Human Performance Laboratory
University of Hartford
West Hartford, Connecticut

James W. Bellew, PT, EdD
Associate Professor
Physical Therapy
Krannert School of Physical Therapy
University of Indianapolis
Indianapolis, Indiana

Shaun G. Boe, BPhEd (Hon), MPT, PhD
Assistant Professor
School of Physiotherapy
Dalhousie University
Halifax, Nova Scotia, Canada

Rafael Escamilla, PhD, PT
Professor
Physical Therapy
Sacramento State University
Sacramento, California

Claudia B. Fenderson, PT, EdD, PCS
Professor
Physical Therapy
Mercy College
Dobbs Ferry, New York

Cynthia K. Flom-Meland, PT, PhD, NCS
Assistant Professor
Physical Therapy
University of North Dakota
Grand Forks, North Dakota

Erin Hussey, DPT, MS, NCS
Clinical Associate Professor
Health Professions–Physical Therapy
University of Wisconsin–La Crosse
La Crosse, Wisconsin

Jennifer A. Mai, PT, DPT, MHS, NCS
Assistant Professor
Physical Therapy
Clarke University
Dubuque, Iowa

Karen McCulloch, PT, PhD, NCS
Professor
Division of Physical Therapy–Allied Health
    Sciences
University of North Carolina–Chapel Hill
Chapel Hill, North Carolina

Stefanie D. Palma, DPT, PT, NCS, CBIS
Chair
Physical Therapy
North Georgia College & State University
Dahlonega, Georgia

E. Anne Reicherter, PT, DPT, PhD, OCS, CHES
Associate Professor
Physical Therapy and Rehabilitation Sciences
University of Maryland School of Medicine
Baltimore, Maryland

Linda J. Tsoumas, PT, MS, EdD
Professor
Physical Therapy
Springfield College
Belchertown, Massachusetts

David Walton, BScPT, MSc, PhD
Assistant Professor
Faculty of Health Sciences
The University of Western Ontario
London, Ontario, Canada

Kevin C. Weaver, PT, DPT, MA, OCS, CEA, CIE
Clinical Assistant Professor
Physical Therapy
New York University
New York, New York

Mark R. Wiegand, PT, PhD
Professor and Program Director
Physical Therapy
Bellarmine University
Louisville, Kentucky

CONTENTS

Anatomy, Physiology, Biomechanics, and Pathophysiology of Peripheral Nerve Injury

Chapter 1

The Anatomy and Physiology of the Peripheral Nerve

STEPHEN J. CARP, PT, PhD, GCS

"Facts are the air of scientists. Without them you can never fly."
—LINUS PAULING (1901–1994)

Objectives

On completion of this chapter, the student/practitioner will be able to:

- Describe the basic anatomical structure of a peripheral nerve.
- Relate the structural and functional anatomy of a peripheral nerve.
- Define the process of wallerian degeneration.
- Compare and contrast the various common nerve classifications.
- Discuss the structural and functional impact of aberrant tensile and compressive forces on peripheral nerves.

Key Terms

- Classification of peripheral nerve injury
- Compression
- Endoneurium
- Epineurium
- Perineurium
- Tension
- Wallerian degeneration

Introduction

Homeostasis (Greek: *homoios,* similar; *histēmi,* to cause to stand still) is the property of an open or closed system that allows regulation of its internal environment.[1] In other words, homeostasis is the physiological and anatomical capacity of an organism to regulate itself by rapidly analyzing and, if aberrant, restoring environmental conditions following a sudden perturbation in the internal or external environment. Such internal or external environmental conditions or "stimuli" initiate electrical impulses in peripheral and central sensory receptors. The impulses travel afferently from the receptors via nerves to the spinal cord and brain where they are analyzed, compared, learned, and coordinated by a process called "integration." Once the afferent information is received and deciphered, the spinal cord and brain convey efferent impulses through nerves to muscles and glands. In an effort to maintain homeostasis, muscles either contract or relax, and glands either secrete or stop secreting their products.

The nervous and endocrine systems are the two major regulatory systems of the body, and both are specialized (and defined) by making appropriate and timely responses to internal or external stimuli. The nervous system, using a combination of electrical potentials and neurotransmitters to communicate messages and tasks, is the faster of the two; the endocrine system depends on a slower transmission system, a chemical system using hormones. Typically, long-term organism growth, metabolic activity, and the reproduction system are controlled by the endocrine system. Faster and immediate tasks such as movement and autonomic regulation are controlled by the neurological system. Although considered two distinct corporal systems, the endocrine and neurological systems are considered a singular regulatory system.

Albeit a unified system peripherally and centrally, the nervous system is typically anatomically defined as having central and peripheral components—the central nervous system (CNS) and the peripheral nervous system (PNS). The CNS consists of the brain and spinal cord. The PNS consists of all neurological tissue outside of the spinal cord and brain.

Failure of the PNS to transmit afferent, efferent, or autonomic data completely or in a timely manner because of illness or trauma is called peripheral neuropathy. Peripheral neuropathy results in possible loss of homeostasis in all corporal systems. Specific neurological illness or trauma leads to impairment of particular functional units of the PNS, defining the scope of impairment and the prognosis for recovery. Along with the broad picture of loss of homeostasis, peripheral neuropathy may lead to functional impairments associated with mobility, balance, and activities of daily living.

The PNS is often simplistically likened to an electrical source such as a generator, a conduction system (wiring), synapse (outlet), or effector organ (appliance such as a vacuum cleaner or electric light). In many ways, this analogy is effective, but our neurological system must accommodate one variable that household wiring does not: mobility. With skilled movements, the PNS is asked to function in a stretched, stationary, mobile, or compressed environment. A skilled observation of a gymnast performing a complicated routine provides ample evidence for this statement. Millesi et al.[2] calculated that the median nerve as measured from axilla to hand is 20% longer in an elbow-extended, wrist-extended compared with an elbow-flexed, wrist-flexed posture. The spinal cord is 5 to 9 cm longer with trunk flexion compared with trunk extension. In addition, nerve trunks must be able to deflect compressive forces directed from extrinsic sources such as an inflated blood pressure cuff and intrinsic sources such as **compression** from a bony prominence (e.g., the ulnar nerve within the olecranon fossa during elbow flexion).

PNS tissues can be divided into conduction and support structures. The conduction structures—nerve fibers and synaptic components such as the dendrites and synaptic cleft—and the support structures—axon sheath, myelin, Schwann cells, and **epineurium** among others—combine to form a quite vigorous and adaptable functional nexus. However, each conduction and support structure is prey to a host of diseases and injuries leading to potentially severe functional impairment.

The nervous system is unique among corporal systems because of its vast complexity and its control, regulation, decoding, transmitting, and action functions. There are 100 billion nerve cells, or neurons, functionally and anatomically specialized to maintain homeostasis. The purpose of this chapter is to present an overall anatomical framework of the PNS, an analysis of the functions of the various entities and subentities of the PNS, and, lastly, a review of the biomechanics of the PNS.

Functional Anatomy of the Peripheral Nervous System

The PNS includes 12 pairs of cranial nerves and 31 pairs of spinal nerves and their terminal branches (Fig. 1-1). The cranial nerves, spinal nerves, and terminal branches are called peripheral nerves. Each spinal nerve is connected to the spinal cord through a posterior root and an anterior root. The two roots combine within the bony intervertebral foramen to form the spinal nerve. The posterior roots contain fibers of sensory neurons, and the anterior roots contain mainly fibers of motor neurons. Immediately after the spinal nerve exits the intervertebral foramen, it divides into

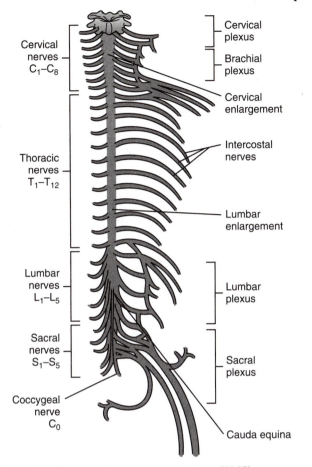

Figure 1-1 The peripheral nervous system (PNS) consists of 12 pairs of cranial nerves and 31 pairs of spinal nerves, which are each denoted by their respective exit from the spinal cord, through the intervertebral foramen, and to their designated destinations (C1–C8, T1–T12, L1–L5, S1–S5). Although there are only seven cerebral vertebrae, there are eight spinal nerves within the cervical region of the spine because the first cervical nerve exits superiorly to C1.

In the figure, labels on the left read: Cervical nerves C_1–C_8; Thoracic nerves T_1–T_{12}; Lumbar nerves L_1–L_5; Sacral nerves S_1–S_5; Coccygeal nerve C_0. Labels on the right read: Cervical plexus; Brachial plexus; Cervical enlargement; Intercostal nerves; Lumbar enlargement; Lumbar plexus; Sacral plexus; Cauda equina.

two branches: the dorsal ramus and the ventral ramus. The dorsal rami typically innervate muscles, skin, and sensory receptors of the head, neck, and back. The ventral rami often unite to form plexus (Greek: *plexi,* to plait or intertwine) before innervating the ventral structures. Proximal peripheral nerves, also known as nerve trunks, consist of blood vessels, connective tissue, and fascicles. The fascicles contain the functional neural element, the neuron. Each of these elements is structurally and strategically required for nerve function, and each element is susceptible to chemotoxic, compressive, and tensile injuries of particular type, force, and duration (Fig. 1-2).

Nerve cells, or neurons (Greek: *neuron,* nerve), are cells that are specially adapted in size and shape to transmit electrical impulses over relatively long distances. Neurons have two unique characteristics: conductivity, the ability to conduct an electrical signal, and excitability, the ability to generate and respond to stimuli. Most neurons consist of three principal parts: the cell body, the cell dendrites, and the axon. Each of these is associated with specific neural functions.

The Cell Body

The cell body, also known as the soma (Greek: *soma,* body) or perikaryon (Greek: *peri,* near, and *karyon,* nut or kernel), may appear microscopically stellate, round, oval, or pyramid-shaped, depending on the function of the particular neuron (Fig. 1-3). The most striking feature of the cell body is the large number of projections or processes that either transmit or receive signals from other cells. Each cell body has a large nucleus that contains a nucleolus as well as additional organelles responsible for growth, production, and reproduction; these include, but are not limited to, the endoplasmic reticulum, neurotubules, neurofilaments, Nissl bodies, lysosomes, mitochondria, neurotubules, and Golgi apparatuses. The neurotubules and neurofilaments are threadlike lipoprotein structures that extend throughout the cell body and process of the neuron and run parallel to the long axis of each process. Neurotubules assist with intracellular transport of chemicals and proteins responsible for cell growth, repair, and conductivity. Neurofilaments provide the scaffolding or endoskeleton of the neuron. Alzheimer disease and senile dementia of Alzheimer type (SDAT) are histologically defined by "tangles" of the neurofilaments and neurotubules in the neurons of the cerebral cortex.[3]

Dendrites

Dendrites and the axon are the two processes extending from the cell body. Dendrites (Greek: *dendron,* tree) are short, threadlike branches that conduct nerve impulses toward the cell body. Typical peripheral nerve cell bodies have up to 300 dendrites.[4]

The structure and branching of a neuron's dendrites as well as the availability and variation in voltage gate ion channels allow neurons to conduct nerve impulses.[5] Voltage-gated ion channels are a class of transmembrane ion channels that are activated by changes in electrical potential differences near the ion channels. These channels strongly influence how the nerve cell responds to the input from other neurons, particularly neurons that input weakly. This integration is both "temporal"—involving the summation of stimuli that arrive in rapid succession—and "spatial"—entailing the aggregation of excitatory and inhibitory inputs from separate branches.[6]

Dendrites were previously believed to convey stimulation passively. The passive cable theory describes how voltage changes at a particular location on a dendrite transmit this electrical signal through a system of converging dendrite segments of different diameters, lengths, and electrical properties. Based on passive

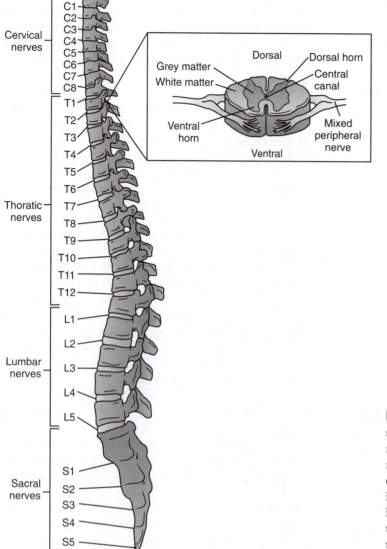

Cervical nerves
- C1
- C2
- C3
- C4
- C5
- C6
- C7
- C8

Thoratic nerves
- T1
- T2
- T3
- T4
- T5
- T6
- T7
- T8
- T9
- T10
- T11
- T12

Lumbar nerves
- L1
- L2
- L3
- L4
- L5

Sacral nerves
- S1
- S2
- S3
- S4
- S5

Grey matter
White matter
Dorsal
Dorsal horn
Central canal
Ventral horn
Mixed peripheral nerve
Ventral

Figure 1-2 Spinal nerves of the peripheral nervous system are connected to the spinal cord by anterior roots (sensory neurons) and posterior roots (motor neurons) within the intervertebral foramen. On exiting the spinal column, the spinal nerve splits into dorsal and ventral rami. Dorsal rami typically innervate muscles, skin, and sensory receptors of the head, neck, and back. Ventral rami often unite to form plexus, such as the brachial plexus before innervating ventral structures.

cable theory, one can track how changes in dendritic morphology of a neuron change the membrane voltage at the soma and thus how variation in dendrite structure impacts the overall output characteristics as well as function of the neuron.[7,8]

Although passive cable theory offers clues regarding input propagation and specificity along dendrite segments, dendrite membranes are host to a variety of proteins that, along with the cable theory, assist with amplification or attenuation of synaptic input. In addition, various calcium, potassium, and sodium ion channels all assist with synaptic modulation. It is hypothesized that each of these channel types has its own biological characteristics relevant to synaptic modulation.[9]

An important feature of dendrites that is allowed by their active voltage-gated conductances is their ability to send action potentials retrograde into the dendritic tree. This retrograde conduction, known as back propagating action potentials, depolarizes the dendritic tree and provides a crucial component toward synapse modulation, long-term propagation, and postsynaptic potentiation. In addition, a train of back propagating action potentials artificially generated at the soma can induce a calcium action potential at the dendritic initiation zone in certain types of neurons. Whether or not this mechanism is of physiological or structural importance remains an open question.[10]

Axon

Most PNS cell bodies have one axon. The axon is a narrow process that extends from the cell body and varies in length depending on the cell from 1 mm to greater than 1 m. Axons, as they travel centrally or peripherally, are often grouped together into bundles, called fascicles. Axons run an undulating course within the fascicles to allow for elongation with articular movements. Functionally, the axon carries the action potential between the cell body and a nerve, gland, receptor, or motor unit. The axon originates from a cone-shaped projection on the cell body called the axon hillock. The axon may have side branches, called collateral branches, that exit the main axon. The axon and collateral branches end in a spray of tiny branches called telodendria. The branches of the telodendria have small bulbs called synaptic boutons. A synapse (Greek: *synapsis*, connection) is where the synaptic boutons interact with the plasma membrane of another neuron (Table 1-1).

The cytoplasm of an axon is called axoplasm, and the plasma membrane is known as the axolemma. The axon may be covered with a laminated shell of myelin (Greek: *myelos*, marrow), which forms an external sheathing called the myelin sheath. A nerve fiber with a myelin sheath is called a myelinated nerve; a nerve fiber without a myelinated sheath is called an unmyelinated nerve. The peripheral nerve myelin sheath is called a neurolemmocyte or Schwann cell. The outermost layer of the Schwann cell is the neurolemma (Greek: *neuri*, nerve; *lemma*, husk). The myelin sheath is classically interrupted at regular intervals by depressions or gaps called neurofibral nodes or, more familiarly, nodes of Ranvier. The distance between nodes is the internodal distance. The myelin is absent at each internode. Myelin appears to increase conduction velocity. Myelinated nerves conduct at velocities between 3 m/sec and 120 m/sec; unmyelinated fibers conduct at velocities of 0.7 to 2.3 m/sec (Fig. 1-4).

Endoneurium

The innermost layer of connective tissue in a peripheral nerve, forming an interstitial layer around each individual fiber outside the neurolemma, is the **endoneurium.** The matrix of tightly bound connective tissue also contains capillaries, mast cells, Schwann cells, and fibroblasts. There is no evidence of lymphatic tissue being present. The endoneurium appears to have two primary functions: to maintain the endoneurial space and fluid pressure and to sustain a homeostatic nerve

Neuron

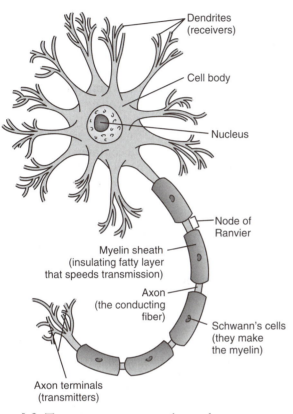

- Dendrites (receivers)
- Cell body
- Nucleus
- Node of Ranvier
- Myelin sheath (insulating fatty layer that speeds transmission)
- Axon (the conducting fiber)
- Schwann's cells (they make the myelin)
- Axon terminals (transmitters)

Figure 1-3 The primary structures that make up neurological tissue consist of the cell bodies, dendrites, and axon fibers. Via saltatory conduction, cell bodies transmit electrical signals down axon fibers to neighboring neurons to communicate sensory or motor information.

Table 1-1	Mammalian Nerve Fiber Type With Functional and Velocity Characteristics				
Fiber Type	Function	Fiber Diameter (μm)	Conduction Velocity (m/sec)	Spike Duration (m/sec)	Absolute Refractory Period
A α	Somatic motor, proprioception	12–20	70–120		
A β	Rapidly adapting touch, pressure	5–12	30–70	0.4–0.5	0.4–1
A λ	Motor to muscle spindle	3–6	5–30		
A δ	Nociception, cold, touch	2–5.0	12–30		
B	Preganglionic autonomic	<3	3–15	1.2	1.2
C dorsal root	Nociception, temperature	5–12	0.5–2	2	2
C sympathetic	Postganglionic sympathetic	0.3–1.3	0.7–2.3	2	2

Data from Millesi H, Zöch G, Reihsner R. Mechanical properties of peripheral nerves. *Clin Orthop.* 1995;314:76–83; Sunderland S. *Nerve Injuries and Their Repair. A Critical Appraisal.* Melbourne: Churchill Livingstone; 1991; Kaye AH. Classification of nerve injuries. In: *Essential Neurosurgery.* London: Churchill Livingstone; 1991:333–334; Seddon H. Nerve injuries. *Med Bull (Ann Arbor).* 1965;31:4–10; and Sunderland S. The anatomy and physiology of nerve injury. *Muscle Nerve.* 1990;13:771–784.

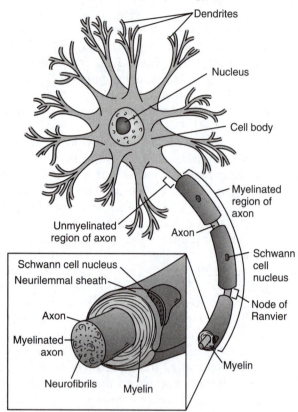

Figure 1-4 Produced by Schwann cells throughout the nervous system, myelin serves as insulation for electrical signals that pass along axonal fibers. Increased myelination of axons increases the nerve fiber diameter and the conduction velocity of the information. Many different types of myelinated or unmyelinated nerves exist that serve multiple purposes within the nervous system.

fiber environment. A slightly positive pressure is maintained within the endoneurial tube. Researchers report an association between endoneurial tube disruption and neural disorganization including neuronal formation and aberrant synapses.[11,12] The collagen within the endoneurial tube is primarily longitudinal, evidence that supports the fact that the endoneurium assists with protecting the neuron from tensile challenges.[11]

Perineurium

Each fascicle is surrounded by a layered sheath known as the **perineurium.** The perineurium has three primary functions:

- To protect the endoneurial tubes from normal articular movement patterns through the tensile and compressive resisted characteristics of the basement collagen fibers and elastin.
- To protect the endoneurial tube from external trauma.
- To serve as a molecular diffusion barrier, keeping certain potentially neurotoxic compounds away from the perineurial and

endoneurial environment via the blood-nerve barrier and the perineurial diffusion barrier (discussed later in this chapter).[11–14]

Along with the aforementioned longitudinal collagen fibers, and in contrast to the endoneurium, there is a rich circular and angled matrix of collagen fibers that protects nerves from "kinking" as they bend in response to articular joint flexion, extension, and rotatory maneuvers.[14]

Epineurium

The **epineurium,** a loose connective tissue, is subdivided into internal and external components. The internal epineurium is the base collagenous tissue that physically separates the fascicles. It provides two basic functions: assisting the external epineurium in providing truncal protection from compressive forces and, more importantly, facilitating gliding between the fascicles. As nerves stretch and rebound, fascicles glide within the base collagen matrix of the nerve trunk. As an anisotropic structure, the peripheral nerve's content of internal epineurium, as a percentage of nerve diameter, varies along the course of the nerve. There is a direct relationship between diameter of the nerve and the volume of epineurium.[15] There is also greater epineurium content in peripheral nerves as they cross joints and as they pass under or near fibrous bands such as the flexor retinaculum at the wrist.[14] The external epineurium surrounds the nerve trunk and provides protection from compressive and tensile forces. The spinal nerves are devoid of epineurium and perineurium, and they may be more susceptible to chronic and acute compressive trauma compared with their terminal branches.[11]

Mesoneurium

The mesoneurium is the outermost tissue around peripheral nerve trunks. It is classified as loose and areolar and is the entry portal for many of the arteries that supply the vasa nervorum, the highly anastomosing venous and arterial network within the nerve trunk.[13] The function of the mesoneurium is not fully understood; however, the "slippery" surface of the mesoneurium limits frictional forces with longitudinal and side-to-side movement of the nerve trunk against local structures. There may also be substantial "sliding" motion between the mesoneurium and the external epineurium facilitating the extensibility characteristics of nerve. The mesoneurium may also provide limited protection from compressive and tensile forces impacting the nerve trunk.[13–16]

Vascular Components

Although possessing only 2% of the body's mass, the CNS and PNS at any given time use 20% of the oxygen carried by the bloodstream.[17] In contrast to some of the less metabolically active tissues such as bone or skin, nerve tissue is especially sensitive to changes to the partial pressure of oxygen (Po_2).[18] The circulatory system within peripheral nerves is known as the vasa nervorum. The blood supply to individual nerves and nerve trunks is well understood. A combination of extrinsic and intrinsic arteries and capillaries provides a redundant supply of oxygenated blood via a rich system of anastomoses. Large external vessels approach a peripheral nerve and run parallel along a section of the course. At intervals, small vessels divide off the main artery and enter the epineurial layer. They immediately divide into ascending and descending branches and anastomose with vessels in the perineurium and endoneurium. Small-vessel injury rarely results in nerve ischemia.[19] Typically, large-vessel injury, such as from atherosclerosis, precipitates nerve ischemia and loss of conduction. In addition, the extrinsic supply of blood to the nerves is designed to allow vessel laxity, which allows uninterrupted blood flow to the nerve in extremes of articular posture.[17] Feeder vessels tend to enter the nerve at locations where there is intrinsically little **tension** with movement, again ensuring uninterrupted blood flow.[19] The intrinsic or intraneural blood supply is extremely redundant (Fig. 1-5).

A slightly positive tissue pressure exists within the fascicle compared with outside the fascicle (+1.5; ± 0.7 mm Hg).[20,21] Research has shown a "mushrooming" of fascicular contents if the perineurium is cut.[21] The relatively positive fascicular pressure is needed to maintain a homeostatic endoneurial environment, facilitating blood flow, nerve conduction, and axoplasmic flow. The blood-nerve barrier and the perineurial diffusion barrier maintain the endoneurial environment. The selective barrier limits toxins crossing from the epineurial blood vessels to the endoneurial vessels. For example, radioactive isotopes and dyes do not cross the barrier. Glucose molecules may cross the barrier, whereas specific nonsteroidal medications do not cross the barrier. Despite the efficient selectivity of the barrier, it is easily broken with acute or chronic nerve trauma. The perineurial diffusion barrier is facilitated by junctions in the perineurial lamellae called "tight cells." With increased intrafascicular pressure, the "tight cells" function to limit bidirectional vascular transport to and from the fascicle. The limitation of bidirectional blood flow is hypothesized to occur to limit the passage of potential local toxins and proinflammatory mediators to the neuron.[22]

Neuron Type: Directional Transport

PNS neurons may be defined by the direction of transport of the action potentials. Neurons transporting action potentials from cortical centers to the periphery or away from the CNS to effector end organs (typically glands, muscles, and blood vessels) are called efferent or motor neurons. Neurons transporting action potential from the periphery to central locations are called afferent or sensory neurons. The afferent neuron cell bodies are located in ganglia that are situated close the CNS. The distal ends of these neurons are typically sensory receptors that are responsive to light touch, pain, sharp, dull, hot, and cold sensations; joint position and movement; and muscle length and state of contraction. Most interneurons rest in the CNS, but a few are distributed between the CNS and the PNS. They carry impulses from sensory neurons to motor neurons, process incoming neural information, and disseminate afferent information to more than one higher center.

Biomechanics of Peripheral Nerves

Peripheral nerves are remarkably complex tissues that not only conduct electrical impulses and communicate chemically and electrically with neighboring nerves, muscles, glands, and receptors but also must bend and stretch to accommodate the movement and potential passive insufficiency that may occur as a result of movements of limb and muscle. To achieve this extensibility, nerves have a complex structure consisting of bundles of neurons packed into fascicles and surrounded by multiple connective tissue layers. Both neural and connective tissue elements of nerve trunks are tethered proximally at the spinal cord and have numerous branch points allowing neurons from a single nerve trunk to synapse with various target organs. Despite some physiological connections—primarily vascular—to surrounding tissue, nerve trunks are largely free to glide along their length within their tissue bed. Frequent intraneural and extraneural anastomoses with blood vessels and a highly redundant vasa nervorum

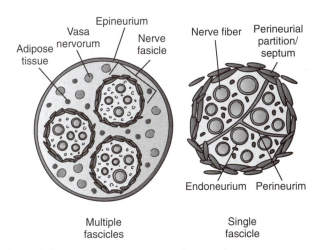

Figure 1-5 The vasa nervorum is the circulatory system within peripheral nerves that, along with intrinsic and extrinsic arteries and capillaries, forms an anastomosis around the nerve. Anastomoses form redundant blood supply pathways that perfuse nervous tissue and help prevent tissue ischemia.

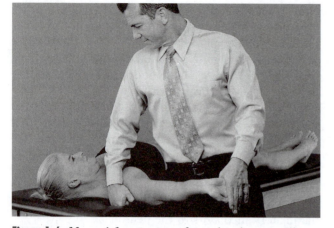

Figure 1-6 Normal functioning of peripheral nerves allows fibers to stretch and slide freely on surrounding tissue. However, after surgical repair or secondary to intraneural fibrosis, limb movement can result in localized increases in tension—leading to a loss of range of motion and function, increased pain and fibrotic tissue, or potential neuropathy. To test the status of the median nerve, the patient is placed in a position such that the median nerve is at its longest length. Severe pain or loss of sensation along the course of the nerve may indicate a possible lesion to the median nerve.

help prevent nerve ischemia with moderated movement patterns and minimal compressive forces. However, the nerve routes through the limbs tend to lie outside the plane of movement of the joints making some degree of length change inevitable during normal function. When this ability of nerves to stretch and glide freely is compromised by adhesion to surrounding tissues, for example, after surgical repair or via intraneural fibrosis secondary to repeated trauma and resultant inflammation, limb movement can result in localized increases in tension leading to loss of range of motion and function, increases in pain and fibrosis, and potentially symptomatic neuropathy (Fig. 1-6).[20,23]

Nerves are strong structures with considerable tensile strength. Numerous studies have been undertaken to define the limits to which nerves can be stretched before their function, structure, and vascular system are compromised. The obvious difficulty in attempting to make generic rules about stretch and the resultant impact on nerve strain and blood flow is the fact that nerve is an anisotropic structure. As a nerve progresses along its length, the ratio of neural to connective tissue and the individual percentage composition of each connective tissue type constantly change. However, it is known that straining nerves beyond the physiological tension range can alter their conduction properties[20,21] and intraneural blood flow[14] with compressive and tensile forces resulting in permanent loss of function. This process is currently understood as a breakdown in integrity of the nerve fiber.[22] Estimates

of maximal elongation of a typical peripheral nerve before reaching the elastic limit are 20% or greater over resting length.[12] Elongation greater than 20% over resting length may lead to decreased perfusion, vascular congestion, and macrophage/monocyte migration leading to intraneural and extraneural fibrosis.[24,25] The development of fibrosis eventually leads to a reduction in nerve stretch capability. With severe tensile-induced trauma, the nerve fibers in the nerve under tension appear to rupture before their endoneurial tubes and perineurium.[26] From a regeneration sense, this is an important finding. In relatively minor injuries, regenerating axons may have intact pathways to follow during their regrowth toward the periphery.

Identifying the maximum tension that nerves can withstand and maintain appropriate conduction properties and understanding the origin of their mechanical resilience are of great functional importance to improving the outcome of surgical nerve gap repairs. As a sutured nerve is stretched, the perineurium tightens. As a result, the endoneurial fluid pressure is increased, and the intraneural capillary bed may become compressed. At a certain stage of tensile force, the microcirculation system fails to function. In studies involving a rat model, an elongation of just 8% over resting length leads to impaired venule flow.[14] As elongation increases above 8%, arteriole flow begins to diminish, stopping entirely at 15% over resting length.[27] The slow growth of space-occupying compressive and tensile lesions of nerves, such as caused by a schwannoma, allows for the development of sufficient vascular collateralization often to prohibit ischemic nerve injury.

Action potential quality under loading is influenced by viscoelasticity. It is dependent on many factors, including the anatomical construction (ratio of each type of connective tissue to each other and the ratio of connective versus neural tissue) of the nerve at the point of tension or compression and the internal and external nerve environment, such as the presence of potentially neurotoxic chemicals or medication concentrations (e.g., lead, chemotherapeutic drugs, or an elevated blood glucose concentration). Additional environmental concerns that are potentially impacted by environmental forces are the internal neuron fluid pressure maintained by the impermeable perineurial membrane[28]; the outer-inner nerve trunk layer integrity[29]; the number, location within the nerve trunk, and arrangement of fascicles[30]; and the molecular structural elements of the extracellular matrix such as collagen and elastin.[25,27,31]

Although understanding the upper limit to which nerves can be safely stretched is such an important clinical variable, the investigation of stretch properties within normal physiological conditions and articular movements has been limited because of the anisotropic property of nerve. In particular, scant information is available on whether increased nerve tension and compression generated by limb flexion, extension, rotation, and distraction is focused around the joint or is dissipated along the full length of the nerve. The anisotropic property of the nerve trunk is often discussed in terms of the contribution of different concentric structural and neural layers to overall mechanical behavior; however, little is known about the presence and impact of the longitudinal variation in these structures. For example, variations in the number of fascicles have been observed along the length of human nerves,[24,30] and increased fasciculation has been suggested to be a protective feature of nerves crossing joints.[32] Such structural variation could possibly result in localized areas of damage and localized areas of sparing with tensile forces.

Classification and Pathophysiology of Peripheral Nerve Injury

A peripheral nerve contains sensory fibers, motor fibers, autonomic fibers, and mixed (sensorimotor) fibers. Typically, the more severe the trauma impacting the peripheral nerve, the more severe the motor, sensory, and autonomic signs and symptoms become. Many classification systems have been developed to aid in diagnosis, prognosis, and intervention strategy.[33–37] Most systems attempt to correlate the degree of injury with symptoms, pathology, and prognosis. In 1943, Seddon[35,36] introduced a classification of nerve injuries based on three main types of nerve fiber injury and whether there is continuity of the nerve (Table 1-2). The three types of nerve injuries are neurapraxia, axonotmesis, and neurotmesis. In 1951, Sunderland[37] expanded Seddon's classification by two and developed an ordinal rather than categorical scale (Table 1-3).

Seddon Classification

Neurapraxia is the mildest form of peripheral nerve injury and results from a temporary interruption in the conduction of the impulse distally along the nerve fiber, without a loss of axonal continuity. The endoneurium, perineurium, and epineurium remain intact. The interruption is physiological and not structural. Recovery takes place from seconds to weeks without **wallerian degeneration** occurring. This is probably a biochemical lesion caused by concussive or shocklike injuries to the

Table 1-2 Seddon Classification of Peripheral Neuropathy

	Neurapraxia	Axonotmesis	Neurotmesis
Pathology			
Anatomical continuity encapsulating structures	Preserved	Preserved	May be lost
Primary damage	None	Nerve fiber interruption	Complete interruption of nerve fiber and encapsulating structures
Clinical			
Motor paralysis	None, partial, or complete	Complete	Complete
Muscle atrophy	None	Progressive	Progressive
Sensory loss	None, partial, or complete	Complete	Complete
Autonomic loss	Usually spared	Complete	Complete
Visual fasciculations	No	Yes	Yes
Electroneuromyography Findings			
Reaction to degeneration	Present	Present	Present
Nerve conduction distal to lesion	Preserved	Absent	Absent
Motor unit action potentials	Absent	Absent	Absent
Fibrillation	Rare	Present	Present
Recovery			
Surgical repair required	Never	Occasionally	Essential
Rate of recovery	Minute to weeks	1–3 mm/day	1–3 mm/day after repair
Quality of recovery	Perfect	Occasionally perfect	Rarely perfect

Data from Sunderland S. *Nerve Injuries and Their Repair. A Critical Appraisal.* Melbourne: Churchill Livingstone; 1991; Seddon H. Advances in nerve repair. *Triangle.* 1968;8:252–259; and Seddon H. Nerve injuries. *Med Bull (Ann Arbor).* 1965;31:4–10.

Table 1-3 Sunderland Classification System of Peripheral Neuropathy

Sunderland Terminology	Equivalent Seddon Terminology	Descriptors
First-degree	Neurapraxia	• Nerve in continuity • Compression or ischemic etiology • Local conduction block • Spontaneous recovery in minutes to weeks
Second-degree	Axonotmesis	• Injury to axon • Encapsulating structures intact • Wallerian degeneration occurs • Recovery 1–3 mm/day • Spontaneous recovery length dependent
Third-degree	Neurotmesis	• Injury to axon • Endoneurium disrupted; epineurium and perineurium intact • Wallerian degeneration occurs • Surgical neurolysis may benefit healing • Spontaneous recovery length dependent
Fourth-degree	Neurotmesis	• Injury to axon • Disruption in all encapsulating elements but with intact epineurium • Wallerian degeneration occurs • Requires surgical intervention for recovery
Fifth-degree	Neurotmesis	• Injury to axon • Disruption in all encapsulating elements • Wallerian degeneration occurs • Requires surgical intervention for recovery

Data from Sunderland S, Lavarack JO, Ray LJ. The caliber of nerve fibers in human cutaneous nerves. *J Comp Neurol.* 1949;91:87–101; Sunderland S. Anatomical features of nerve trunks in relation to nerve injury and nerve repair. *Clin Neurosurg.* 1970;17:38–62; Sunderland S. *Nerve Injuries and Their Repair. A Critical Appraisal.* Melbourne: Churchill Livingstone; 1991; Seddon H. Advances in nerve repair. *Triangle.* 1968;8:252–259; and Seddon H. Nerve injuries. *Med Bull (Ann Arbor).* 1965;31:4–10.

fiber as a result of compressive, tensile, or chemotoxic insult. There is frequently greater involvement of motor than sensory function with autonomic function typically being retained. Symptoms typically occur distal to the lesion. Nerve conduction examination is normal in the proximal segment and the distal segment but not across the area of injury. Electroneuromyography (using an electromyography [EMG] needle) examination is typically benign with no fibrillation potential or positive sharp waves noted (Fig. 1-7).[35]

Axonotmesis involves a loss of the relative continuity of the axon and its covering of myelin but preservation of the connective tissue framework of the nerve (the encapsulating Schwann cells, epineurium, and perineurium are preserved). Because axonal continuity is lost, wallerian degeneration occurs. EMG examination performed 2 to 3 weeks after injury shows fibrillations and denervation potentials in musculature distal to the injury site. Loss in myotomal and dermatomal distributions is more complete and pervasive with axonotmesis than with neurapraxia, and recovery occurs only through regeneration of the axons, which requires substantial time. Axonotmesis is usually the result of a more severe crush, traction, or contusion injury than neurapraxia. There is usually an element of retrograde proximal degeneration of the axon, and for regeneration to occur, this loss must first be overcome. The regeneration fibers must cross the injury site and regenerate through the proximal or retrograde area of degeneration. This may require several weeks. The regenerating neuron progresses down the distal site, such as the wrist or hand. Proximal lesions may grow distally 2 to 3 mm per day; distal lesions may grow only 1.5 mm per day.[36] Various factors, including local rest versus activity, neural tension, and the presence or absence of neurotoxic chemicals such as chemotherapy medications or elevated blood glucose concentrations, may impact regeneration times.[36–38] Surgical intervention sometimes is required to assist healing secondary to extraneural and intraneural scarring.

Neurotmesis, as described by Seddon,[35] is the most severe lesion involving peripheral nerves based on the quality and quantity of trauma to the nerve and the impact of the damage on regeneration and recovery. Etiologies include laceration, a severe compression, or tension injury affecting the nerve. Similar to axonotmesis, the axon is injured. In addition, the encapsulating connective tissues lose their continuity. Denervation changes recorded by EMG are the same as changes seen with axonometric injury. There is usually a complete loss of motor, sensory, and autonomic function. However, partial function may be retained if there is

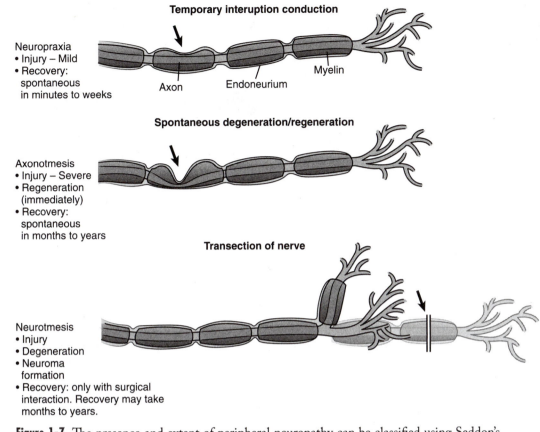

Temporary interruption conduction

Neuropraxia
• Injury – Mild
• Recovery:
  spontaneous
  in minutes to weeks

Axon   Endoneurium   Myelin

Spontaneous degeneration/regeneration

Axonotmesis
• Injury – Severe
• Regeneration
  (immediately)
• Recovery:
  spontaneous
  in months to years

Transection of nerve

Neurotmesis
• Injury
• Degeneration
• Neuroma
  formation
• Recovery: only with surgical
  interaction. Recovery may take
  months to years.

Figure 1-7 The presence and extent of peripheral neuropathy can be classified using Seddon's terminology. Recognizing pathological, clinical, recovery-based, and electromyogram-observed characteristics of neurapraxia, axonotmesis, and neurotmesis helps in the proper diagnosis of peripheral neuropathy.

dual myotomal or dermatomal innervation through an undamaged nerve. Neurotmesis always requires surgical intervention if there is to be hope of regeneration. Sunderland's classification divides Seddon's neurotmetic lesion into degrees.[33]

Sunderland Classification

In 1951, Sunderland expanded Seddon's classification to five degrees of peripheral nerve injury.[33,34,37] A first-degree, or, as per the later nomenclature, class 1, nerve lesion is analogous to Seddon's definition of neurapraxia. Second-degree, or class 2, corresponds to Seddon's definition of axonotmesis. Sunderland's third-, fourth-, and fifth-degree lesions, all termed class 3, correspond to Seddon's neurotmetic nerve injury. Third-degree describes a nerve fiber interruption. There is a disruption of the endoneurium, but the epineurium and perineurium remain intact. Recovery from a third-degree injury is possible but rare without surgical intervention. Sunderland's fourth-degree lesion results in only the epineurium remaining intact; all encapsulated structures are disrupted. A fifth-degree lesion is a complete transection of the peripheral nerve. Fourth- and fifth-degree injuries require surgical intervention.

Wallerian Degeneration

Wallerian degeneration is a process that follows axonotmetic and neurotmetic (Sunderland classification second- to fifth-degree) peripheral nerve injuries.[33] When a nerve fiber is cut, crushed, severely tensioned, or chemotoxically damaged resulting in axonotmesis or neurotmesis, the axon, separated from the neuron's cell nucleus, degenerates. Wallerian degeneration occurs after axonal injury in both the PNS and the CNS. It occurs in the axon stump distal to a site of injury and usually begins within 24 to 36 hours of a lesion.[38,39] Before degeneration, distal axon stumps tend to remain electrically excitable. After injury, the axonal skeleton disintegrates, and the axonal membrane breaks apart. The axonal degeneration is followed by degradation of the myelin sheath and infiltration by macrophages. The macrophages, accompanied by Schwann cells, serve to clear the debris from the degeneration.[39–42]

Although most injury responses include a calcium influx signaling to promote resealing of severed parts, axonal injuries initially lead to acute axonal degeneration (AAD), which is rapid separation of the proximal part and distal ends within 30 minutes of injury.[42] Degeneration follows with swelling of the axolemma eventually leading to a beadlike formation. The process takes roughly 24 hours in the PNS and longer in the CNS. The signaling pathways leading to axolemma degeneration are currently unknown. However, research has shown that this AAD process is calcium-independent.[43,44]

Granular disintegration of the axonal cytoskeleton and inner organelles occurs after axolemma degradation. Early changes include accumulation of mitochondria in the paranodal regions at the site of injury. The endoplasmic reticulum degrades, and mitochondria swell up and eventually disintegrate. The depolymerization of microtubules occurs and is soon followed by degradation of the neurofilaments and other cytoskeleton components. The rate of degradation depends on the type of injury and is also slower in the CNS than in the PNS. Another factor that affects degradation rate is the diameter of the axon—larger axons require a longer time for the cytoskeleton to degrade and take a longer time to degenerate.[45]

The neurolemma of the nerve fiber does not degenerate and remains as a hollow tube. Within 96 hours of the injury, the proximal end of the nerve fiber sends out sprouts toward those tubes, and these sprouts are attracted by growth factors produced by Schwann cells within the tubes. If a sprout reaches the tube, it grows into it and advances about 1 mm per day, eventually reaching and reinnervating the target tissue. If the sprouts cannot reach the tube—for instance, because the gap is too wide or scar tissue has formed—surgery can help to guide the sprouts into the tubes.[45,46]

Schwann cells have been observed to recruit macrophages via the release of proinflammatory cytokines and chemokines after sensing of axonal injury. The recruitment of macrophages helps improve the clearing rate of myelin debris. The resident macrophages present in the nerves release further chemokines and cytokines to attract further macrophages. The degenerating nerve also produces macrophage chemotactic molecules. Another source of macrophage recruitment factors is serum.[46]

Murinson et al.[47] observed that nonmyelinated or myelinated Schwann cells in contact with an injured axon enter the cell cycle, leading to proliferation. Observed time duration for Schwann cell divisions were approximately 3 days after injury.[48] Schwann cells emit growth factors that attract new axonal sprouts growing from the proximal stump after complete degeneration of the injured distal stump. This leads to possible reinnervation of the target cell or organ. However, the reinnervation is not perfect because misleading can occur during reinnervation of the proximal axons to target cells.[47,48]

A related process known as "wallerian-like degeneration" occurs in many neurodegenerative diseases, especially diseases where axonal transport is impaired. Primary culture studies suggest that a failure to deliver sufficient quantities of the essential axonal protein NmnAT2 is a key initiating event.[49,50]

CASE STUDY

Jack is an 18-year-old high school football player. He plays the position of running back. On a play late in the first half, the quarterback handed the ball off to Jack who sprinted toward the sidelines, attempting to turn up field for a large gain. As he was making his turn, the defender launched himself at Jack attempting to tackle him. The defender's helmet hit Jack square in the left upper arm. Jack felt an immediate stabbing pain in his upper arm as he tumbled out of bounds. He could not lift his left arm above 90°.

Jack was taken to the emergency department, and x-rays were taken. The x-rays revealed no fractures or dislocations of left humerus, scapula, clavicle, or cervical spine. On physical examination at the hospital, Jack still could not lift the arm greater than 90°, and a small patch, approximately 4 cm × 4 cm of skin over the left middle deltoid, was unable to perceive tactile sensation.

Jack's left arm was placed in a sling, and he was referred to an orthopedist. The next day when Jack saw the orthopedist, the clinical signs were unchanged. The orthopedist referred Jack for an electroneuromyogram to be performed in 2 weeks and for physical therapy.

Case Study Questions

1. Based on the history given, the most likely etiology for Jack's clinical signs is which tissue?
   a. Bone
   b. Muscle
   c. Tendon
   d. Nerve

2. Based on the history given, which of the following nerves is most likely involved?
   a. Axillary
   b. Radial
   c. Median
   d. Ulnar

3. If the electroneuromyography study found positive sharp waves and denervation potentials in the deltoid, and considering the mechanism of injury, the most likely Seddon classification for this injury would be which of the following?
   a. Neurapraxia
   b. Neurotmesis
   c. Axonotmesis
   d. Bruising

4. The electroneuromyography examination will most likely reveal similar findings with which muscle in addition to the deltoid?

a. Biceps

b. Teres minor

c. Extensor carpi ulnaris

d. Subscapularis

5. If the diagnosis is an axonotmetic lesion of the left axillary nerve, what would be the expected approximate length of time for healing?

a. 2 days

b. 1 week

c. 2 months

d. 2 years

References

1. Sunderland S. A classification of peripheral nerve injuries producing loss of function. *Brain*. 1951;74:491–516.
2. Millesi H, Zöch G, Rath T. The gliding apparatus of peripheral nerve and its clinical significance. *Ann Hand Surg*. 1990;9:87–97.
3. Yamamoto T, Hirano A. Nucleus raphe dorsalis in Alzheimer's disease: Neurofibrillary tangles and loss of large neurons *Ann Neurol*. 1985;17:573–577.
4. Glees P. Observations on the connective tissue sheaths of peripheral nerves. *J Anat*. 1942;77:153–159.
5. Jordan PC. Semimicroscopic modeling of permeation energetics in ion channels. *IEEE Trans Nanobioscience*. 2005;4:94–101.
6. Ahern CA, Horn R. Specificity of charge carrying residues in the voltage sensor of potassium channels. *J Gen Physiol*. 2004;123:204–216.
7. Rall W, Agmon-Snir H. Cable theory for dendritic neurons. In: Koch C, Segev I, eds. *Methods in Neuronal Modeling*. 2nd ed. Cambridge, MA: MIT Press; 1998:27–92.
8. Jack JJB, Noble D, Tsien RW. *Electric Current Flow in Excitable Cells*. Oxford: Calderon Press; 1975.
9. Rall W. Cable theory for neurons. In: Kandel ER, Brookhardt JM, Mountcastle VB, eds. *Handbook of Physiology: The Nervous System*. Vol 1. Baltimore: Williams & Wilkins; 1977:39–98.
10. Hartzell HC, Kuffler SW, Yoshikami D. Post-synaptic potentiation: Interaction between quanta of acetylcholine at the skeletal neuromuscular synapse. *J Physiol*. 1975;251:427–463.
11. Tassler PL, Dellon AL, Canoun C. Identification of elastic fibers in the peripheral nerve. *J Hand Surg (Br Eur)*. 1994;19B:48–54.
12. Sunderland S, Bradley KC. The cross-sectional area of peripheral nerve trunks devoted to nerve fibres. *Brain*. 1949;72:428–449.
13. Driscoll PJ, Glasby MA, Lawson GM. An *in vivo* study of peripheral nerves in continuity: Biomechanical and physiological responses to elongation. *J Orthop Res*. 2002;20:370–375.
14. Lundborg G, Rydevik B. Effects of stretching the tibial nerve of the rabbit. A preliminary study of the intraneural circulation and the barrier function of the perineurium. *J Bone Joint Surg Br*. 1973;55:390–401.
15. Salvador-Sanz JF, Torres AN, Calpena FT, Sanz-Gimenez-Rico JR, Lopez SC, Barraquer EL. Anatomical study of the cutaneous perforator arteries and vascularisation of the biceps femoris muscle. *Br J Plast Surg*. 2005;58(8):1079-1085.
16. Sarikcioglu L, Demirel BM, Demir N, Yildirim FB, Demirtop A, Oguz N. Morphological and ultrastructural analysis of the watershed zones after stripping of the vasa nervorum. *Int J Neurosci*. 2008;118:1145–1155.
17. Myers RR, Powell HC, Heckman HM, Costello ML, Katz J. Biophysical and pathological effects of cryogenic nerve lesion. *Ann Neurol*. 1981;10:478–485.
18. Powell HC, Costello ML, Myers RR. Endoneurial fluid pressure in experimental models of diabetic neuropathy. *J Neuropathol Exp Neurol*. 1981;40:613–624.
19. Dunn JS, Wyburn GM. The anatomy of the blood brain barrier: A review. *Scott Med J*. 1972;17:21–36.
20. Hunter JM. Recurrent carpal tunnel syndrome, epineurial fibrous fixation, and traction neuropathy. *Hand Clin*. 1991;7:491–504.
21. Kwan MK, Wall EJ, Massie J, Garfin SR. Strain, stress and stretch of peripheral nerve. Rabbit experiments *in vitro* and *in vivo*. *Acta Orthop Scand*. 1992;63:267–272.
22. Haftek J. Stretch injury of peripheral nerve. Acute effects of stretching on rabbit nerve. *J Bone Joint Surg Br*. 1970;52:354–365.
23. Millesi H, Zöch G, Reihsner R. Mechanical properties of peripheral nerves. *Clin Orthop*. 1995;314:76–83.
24. Sunderland S, Lavarack JO, Ray LJ. The caliber of nerve fibers in human cutaneous nerves. *J Comp Neurol*. 1949;91:87–101.
25. Rydevik BL, Kwan MK, Myers RR, Brown RA, Triggs KJ, Woo SL, Garfin SR. An *in vitro* mechanical and histological study of acute stretching on rabbit tibial nerve. *J Orthop Res*. 1990;8:694–701.
26. Sunderland S. Anatomical features of nerve trunks in relation to nerve injury and nerve repair. *Clin Neurosurg*. 1970; 17:38–62.
27. Miyamoto Y. Experimental studies on repair for peripheral nerves—relationship between circulatory disturbances at nerve stumps caused by tension at the suture line and axon regeneration. *Hiroshima J Med Sci*. 1979;28:87–93.
28. Low P, Marchand G, Knox F, Dyck PJ. Measurement of endoneurial fluid pressure with polyethylene matrix capsules. *Brain Res*. 1977;122:373–377.
29. Walbeehm ET, Afoke A, de Wit T, Holman F, Hovius SE, Brown RA. Mechanical functioning of peripheral nerves: Linkage with the mushrooming effect. *Cell Tissue Res*. 2004;316:115–121.
30. Sunderland S, Bradley KC. Stress-strain phenomena in human peripheral nerve trunks. *Brain*. 1961;84:102–119.
31. Wall EJ, Massie JB, Kwan MK, Rydevik BL, Myers RR, Garfin SR. Experimental stretch neuropathy. Changes in nerve conduction under tension. *J Bone Joint Surg Br*. 1992;74:126–129.
32. Sunderland S. *Nerve Injuries and Their Repair. A Critical Appraisal*. Melbourne: Churchill Livingstone; 1991.
33. Kaye AH. Classification of nerve injuries. In: *Essential Neurosurgery*. London: Churchill Livingstone; 1991:333–334.
34. Greenberg MS. Injury classification system. In: *Handbook of Neurosurgery*. 3rd ed. Lakeland, FL: Greenberg Graphics; 1994:411–412.
35. Seddon H. Advances in nerve repair. *Triangle*. 1968; 8:252–259.
36. Seddon H. Nerve injuries. *Med Bull (Ann Arbor)*. 1965; 31:4–10.
37. Sunderland S. The anatomy and physiology of nerve injury. *Muscle Nerve*. 1990;13:771–784.
38. Wall EJ, Kwan MK, Rydevik BL, Woo SL, Garfin SR. Stress relaxation of a peripheral nerve. *J Hand Surg (Am)*. 1991;16:859–863.
39. Coleman MP, Freeman MF. Wallerian degeneration WldS and Nmnat. *Ann Rev Neurosci*. 2010; 33:245–267.

40. Liu HM, Yang LH, Yang YJ. Schwann cell properties: 3. C-fos expression, bFGF production, phagocytosis and proliferation during Wallerian degeneration. *J Neuropathol Exp Neurol.* 1995;54:487–496.

41. Coleman MP, Conforti M, Buckmaster AE, Tarlton A, Ewing RM, Brown MC, et al. An 85-kb tandem triplication in the slow wallerian degeneration (Wlds) mouse. *Proc Natl Acad Sci U S A.* 1998;95:9985–9990.

42. Kerschensteiner M, Schwab ME, Lichtman JW, Misgeld T. In vivo imaging of axonal degeneration and regeneration in the injured spinal cord. *Nat Med.* 2005;11:572–577.

43. Vargas ME, Barres BA. Why is wallerian degeneration in the CNS so slow. *Annu Rev Neurosci.* 2007;30:153–179.

44. Zimmerman UP, Schlaepfer WW. Multiple forms of Ca-activated protease from rat brain and muscle. *J Biol Chem.* 1984;259:3210–3218.

45. Guertin AD, Zhang DP, Mak KS, Alberta JA, Kim HA. Microanatomy of axon/glial signaling during Wallerian degeneration. *J Neurosci.* 2005;25:3478–3487.

46. Vargas ME, Singh SJ, Barres BA. Why is Wallerian degeneration so slow in the CNS? *Soc Neurosci.* 2005;Program No. 439.2

47. Murinson BB, Archer DR, Li Y, Griffin JW. Degeneration of myelinated efferent fibers prompts mitosis in Remak Schwann cells of uninjured C-fiber afferents. *J Neurosc.* 2005;25:1179–1187.

48. Liu HM, Yang LH, Yang YJ. Schwann cell properties: 3. C-fos expression, bFGF production, phagocytosis and proliferation during Wallerian degeneration. *J Neuropathol Exp Neurol.* 1995;54:487–496.

49. Coleman MP, Freeman MF. Wallerian degeneration, WldS and Nmnat. *Annu Rev Neurosci.* 2010;33:245–267.

50. Gilley J, Coleman MP. Endogenous Nmnat2 is an essential survival factor for maintenance of healthy axons. *PLOS Biol.* 2010;8:27–47.

Chapter 2

The Biomechanics of Peripheral Nerve Injury

STEPHEN J. CARP, PT, PHD, GCS

"Seize the moment of excited curiosity on any subject to solve your doubts; for if you let it pass, the desire may never return and you may remain forever in ignorance."
—WILLIAM WIRT (1772–1834)

Objectives

On completion of this chapter, the student/practitioner will be able to:

- Develop an evidenced-based evaluative algorithm for the assessment of suspected peripheral neuropathy.
- Develop sufficient knowledge of the cognitive components of the peripheral neuropathy evaluation to enable the development of the psychomotor components of the evaluation.
- Identify important signs and symptoms that may relate to peripheral neuropathy.

Key Terms

- Epineurium
- Lower motor neuron
- Mesoneurium
- Perineurium
- Vasa nervorum

Introduction

The peripheral nerve is a functional component of an intricate intrinsic conduction system that serves as a mediator for bidirectional transport between the central nervous system (CNS) and the peripheral nervous system (PNS). Peripheral nerves extend to distal tissues to aid in system regulation, homeostasis, repair, function, learning, posture, reproduction, mobility, and protection. For descriptive purposes, the peripheral nerves may be classified via segmental and peripheral nomenclature according to their function and site of CNS origin: The cranial nerves emerge from the base of the brain, the spinal nerves originate in the spinal cord, and the autonomic system is intimately associated with the cranial and spinal nerves but differs in function and in the details of structure and distribution.

Efferent, Afferent, and Autonomic Pathways

The bidirectional movement of action potentials along the peripheral nerve serves as afferent pathways, efferent pathways, and autonomic pathways. The afferent pathways are primarily sensory. A wide spectrum of sensory modalities exist: vision, hearing, smell, taste, rotational acceleration, linear acceleration, verticality, touch, pressure, warmth, cold, pain, proprioception, kinesthesia, muscle length, muscle tension, arterial blood pressure, central venous pressure, inflation of lung, temperature of blood in the head, osmotic pressure of plasma, and arteriovenous blood glucose difference. A loss or diminished function in any of these modalities may have devastating homeostatic and functional consequences. The signs and symptoms of loss are directly related to the specific sensory modality that is compromised. Positive signs of sensory nerve injury are typically described as sensations additive to normal perception, such as burning, formication, tingling, hyperalgesia, pain, or a feeling of temperature change. Negative signs are a reduction in sensory perception, such as numbness, ataxia, orthostasis, loss of visual acuity and tracking, deafness, movement degradation, and dyskinesia. In higher level animals, there is a redundancy of sensory modalities that allows for continued, albeit diminished, function with the loss of specific sensory modalities. An example of redundancy in humans is balance. The visual, vestibular, and sensorimotor systems all contribute to balance control. Functional performance with loss of one or more of these systems has been extensively studied.[1-6]

The efferent pathways are primarily motoric. Motion is a fundamental property required for most organisms to maintain life. Unicellular organisms achieve motion through accessory organs such as cilia and flagella. High-level, multicellular organisms have a much more complicated motoric system requiring a complex variety and interaction of afferent and efferent neural tissues, in addition to both contractile and noncontractile connective tissues. These elements work in harmony to provide coordinated movement patterns and locomotion.

The **lower motor neuron,** also called the final common pathway, consists of a cell body located in the anterior gray column of the spinal cord or the brainstem and an axon passing via the peripheral nerve to the motor end plates within the muscles. It is called the final common pathway because it is acted on by the rubrospinal, olivospinal, vestibulospinal, corticospinal, and tectospinal tracts and their associated intersegmental and intrasegmental reflex neurons and is the ultimate pathway through which neural impulses reach the muscle. Motor disturbances associated with peripheral nerve injury may consist of weakness, dyskinesia, obligatory posturing, and tonal change. Such disturbances may be the result of lesions within the muscle, at the myoneural junction, within the peripheral nerve, or within the CNS. The specific nature of the patient's presenting signs and symptoms may lead an astute clinician to the specific etiology of the observed weakness and serve to guide future intervention.

The predominant clinical sign of a lower motor neuron injury is weakness. The spectrum of involvement ranges from subclinical weakness to complete paralysis. Movement disorders such as dyskinesia may also occur. Depending on the site of injury, one muscle or a patterned group of muscles may be involved. Typically, there is a concurrent decrease in or absent deep tendon reflex. Myalgias, or muscle-specific pain and cramping, may also accompany the weakness.

The second type of motor (efferent) system that may be affected by injury to the peripheral nerve is the autonomic nervous system (ANS). The ANS is a division of the PNS that is distributed to glands and smooth muscle. Most functions of the ANS are carried out below the level of conscious input. The cell body of the preganglionic or presynaptic neuron, located within the CNS, sends out its axon to one of the outlying ganglia from where the postganglionic axon extends to its terminal distribution. Cell bodies of presynaptic sympathetic nerve fibers lie in the ventral horn from cord segments T1–L3. Postganglionic fibers arise from the sympathetic trunk. The ANS is divided into the sympathetic and parasympathetic systems. With injury to a peripheral nerve, signs and symptoms related to an autonomic dysfunction may appear. These include, but are not limited to, aberrations in vascular flow, skin moisture, and hair growth; trophic changes; nail loss; and delayed wound healing.

Structure of the Peripheral Nerve

The nerve fiber represents the greatly elongated process of a nerve cell whose body lies within the CNS or one of the outlying ganglia. The nerve cell, or neuron, consists of a cell body and all of its processes. The nucleus-containing cell body is the vital center controlling the metabolic activity of the cell. Injury to the nerve cell or fiber results in degeneration of the distal segment (Fig. 2-1).

A typical spinal motor neuron has many processes, called dendrites, which extend out from the cell body and arborize. The spinal neuron has a long axon that originates from an area of the cell body called the axon hillock. Near its origin, the typical motor neuron develops a sheath of myelin composed of a multilayered, lipoprotein complex. The myelin sheath envelops the axon except at its ending and at periodic constrictions,

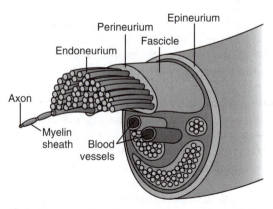

Figure 2-1 Cross-sectional representation of a peripheral nerve. Note the complexity of the protective elements surrounding the functional components.

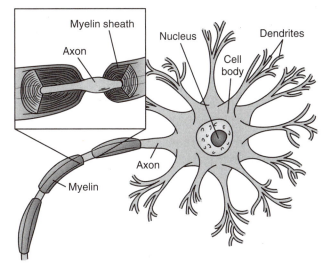

Figure 2-2 Representation of a myelinated peripheral neuron. The myelin sheath protects the neuron and increases the velocity of conduction.

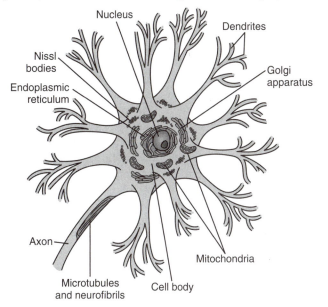

Figure 2-3 Schematic representation of a cell body.

which are approximately 1 mm apart. This arrangement of the myelin sheath is known as the nodes of Ranvier. The discontinuity in the myelin sheath allows rapid impulse conduction as the action potential leaps from one node to the next. In nonmyelinated fibers, one Schwann cell is associated with many axons, whereas in the myelinated fibers, the ratio is one Schwann cell per axon. Unmyelinated axons are enveloped by Schwann cell cytoplasm and plasma membrane but do not have the multiple wrappings of Schwann cell plasma membranes similar to myelinated axons (Fig. 2-2).

The dendritic zone is the term used to refer to the receptor membrane of a neuron. The axon is a single elongated protoplasmic neuronal process with the specialized function of moving impulses away from the dendritic zone and ends in numerous terminal buttons or axon telodendra. Typically, the cell body is located at the dendritic zone, but it may occasionally be located within the axon or attached to the side of the axon (Fig. 2-3).

The nerve fiber, which is the functional component of the peripheral nerve, is surrounded by connective tissues similar to those found in muscle or ligament. Together, these connective tissues provide protection to the nerve fibers through their combined abilities to resist compressive and tensile forces and, in some cases, chemotoxic elements. Axons and the bundled nerve fibers, called fascicles, run an undulated course through the peripheral nerve that serves to resist tensile forces (Fig. 2-4). In the peripheral nerve, fascicle number is greater proximally than distally.[7,8]

The **mesoneurium** is a loose areolar tissue that surrounds peripheral nerve trunks. The function of the mesoneurium is unclear; however, the mesoneurium

Connective tissue components

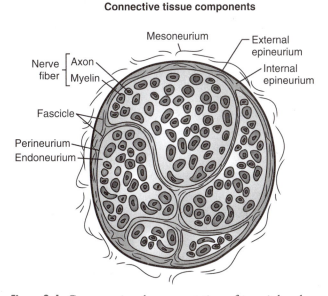

Figure 2-4 Cross-sectional representation of a peripheral nerve focusing on the connective tissue components.

likely provides friction relief between the nerve and adjacent structures such as bone, ligament, or muscle.[9–11] There may also be some sliding of the fascicles inside the mesoneurium.[10,11]

The **epineurium** is the outermost connective tissue of the fascicles.[12] Collagen bundles in the epineurium are arranged longitudinally. External epineurium provides a definitive sheath among the fascicles.[13] Internal epineurium helps keep the fascicles apart and assists gliding between fascicles, a necessary adjunct to movement, especially when the nerve is asked to move about a joint.[14] The epineurium also supports a well-developed intrinsic circulation. A lymphatic capillary network exists in the epineurium, drained by channels accompanying the arteries of the nerve trunk.[15] The epineurial layer includes bundles of type I and type III collagen fibrils and elastic fibers as well as fibroblasts, mast cells, and fat cells.[14,15]

A thin sheath, called the **perineurium,** surrounds bundles of nerve fibers; microscopically, the perineurium is lamellar in design with up to 15 layers present in the larger nerve trunks.[16] Lundborg[17–21] described the role of the perineurium as protecting the contents of the endoneural tubes, acting as mechanical barriers to external forces, and serving as a diffusion barrier by keeping certain substances out of the intrafascicular environment. With a high ratio of elastin to collagen, the perineurium is thought to prevent neural damage from tensile forces more so than protecting the nerve from compressive forces.[22] Lundborg et al.[20,21] described the perineurium as having elastin fibers running parallel to the nerve and, to a lesser extent, oblique fibers running at an angle to the longitudinal fibers. It is hypothesized that the oblique fibers may assist in the prevention of kinking of the nerve as it flexes at the interior surfaces of joints.

The endoneurium, with its longitudinally arranged collagen fibers, is the membrane associated with the neural tube and serves to establish a constant nerve fiber environment by maintaining a slightly positive pressure around the neuron.[20] The endoneurium consists of fibroblasts, capillaries, mast cells, and Schwann cells.[15] Cutaneous nerves have a greater percentage of endoneurium than motor nerves; this is due to the extra protection a cutaneous nerve requires because of its more superficial location.[16,17]

The blood supply of the PNS is called the **vasa nervorum.** Vessels extrinsic to the nerve supply feed arteries to the multiple neural layers. Once inside the nerve, there is a rich anastomotic intrinsic blood supply. The redundant blood supply to the nerve, necessary because of the high metabolic demands of neural tissue[23] and the mobility of the PNS,[24,25] provides for excellent perfusion even with significant intrinsic arteriole or extrinsic artery injury. The intrinsic arteriole system is quite extensive, linking the mesoneurium, endoneurium, and perineurium. Intraneural blood vessels have autonomic innervation[25] that most likely allows for an adjustable blood supply required for the functional demands of the nerve.

Various mammalian receptor and effector neurons are associated with the PNS, which allow for the appreciation of sensation. Specialized cells for detecting particular changes in the environment are called receptors. Exteroceptors include receptors affected by changes in the external environment. Teleceptors are receptors sensitive to distant stimuli. Proprioceptors receive impulses directly from muscle spindles, Golgi tendon organs, tendons, and periarticular tissues. Interoceptors are sensitive to changes within visceral tissues and blood vessels.

Peripheral Nerve Response to Injury

The inflammatory acute phase response to peripheral nerve tissue injury is thoroughly explained in Chapter 3. From a clinical point of view, there are three basic ways nerve fibers may respond to injury. These categories of nerve injury were initially described by Seddon[26,27] and expanded on by Sunderland.[28–39] Nerves are not homogeneous structures, but rather are considered to be anisotropic with varying diameter, length, level of myelination, blood supply, percentages of surrounding protective tissue types, and distance from the cell body.[40–42] Most nerve injuries result in a combination of the three primary categories of nerve injury: neurapraxia, neurotmesis, and axonotmesis.[30–32]

Neurapraxia is defined as a segmental block of axonal conduction. The nerve can conduct an action potential above and below the blockage but not across the blockage. The nerve is in continuity but does not function. This phenomenon is due to a focal region of demyelination of the nerve. The conduction block is due to a physiological process without histological change. No wallerian degeneration is present in neurapraxia.[33] Etiologies include mild blunt trauma, prolonged mild compression, repetitive strain, and stretch. Stimulation proximal to the injury often fails to produce a muscle contraction; however, stimulation distal to the injury provokes a muscle contraction. Neurapraxia typically affects larger, myelinated fibers, and fine fibers innervating pain and autonomic function are often spared. Recovery is usually uncomplicated and can occur minutes to months after injury.[30–32]

Axonotmesis is defined as a loss of continuity of the nerve axon with maintenance of the continuity of the connective sheaths. Axonotmesis leads to wallerian degeneration of the distal part of the nerve. Electromyography (EMG) performed 2 to 3 weeks after injury shows fibrillations and denervation potentials in the musculature distal to the injury site[32] with a concomitant normal response in muscles proximal to the injury site. Loss of motor and sensory function is typically more advanced than that observed with neurapraxia. Recovery occurs only through regeneration of the axon. The etiology of axonotmesis is similar to the etiology of neurapraxia with the difference being the intensity of the injury. There is usually an element of additional retrograde nerve injury that must be overcome for complete recovery to occur.[34] The rate of axonal regeneration varies according to the presence of comorbidities (especially conditions implicated in the cause of the neuropathy), physical activity impacting the site of the injury, and the distance between the injury site and the CNS.[36] Uncomplicated recovery rates range from 1.5 to 3 mm/day.[30–32]

Neurotmesis, similar to axonotmesis, involves destruction of the axons. The connective supporting tissues of the axon are injured as well. Neurotmesis is caused by a severe contusion, stretch, avulsion, laceration, or chemotaxis. There are three basic types of neurotmesis[36–38]: The first type is a loss of the continuity of the axons and endoneurium with an intact perineurium; the second type is loss of the continuity of the axons, endoneurium, and perineurium with an intact epineurium; and the third type is a complete transection of the nerve. EMG examination of neurotmesis typically reveals the same findings that are seen with axonotmetic injury.[42] Stimulation above and below the injury site does not produce a muscle contraction. Spontaneous repair and recovery of function is much less likely to occur compared with axonotmetic injury because the regeneration axons become entangled in a swirl of collagen and fibroblasts. This phenomenon creates a disorganized, impenetrable repair site.[34–36]

Regenerating axons may not function even after reaching distal end organs, unless they arrive close to their original sites.[20] Cutaneous fibers do not cross certain boundaries even for sensory reinnervation. In addition, ulnar and median motor fibers that have undergone regeneration have seldom been found to return to normal function.[43] A similar inability to return to normal function is seen with the synkinesis of the muscles of facial expression after facial nerve injury.[44,45]

Histological changes typically occur in the denervated muscles by the 3rd week. The muscle fibers kink, and their cross striations decrease. With continued denervation and lack of movement or extrinsic muscle stimulation, the entire muscle may be replaced by fat or fibrous tissue within 2 to 3 years.[29,30]

Physiological Basis for Biomechanical and Chemotoxic Nerve Injury

The three primary etiologies of neuropathy include mechanical, ischemic, and metabolic factors. The forces that contribute to mechanical nerve injury typically include any combination of compression, traction, friction, shear, contusion, or laceration. Although consensus exists regarding the mechanical factors that result in peripheral nerve injury, confusion remains regarding the magnitude of the injurious force and the significance of the injury. Much of this confusion relates directly to the fact that peripheral nerve tissue is an anisotropic structure, consisting of a combination of neural and nonneural connective tissue with composition percentages varying with location along the nerve. In other words, forces that may result in severe injury at one location along a peripheral nerve as measured by functional examination, electroneuromyography examination, and biomarker examination may result in no measurable injury at a different location along the same nerve. In addition, the location of extrinsic ancillary structures such as bone, ligament, or retinaculum may predispose a particular nerve location to injury in the presence of mechanical insult.

Nerves are elastic structures with substantial ability to resist tensile forces. However, the tensile demands on peripheral nerve tissue often produce symptoms before histological or gross changes within the nerve and nerve sheaths.[45] With the application of a small tensile force, the intact nerve reacts with characteristics of an elastic material. As the linear limit is reached, the nerve fibers begin to rupture within the endoneurial tube. The epineurium and perineurium begin to rupture with the ever-increasing load of force and there is disintegration of the elastic properties of the nerve, and the nerve begins to react more like a plastic material.[46,47] Sunderland[31] estimated that the elastic limit of a nerve is resting length plus 20% of resting length and that maximum elongation before rupture is resting length plus 30% resting length.

Sunderland[31] reported that the median nerve at the level of the wrist can withstand 70 to 220 N of traction before complete transection occurs. Ochs et al.[48] reported an in vivo complete action potential block after 30 minutes of mild stretch with no apparent histological changes. These authors postulated that the nerve block was due to vascular ischemia. Sunderland[31] believed that most of the tensile resistance of the nerve is due to the perineurium. As long as the perineurium remains intact, the tensile resisting function of the nerve remains sufficient.

Thomas and Olson[49] assessed structural changes of nerves during compression of peroneal nerves in rats. The nerves were compressed at different pressures for various amounts of time. The initial event of injury is the expression of endoneurial fluid, followed by compression of the outflow of axoplasm, and cleavage and displacement of myelin. Clinically, the fact that nerve fiber rupture occurs before epineurial and perineurial rupture indicates that after a moderate stretch injury, the axons may have intact pathways to follow to their respective end organ; this bodes well for the recovery of normal functioning. As seen with chronic nerve compression and tension, epineurial and perineurial scarring may result in loss of nerve elasticity, resulting in early rupture. One must also question the effect of epineurial and perineurial scarring on blood flow. Such scarring may limit oxygen and nutrient uptake by the neural components, leading to a worsening of the injury and slower healing.

Cornefjord et al.[50] used a porcine model to investigate the effects of chronic nerve compression. They identified inflammatory cells, nerve fiber damage, endoneurial hyperemia, and bleeding at the site of compression. Barr et al.[51] reported similar findings using a rat model of work relating nerve compression to musculoskeletal disorder. Typically, the relationship between force of compression and time of compression is significant in defining the extent of the nerve injury. In a rat model, pressures of 30 mm Hg have been shown to cause functional loss and intraneural edema with epineurial scarring. It was found that 80 mm Hg of pressure immediately caused local ischemia. Pressures of 80 mm Hg resulted in a fourfold increase of edema compared with 30 mm Hg of pressure, indicating a force/trauma relationship to injury. In addition, a threefold increase in edema was found at both 80 mm Hg and 30 mm Hg at 8 hours compared with 4 hours, indicating a time/trauma relationship to injury. Such an increase in endoneurial fluid pressure may interfere with intrafascicular capillary flow, constituting an important pathological mechanism for the development of compressive neuropathies. In a related study, indirect compression at very high pressures caused less of a functional loss than direct compression at much lower pressures.[50] This finding suggests that direct compressive trauma to a nerve, as seen with bony abnormalities from arthritis, compression from the transverse carpal tunnel ligament, or compressive forces in response to local tumor infiltration, may have a significant functional impact on nerve function.

Compared with other tissues, peripheral nerves are relatively resistant to direct or indirect ischemic injury because of their abundant circulation. In addition to a rich intraneural network of vasa nervorum, there are extensive anastomotic connections with the nutrient arterial supply to the nerve. Impulse propagation is directly related to local oxygen supply.[52-54] For that reason, the vasa nervorum has a large reserve capacity. Large vessels approach the peripheral nerve along the course of the nerve. These large vessels divide into ascending and descending branches. The ascending and descending branches run longitudinally and frequently join with vessels in the perineurium and endoneurium. Each fascicle has a longitudinally oriented capillary plexus with loop formations at various levels. This rich anastomosis provides a wide safety margin in the presence of a nerve transection. Lundborg et al.[21] dissected the regional nutrient vessels from a 15-cm section of rabbit sciatic nerve and found no reduction in the intrafascicular blood flow.

From a clinical standpoint, several scenarios of vascular compromise may result in neuropathic signs and symptoms secondary to ischemia. Lundborg et al.[19] showed that elongation of just 8% of resting length results in impaired venular flow. At elongations greater than 8% of resting nerve length, there was impaired arteriole flow, and all arteriole flow stopped completely at 15% greater than resting nerve length. Studies of the rat sciatic nerve demonstrated that blood flow is reduced by 50% with a strain of 11% and 100% with a sustained strain of 15.7%.[55] This strain may impact the quality of repair after epineurial repair, especially if the trauma resulted in a gap between the two ends. From a therapist standpoint, care must be taken during passive stretching maneuvers that result in neurological symptoms so as not to interfere with normal healing.

Long-term usage of handheld vibratory tools such as sanders, jackhammers, and dental tools can induce changes in peripheral circulation and tissue oxygen levels as well as sensory disturbances, motor weakness, and injury.[56,57] Loss of tactile and position sense may be associated with long-term inflammatory changes within the median and ulnar nerves at the level of the wrist and hand.[58,59] In addition, injuries to nearby structures such as skin receptors and nerve cell bodies have been implicated as a potential cause for the sensory loss.[60]

Space-occupying lesions may also result in significant biomechanical changes causing peripheral nerve injury. Bony exostoses caused by trauma have been associated with neuropathy.[61] Tumors may also impinge on peripheral nerves leading to injury.[62] For instance, Pancoast tumors of the lung may affect the lower trunks of the brachial plexus with initial symptoms of tumor development being hand weakness and paresthesias. Degenerative arthropathies caused by connective tissue disorders may result in elongation or compression neuropathies.

In addition to biomechanical factors, a host of infectious and chemotoxic etiologies may result in direct or indirect peripheral nerve injury. Diabetes mellitus is the most common cause of peripheral neuropathy. Objective evidence of a sensory or motor neuropathy is present in 59% of patients with type 2 diabetes and 66% of patients with type 1 diabetes.[63] Although intervention is available for diabetic neuropathy, prevention of complications from diabetes through tight glycemic control from the onset of diagnosis is the most effective therapy.

Diabetes mellitus may result in focal and multifocal neuropathies. Nerves in patients with diabetes are more susceptible to tensile and compressive forces than nerves in individuals without diabetes.[63] Common nerve injuries include injuries to the third and sixth cranial nerves, the median nerve at the wrist, the ulnar nerve at the elbow, the lateral femoral cutaneous nerve, and the common peroneal nerve at the head of the fibula as well as truncal sensory neuropathy.

Diabetic polyneuropathy is a systemic complication usually beginning at the feet and moving proximally. The hands are often involved as well. Initially, there may be complaints of severe paresthesias and pain, which eventually change to complaints of numbness.

Often there are complaints of residual pain, which is frequently paroxysmal in nature. Atrophy and intrinsic motor weakness eventually develop. Autonomic symptoms and signs may appear as well, including cardiovascular manifestations such as postural hypotension or altered heart rate. Neurological impotence may also occur, which consists of an atonic bladder, hyperhydrosis or hypohydrosis of the skin, diarrhea, and gastric paresis. Richardson[63] discussed three important clinical signs as a prediction model for diagnosing diabetic peripheral neuropathy: an absent Achilles reflex even with Jendrassik maneuver, diminished vibratory sense, and diminished proprioception. The etiology of focal and patterned neuropathy related to diabetes mellitus is unclear. The two major theories of nerve injury related to diabetes include metabolic and vascular abnormalities. The variability of glycemic control also affects the development of neuropathy.

Guillain-Barré syndrome (GBS) typically consists of a variety of disorders—all are acute PNS disorders that are monophasic, with peak neurological deficit reached in most cases within 2 weeks—and is frequently preceded by an antecedent event. Antecedent events include acute infections such as with Epstein-Barr or influenza virus, systemic illnesses such as sarcoidosis and Hodgkin disease, and other medically invasive conditions such as surgical procedures and immunizations. The diseases are presumed to be immune-mediated, have albuminocytological dissociation in the spinal fluid, and are generally associated with spontaneous recovery in most cases.[64] In almost 85% of patents, symptom presentation follows a pattern of "classical" GBS.[64,65] Initial symptoms are typically sensory dysfunction in the extremities with associated arthralgias and myalgias. The pain typically begins in the low back and extends down the thighs to the calves. Weakness follows the sensory manifestations, beginning in the legs and extending proximally to the trunk and arms. Electrodiagnostic guidelines for the identification of peripheral nerve demyelination in patients with GBS have been established.[64]

Peripheral neuropathies may also be associated with connective tissue diseases, such as systemic lupus erythematosus, scleroderma, rheumatoid arthritis and Sjögren syndrome. These connective tissue diseases represent a diverse group of disorders.[66,67] A hallmark is the related presentation of trigeminal sensory neuropathy. This entity appears to be associated with a lesion of the sensory ganglion of the fifth cranial nerve. Almost all of the connective tissue disorders are associated with a length-dependent sensorimotor neuropathy. Other, less common illnesses that may result in peripheral neuropathy include HIV infection, familial amyloid polyneuropathy, leprosy, organ transplantation, cancer, and radiation-induced plexopathies.

Because of the incredible spectrum of possible etiologies and functional impairments, the importance of the clinical examination of a patient with suspected peripheral neuropathy cannot be overemphasized. An accurate clinical examination, correlated with relevant radiographic, electrophysiological, and laboratory diagnostic studies, allows the therapist to develop an accurate functional and clinical diagnosis. Only with the correct clinical diagnosis can an effective intervention program be developed.

References

1. Bucci MP, Le TT, Wiener-Vacher S, Bremond-Gignac D, Bouet A, Kapoula Z. Poor postural stability in children with vertigo and vergence abnormalities. *Invest Ophthalmol Vis Sci.* 2009;50(10):4678–4684.
2. Glasauer S, Schneider E, Jahn K, Strupp M, Brandt T. How the eyes move the body. *Neurology.* 2005;65(8):1291–1293.
3. Guo X, Chau WW, Hui-Chan CW, Cheung CS, Tsang WW, Cheng JC. Balance control in adolescents with idiopathic scoliosis and disturbed somatosensory function. *Spine (Phila Pa 1976).* 2006;31(14):E437–440.
4. Horak FB. Postural compensation for vestibular loss. *Ann N Y Acad Sci.* 2009;1164:76–81.
5. Horlings CG, Kung UM, Honegger F, et al. Vestibular and proprioceptive influences on trunk movements during quiet standing. *Neuroscience.* 2009;161(3):904–914.
6. Swanenburg J, de Bruin ED, Favero K, Uebelhart D, Mulder T. The reliability of postural balance measures in single and dual tasking in elderly fallers and non-fallers. *BMC Musculoskelet Disord.* 2008;9:162.
7. Grinberg Y, Schiefer MA, Tyler DJ, Gustafson KJ. Fascicular perineurium thickness, size, and position affect model predictions of neural excitation. *IEEE Trans Neural Syst Rehabil Eng.* 2008;16(6):572–581.
8. Sekiya S, Suzuki R, Miyawaki M, Chiba S, Kumaki K. Formation and distribution of the sural nerve based on nerve fascicle and nerve fiber analyses. *Anat Sci Int.* 2006;81(2):84–91.
9. Burge PD, Shewring DJ. Vascularized pedicle graft of the lower trunk for reconstruction of the branchial plexus. *J Hand Surg Br.* 1995;20(2):215–217.
10. Starkweather RJ, Neviaser RJ, Adams JP, Parsons DB. The effect of devascularization on the regeneration of lacerated peripheral nerves: an experimental study. *J Hand Surg Am.* 1978;3(2):163–167.
11. Tazaki K. Experimental study on the repair of peripheral nerve lesions—subacute compression neuropathy and neurolysis. *Nihon Seikeigeka Gakkai Zasshi.* 1983;57(12):1821–1833.
12. Biers SM, Brading AF. Nerve regeneration: might this be the only solution for functional problems of the urinary tract? *Curr Opin Urol.* 2003;13(6):495–500.
13. Dagum AB. Peripheral nerve regeneration, repair, and grafting. *J Hand Ther.* 1998;11(2):111–117.
14. Johnson EO, Charchanti A, Soucacos PN. Nerve repair: experimental and clinical evaluation of neurotrophic factors in peripheral nerve regeneration. *Injury.* 2008;39(suppl 3):S37–42.
15. Kuntzer T, Antoine JC, Steck AJ. Clinical features and pathophysiological basis of sensory neuronopathies (ganglionopathies). *Muscle Nerve.* 2004;30(3):255–268.
16. Elsohemy A, Butler R, Bain JR, Fahnestock M. Sensory protection of rat muscle spindles following peripheral nerve injury and reinnervation. *Plast Reconstr Surg.* 2009;124(6):1860–1868.
17. Kanda T. Peripheral neuropathy and blood-nerve barrier. *Rinsho Shinkeigaku.* 2009;49(11):959–962.

18. Lundborg G. Regeneration after peripheral nerve injury—a biological and clinical problem. *Lakartidningen*. 1982; 79(20):2013–2017.

19. Lundborg G, Dahlin LB, Danielsen N, et al. Nerve regeneration in silicone chambers: influence of gap length and of distal stump components. *Exp Neurol*. 1982; 76(2):361–375.

20. Lundborg G, Dahlin LB, Danielsen N, Nachemson AK. Tissue specificity in nerve regeneration. *Scand J Plast Reconstr Surg*. 1986;20(3):279–283.

21. Lundborg G, Gelberman RH, Minteer-Convery M, Lee YF, Hargens AR. Median nerve compression in the carpal tunnel—functional response to experimentally induced controlled pressure. *J Hand Surg Am*. 1982;7(3):252–259.

22. Rigoard P, Lapierre F. Review of the peripheral nerve. *Neurochirurgie*. 2009;55(4-5):360–374.

23. Salvador-Sanz JF, Torres AN, Calpena FT, Sanz-Gimenez-Rico JR, Lopez SC, Barraquer EL. Anatomical study of the cutaneous perforator arteries and vascularisation of the biceps femoris muscle. *Br J Plast Surg*. 2005;58(8):1079–1085.

24. Sarikcioglu L, Demirel BM, Demir N, Yildirim FB, Demirtop A, Oguz N. Morphological and ultrastructural analysis of the watershed zones after stripping of the vasa nervorum. *Int J Neurosci*. 2008;118(8):1145–1155.

25. Yang HJ, Gil YC, Lee HY. Topographical anatomy of the transverse facial artery. *Clin Anat*. 2010;23(2):168–178.

26. Seddon H. Advances in nerve repair. *Triangle*. 1968;8(7):252–259.

27. Lee SK, Wolfe SW. Peripheral nerve injury and repair. *J Am Acad Orthop Surg*. 2000;8(4):243–252.

28. Leffert RD, Seddon H. Infraclavicular plexus injuries. *J Bone Joint Surg Br*. 1965;31:9–22.

29. Seddon H. Nerve injuries. *Med Bull (Ann Arbor)*. 1965; 31:4–10.

30. Sunderland S. Anatomical features of nerve trunks in relation to nerve injury and nerve repair. *Clin Neurosurg*. 1970; 17:38–62.

31. Sunderland S. A classification of peripheral nerve injuries producing loss of function. *Brain*. 1951;74(4):491–516.

32. Sunderland S. Rate of regeneration of sensory nerve fibers. *Arch Neurol Psychiatry*. 1947;58(1):1–6.

33. Sunderland S. Observations on the treatment of traumatic injuries of peripheral nerves. *Br J Surg*. 1947;35(137):36–42.

34. Sunderland S. Rate of regeneration in human peripheral nerves: analysis of the interval between injury and onset of recovery. *Arch Neurol Psychiatry*. 1947;58(3):251–295.

35. Sunderland S. The effect of rupture of the perineurium on the contained nerve-fibres. *Brain*. 1946;69:149–152.

36. Mackinnon, SE, Jost S. FK506 promotes functional recovery in crushed rat sciatic nerve. *Muscle Nerve*. 2000;4:633–640.

37. Sunderland S, Bradley KC. The cross-sectional area of peripheral nerve trunks devoted to nerve fibers. *Brain*. 1949;72(3):428–449.

38. Sunderland S, Lavarick J, Ray LJ. The caliber of nerve fibers in human cutaneous nerves. *J Comp Neurol*. 1949;91(1):87–101.

39. Sunderland S, Ray LJ. The intraneural topography of the sciatic nerve and its popliteal divisions in man. *Brain*. 1948;71(pt 3):242–273.

40. de Campos Vidal B, Mello ML, Caseiro-Filho AC, Godo C. Anisotropic properties of the myelin sheath. *Acta Histochem*. 1980;66(1):32–39.

41. Kuroiwa T, Ueki M, Chen Q, Ichinose S, Okeda R. Is the swelling in brain edema isotropic or anisotropic? *Acta Neurochir Suppl (Wien)*. 1994;60:155–157.

42. Shinar H, Seo Y, Navon G. Discrimination between the different compartments in sciatic nerve by 2H double-quantum-filtered NMR. *J Magn Reson*. 1997;129(1):98–104.

43. Charness ME, Ross MH, Shefner JM. Ulnar neuropathy and dystonic flexion of the fourth and fifth digits: clinical correlation in musicians. *Muscle Nerve*. 1996;19(4):431–437.

44. Furlong R. Peripheral pain in the arm. *Lond Clin Med J*. 1970;11(2):17–21.

45. Davis DS, Anderson JB, Carson MG, Elkins CL, Stuckey LB. Upper limb neural tension and seated slump tests: the false positive rate among healthy young adults without cervical or lumbar symptoms. *J Man Manip Ther*. 2008;16(3):136–141.

46. Lundborg G, Rydevik B. Effects of stretching the tibial nerve of the rabbit. A preliminary study of the intraneural circulation and barrier function of the perineurium. *J Bone Joint Surg Br*. 1973;55:3390–3401.

47. Haftek J. Stretch injury to peripheral nerves. Acute effects of stretching rabbit nerve. *J Bone Joint Surg Br*. 1970;52:354.

48. Ochs S Pourmand R, Si K, Friedman RN. Stretch of mammalian nerve in vitro: effect on compound action potential. *J Peripher Nerv Syst*. 2000;5:227–235.

49. Thomas PK, Olson Y. Microscopic anatomy and the function of the connective tissue components of the peripheral nerve. In: Dyck PJ, Thomas PK, Lambert EH, Bunge R, eds. *Peripheral Neuropathy*. 2nd ed. Philadelphia: Saunders; 2001:128–143.

50. Cornefjord M, Sato K, Olmarker K, Rydevik B, Nordborg CA. Model for chronic nerve root compression studies. Presentation of a porcine model for controlled, slow-onset compression with analyses of anatomic aspects, compression onset rate, and morphological and neurophysiologic effects. *Spine*. 1997;22:946–957.

51. Barr AE, Amin M, Barbe MF. Dose response relationship between reach repetition and indicators of inflammation and movement dysfunction in a rat model of work-related musculoskeletal disorder. Proceedings of the Human Factors and Ergonomics Society 46th Annual Meeting; Baltimore, MD. September 30–October 4, 2002.

52. Barbe MF, Safadi FF, Rivera-Nieves EI, Montara TE, Popoff SN, Barr AE. Expression of ED1, ED2, IL-1 and COX2 in bone and in the rat model of cumulative trauma disorder (CTD). *Journal of Bone and Mineral Research*. 1999;14 (suppl.1): 1099–1115.

53. Barr AE, Barbe MF. Inflammation reduces physiological tissue tolerance in the development of work-related musculoskeletal disorders. *J Electromyogr Kinesiol*. 2004;14:77–85.

54. Appenzeller O, Dithal KK, Dowan T, Burnstock G. The nerves to blood vessels supplying blood nerves: the innervation of the vasa nervorum. *Brain Res* 1984;304:383–386.

55. Ogata K, Naito M. Blood flow of the peripheral nerve effects of dissection, stretching and compression. *J Hand Surg Br*. 1986;18:149–155.

56. Lundborg G, Sollerman C, Stromberg T, Pyykko I, Rosen B. A new principle for assessment of vibrotactile sense in vibration induced neuropathy. *Scand J Work Environ Health*. 1987;13:375–379.

57. Farkkilii M. Grip force in vibration disease. *Scand J Work Environ Health*. 1978;4:159–166.

58. Rosen I, Stromberg T, Lundborg G. Neurophysiological investigation of hands damaged by vibration: comparison with idiopathic carpal tunnel syndrome. *Scand J Plast Reconstr Surg Hand Surg*. 1993;27:209–216.

59. Hjortsberg U, Rosen I, Orback P, Lundborg G, Balough I. Finger receptor dysfunction in dental technicians exposed to high frequency vibration. *Scand J Work Environ Health*. 1989;15:339–344.

60. McLain RF, Weinstein JN. Nuclear cleft in dorsal ganglion neurons: a response to whole body vibration. *J Comp Neurol*. 1992;322:538–547.

61. Maquirriain J. Posterior ankle impingement syndrome. *J Am Acad Orthop Surg*. 2005;6:365–371.

62. Carp S, Eddy L, Whitenack S. Complete excision of the lower trunk and C8 and T1 nerve roots in a patient with Pancoast tumor with a resulting fully functional hand. *Physiother Res Int*. 1997;1:51–55.

63. Richardson JK. The clinical identification of peripheral neuropathy among older persons. *Arch Phys Med*. 2002;83:1553–1558.

64. Hadden RD, Cornblath DR, Hughes RA, et al. Electrophysiological classification of Guillain-Barré syndrome: clinical associations and outcomes. Plasma Exchange/Sandoglobulin Guillain-Barré Syndrome Trial Group. *Ann Neurol*. 1998;44:780–788.

65. Zhang Q, Gu Z, Jiang J, et al. Orthostatic hypotension as a presenting symptom of the Guillain-Barre syndrome. *Clin Auton Res*. 2010;20:209–210.

66. Cortes S, Chambers S, Jeronimo A, Isenberg D. Diabetes mellitus complicating systemic lupus erythematosus—analysis of the UCL lupus cohort and review of the literature. *Lupus*. 2008;17(11):977–980.

67. Mellgren SI, Goransson LG, Omdal R. Primary Sjogren's syndrome associated neuropathy. *Can J Neurol Sci*. 2007;34(3):280–287.

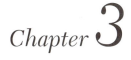

Chapter 3

Pathophysiology of Peripheral Nerve Injury

Mary F. Barbe, PhD, and Ann E. Barr, DPT, PhD

"To kill an error is as good a service as, and sometimes even better than, the establishing of a new truth or fact."
—Charles Darwin (1809–1882)

Objectives

On completion of this chapter, the student/practitioner will be able to:

- Relate the structural anatomy of the peripheral nerve to the etiologies of injury.
- Outline the role of cytokines in the inflammatory cascade of peripheral nerve injury.
- Define spinal cord sensitization as it relates to peripheral nerve injury.
- Define the local and systemic impact of peripheral nerve inflammation.
- Define "fibrosis" as it relates to peripheral nerve injury.

Key Terms

- Fibrosis
- Inflammation
- Neuropathy
- Overuse

Introduction

Neuropathies can result from mechanical trauma, such as shear or compressive forces on the nerve, particularly if repeated, and have been linked to the following risk factors: gender (female), advanced age, and reduced fitness.[1-4] Patients with median nerve **neuropathy** report symptoms such as pain in the hands and wrists or fingers that may travel into the forearm, elbow, and shoulder; paresthesias; numbness; and weakness.[5] An objective diagnosis of median nerve dysfunction is typically based on electrophysiological evidence of slowed median nerve conduction localized to the wrist, although the combination of electrodiagnostic findings and symptom characteristics is reported to provide the most accurate diagnosis of carpal tunnel syndrome (CTS).[2]

Peripheral Nerve Damage and Inflammation With Overuse

Risk factors for the development of neuropathies include the performance of jobs characterized by repetitiveness, forcefulness, or awkward postures.[1,3,6,7] A relationship between advancing age and susceptibility to other risk factors for neuropathies has also been reported,[3,5,6,8] albeit one longitudinal study suggested that slowing of conduction in the median nerve occurs naturally with increasing age.[4] CTS has the highest incidence rate of all occupation-related peripheral neuropathies, with 10,780 combined cases reported to the U.S. Occupational Safety and Health Administration in 2009 by private industry and state and local government, resulting in a median of 21 lost workdays per case. The overall CTS incidence rate affects 1 in 10,000 workers. Among female workers, CTS affects 1.5 in 10,000 workers, whereas among men, CTS affects 0.7 in 10,000 workers. The incidence rate for CTS was highest among workers 45 to 64 years old (1.5 in 10,000) compared with rates of 0.3 in 10,000 for workers 20 to 24 years old and 0.7 in 10,000 for workers 25 to 34 years old.[6] In a 3-year prospective study of incidence in newly hired workers in computer-intensive jobs, computer operators older than age 30 showed an increased risk of developing neck, shoulder, arm, and hand symptoms, such as pain, aching, burning, numbness, or tingling.[8] The most common disorder identified by the study relative to this population was somatic pain syndrome. Our laboratory has reported that patients with upper extremity **overuse** injuries have increased frequency of local signs of pain and tenderness, peripheral nerve irritation and weakness, and increased frequency of these symptoms at multiple anatomical sites (mean age = 45 years; age range, 19 to 74 years; 23 of 31 subjects older than 30). These findings correlated with increased serum inflammatory cytokines.[9,10]

Effects of Overuse on Nerves in Human Subjects

Human studies examining tissue biopsy specimens in patients with long-term chronic overuse syndromes found evidence of nerve compression and injury, **inflammation, fibrosis,** and degeneration. Freeland et al.[11] detected increased tenosynovium interleukin (IL)-6, an inflammatory cytokine, and increased serum malondialdehyde, a cell injury biomarker and a reactive oxygen species that initiates arachidonic acid metabolism into products (e.g., prostaglandin E_2), in patients with CTS. As mentioned earlier, increased inflammatory cytokines have also been detected in serum of patients with early onset of moderate to severe symptoms of upper limb overuse injury,[9] presumably as a result of increased cytokines in injured or inflamed tissues. However, despite numerous epidemiological studies demonstrating a positive relationship between exposure to repetitive or forceful motion and the prevalence of overuse injuries,[1] the mechanisms of pathophysiology are incompletely understood. Animal models provide an opportunity to examine such tissue effects at a much earlier time point and under experimental conditions in which exposure can be controlled. In an effort to understand the underlying mechanisms of these disorders, we and numerous other authors have developed animal models of overuse injuries.[2,12–17]

Rat Model of Overuse Injury

Whishaw[18,19] quantified the similarities between rats and humans in targeted reach submovements of the

Table 3-1 Repetitive Task Group Parameters of the Barbe and Barr Rat Model of Overuse

Group	Target Reach Rate (Reaches/min)	Actual Reach Rate (Reaches/min)	Reach Force (% of Maximum Pull Force)
HRHF	8	12	60 ± 5
MRHF	4	9.4	60 ± 5
HRLF	8	12	15 ± 5
HRNF = MRNF	4	8	<5[a]
LRNF	2	3.3	<5[a]

HRHF = high repetition high force; MRHF = moderate repetition high force; HRLF = high repetition low force; HRNF = high repetition negligible force, redefined as MRNF based on the repetition rate; LRNF = low repetition negligible force.
[a]The negligible force rats retrieved a 45-mg food pellet, which was estimated to be less than 5% maximum pulling force.

upper extremity. Also, Viikari-Juntura[20,21] stated that laboratory studies of animals examining the effects of repetitive loading on tissue function may be extrapolated to human exposures and responses. We developed a unique rat model of voluntary repetitive reaching in which rats can be trained to perform an upper limb repetitive hand and wrist–intensive task. Reach rate and force levels used in our model, which are shown in Table 3-1, were derived from investigations of industrial workers by Silverstein et al.[22,23] They defined risk levels for repetitiveness to be high when reaching and grasping motions are performed faster than 30 sec/cycle. Force is considered negligible to low if less than 15% of maximum voluntary contraction (MVC) is required and high if it is greater than 50% of MVC. Our rat model of a paced reaching and grasping task may be generalized to humans in terms of both behavioral and tissue responses for some types of physically constrained and paced occupational tasks, as explained further elsewhere.[24,25] An example of such a paced task would be packing, in which a worker repeatedly places small objects presented on a conveyor belt into a package crate.

In our model, rats are placed into operant test chambers for rodents with a portal located in one wall, as described previously.[26–29] They are trained to perform a repetitive reaching task in which they reach through the portal to grasp and retrieve a food pellet or to grasp and isometrically pull a force handle that is attached to a force transducer, until a predetermined force threshold is reached and held for at least 50 msec. On successful achievement of reach force and time criteria, the rat releases the handle and retrieves a food pellet reward by mouth from a food trough. Using this apparatus, the short-term effects (3 to 12 weeks) of a voluntary low force task performed at low, moderate, or high reach rates, with force requirements of low or high (see details in Table 3-1), on sensorimotor behavior, forelimb musculoskeletal and nerve tissues, spinal cord, and brain have been determined.[26–41] With regard to the peripheral nerve, the short-term effects of repetitive or forceful tasks on nerve pathophysiology have been characterized, focusing on injury, inflammation, inflammation-induced catabolic changes, and fibrotic changes that might contribute to peripheral nerve injury and degeneration. Inflammation-induced central nervous system changes that might contribute to sensorimotor behavior changes, such as the development of pain behaviors as a result of spinal cord sensitization or the development of reduced fine motor control as a result of sensory and motor cortex reorganization, have also been investigated in our model.

Nerve Injury, Inflammation, and Fibrosis Induced by Overuse

A peripheral nerve injury mechanism has been identified in our overuse model. We have observed demyelination and focal axonal swelling in the median nerve at the level of the wrist, suggestive of focal nerve injury, in combination with increased extraneural connective tissue and fibroblasts, suggestive of nerve fibrosis (Fig. 3-1A–D).[27,28,35,36] These tissue changes were accompanied by a decrease in nerve conduction velocity (Fig. 3-1E) as well as changes in forepaw sensation and a decrease in grip strength, both significantly correlating with the declines in nerve conduction velocity (Fig. 3-2). This correlation strongly indicates that nerve compression injury is contributing to these behavioral declines. The declines in median nerve conduction were exposure-dependent with reductions ranging from 9% to 23% depending on the level of task intensity and the age of the rat, with greater losses with high repetition high force tasks and in aged rats. Chronic inflammatory responses were also induced by task performance, such as persistently increased macrophages and proinflammatory cytokines in nerves and serum (Fig. 3-1F).[26–28,30,31,40,42–44] Increased fibrotic

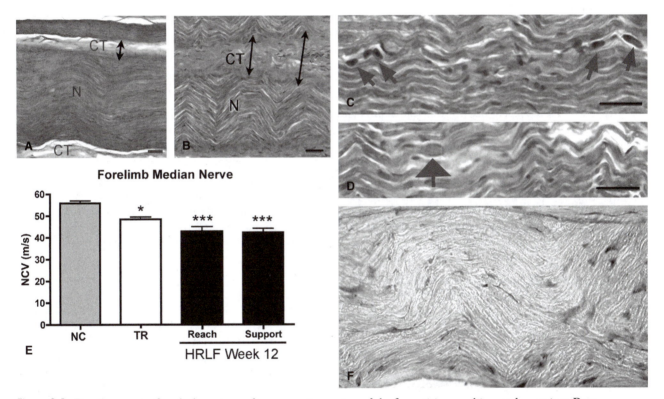

Figure 3-1 Development of pathology in median nerve in a rat model of repetitive reaching and grasping. Rats performed a high repetition low force (HRLF) task for 12 weeks. A, Median nerve of a normal control rat. B, Median nerve from 12-week HRLF rat showing an increase in connective tissue (CT), indicative of nerve fibrosis. C, Median nerve from 12-week HRLF rat showing increased inflammatory cells (arrows) within the median nerve. D, Median nerve from 12-week HRLF rat showing presence of axonal swelling (arrow), indicative of nerve injury. Scale bars = 5 μm. E, Bar graph showing decreased nerve conduction velocity (NCV) in median nerve of 12 week HRLF rats compared with normal control rats (NC) and rats that underwent the initial training only (TR). *$P < 0.05$ compared with NC. ***$P < 0.001$ compared with NC. F, Median nerve of 12-week HRLF rat showing presence of tumor necrosis factor (TNF)-α, a key proinflammatory cytokine. *(Used by permission from Elliott MB, Barr AE, Clark BD, Wade CK, Barbe MF. Performance of a repetitive task by aged rats leads to median neuropathy and spinal cord inflammation with associated sensorimotor declines. Neuroscience. 2010;170:929–941.)*

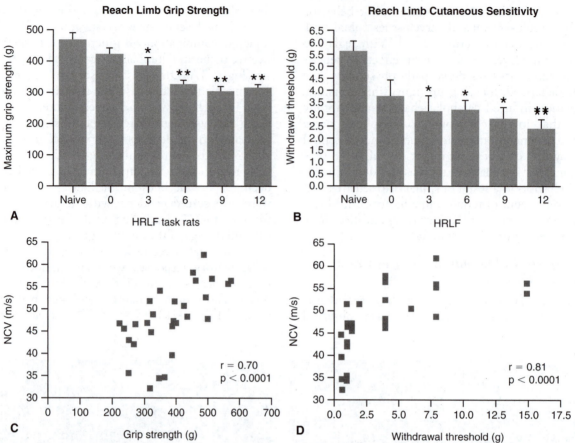

Figure 3-2 Development of grip strength declines and cutaneous hypersensitivity in the reach forelimbs of rats performing a high repetition low force (HRLF) task for 12 weeks. A, Grip strength declines from naïve levels with continued task performance. B, Cutaneous hypersensitivity develops, shown as a reduction in Von Frey hair size (threshold) needed to induce a forelimb withdrawal response with continued task performance. C, Scatterplot showing positive correlation between median nerve conduction velocity (NCV) and grip strength by Spearman's r test. D, Scatterplot showing positive correlation between median nerve conduction velocity (NCV) and withdrawal threshold by Spearman's r test. *$P < 0.05$ compared with NC. **$P < 0.01$ compared with NC. *(Used by permission from Elliott MB, Barr AE, Clark BD, Wade CK, Barbe MF. Performance of a repetitive task by aged rats leads to median neuropathy and spinal cord inflammation with associated sensorimotor declines. Neuroscience. 2010;170:929–941.)*

tissue changes were observed in the synovial sheaths of adjacent flexor digitorum tendons,[38] which likely also contributed to compression of the median nerve.

Spinal Cord Neuroplastic Changes Induced by Peripheral Nerve Inflammation

Several studies have found phenotypic changes in dorsal root ganglion neurons in which the expression of proteins, receptors, neurotransmitters, and neurotrophic factors was altered.[45,46] For example, substance P increases in spinal cord dorsal horns following chronic constriction injury from partial nerve ligation, peripheral nerve injury, or inflammation.[46,47] This increase may be due to inflammation-induced increases in afferent synaptic input to the spinal cord through an increased rate of discharge, increased peptide production by the dorsal root ganglion, or afferent fiber

phenotype alterations that favor substance P expression.[48,49] Schaible et al.[50] described this type of afferent influx of excitatory transmitters into the spinal cord dorsal horn after injury as the presynaptic component of central sensitization. An increase in neurokinin 1, a key receptor for substance P, occurs in the postsynaptic spinal cord neurons and most likely occurs as a response to the increased release of substance P from nociceptive afferent terminals.[49]

It was not a surprise to see increased substance P and neurokinin 1 in dorsal horns in cervical spinal cord regions with performance of low and moderate repetitive tasks with or without high force (Fig. 3-3).[34-37] This neurochemical response was associated temporally with a peripheral tissue macrophage or inflammatory cytokine response. This association supports the hypothesis that task-induced peripheral tissue injury

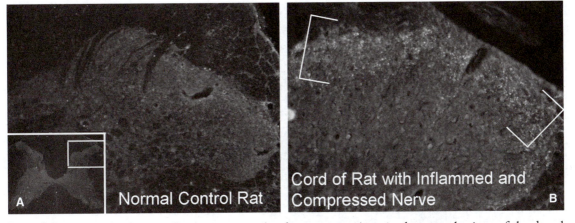

Figure 3-3 Increased substance P, a nociceptor-related neurotransmitter, in the upper laminae of the dorsal horn of cervical spinal cord segments in a rat model of repetitive reaching and grasping. Rats performed a high repetition low force (HRLF) task for 12 weeks. A, The dorsal horn of the untrained side (i.e., the support limb side), showing only a small amount of substance P immunoreactivity (dark staining; HRP-DAB reaction product) in the bracketed area. B, The dorsal horn of the trained side (i.e., the reach limb side), showing an increase of substance P immunoreactivity in the bracketed area.

and inflammation drives a spinal cord neurochemical response from nociceptive afferent terminals. Such increases in substance P and neurokinin 1 are temporally associated with mechanical hypersensitivity[47,51] and behavioral changes (see Fig. 3-2). These studies combined provide evidence that spinal cord sensitization associated with injury and inflammatory conditions may contribute to chronic pain conditions in patients with overuse injury.

Numerous studies show spinal cord inflammatory responses after unilateral peripheral nerve injury as well. For example, peripheral nerve crush or ligation leads to an increase in activated microglia and increased production of proinflammatory cytokines in neurons and glial cells in spinal cord segments innervating that nerve.[51-55] We observed increased interleukin (IL)-1β and tumor necrosis factor (TNF)-α immunoexpression in neurons within the dorsal horn superficial lamina in aged rats that had performed a moderate demand task (HRLF) for 12 weeks compared with normal control rats (Fig. 3-4A).[36]

Cortical Brain Neuroplastic Changes Induced by Repetitive Strain Injury

The possibility that both peripheral inflammatory and central cortical neuroplastic change mechanisms coexist with altered motor performance has been studied only more recently.[32] We examined primary somatosensory cortical (S1) and primary motor cortical (M1) changes in rats performing a reaching and grasping task with moderate repetition and negligible force demands for 2 hours per day, 3 days per week for 8 weeks. We found repetitive task-induced degradation of S1 neuronal properties, such as increased cortical receptive fields that represented several forepaw subdivisions (i.e., several digits or palmar pads rather than a single digit or pad), increased receptive fields that represented both glabrous and hairy surfaces, and increased cortical responsiveness to light tactile stimulation. In addition, the receptive fields located on the glabrous forepaw were significantly larger in rats performing repetitive tasks than in control rats. Also, the forepaw representation in the S1 cortical map was patchy and disrupted in rats performing repetitive tasks relative to control rats. In the aforementioned study, the enlargement of S1 receptive fields and the emergence of large receptive fields that encompassed the whole forepaw (digits and palmar pads) or dorsal hand and wrist or forearm correlated statistically with a reduction in successful reaches, an increase in the inefficient raking food retrieval pattern, and an increase in reach time. These findings support our hypothesis that ambiguous interpretation of tactile cues results in reduced motor performance, particularly with fine motor skills. These data confirm and extend data found in primates in which repetitive, rewarded hand grasp led to a dedifferentiation of the finger maps in the S1 cortex, characterized by enlarged, overlapping receptive fields; the emergence of multidigit and hairy-glabrous receptive fields; and abnormal somatosensory maps in the thalamus.[56-58]

In the motor (M1) cortex, performance of a moderate repetitive task in our model drastically increased the size of the M1 forepaw maps, especially the movement representation of the digits, digits-arm, and elbow-wrist specifically involved in the behavioral task.[32] The

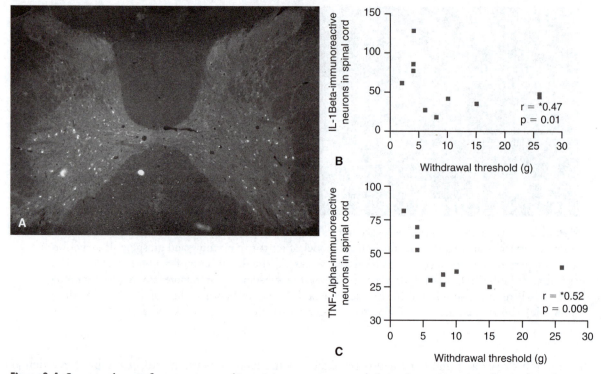

Figure 3-4 Increased proinflammatory cytokines in neurons scattered throughout the cervical spinal cord segments in a rat model of repetitive reaching and grasping. Rats performed a high repetition low force (HRLF) task for 12 weeks. A, Low-power micrograph showing increased tumor necrosis factor (TNF)-α (white staining), a key proinflammatory cytokine, in neurons throughout the spinal cord gray matter. B, Scatterplot showing negative correlation between interleukin (IL)-1β immunoreactivity in neurons and withdrawal threshold by Pearson's *r* test. C, Scatterplot showing negative correlation between TNF-α immunoreactivity n neurons and withdrawal threshold by Pearson's *r* test. *(From data generated for Elliott MB, Barr AE, Clark BD, Wade CK, Barbe MF. Performance of a repetitive task by aged rats leads to median neuropathy and spinal cord inflammation with associated sensorimotor declines. Neuroscience. 2010;170:929–941.)*

movement representation area of the elbow-wrist multijoint responses tripled, and the arm-digits multijoint areal extent was 17 times larger than in untrained rats. The cortical increase in the multijoint movement representation for elbow-wrist, arm, and arm-digits correlated strongly with the increased prevalence of a degraded reaching and grasping strategy. Unexpectedly, but interesting to consider here as well, task-induced peripheral increases in inflammatory cytokines in muscles and nerves of rats performing repetitive tasks had a strong negative correlation with not only grip strength but also with the amount of current required to evoke movements of the wrist, elbow-wrist, and arm-digits multijoints in the primary motor cortex. The higher the inflammation in flexor muscles and nerves specifically involved in the task, the lower the threshold required to elicit arm-digits movements, which was decreased in trained rats relative to controls. This latter finding suggests that the peripheral inflammatory responses are altering the cortical maps negatively and altering, in this indirect manner, the ability to perform fine motor tasks.

Links Between Pain Behaviors and Peripheral or Central Neural Changes

Peripheral Nerve Sensitization

Heightened pain sensitivity is a known consequence of increased inflammatory mediators, particularly TNF-α. Proinflammatory cytokines activate and sensitize peripheral terminals of nociceptors both directly (e.g., within the nerve) and indirectly (e.g., in surrounding tissues), leading to hypersensitivity.[59,60] We reported a correlation between increased inflammatory cytokines in the median nerve and forepaw mechanical hypersensitivity.[36] Alternatively, a task-induced systemic cytokine response may also be associated with the widespread mechanical hypersensitivity found in our rat model. We previously observed a significant correlation between reduced grip strength and task-induced increases in serum inflammatory cytokines[30,36] as well as a significant correlation between cutaneous hypersensitivity and task-induced increases in spinal cord inflammatory cytokines (Fig. 3-4B and C).[36] These findings combined suggest that inflammation-driven peripheral sensitization contributes to sensorimotor changes with performance of repetitive tasks.

Spinal Cord Central Sensitization

The phenomenon of central sensitization is characterized by adaptations in neurons and glial cells, such as changes in neuronal structure, protein production, function, and survival within the central nervous system, which contribute to abnormal pain behaviors.[61] For example, it has been proposed that spinal cytokines released in the dorsal horn nerve terminal region ipsilateral to the affected peripheral nerve spread to nearby spinal nerve terminals and affect uninvolved peripheral nerves and central sensory processing.[62] These changes may elicit remote and contralateral sensitization effects. We have observed forepaw hypersensitivity bilaterally in our model.[25,36] However, we also showed that the nonreach limb is used as a support limb in our model.[38] The bilateral hypersensitivity responses in our study are not a type of "mirror allodynia" sometimes seen after unilateral nerve ligation, in which there is a contralateral spread of symptoms via spinal cord mechanisms,[52,62,63] but rather are due to bilateral use of the forelimbs in performing the task and then bilateral changes in the median nerves.

We have also reported the presence of hind paw mechanical hypersensitivity in our model[25,36] in limbs not involved with performing an upper extremity repetitive task. We observed hind paw mechanical hypersensitivity in aged rats performing a HRLF task for 12 weeks[36] and an early increase in hind paw sensitivity at 3 weeks in young rats performing a high repetition high force (HRHF) task (before the development of hyposensation in these latter rats). These findings are suggestive of an extraterritorial spread of symptoms via central sensitization mechanisms that may contribute to pain behaviors with overuse injuries. Studies showing mirror allodynia (mechanical hypersensitivity) or extraterritorial hyperalgesia in cases of unilateral nerve injury provide evidence of nerve injury–induced mechanisms of central sensitization.[62] We suggest that the hypersensitivity in the uninvolved hind paws in our model may be due to increased proinflammatory cytokines in cervical spinal cord affecting cells or processing in distal spinal cord segments (see Fig. 3-4).

Does Sensitization Result From Both Peripheral and Central Changes?

Signs of injury and inflammation occurring in the median nerve in addition to the spinal cord inflammatory response prevent us from separating peripheral versus central mechanisms contributing to observed cutaneous sensation changes in forepaws. Proinflammatory cytokines have been shown to sensitize peripheral terminals of nociceptors both directly and indirectly, leading to hypersensitivity.[59,60] We reported the presence of inflammatory cytokines in peripheral nerves, in musculoskeletal tissues, and widely circulating in serum in our model (see Fig. 3-1F).[25,26,30,33,38,40,44] We also reported statistical correlation between these cytokine increases, hypersensitivity, and declines in grip strength in several studies, suggesting a link between increased peripheral cytokines and pain-related behaviors with overuse injuries.

Nerve compression can be initially irritating to nerves, resulting in cutaneous hypersensitivity. Our findings of mechanical hypersensitivity in the presence of decreased nerve conduction velocity and histological findings of increased extraneuronal connective tissue and axonal swelling in the median nerve are suggestive of nerve compression with long-term repetitive task performance, particularly HRHF tasks. Hand and arm pain in the distribution of the median nerve is a common symptom in patients with electrophysiologically diagnosed CTS, particularly in patients who engage in full-time intensive manual work.[64]

With regard to central sensitivity, we can only point to numerous other studies showing spinal cord inflammatory responses after unilateral peripheral nerve injury (e.g., increased spinal cord cytokines produced by neurons and glia, increases that are temporally associated with mechanical hypersensitivity).[52,53,65-69] The contribution of central sensitization to repetition-induced hypersensitivity is also suggested by studies from our laboratory showing increased substance P and neurokinin-1 receptors in spinal cord dorsal horns.[34-37] These increases in substance P correlated statistically with declines in forelimb grip strength[34] and coincided with degraded forelimb movement patterns.[37] We have also observed increased substance P in forelimb tendons with HRHF task performance—changes that correlate strongly with declines in grip strength[38] and bring us back to a potential peripheral sensitization mechanism. We hypothesize that both mechanisms are at work in our model as well as in cases of overuse injury in which chronic pain is present.

Our data from a rat model of overuse injury show that peripheral nerve injury, peripheral inflammatory responses, spinal cord sensitization, and central neuroplastic mechanisms coexist. Each of these factors appears to contribute to motor behavior declines and the development of pain-related behaviors. What was previously unknown was whether peripheral inflammation was primarily responsible for the movement performance deficits that emerge in these rats over time or whether cortical degradation was responsible for the movement defects.[56] It is clear from our studies that *both* sensorimotor cortical reorganization and peripheral inflammation and injury mechanisms contribute to declines in movement performance and changes in movement patterns in the progression of the overuse injury.

References

1. Bernard B. *Musculoskeletal Disorders and Workplace Factors.* NIOSH Report 97-141. Cincinatti: National Institute for Occupational Safety and Health; 1997.

2. Rempel DM, Diao E. Entrapment neuropathies: pathophysiology and pathogenesis. *J Electromyogr Kinesiol.* 2004;14:71–75.

3. Zambelis T, Tsivgoulis G, Karandreas N. Carpal tunnel syndrome: associations between risk factors and laterality. *Eur Neurol.* 2010;63:43–47.

4. Nathan PA, Keniston RC, Myers LD, Meadows KD, Lockwood RS. Natural history of median nerve sensory conduction in industry: relationship to symptoms and carpal tunnel syndrome in 558 hands over 11 years. *Muscle Nerve.* 1998;21:711–721.

5. Gerr F, Marcus M, Monteilh C. Aerobic exercise, median nerve conduction, and the reporting of study results. *J Occup Environ Med.* 2002;44:303.

6. Bureau of Labor Statistics. *Nonfatal Occupational Injuries and Illnesses Requiring Days Away From Work.* Washington, D.C.: U.S. Department of Labor; 2010.

7. Szabo RM. Carpal tunnel syndrome as a repetitive motion disorder. *Clin Orthop Relat Res.* 1998;(351):78–89.

8. Gerr F, Marcus M, Ensor C, et al. A prospective study of computer users: I. study design and incidence of musculoskeletal symptoms and disorders. *Am J Ind Med.* 2002;41:221–235.

9. Carp SJ, Barbe MF, Winter KA, Amin M, Barr AE. Inflammatory biomarkers increase with severity of upper-extremity overuse disorders. *Clin Sci (Lond).* 2007;112:305–314.

10. Carp SJ, Barr AE, Barbe MF. Serum biomarkers as signals for risk and severity of work-related musculoskeletal injury. *Biomark Med.* 2008;2:67–79.

11. Freeland AE, Tucci MA, Barbieri RA, Angel MF, Nick TG. Biochemical evaluation of serum and flexor tenosynovium in carpal tunnel syndrome. *Microsurgery.* 2002;22:378–385.

12. Topp KS, Byl NN. Movement dysfunction following repetitive hand opening and closing: anatomical analysis in Owl monkeys. *Mov Disord.* 1999;14:295–306.

13. Hollander MS, et al. Effects of age and glutathione levels on oxidative stress in rats after chronic exposure to stretch-shortening contractions. *Eur J Appl Physiol.* 2010;108:589–597.

14. Baker BA, Hollander MS, Mercer RR, Kashon ML, Cutlip RG. Adaptive stretch-shortening contractions: diminished regenerative capacity with aging. *Appl Physiol Nutr Metab.* 2008;33:1181–1191.

15. Stauber WT, Willems ME. Prevention of histopathologic changes from 30 repeated stretches of active rat skeletal muscles by long inter-stretch rest times. *Eur J Appl Physiol.* 2002;88:94–99.

16. Willems ME, Miller GR, Stauber FD, Stauber WT. Effects of repeated lengthening contractions on skeletal muscle adaptations in female rats. *J Physiol Sci.* 2010;60:143–150.

17. Sommerich CM, Lavender SA, Buford JA, J Banks J, Korkmaz SV, Pease WS. Towards development of a nonhuman primate model of carpal tunnel syndrome: performance of a voluntary, repetitive pinching task induces

18. Sacrey LA, Alaverdashvili M, Whishaw IQ. Similar hand shaping in reaching-for-food (skilled reaching) in rats and humans provides evidence of homology in release, collection, and manipulation movements. *Behav Brain Res.* 2009; 204:153–161.

19. Whishaw IQ, Pellis SM, Gorny BP. Skilled reaching in rats and humans: evidence for parallel development or homology. *Behav Brain Res.* 1992;47:59–70.

20. Viikari-Juntura ER. The scientific basis for making guidelines and standards to prevent work-related musculoskeletal disorders. *Ergonomics.* 1997;40:1097–1117.

21. Viikari-Juntura E, Silverstein B. Role of physical load factors in carpal tunnel syndrome. *Scand J Work Environ Health.* 1999;25:163–185.

22. Silverstein BA, Fine LJ, Armstrong TJ. Hand wrist cumulative trauma disorders in industry. *Br J Ind Med.* 1986;43:779–784.

23. Silverstein BA, Fine LJ, Armstrong TJ. Occupational factors and carpal tunnel syndrome. *Am J Ind Med.* 1987;11:343–358.

24. Barr AE, Barbe MF. Pathophysiological tissue changes associated with repetitive movement: a review of the evidence. *Phys Ther.* 2002;82:173–187.

25. Barr AE, Barbe MF, Clark BD. Systemic inflammatory mediators contribute to widespread effects in work-related musculoskeletal disorders. *Exerc Sport Sci Rev.* 2004;32:135–142.

26. Barbe MF, Barr AE, Gorzelany I, Amin M, Gaughan JP, Safadi FF. Chronic repetitive reaching and grasping results in decreased motor performance and widespread tissue responses in a rat model of MSD. *J Orthop Res.* 2003;21:167–176.

27. Clark BD, Al-Shatti TA, Barr AE, Amin M, Barbe MF. Performance of a high-repetition, high-force task induces carpal tunnel syndrome in rats. *J Orthop Sports Phys Ther.* 2004;34:244–253.

28. Clark BD, Barr AE, Safadi FF, et al. Median nerve trauma in a rat model of work-related musculoskeletal disorder. *J Neurotrauma.* 2003;20:681–695.

29. Rani S, Barbe MF, Barr AE, Litivn J. Role of TNF alpha and PLF in bone remodeling in a rat model of repetitive reaching and grasping. *J Cell Physiol.* 2010;225:152–167.

30. Barbe MF, Elliott MB, Abdelmagid SM, et al. Serum and tissue cytokines and chemokines increase with repetitive upper extremity tasks. *J Orthop Res.* 2008;26:1320–1326.

31. Barr AE, Safadi FF, Gorzelany I, Amin M, Popoff SN, Barbe MF. Repetitive, negligible force reaching in rats induces pathological overloading of upper extremity bones. *J Bone Miner Res.* 2003;18:2023–2032.

32. Coq JO, Barr AE, Strata F, et al. Peripheral and central changes combine to induce motor behavioral deficits in a moderate repetition task. *Exp Neurol.* 2009;220:234–245.

33. Driban JB, Barr AE, Amin M, Sitler MR, Barbe MF. Joint inflammation and early degeneration induced by high-force reaching are attenuated by ibuprofen in an animal model of work-related musculoskeletal disorder. *J Biomed Biotechnol.* 2011;2011:691412.

34. Elliott MB, Barr AE, Barbe MF. Spinal substance P and neurokinin-1 increase with high repetition reaching. *Neurosci Lett.* 2009;454:33–37.

35. Elliott MB, Barr AE, Clark BD, Amin M, Amin S, Barbe MF. High force reaching task induces widespread inflammation, increased spinal cord neurochemicals and neuropathic pain. *Neuroscience.* 2009;158:922–931.

36. Elliott MB, Barr AE, Clark BD, Wade CK, Barbe MF. Performance of a repetitive task by aged rats leads to median neuropathy and spinal cord inflammation with associated sensorimotor declines. *Neuroscience.* 2010;170:929–941.

37. Elliott MB, Barr AE, Kietrys DM, Al-Shatti T, Amin M, Barbe MF. Peripheral neuritis and increased spinal cord neurochemicals are induced in a model of repetitive motion injury with low force and repetition exposure. *Brain Res.* 2008;1218:103–113.

38. Fedorczyk JM, Barr AE, Rani S, et al. Exposure-dependent increases in IL-1beta, substance P, CTGF, and tendinosis in flexor digitorum tendons with upper extremity repetitive strain injury. *J Orthop Res.* 2010;28:298–307.

39. Rani S, Barbe MF, Barr AE, Litvin J. Induction of periostin-like factor and periostin in forearm muscle, tendon, and nerve in an animal model of work-related musculoskeletal disorder. *J Histochem Cytochem.* 2009;57:1061–1073.

40. Xin DL, Harris MY, Wade CK, Amin M, Barr AE, Barbe MF. Aging enhances serum cytokine response but not task-induced grip strength declines in a rat model of work-related musculoskeletal disorders. *BMC Musculoskelet Disord.* 2011;12:63.

41. Rani S, Barbe MF, Barr AE, Litvin J. Periostin-like-factor and Periostin in an animal model of work-related musculoskeletal disorder. *Bone.* 2009;44:502–512.

42. Elliott MB, Barr AE, Clark BD, Amin M, Amin S, Barbe MF. High force reaching task induces widespread inflammation, increased spinal cord neurochemicals and neuropathic pain. *Neuroscience.* 2009;158:922–931.

43. Fedorczyk JM, Barr AE, Rani S, et al. Exposure-dependent increases in IL-1beta, substance P, CTGF, and tendinosis in flexor digitorum tendons with upper extremity repetitive strain injury. *J Orthop Res.* 2010;28:298–307.

44. Al-Shatti T, Barr AE, Safadi FF, Amin M, Barbe MF. Increase in inflammatory cytokines in median nerves in a rat model of repetitive motion injury. *J Neuroimmunol.* 2005;167:13–22.

45. Hammond DL, Ackerman L, Holdsworth R, Elzey B. Effects of spinal nerve ligation on immunohistochemically identified neurons in the L4 and L5 dorsal root ganglia of the rat. *J Comp Neurol.* 2004;475:575–589.

46. Chao T, Pham K, Steward O, Gupta R. Chronic nerve compression injury induces a phenotypic switch of neurons within the dorsal root ganglia. *J Comp Neurol.* 2008;506: 180–193.

47. Rothman SM, Winkelstein BA. Chemical and mechanical nerve root insults induce differential behavioral sensitivity and glial activation that are enhanced in combination. *Brain Res.* 2007;1181:30–43.

48. Neumann S, Doubell TP, Leslie T, Woolf CJ. Inflammatory pain hypersensitivity mediated by phenotypic switch in myelinated primary sensory neurons. *Nature.* 1996;384: 360–364.

49. Pitcher GM, Henry JL. Nociceptive response to innocuous mechanical stimulation is mediated via myelinated afferents and NK-1 receptor activation in a rat model of neuropathic pain. *Exp Neurol.* 2004;186:173–197.

50. Schaible HG, Ebersberger A, Von Banchet GS. Mechanisms of pain in arthritis. *Ann N Y Acad Sci.* 2002;966:343–354.

51. Winkelstein BA, Rutkowski MD, Sweitzer SM, Pahl JL, DeLeo JA. Nerve injury proximal or distal to the DRG induces similar spinal glial activation and selective cytokine expression but differential behavioral responses to pharmacologic treatment. *J Comp Neurol.* 2001;439:127–139.

52. DeLeo JA, Colburn RW, Rickman AJ. Cytokine and growth factor immunohistochemical spinal profiles in two animal models of mononeuropathy. *Brain Res.* 1997;759:50–57.

53. Hunt JL, Winkelstein BA, Rutkowski MD, Weinstein JN, DeLeo JA. Repeated injury to the lumbar nerve roots produces enhanced mechanical allodynia and persistent spinal neuroinflammation. *Spine (Phila Pa 1976).* 2001;26:2073–2079.

54. Rutkowski MD, Winkelstein BA, Hickey WF, Pahl JL, DeLeo JA. Lumbar nerve root injury induces central nervous system neuroimmune activation and neuroinflammation in the rat: relationship to painful radiculopathy. *Spine (Phila Pa 1976).* 2002;27:1604–1613.

55. Winkelstein BA, Rutkowski MD, Weinstein JN, DeLeo JA. Quantification of neural tissue injury in a rat radiculopathy model: comparison of local deformation, behavioral outcomes, and spinal cytokine mRNA for two surgeons. *J Neurosci Methods.* 2001;111:49–57.

56. Byl NN, Melnick M. The neural consequences of repetition: clinical implications of a learning hypothesis. *J Hand Ther.* 1997;10:160–174.

57. Byl NN, Merzenich MM, Cheung S, Bedenbaugh P, Nagarajan SS, Jenkins WM. A primate model for studying focal dystonia and repetitive strain injury: effects on the primary somatosensory cortex. *Phys Ther.* 1997;77:269–284.

58. Byl NN, Merzenich MM, Jenkins WM. A primate genesis model of focal dystonia and repetitive strain injury: I. learning-induced dedifferentiation of the representation of the hand in the primary somatosensory cortex in adult monkeys. *Neurology.* 1996;47:508–520.

59. Moalem G, Tracey DJ. Immune and inflammatory mechanisms in neuropathic pain. *Brain Res Rev.* 2006;51:240–264.

60. Schafers M, Sorkin L. Effect of cytokines on neuronal excitability. *Neurosci Lett.* 2008;437:188–193.

61. Woolf CJ, Salter MW. Neuronal plasticity: increasing the gain in pain. *Science.* 2000; 288:1765–1769.

62. Chacur M, Milligan ED, Gazda LS, et al. A new model of sciatic inflammatory neuritis (SIN): induction of unilateral and bilateral mechanical allodynia following acute unilateral peri-sciatic immune activation in rats. *Pain.* 2001;94:231–244.

63. Kelly S, Dunham JP, Donaldson LF. Sensory nerves have altered function contralateral to a monoarthritis and may contribute to the symmetrical spread of inflammation. *Eur J Neurosci.* 2007;26:935–942.

64. Bonfiglioli R, Mattioli S, Violante FS. Relationship between symptoms and instrumental findings in the diagnosis of upper limb work-related musculoskeletal disorders. *Med Lav.* 2007;98:118–126.

65. Hatashita S, Sekiguchi M, Kobayashi H, Konno S, Kikuchi S. Contralateral neuropathic pain and neuropathology in dorsal root ganglion and spinal cord following hemilateral nerve injury in rats. *Spine (Phila Pa 1976).* 2008;33:1344–1351.

66. Hubbard RD, Winkelstein BA. Transient cervical nerve root compression in the rat induces bilateral forepaw allodynia and spinal glial activation: mechanical factors in painful neck injuries. *Spine (Phila Pa 1976).* 2005;30:1924–1932.

67. Schafers M, Svensson CI, Sommer C, Sorkin LS. Tumor necrosis factor-alpha induces mechanical allodynia after spinal nerve ligation by activation of p38 MAPK in primary sensory neurons. *J Neurosci.* 2003;23:2517–2521.

68. Ohtori S, Takahashi K, Moriya H, Myers RR. TNF-alpha and TNF-alpha receptor type 1 upregulation in glia and neurons after peripheral nerve injury: studies in murine DRG and spinal cord. *Spine (Phila Pa 1976).* 2004;29:1082–1088.

69. Shubayev VI, Myers RR. Anterograde TNF alpha transport from rat dorsal root ganglion to spinal cord and injured sciatic nerve. *Neurosci Lett.* 2002;320:99–101.

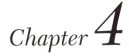

Chapter *4*

Peripheral Neuropathy and Vasculitic, Connective Tissue, and Seronegative Spondyloarthropathic Disorders

Stephen J. Carp, PT, PhD, GCS

"A merry heart doeth good like medicine."
—Socrates (469 b.c.–399 b.c.)

Objectives

On completion of this chapter, the student/practitioner will be able to:

- Develop an evidenced-based understanding of vasculitic, connective tissue, and spondyloarthropathic disorders as they relate to neuropathic signs and symptoms.
- Identify on the physical examination potential neuropathic impairments related to vasculitic, connective tissue, and seronegative spondyloarthropathic disorders.
- Develop a goal-oriented treatment plan for vasculitic, connective tissue, and seronegative spondyloarthropathic disorders.

Key Terms

- Connective tissue disorders
- Seronegative spondyloarthropathies
- Vasculitic disorders

Introduction

The group of disorders comprising the vasculitides, **connective tissue disorders,** and **seronegative spondyloarthropathies** produces impairments related to most corporal systems, including respiratory, musculoskeletal, renal, cardiac, gastrointestinal, integument, and neurological. **Vasculitic disorders** affect primarily the vasculature resulting in "downstream" impairments related to perfusion issues and inflammation. On a system-wide scale, connective tissue disorders and seronegative spondyloarthropathies (SpAs) affect multiple tissue types. In many of these disorders, peripheral neuropathy is a common, although often secondary, manifestation. In addition, many of the interventions currently indicated for these disorders—immunomodulating drugs, biologicals, steroids, and nonsteroidal anti-inflammatory drugs (NSAIDs)—may produce signs and symptoms that may require rehabilitation services interventions.

Vasculitic Diseases

Knowledge of vasculitic neuropathy is important for clinicians for three reasons: (1) Once diagnosed, vasculitic diseases are often treatable with immunosuppressive medications and therapies, especially when the disease is identified in its early stages. (2) Neuropathy is often the presenting sign of vasculitic disease. (3) The neuropathic signs are often present in the well-recognized pattern of multifocal motor, sensory, and autonomic neuropathy.

Vasculitis is a local or systemic inflammation of the vasculature, including the arteries, capillaries, and veins. Typically, lymph vessels are spared. Inflammation of the blood vessels is characterized by leukocyte and macrophage infiltration of the vessel walls resulting in edema, angiogenesis, scarring and potential vascular necrosis, clot, and hemorrhage.[1-3] Local inflammation, if of sufficient magnitude, may produce systemic signs of inflammation, such as cachexia, anemia of chronic disease, depression, and sickness behavior.[4-6]

Although there are many theories regarding the etiology of vasculitic disorders, the exact pathogenesis is not fully understood. Some vasculitides are thought to be an allergic-type reaction, and others are thought to be autoimmune-mediated. This inflammation and the body's subsequent inflammatory cascade reactions may cause the vessels to become weakened and may impair the integrity of the vessel walls, which can prevent adequate flow of blood through the affected vessels. Ischemia of the organ and body tissues perfused by the blood supply may result. The resultant ischemia is the cause for many of the problems that the different types of vasculitis can cause.[7-9]

Vasculitides can also be secondary to other conditions (secondary vasculitis), such as infections, malignancy, reactions to certain medications, complications after organ transplant, connective tissue disease, or others. Vasculitis can also be a primary disease that is not associated with another disease process. The different types of vasculitis are usually first categorized by size of blood vessels involved. Large vessels are involved in temporal arteritis (also called giant cell arteritis) and Takayasu arteritis. Medium-sized vessels are affected in polyarteritis nodosa and Kawasaki disease. Diseases such as Wegener's granulomatosis, Churg-Strauss syndrome, and Henoch-Schönlein purpura affect small vessels.[8,9]

In some diseases, vasculitis is the most overt disease manifestation (e.g., in temporal arteritis), but it may manifest in varying intensities in other diseases (e.g., systemic lupus erythematosis).[8] In general, most types of primary vasculitis are uncommon. For example, Wegener's granulomatosis affects 1 to 5 people per 100,000.[10] Henoch-Schönlein purpura affects up to 10 people per 100,000.[11] Temporal arteritis affects around 50 people per 100,000.[11] Some diseases affect certain populations more than others. Temporal arteritis is usually a disease of older individuals, whereas Henoch-Schönlein purpura usually affects children 5 to 15 years old. Some ethnic groups have much higher incidences of certain diseases; for example, Kawasaki disease affects up to 1 in 1000 children in Japan.

The symptoms of vasculitis stem from the general inflammatory process as well as from complications of ischemia to the specific organ system affected. There are usually some nonspecific systemic complaints such as fever, weakness, or body aches as well as specific symptoms depending on the end-organ system compromised. The nonspecific symptoms are most likely related to the systemic impact of the proinflammatory mediators such as tumor necrosis factor (TNF)-α and interleukin (IL)-1β produced by the macrophages. Patients with Henoch-Schönlein purpura typically present with the triad of abdominal pain; palpable purpura; and periarticular inflammation, swelling, and tenderness.[11] Wegener's granulomatosis can affect the lungs and the kidneys, so patients may complain of symptoms related to these organ systems, such as respiratory issues related to lung involvement and metabolic impairments secondary to renal failure.[10]

The fact that there are many different kinds of vasculitides that affect different organs and cause different symptoms in different patients often makes the diagnosis of vasculitis difficult. Vasculitis is usually suspected in patients with some systemic symptoms as well as a specific organ involved (e.g., the skin, lungs, kidneys). Screening blood tests to assess the function of organ systems are needed. Other blood tests, such as a test for antineutrophil cytoplasmic antibodies (ANCA), are abnormal in certain types of vasculitis and can aid in the diagnosis. However, a biopsy of the most affected organ is usually needed to identify vessel inflammation and to verify the diagnosis.[2]

Although making a definitive diagnosis of vasculitis is difficult, early diagnosis is important because these diseases do respond to appropriate treatments. For example, untreated Wegener's granulomatosis has 100% mortality with an average survival of only 5 months. However, aggressive treatment of this disease achieves remission in 80% to 90% of patients, and the 5-year survival is approximately 75% with treatment. This example illustrates the importance of being persistent in obtaining a definitive diagnosis in patients with possible vasculitis.[12,13]

The American College of Rheumatology has developed a classification rubric based on symptoms to help identify the type of vasculitis a patient has, and this rubric is useful in determining which treatments may be most appropriate and in aiding with prognosis. However, this classification system is more of a screening tool; a biopsy of the most involved organ is considered necessary for a definitive diagnosis, prognosis, and intervention.[14–16]

Because the vasculitides are primarily immune-related inflammatory diseases, the treatments are often steroid-type medications to combat the inflammation as well as other immune system–modifying medications. Long-term use of these medications is typically required for many types of vasculitis, but their use is not without a downside. People who die of the disease usually die as a result of direct complications (e.g., failure of the affected organ), but they often exhibit severe complications related to the immune suppression and other complications of the medications used to treat the disease. Because discontinuing the medications may result in acute disease flare, the balance between the complications from the disease and the potential complications from the treatments can be difficult.

In vasculitic neuropathy, a relatively common disease complication, the target anatomy of the disease is the vasa nervorum, the intraneuronal vasculature system. The vasa nervorum and the nerve tissues downstream are supplied with nutrient blood via numerous small artery anastomoses with larger trunk vessels entering the nerve periodically along its course to and from the central nervous system (CNS) to its target organ. When inside the epineurium and perineurium of the peripheral nerve, the vascular branches anastomose frequently, establishing a complex and rich collateralization of blood flow within the nerve. The frequent anastomoses with larger, extraneural blood vessels and the collateralization within the nerve often prevent focal neuropathic ischemic injury secondary to trauma or atherosclerotic processes involving the larger trunk vessels. However, processes such as vasculitis damage smaller blood vessels ranging in diameter from 50 to 300 μm, which leads to focal nerve necrosis: neurapraxia, neurotmesis, and potentially axonotmesis. The signs and symptoms related to vasculitic neuropathy are directly related to which portion of the nerve is injured. Motor, sensory, and autonomic nerve injuries—alone or in combination with varying levels of severity—have been reported.[17–20] Table 4-1 lists common vasculopathies with the relative frequency of associated peripheral neuropathy.

Table 4-1 Classification of Vasculitic Syndromes and Relative Frequency of Neuropathy	
Syndrome	**Relative Frequency of Neuropathy[a]**
Polyarteritis Group	
Classic polyarteritis nodosa	+++
Allergic granulomatosis of Churg-Strauss syndrome	+++
Polyangiitis	+++
Microscopic polyangiitis	+++
Hypersensitivity vasculitis	
Serum sickness	
Drug-induced vasculitis	
Infectious disease–associated	+
Henoch-Schönlein purpura	
Essential mixed cryoglobulinemia	++
Malignancy-associated vasculitis	+
Vasculitis associated with connective tissue disease	+++
Vasculitis associated with congenital deficiencies of complement	
Wegener's granulomatosis	+++
Giant cell arteritis	
Temporal arteritis	+
Takayasu's arteritis	
Other Vasculitic Syndromes	
Kawasaki disease	
Isolated CNS vasculitis	
Isolated PNS vasculitis	+++
Adamantiades-Behçet disease	
Buerger's disease	
Polymyalgia rheumatica	+
Rheumatoid vasculitis	++

CNS = central nervous system; PNS = peripheral nervous system.
[a]+ indicates neuropathy complication infrequent; ++ indicates neuropathy complication moderately frequent; +++ indicates neuropathy complication very frequent.

Connective Tissue Disorders

Many diseases in rheumatological classifications are associated with peripheral motor, sensory, and autonomic neuropathies. For the diagnosing rheumatologist or neurologist, there is often confusion if the presenting symptoms are those of a connective tissue disease or multiple sclerosis (MS). Clinically, in the early stages of the disease, differentiation of autoimmune disease and MS is difficult. Autoantibodies, such as antinuclear antibody (ANA), are typically present in these diseases but may also be present in MS, increasing the confusion. An acute isolated peripheral nervous system (PNS) or CNS sign identified on magnetic resonance imaging (MRI) manifesting with a functional impairment or musculoskeletal or neurological symptom presents the biggest diagnostic problem: differentiating between the etiology of MS and connective tissue disease.[21] Later in the course of the disease, the clinical presentation and MRI are much more sensitive in disease identification compared with tests performed at the time of disease presentation.

Central and peripheral neuropathies are strongly associated with rheumatological diseases. The etiology of the peripheral neuropathies may be compressive or tensile secondary to space-occupying lesions or abnormal biomechanics, direct vasculitic injury resulting in nerve injury related to the disease process, and complications related to therapies.

Rheumatoid Arthritis

Rheumatoid arthritis (RA) is an inflammatory polyarthritis often leading to pain, stiffness, joint destruction, deformity, and eventually loss of function. Additive, progressive, and symmetrical swelling of peripheral joints, often worse in the morning, is the hallmark of the disease. Extra-articular features and systemic symptoms such as malaise, myalgia, and fever can commonly occur and may antedate the onset of joint symptoms. Chronic pain, disability, and excess morbidity and mortality are sequelae.

RA has a worldwide distribution with an estimated prevalence of 1% to 2%. Prevalence increases with age and is almost 5% in women older than age 55. The average annual incidence in the United States is about 70 per 100,000 annually. Both incidence and prevalence of RA are two to three times greater in women than in men. Although RA may manifest at any age, patients most commonly are first affected in the third to sixth decades.[22,23]

There are three broad classifications of peripheral neuropathy associated with rheumatological conditions. These include the relatively uncommon vasculitic component of specific rheumatological diseases. Space-occupying lesions related to subcutaneous nodules, joint deformity, synovitis, edema, and bony changes may result in tensile or compressive neuropathies. Lastly, medications directed at modifying the rheumatological disease may result in injury to the peripheral nerve.

Rheumatoid vasculitis (RV), a relatively rare complication of RA, results in inflammatory disease in small and medium-sized blood vessels. RV most commonly occurs in the skin as venulitis or capillaritis, but it may occur in other organ systems. RV occurs in approximately 3% to 5% of patients who have RA.[24] It is unclear why RV develops in some patients with RA and not others. Genetic factors may be involved. Viral infections and drug reactions have been suggested as causes of RV, but there is little research to support this. Some research suggests that the prolonged use of medications such as corticosteroids, gold compounds, penicillamine, and azathioprine that are currently prescribed or were prescribed in the past to treat RA can cause the development of RV. However, this cause may be difficult to determine because the accelerated use of these drugs is probably due to severe or long-standing RA, and either severe or long-standing RA may be associated with the development of RV.[24,25]

RV typically occurs in patients who have had RA for longer than a decade.[25] In one study, the average time between the diagnosis of RA and the onset of RV symptoms was 13.6 years. Patients with RA seem more likely to develop RV when high rheumatoid factor (RF) levels are present. Men with RA are two to four times more likely than women with RA to develop RV.[26]

The clinical manifestations of RV can involve many organs of the body, including the skin, nerves to the hands and feet, blood vessels of the fingers and toes, and the eyes. The most common clinical manifestations of vasculitis are small digital infarcts along the nail beds. These can occur in 90% of patients with the complication of RV. The abrupt onset of an ischemic sensory or motor mononeuropathy (mononeuritis multiplex) or progressive scleritis is typical of RV. Ischemia induced by a vasculitis may also lead to skin necrosis.[27–31] Limited data are available concerning the functional outcome of patients with RV and specific therapies, although this cohort of patients with RA usually has worse and more ongoing symptoms than patients with RA who do not have RV.[26]

Rheumatoid nodules are firm, flesh-colored cutaneous lumps that grow close to the affected joints. Typical locations include the hands, fingers, knuckles, elbows, and heels. Rheumatoid nodules can range in size from as large as a walnut to as small as a pea. The nodules may be fixed or movable. Fixed nodules are typically connected to tendons or fascia.[32,33] Nodules are found in 25% to 35% of adults with RA.[32] Other factors may increase the risk of RA nodules. One study positively correlated cigarette smoking and the presence of nodules in patients with RA.[32] Methotrexate, a

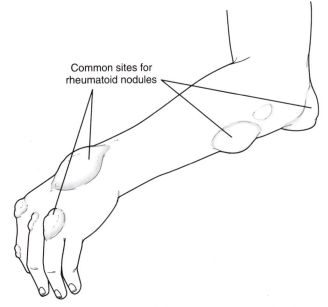

Common sites for rheumatoid nodules

Figure 4-1 Rheumatoid nodules, a common complication of rheumatoid arthritis, not only may result in pain and disfigurement but also may lead to compressive neuropathy secondary to pressure on superficial peripheral nerves. The nodules vary in size from a pea to a walnut and are commonly found in the metacarpophalangeal region of the hand, the wrist, and the elbow. Nodules may be functionally benign or may cause pain (especially over weight-bearing areas), become infected, or lead to tensile or compressive neuropathies if located along the path of a peripheral nerve.

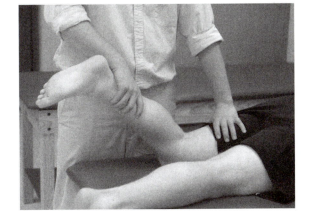

Figure 4-2 Aseptic synovitis in a child with juvenile idiopathic arthritis. With synovitis, the knee tends to rest in the open-packed position resulting in periarticular scarring and eventually a 20° knee flexion contracture. Functionally, the contracture results in an apparent leg-length discrepancy leading to a shortened leg gait pattern.

commonly used RA therapy, has also been linked to increased development of rheumatoid nodules (Fig. 4-1).[33]

Rheumatoid nodules can also form on the vocal cords, causing hoarseness. Nodules may appear in the lungs, heart, and other internal organs. Most nodules do not produce pain or symptoms. However, some patients find the nodules to be painful, especially if the nodules are located on weight-bearing surfaces of the buttocks, feet, elbows, or hands. The size and location of nodules may have a direct impact on activities of daily living by interfering with grasp, limiting joint range of motion, or limiting weight bearing. There is evidence in the literature of compressive and tensile neuropathies directly attributable to the location of the nodule near a peripheral nerve.[31–33]

Nodules may be treated by disease-modifying anti-rheumatic drugs (DMARDs). DMARDs can reduce the size of the nodules. If nodules are thought to be a result of methotrexate treatment, a change in medication regimen may help; however, this decision must be made carefully on an individual basis. Injections of glucocorticoids may help shrink nodules. Surgery sometimes is necessary if rheumatoid nodules become infected, result in progressive symptoms, or are

shown via electroneuromyographic evidence to result in neuropathy.[30–33]

Juvenile Idiopathic Arthritis

The term juvenile idiopathic arthritis (JIA) is used to describe arthritis with onset before 16 years of age. Previously called juvenile RA, the name was changed to reflect the difference between the juvenile (childhood) forms of arthritis and adult forms of arthritis. Although JIA is idiopathic, it is likely the result of a combination of genetic, infectious, and environmental factors. Because arthritis in children may resemble the joint pain associated with infections, cancer, bone disorders, and other inflammatory disorders, these potential causes must be excluded before the diagnosis of JIA can be made.[34,35]

Symptoms of JIA include morning stiffness; pain, swelling, and tenderness of joints; and gait dysfunction—typically antalgic gait or shortened leg gait as a result of hip or knee flexion contracture (Fig. 4-2). Nonspecific complaints of fever, rash, malaise, weight loss, fatigue, and irritability often manifest as the first symptoms. Aseptic conjunctivitis and complaints of blurred vision often are present.

JIA is the most common type of arthritis in children. It affects about 1 in 1000 children, or about 300,000 children in the United States.[34] The American College of Rheumatology classifies juvenile RA into three distinct subtypes: pauciarticular juvenile RA, polyarticular juvenile RA, and systemic juvenile RA. Other childhood arthritides, such as juvenile ankylosing spondylitis (AS) and psoriatic arthritis (PsA), are classified under SpAs (Box 4-1).[34,35]

The etiology and progression of JIA are not completely understood. An external factor (e.g., bacterial

Box 4-1

Classification System of Juvenile Idiopathic Arthritis

Systemic arthritis: Also called Still's disease, this type occurs in about 10%–20% of children with JIA. A systemic illness is one that can affect the entire person or many body systems. Systemic JIA usually causes a high fever and a rash, which most often appears on the trunk, arms, and legs. Multiple organ systems are involved. The heart, liver, spleen, and lymph nodes may be symptomatic. Systemic arthritis typically affects boys and girls equally and rarely affects the ocular system.

Oligoarthritis: This type of JIA affects fewer than five joints in the first 6 months of disease, most often the knee, ankle, and wrist joints. Ocular symptoms are common including uveitis, iridocyclitis, or iritis. About half of all children with JIA have this type, and it is more common in girls than in boys. Symptoms diminish by adulthood.

Polyarthritis: This type of JIA affects five or more joints in the first 6 months, often the same joints on each side of the body. Polyarthritis can also affect the neck and jaw joints and small joints such as those in the hands and feet. It is more common in girls than in boys.

Psoriatic arthritis: This type of arthritis affects children who have arthritis associated with psoriasis. Nail changes are common. The arthritis can precede the rash by many years or vice versa.

Enthesitis-related arthritis: This type of arthritis often affects the spine, hips, and enthesis and occurs mainly in boys older than 8 years. The eyes are often affected in this type of arthritis. There is often a family history of arthritis of the back (spondylitis) in male relatives.

Data compiled from Carbajal-Rodriguez L, Perea-Martinez A, Loredo-Abdala A, Rodriguez-Herrera R, del Angel-Aguilar A, Reynes-Manzur JN. Neurologic involvement in juvenile rheumatoid arthritis. *Bol Med Hosp Infant Mex.* 1991;48:502–508; El-Sayed ZA, Mostafa GA, Aly GS, El-Shahed GS, El-Aziz MM, El-Emam SM. Cardiovascular autonomic function assessed by autonomic function tests and serum autonomic neuropeptides in Egyptian children and adolescents with rheumatic diseases. *Rheumatology (Oxford).* 2009;48:843–848; Lindehammar H, Lindvall B: Muscle involvement in juvenile idiopathic arthritis. *Rheumatology (Oxford).* 2004;43:1546–1554; Pineda Marfa M. Neurological involvement in rheumatic disorders and vasculitis in childhood. *Rev Neurol.* 2002;35:290–296; Quartier P, Taupin P, Bourdeaut F, et al. Efficacy of etanercept for the treatment of juvenile idiopathic arthritis according to the onset type. *Arthritis Rheum.* 2003;48:1093–1101; and Ayaz NA, Ozen S, Bilginer Y, et al. MEFV mutations in systemic onset juvenile idiopathic arthritis. *Rheumatology (Oxford).* 2009;48:23–25.

or viral infection, trauma) triggering an autoimmune cascade and leading to synovial hypertrophy and chronic joint inflammation along with the potential for extra-articular manifestations is theorized to occur in genetically susceptible individuals. JIA is a genetically complex trait in which multiple genes are important for disease onset and manifestations. The *IL2RA/CD25* gene has been implicated as a JIA susceptibility locus, as has the *VTCN1* gene.[35–37]

The pathogenesis of JIA involves humoral and cell-mediated immunity. T lymphocytes and macrophages/monocytes have a central role, releasing local and systemic proinflammatory cytokines (e.g., TNF-α, IL-6, IL-1) and favoring a type 1 helper T-lymphocyte response. A complex interaction between type 1 and type 2 T-helper cells has been postulated. Studies of T-cell receptor expression confirm recruitment of T lymphocytes specific for synovial nonself antigens. Evidence for abnormalities in the humoral immune system includes the increased presence of autoantibodies (especially ANAs), increased serum immunoglobulins, presence of circulating immune complexes, and complement activation.[36]

Chronic inflammation of synovium is characterized by B-lymphocyte infiltration and expansion. Macrophages and T-cell invasion are associated with the release of cytokines, which evoke synoviocyte proliferation, angiogenesis, and interarticular and periarticular scarring. A study by Scola et al.[37] found synovium to contain messenger RNA for vascular endothelial growth factor, angiopoietin 1, and their respective receptors, suggesting that induction of angiogenesis by products of lymphocytic infiltration may be involved in persistence of disease.[38]

Systemic-onset JIA may be more accurately classified as an autoinflammatory disorder, such as familial Mediterranean fever (FMF) or cryopyrin-associated periodic fever syndromes, than other subtypes of JIA. This theory is supported by work demonstrating similar expression patterns of a phagocytic protein (S100A12) in systemic-onset JIA and FMF as well as the same marked responsiveness to IL-1 receptor antagonists. FMF is associated with mutations in the *MEFV* gene. These mutations are associated with activation of the IL-1β pathway, resulting in inflammation.[38] A study by Ayaz et al.[39] of Turkish children with a diagnosis of systemic JIA found an increased frequency of *MEFV* mutations; this study has not been replicated in other populations.

Peripheral neurological complications associated with JIA are relatively rare. The complication of visual loss or decreased vision is associated with iridocyclitis or uveitis rather than direct involvement with the optic nerve. Peripheral neurological manifestations are typically secondary to tension or compressive neuropathies associated with synovitis, joint instability or contracture, reduction via arthroplasty of long-joint contractures with concomitant adaptive shortening of the peripheral nerve, or abnormal biomechanics.[34–38]

Systemic Lupus Erythematosus

Systemic lupus erythematosus (SLE) is a multisystem autoimmune disease with protean manifestations characterized by acute and chronic inflammation of various tissues of the body. SLE may result in disease of the skin, heart, lungs, kidneys, joints, or nervous system.

When only the skin is involved, the condition is called lupus dermatitis or cutaneous lupus erythematosus. Discoid lupus is a form of lupus dermatitis that can be isolated to the skin, without internal disease. When internal organs are involved, the condition is referred to as SLE. Both discoid lupus and SLE are more common in women than men (about eight times more common).[40] The disease can affect individuals of all ages but most commonly manifests in individuals 20 to 45 years old. Statistics demonstrate that lupus is more frequent in African Americans and people of Chinese and Japanese descent.[40]

Genetic factors increase the likelihood of developing autoimmune diseases, and autoimmune diseases such as lupus, RA, and autoimmune thyroid disease are more common among relatives of people with lupus than the general population. Some researchers hypothesize that the immune system in lupus is more easily stimulated by external factors such as viruses or ultraviolet light.[40,41] Symptoms of lupus sometimes can be precipitated or aggravated by only a brief period of sun exposure or the onset of the menstrual period. More recently, research has demonstrated evidence that failure of a key enzyme to dispose of dying cells may contribute the development of SLE. The enzyme, DNase1, normally eliminates what is called "garbage DNA" and other cellular debris by chopping them into tiny fragments for easier disposal. In DNase1 knockout mice, the mice appeared healthy at birth, but after 6 to 8 months, most mice without DNase1 showed signs of SLE.[42]

Neurological impairments, symptoms, and signs are quite common in SLE. Neuropsychiatric signs are present in 60% of persons with SLE.[40] Demyelinating syndrome and myelopathy are 2 of the 19 defined syndromes associated with neuropsychiatric SLE.[40–42] The term lupoid sclerosis is used to describe the manifestation of neurological signs and symptoms of SLE similar to those of multiple sclerosis (MS). Presenting complaints of lupoid sclerosis are often indistinguishable from presenting complaints of early MS. Signs and symptoms of lupoid sclerosis include neuropsychiatric disorders such as bipolar disorder, generalized anxiety disorder, and depression; headache; gait dysfunction; paresthesia; and seizure. MRI offers the best combination of sensitivity and specificity to confirm or rule out MS. ANA, previously considered a strong differentiator between lupoid sclerosis and MS, has been found not to be sufficiently specific; ANAs were found in patients with MS at a frequency of 2.5% to 81%, although no correlation between the presence of ANA and symptoms of SLE was established in many studies.[43] Despite these results, clinically, when ANA titers are high and persistent and appear in the context of other autoimmune diagnostic signs, a diagnosis of SLE should be strongly considered. Visual evoked potentials are rarely typically normal in patients with MS and act as a differentiator between MS and SLE.[44]

Involvement of the CNS, PNS, and autonomic nervous system (ANS) in SLE is common. CNS lupus may manifest with a spectrum of signs and symptoms including headache, cognitive loss, fatigue, depression, anxiety, seizure, stroke, central vision loss, and variability in mood. Adding confusion is the fact that medications used to treat SLE—NSAIDs, corticosteroids, immune-modulating drugs, and antihypertensives—may have similar side effects.[45] CNS vasculitis, a rare but potentially lethal complication, is characterized by high fevers, seizures, psychosis, and meningitis-like stiffness of the neck. CNS vasculitis is the most dangerous form of lupus involving the nervous system and usually requires recurrent hospitalizations and high doses of corticosteroids to suppress the inflammation.[46–48]

PNS lupus may be caused by direct trauma to peripheral nerves related to expansive articular or muscle edema or due to generalized systemic inflammation. Compressive and tensile neuropathies such as tarsal tunnel syndrome, carpal tunnel syndrome, and cervical or lumbosacral radiculopathy are common. Cranial nerve symptoms may include loss of visual acuity, diplopia, trigeminal neuralgia, tinnitus, vertigo, and ptosis.[47]

ANS lupus is typically the result of nonspecific nerve inflammation. Aberrant resting and exercise heart rate, blood pressure, and positional responses such as orthostatic hypotension are common. Perceptions of abnormal corporal coldness or warmth have been reported. Gastric motility issues are common including constipation, vomiting, and diarrhea. Incontinence or inability to void is often reported. The "fishnet" appearance on the arms and legs are a common sign of livedo reticularis and palmar erythema commonly seen with ANS lupus.[48] Raynaud's phenomenon is a common complaint of patients with ANS lupus (Fig. 4-3).

Symptoms of cognitive dysfunction, often referred to in the lay literature as "lupus fog," are described by 50% of patients with SLE. Symptoms include confusion, fatigue, memory loss, and difficulty expressing thoughts and needs. Cognitive dysfunction most often affects patients with mild to moderately active lupus. Cognitive symptoms are variable.[45,46,49] Compared with the general population, patients with lupus are twice as likely to experience migraine headaches, commonly known as "lupus headaches." The features of lupus headaches are similar to migraines and may be seen more often in patients who also have Raynaud's phenomenon. However, headaches can also be caused by vasculitis.[46]

Primary Sjögren's Syndrome

Sjögren's syndrome (SS), also known as sicca syndrome and Mikulicz disease, is a chronic autoimmune exocrinopathy, which, in addition to the two most common characteristics of xerostomia (dry mouth) and dry eyes,

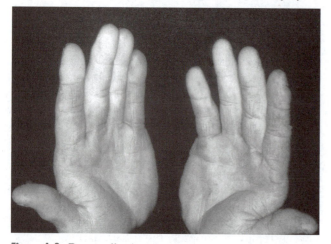

Figure 4-3 Raynaud's phenomenon is a vasospastic disorder of the hands and feet. When exposed to cold, the arteries in the fingers, toes, earlobes, and occasionally other parts of the body constrict, severely limiting blood flow. Often a complication of rheumatological disease, Raynaud's phenomenon is an autonomic nervous system impairment resulting in a permanent or intermittent diminished blood flow primarily to the distal hands and feet resulting in loss of tactile sensation and a feeling of "coldness." Blood flow may be so impaired as to lead to ischemic skin lesions.

may have extraglandular manifestations in various organ systems. Approximately 4 million Americans have SS. Women account for 9 out of 10 patients.[50]

SS may occur alone or in the presence of another autoimmune connective tissue disease such as RA, lupus, or scleroderma. When SS occurs alone, it is referred to as primary SS. When it occurs with another connective tissue disease, it is referred to as secondary SS.

Because symptoms of SS mimic other conditions and diseases, it can often be overlooked or misdiagnosed. On average, it takes nearly 7 years to make a diagnosis of SS.[50] SS often goes unrecognized because of the spectrum and varying intensity of signs and symptoms.

The diagnosis of SS involves detecting the features of dryness of the eyes and mouth. The dryness of the eyes can be determined by testing the ability of the eye to wet a small testing paper strip placed under the eyelid (Schirmer's test using Schirmer tear test strips). More sophisticated testing can be performed by an ophthalmologist.

Salivary glands can become larger and harden or become tender. Salivary gland inflammation can be detected by nuclear medicine salivary scans. Also, the diminished ability of the salivary glands to produce saliva can be measured with salivary flow testing. The diagnosis of SS is strongly supported by abnormal findings of a biopsy of salivary gland tissue. The glands of the lower lip are often used to obtain a biopsy sample of the salivary gland tissue.[50,51]

Patients with SS typically produce various autoantibodies, including ANAs, which are present in nearly all patients. Typical antibodies that are found in most, but not all, patients are SS-A and SS-B antibodies (SS A and B antibodies), RF thyroid antibodies, and others. Anemia and an elevated erythrocyte sedimentation rate are typical findings in patients with SS. The absence of antibodies (ANA, anti-La, RF) does not automatically exclude a diagnosis of SS, although most patients with SS do have the antibodies.[50,51]

Neurological signs and symptoms have been reported in 20% to 35% of patients with SS.[51] However, some studies report a strongly negative association. Neuropathies are characterized by paresthesias, which can comprise numbness and tingling or painful dysesthesias such as burning and aching. The neurological examination may be normal despite clinical complaints because of involvement of small fibers. The lower extremities are more involved than the upper extremities.[52]

Types of possible neuropathies include sensory neuropathy or dorsal root ganglioneuropathy. Patients may present with a history of a fall, ataxia, loss of vibration and position sense, or hyperalgesia. There also may be alterations in appreciation of pain and temperature with hypoesthesia. Reflexes may be absent, especially in the lower extremities.[53]

Motor involvement can occur along with sensory involvement. Weakness, if present, is typically subacute and symmetrical. There can also be a rapidly progressive course of weakness to include a mononeuritis multiplex. Asymmetrical findings as well as stocking-glove distribution of motor weakness have also been reported.[53]

Polyradiculoneuropathy may be present. Polyradiculoneuropathy associated with SS is characterized by findings mimicking disc abnormalities with nerve root pain and weakness in a radicular distribution.

Trigeminal sensory neuropathy can occur and may be characterized by progressive sensory complaints involving the face. These sensations are generally spontaneous and nonlancinating. They typically begin unilaterally and subsequently become bilateral. They may be progressive over months to years. Motor involvement of the fifth cranial nerve with associated impairment of chewing and jaw movements is uncommon. There can be tissue destruction around the nostrils because of picking and scratching secondary to abnormal sensations, corneal ulcerations, lingual ulcerations, and alteration of taste and smell.[53] Other cranial nerves can be involved, such as the second cranial nerve, resulting in signs associated with optic neuritis.[54] In some patients, the optic signs occurred before the diagnosis of SS. SS should be considered in any patient with unexplained optic neuropathy and serological abnormalities suggestive of a connective tissue disorder.[54]

Multiple mononeuropathies, such as carpal tunnel syndrome, ulnar neuropathy, or tarsal tunnel syndrome, can occur. There can be autonomic neuropathy with anhydrosis, postural hypotension, and bradycardia leading to light-headedness and dizziness with change of body position.[54]

Adamantiades-Behçet Disease

Adamantiades-Behçet disease (ABD), often referred to as Behçet disease, is an inflammatory, multisystem disorder affecting primarily arteries and veins and characterized by erythema nodosum—skin lesions involving the dermis, oral mucosa, and genitalia—and uveitis.[55] The incidence is highest in people living around the Mediterranean basin and in Japan.[56] The mean age at onset is the third decade of life.[57] Children are rarely affected, and few neonatal cases have been reported. In large series of patients, the incidence is greater in men than in women.[56] Infectious agents, immune mechanisms, and genetic factors are implicated in the etiopathogenesis of the disease, which remains to be determined. The pathology of the lesions consists of widespread vasculitis; eyes, skin, joints, the oral cavity, blood vessels, and CNS are usually involved, although less frequently the heart, lung, kidney, genital system, gastrointestinal tract, and PNS may be affected. The prognosis of the disease is improved with early diagnosis and suitable treatment. Treatment comprises local therapies and systemic administration of colchicine, corticosteroids, immunosuppressives, and other agents (Fig. 4-4).[57,58]

Neurological manifestations are present in 10% to 50% of patients.[56] Most are late manifestations of the disease; manifestations occur 1 to 8 years after diagnosis. As is the case with many connective tissue diseases and vasculopathies, there is often early diagnostic confusion with MS. Multiple hemispheric white matter lesions seen on MRI resemble lesions found in MS. In end-stage ABD, atrophy of the brainstem rather than cortical atrophy is a classic finding, which differs from MS. Patients with ABD also have different serum and cerebrospinal fluid cytokine and chemokine profiles and concentrations than typically seen with MS. Progression of impairment in MS tends to be polyphasic, whereas impairments with ABD tend to be slow-progressive.[57]

Clinical manifestations of ABD include optic pathology primarily secondary to necrosis and perivascular demyelination with macrophage/monocyte infiltration of the optic nerves and cognitive and focal motor signs. Motor signs, especially tonal changes, are typically present whether the involvement is central or peripheral. Sensory impairment is rarely seen even with fairly dense motor neuropathy.[58,59] Memory tends to be affected in most cases, particularly affecting recall and learning. Orientation (time, place, person) and calculative math skills appear unaffected. Behavioral changes, primarily apathy, depression, or disinhibition, occur in 54% of cases.[59]

Seronegative Spondyloarthropathies

Seronegative SpAs include AS, reactive arthritis (ReA), PsA, arthritis associated with ulcerative colitis, and Crohn's disease, plus other forms that do not meet the criteria for definite categories and are labeled as undifferentiated seronegative SpAs. Two sets of classification criteria have been proposed more recently for the entire group including undifferentiated forms: the European Spondyloarthropathies Study Group and the Amor criteria.[60]

SpAs, or spondyloarthritides as proposed more recently, represent a group of distinct diseases with similar clinical features and a common genetic predisposition. The five major subtypes are AS, PsA, ReA, inflammatory bowel disease–associated SpA (IBD-SpA), and undifferentiated SpA. The main recognized genetic association is with HLA-B27, but it is clear that there are other genes involved.

According to the European Spondyloarthropathy Study Group (ESSG) criteria, IBD is a criterion of SpA; psoriasis or enteric infections are two other manifestations included in the ESSG criteria for identifying patients with PsA and ReA. Patients with IBD presenting with inflammatory back pain or synovitis (predominantly of the lower limbs) are given a diagnosis of SpA. The ESSG criteria, designed to be applicable without radiological examination and laboratory testing, have good sensitivity (75%) and specificity (87%), at least in established disease. An alternative classification scheme was suggested by Amor et al., which is more complicated but has improved sensitivity (85%) and specificity (90%) owing to the incorporation of common extra-articular manifestations of disease, including enthesopathy, dactylitis, eye disease,

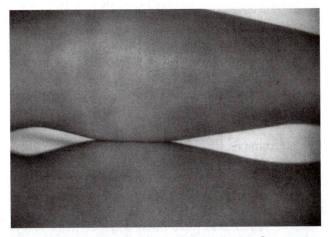

Figure 4-4 Adamantiades-Behçet disease is an inflammatory, multisystem disorder primarily affecting the vasculature and often characterized by erythema nodosum—skin lesions involving the dermis, oral mucosa, and genitalia.

and HLA-B27 positivity. The basic concepts underlying each classification set are similar.[60]

The prevalence of SpAs is directly correlated with the prevalence of the HLA-B27 antigen in the population. The highest prevalence of AS (4.5%) has been found in Canadian Haida Indians[61]; 50% of this population is HLA-B27–positive. Among Europeans, the frequency of the HLA-B27 antigen in the general population ranges from 3% to 13%, and the prevalence of AS is estimated to be 0.1% to 0.23%.

Seronegative SpAs have common clinical and radiological manifestations, including inflammatory spinal pain, sacroiliitis, chest wall pain, peripheral arthritis, peripheral enthesitis, dactylitis, lesions of the lung apices, conjunctivitis, uveitis, and aortic incompetence together with cardiac conduction disturbances. These symptoms may occur in tandem or groups or in isolation.[62]

Ankylosing Spondylitis

The term ankylosing spondylitis derives from the Greek roots *ankylos* (crooked or bent) and *spondylos* (facet joint of the back). The name of the disease is evocative of the severely kyphotic, forward head posture exhibited by patients with advanced cases of AS. This disease is also known as rheumatoid spondylitis, Bechterew syndrome, and Marie-Strümpell spondylitis. AS is a progressive inflammatory disorder of the facet joints that may also affect extra-articular connective tissues and is the principal example of the seronegative SpAs. The hallmark initial symptoms of inflammatory low back and joint stiffness usually first appear insidiously in late adolescence or early adulthood—80% of the time before age 30—and affect men about twice as often as women (Fig. 4-5).[63]

The most common initial symptoms are low back pain and joint stiffness occurring primarily in the early morning.[63–65] The low back pain and joint stiffness are worsened by rest and relieved by activity. Articular pain may spread to the chest and buttocks or may first appear appendicularly (especially in the hips or shoulders), rather than axially, in one fifth of patients. Initially, radiating pain to one buttock may be mistaken as a symptom of thoracic, lumbar, or sacral radiculopathy; however, the buttock pain eventually becomes bilateral and is not accompanied by motor or sensory symptoms or signs. Reflexes are typically preserved. Over years to decades, the axial and appendicular articular symptoms become more pronounced. In a few patients, the axial articular manifestations may eventually reach the point where the entire spine is effectively fused into a single, markedly kyphotic unit, resulting in spinal immobility.[66]

Extra-articular symptoms of AS manifest as the disease evolves. Enthesitis frequently ensues, especially at sites of greater physical stress, and results in considerable extra-articular tenderness and pain.

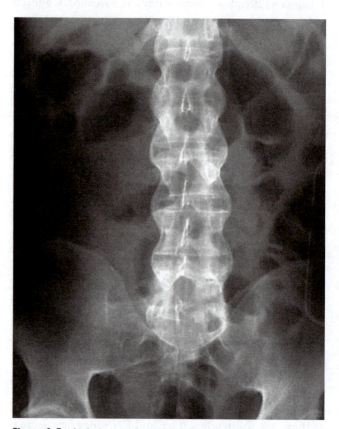

Figure 4-5 Ankylosing spondylitis is a progressive inflammatory disorder of the facet joints that may also affect extra-articular connective tissues. Initial complaints are early morning stiffness that is relieved by activity. Eventually, intra-articular scarring leads to an immobile spine.

Osteoporosis is another widespread extra-articular feature of the disease.[63–65] Patients commonly experience fatigue, which is often the product of muscle imbalance and the need to expend energy to maintain an upright posture, and may be prone to other constitutional symptoms such as weight loss and low-grade fevers. Risk of falling is common. AS may affect the eyes, digestive tract, heart, kidney, lungs, or nervous system (Box 4-2).

Reactive Arthritis

Previously known as Reiter's syndrome, reactive, RF-seronegative, HLA-B27–linked SpA arthritis, is an autoimmune disorder that develops in response to an infection—hence the adjective "reactive" in its name.[67,68] ReA is also known as arthritis urethritica, venereal arthritis, and polyarteritis enterica. The former name Reiter's syndrome, after German physician Hans Conrad Reiter, was discredited when Reiter's history of eugenics, Nazi party membership, human experiments in the Buchenwald concentration camp, and prosecution in Nuremburg as a war criminal came to light.[69]

Box 4-2

Organ-Specific Extraskeletal Manifestations or Associations of Ankylosing Spondylitis

Eyes
  Acute anterior uveitis
Gastrointestinal
  Crohn's disease
Heart/vascular
  Aortic inflammation
  Aortic valve incompetence
  Arrhythmia
  Cardiomegaly
  Pericarditis
  Vertebrobasilar artery insufficiency
Kidneys
  IgA nephropathy
  Amyloidosis
Lungs
  Apical lobe fibrosis
  Reduced tidal volume
  Reduced maximum oxygen
  Restrictive lung disease
Nervous system
  Radiculopathy
  Cauda equina syndrome
  Myelopathy
  Vertebrobasilar insufficiency
  Peripheral neuropathy

Data compiled from Nanke Y, Kotake S, Goto M, Matsubara M, Ujihara H. A Japanese case of Behcet's disease complicated by recurrent optic neuropathy involving both eyes: a third case in the English literature. *Mod Rheumatol.* 2009;19:334–337; Rudwaleit M, van der Heijde D, Landewé R, et al. The development of assessment of Spondyloarthritis International Society classification criteria for axial spondyloarthritis (part II): validation and final selection. *Ann Rheum Dis.* 2009;68:777–783; Olivieri I, Barozzi L, Padula A, De Matteis M, Pavlica P. Clinical manifestations of seronegative spondylarthropathies. *Eur J Radiol.* 1998;27(Suppl 1):S3–6; Barozzi L, Olivieri I, De Matteis M, Padula A, Pavlica P. Seronegative spondylarthropathies: imaging of spondylitis, enthesitis and dactylitis. *Eur J Radiol.* 1998;27(Suppl 1): S12–17; and Rehart S, Kerschbaumer F, Braun J, Sieper J. Modern treatment of ankylosing spondylitis. Orthopade. 2007;36:1067–1078.

Table 4-2 Percent Sensitivity and Specificity of Criteria for Typical Reactive Arthritis

Method of Diagnosis	Sensitivity (%)	Specificity (%)
1. Episode of arthritis of more than 1 month with urethritis or cervicitis or both	84.3	98.2
2. Episode of arthritis of more than 1 month and either urethritis or cervicitis or bilateral conjunctivitis	85.5	96.4
3. Episode of arthritis, conjunctivitis, and urethritis	50.6	98.8
4. Episode of arthritis of more than 1 month, conjunctivitis, and urethritis	48.2	98.8

The "trigger" infection is often healed or is in remission making determination of the etiological microbe difficult. The most common triggers are sexually transmitted chlamydial infection and, perhaps less commonly, gonorrhea. *Salmonella, Shigella,* and *Campylobacter* intestinal infections have also been implicated. ReA has also been reported to occur after tetanus and rabies vaccinations. ReA usually manifests about 1 to 3 weeks after a known infection (Table 4-2).[70–72]

ReA most commonly affects individuals 20 to 40 years old, is more common in men than in women, and is more common in white men than in black men. The last-mentioned is due to the fact that white individuals are more likely to have tissue type HLA-B27 than black individuals. Persons who are HIV-positive have an increased risk of developing ReA.[73]

The manifestations of ReA include a combination of three seemingly unlinked disorders: an inflammatory polyarthritis of large joints, often including the spine; conjunctivitis or uveitis of the eyes; and urethritis in men or cervicitis in women. A useful mnemonic is "the patient can't see, can't pee, can't bend the knee" or "can't see, can't pee, can't climb a tree."[73] A fourth, relatively common manifestation is a complex of psoriasis-like skin lesions, including the rashes circinate balanitis and keratoderma blennorrhagicum (Fig. 4-6). The pathogenesis and broad spectrum of symptoms and signs of ReA may result from the complex interplay of genetic factors (HLA-B27) and environmental factors—molecular mimicry between bacterial fragments in synovial fluid and the HLA-B27 molecule. Most patients (75% to 85%) with ReA are positive for HLA-B27 compared with 7% in the general population. The arthritis may be induced by the manifestation of cytotoxic T lymphocytes by microbial fragments in the joints, but these cytotoxic lymphocytes have specificity for the HLA-B27 cells. The presence of HLA-B27 may allow for more persistent and destructive axial and appendicular skeletal infections.[74,75]

Nervous system involvement in ReA is extremely rare. The literature documents a few cases of patients who initially presented with progressive cervical myelopathy and were diagnosed as having ReA 2 years later. The myelopathy was stable after treatment with methotrexate and sulfasalazine. These cases suggest that ReA can manifest as progressive myelopathy and should be considered in the differential diagnosis of

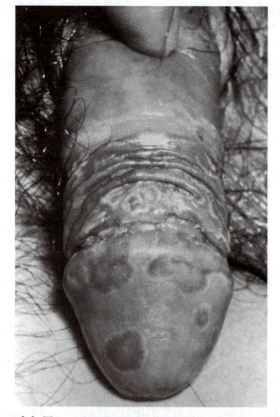

Figure 4-6 This patient presented with what was diagnosed as reactive arthritis with accompanying circinate balanitis of the glans penis. In reactive arthritis, a useful mnemonic is "the patient can't see, can't pee, can't bend the knee" or "can't see, can't pee, can't climb a tree" (73). A fourth, relatively common manifestation is a complex of psoriasis-like skin lesions, including rashes termed circinate balanitis and keratoderma blennorrhagicum.

treatable myelopathies. There have also been fragmentary reports of polyneuropathy—primarily small-fiber sensory, cranial nerve palsy and myelopathy.[75]

Psoriatic Arthritis

PsA is a multigenic autoimmune disease that involves synovial tissue, entheseal sites, and skin, and often results in significant appendicular joint damage. Although there are no diagnostic tests for PsA, research has identified consistent features that help to distinguish the condition from other common rheumatic and connective diseases. Comparison of HLA-B and HLA-C regions in patients with PsA with these regions in patients with psoriasis without joint involvement demonstrates significant differences, and PsA cannot be viewed simply as a subset of genetically homogeneous psoriasis.[76] T-cell receptor phenotypic studies have failed to identify antigen-driven clones, and an alternative hypothesis for CD8 stimulation involving innate immune signals is proposed. There is increasing evidence that PsA is an autoimmune disease

Box 4-3

Presentations of Psoriatic Arthritis

Arthritis mutilans: This extremely severe form of chronic psoriatic arthritis and rheumatoid arthritis is characterized by resorption of bones and the consequent collapse of soft tissue; when this affects the hands, it can cause a phenomenon sometimes referred to as "telescoping fingers." Similar changes can occur in the feet.

Asymmetric psoriatic arthritis: The mildest form of psoriatic arthritis typically affects joints on only one side of the body or different joints on each side hip, knee, ankle, or wrist joints. Fewer than five joints are generally involved. When asymmetric arthritis occurs in the hands and feet, swelling and inflammation in the tendons can cause fingers and toes to resemble small sausages (dactylitis).

Distal interphalangeal joint–predominant arthritis: Distal interphalangeal joint–predominant psoriatic arthritis occurs in only about 5%–10% of patients with psoriatic arthritis. The primary features are involvement of the distal joints of the fingers and toes (the joint closest to the nail) and evidence of nail changes.

Spondylitis: Spondylitis can cause inflammation in the facet joints of the vertebral spine and the sacroiliac joints. Inflammatory changes can also occur at the insertion of ligaments and tendons on the spine. As the disease progresses, movement tends to become increasingly painful, and range of motion becomes limited.

Symmetric psoriatic arthritis: Symmetric psoriatic arthritis usually affects five or more of the same joints on both sides of the body. More women than men have symmetric psoriatic arthritis, and psoriasis associated with this condition tends to be severe.

Data compiled from Narayanaswami P, Chapman KM, Yang ML, Rutkove SB. Psoriatic arthritis-associated polyneuropathy: a report of three cases. *J Clin Neuromuscul Dis.* 2007;9:248–251; Rothenberg RJ, Sufit RL. Drug-induced peripheral neuropathy in a patient with psoriatic arthritis. *Arthritis Rheum.* 1987;30:221–224; and Kane D, Stafford L, Brenihan B, Fitzgerlad O. A prospective, clinical and radiological study of early psoriatic arthritis: an early synovitis clinic experience. *Rheumatology.* 2003;42:1460–1468.

in which the CD8+ T cell plays a central role. Finally, in contrast to RA, imaging and cytokine studies have demonstrated entheseal involvement in PsA, and it is possible that entheseal-derived antigens may trigger an immune response that is critically involved in the disease pathogenesis and progression (Box 4-3).[77]

In contrast to most other rheumatic diseases, heredity influence plays a strong role in the development of PsA. About 15% of the relatives of a patient with PsA also have PsA, and an additional 30% to 45% have psoriasis. The presence of either psoriasis or PsA in a family member of a patient with signs and symptoms suggestive of PsA provides support for the diagnosis.[78]

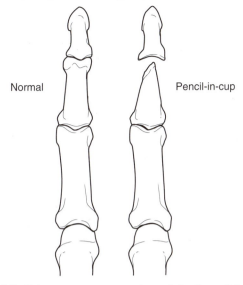

Normal   Pencil-in-cup

Figure 4-7 Schematic representation of the "pencil-in-cup" interdigital deformity associated with psoriatic arthritis.

The classic radiological features of PsA include new bone formation at entheseal sites; bone resorption or osteolysis; sacroiliitis, which is often asymmetrical; and the hallmark "pencil-in-cup" deformity of the interphalangeal and metacarpophalangeal or tarsophalangeal joints (Fig. 4-7), which results from a combination of new bone formation and osteolysis. These features sometimes have diagnostic utility, but none are specific, and more often the radiological features in PsA are either minimal or nonspecific. For example, erosions occur in PsA but less frequently than in RA, and the rate of development of new erosions is much slower. In one study of patients with early PsA, 47% of patients had developed erosive disease at 2 years, but the number of erosions increased from a mean of 1.2 (±2.9) to a mean of only 3 (±5.2). Although this increase was significant ($P = 0.002$), the number of new erosions over a similar time frame is fewer than described in RA.[79] In contrast, new bone formation is not a feature of RA. The use of MRI in PsA has emphasized the importance of enthesitis with bone marrow edema occurring at entheseal sites.[80] As a result of these observations, it has been proposed that involvement of the enthesis is the primary event in PsA, with synovial involvement occurring later and in a nonspecific manner.[80]

Neurological symptoms associated with PsA are relatively rare compared with RA and are associated with the more severe and progressive forms of PsA: spondylitis and arthritis mutilans. Symptoms are typically related to compression or tension of a peripheral nerve—related to articular and osteogenic changes affecting the local nerve and nerve trunk. Motor, sensory, and autonomic nerve involvement is possible.[77,78]

Enteropathic Arthritis

Inflammation of axial or peripheral joints is one of the most frequent extraintestinal manifestations complicating the clinical course and therapeutic approach in IBD. Musculoskeletal manifestations occur in 20% to 50% of patients with IBD.[81-83] The frequency of these complications seems to be similar for both Crohn's disease and ulcerative colitis. Arthritis associated with IBD belongs to the category of SpAs. Axial involvement ranges from isolated inflammatory back pain to AS, whereas peripheral arthritis is noted in periarticular and polyarticular disease. Asymptomatic radiological involvement of the sacroiliac joints is reported to occur in 50% of patients.[83] Other musculoskeletal manifestations, such as buttock pain, dactylitis, calcaneal enthesitis, and thoracic pain, are frequently underdiagnosed and consequently are not treated appropriately. Several diagnostic approaches and criteria have been proposed over the past 40 years in an attempt to classify and diagnose such manifestations correctly. The correct recognition of SpAs requires an integrated multidisciplinary approach to identify common therapeutic strategies, especially in the era of the new biological therapies.[84]

The recognition of this entity is based on clinical diagnosis (e.g., joint swelling and tenderness) but may be confirmed by ultrasound examination[83] or MRI,[84,85] whereas conventional radiographs usually are not helpful. Enthesitis is inflammation at the site of the tendon, ligament, and joint capsule insertion to bone. The most frequent clinical expressions are Achilles tendinitis, plantar fasciitis, and pain and swelling of the tibial tubercle.[86]

Two subtypes of peripheral arthritis are recognized.[86] Type 1 involves fewer than five joints and is clinically characterized by acute self-limiting attacks of less than 10 weeks' duration often paralleling intestinal inflammatory activity. It is also strongly associated with other extraintestinal manifestations of IBD such as erythema nodosum. Type 2 peripheral arthritis is polyarticular, involving five or more joints with symptoms that persist for months and years running independently from IBD flares. This type is associated with uveitis but not with other extraintestinal manifestations. Both types are seronegative, usually nonerosive and nondeforming, but may become chronic and erosive in 10% of patients. In addition, no significant association has been shown between peripheral arthropathies and HLA-B27 in IBD. A type 3 peripheral arthritis has been proposed, which includes patients with both axial involvement and peripheral arthritis.[87]

Dactylitis is characterized by inflammatory swelling of one or more fingers ("sausage" fingers) or toes caused by tenosynovitis of the flexor tendons and sheaths. Metacarpophalangeal or proximal interphalangeal joint arthritis may also be present (Fig. 4-8). Thoracic

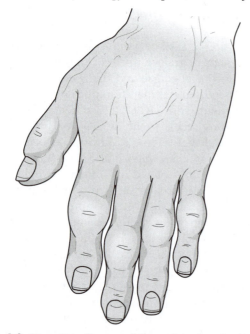

Figure 4-8 Dactylitis ("sausage" fingers) is characterized by inflammatory swelling of one or more fingers or toes secondary to tenosynovitis of the flexor tendons and sheaths. One of the many causes of dactylitis is enteropathic arthritis.

pain results from enthesitis of costovertebral, costosternal, or manubriocostal articulations; is exacerbated by cough and deep inspirations; limits respiratory expansion; and has episodes of variable duration. Buttock pain is part of the IBD, irradiates to the sacrum, and may be alternating; it is related to inflammation of sacroiliac joints.

Extra-articular features include uveitis (25%), aortic insufficiency (4% to 10%), and cardiac conduction disturbances (3% to 9%).[88] These latter cardiac complications seem to be related to disease duration and are associated with HLA-B27.

Celiac Disease

The symptoms of celiac disease can vary significantly from patient to patient. The spectrum of symptoms may vary from constipation to diarrhea, to abdominal pain to bloating, to cramps to no pain, and this is part of the reason the diagnosis is frequently delayed. Additional symptoms may include unexpected weight loss, lactose intolerance, nausea and vomiting, and decreased appetite. Nonintestinal symptoms include anemia, bone and joint pain, osteoporosis, ecchymoses, dental enamel defects, alopecia, mouth ulcers, vitamin deficiency impairments, and fatigue.[89–92]

Celiac disease is treated primarily by following a gluten-free diet. This diet allows the diseased intestinal villi to heal. In addition, vitamin and mineral supplements are typically used to correct deficiencies. Short-term or long-term corticosteroids may be prescribed for refractory disease.

The exact cause of celiac disease is unknown. The intestines contain projections (called villi) that absorb nutrients. In undiagnosed or untreated celiac disease, these villi become flattened, which affects the ability to absorb nutrients properly. The disease can develop at any point in life, from infancy to late adulthood. People with a family member with celiac disease are at greater risk for developing the disease. The disorder is most common in Caucasians and those of European ancestry. Women are affected more commonly than men.[89]

Symptoms of peripheral neuropathy associated with celiac disease are often related to osteoporosis. In one study, anemia was the most common manifestation accounting for 66% of patients.[89] Less than half of the patients had any of the classic symptoms of celiac disease, and 25% had none of the classic symptoms at presentation.[90] Anti-gliadin antibodies, anti-endomysial antibody, and anti–tissue transglutaminase showed 75%, 68%, and 90% sensitivity. In combination, serology results were 100% sensitive as screening tests for adult celiac disease. Either osteoporosis or osteopenia was present in 59% of patients. There were no malignant complications observed during the follow-up of our patients.[91]

CASE STUDY

Chris is a 67-year-old corporate executive in whom rheumatoid arthritis was diagnosed 20 years ago. Surgeries related to the rheumatoid arthritis include a left total knee arthroplasty and a right hip arthroplasty. The disease is relatively stable with methotrexate and occasional nonsteroidal medications. Recently, Chris has been complaining of progressive numbness in his right hand and weakness of his thumb. He was referred to a physical therapist for evaluation and treatment.

On examination, the physical therapist noted moderate right wrist edema and tenosynovitis. Finger and thumb range of motion was functional and painless, but the wrist tended to rest in 45° of ulnar deviation with −10° of passive radial deviation. Wrist flexion and extension range of motion were full and painless. Elbow range of motion was normal. The therapist noted a large rheumatoid nodule 10 cm proximal to the radial styloid. Sensory examination revealed loss of tactile sense of the palmar side of the thumb, fore, middle, and ring fingers. Pinch assessments revealed a 40% decrease in strength compared with the uninvolved side.

Case Study Questions

1. Possible etiologies of the neuropathy include which of the following?
  a. A traction-induced median neuropathy caused by the static ulnar deviated posture of the wrist
  b. A compressive neuropathy of the median nerve secondary to pressure from the rheumatoid nodule
  c. A compressive neuropathy of the median nerve secondary to the tenosynovitis at the wrist
  d. All of the above

2. Which of the following tests is the most effective test for determining location and severity of the neuropathy?
  a. Tinel
  b. Filament sensory testing
  c. Electroneuromyogram
  d. X-ray

3. Which orthosis may be most indicated for this patient?
  a. A functional wrist splint placing the wrist in a neutral radial/ulnar deviation posture
  b. An elbow pad
  c. A shoulder sling
  d. A cervical collar

4. Along with orthoses, other interventions for this patient, before a definitive diagnosis, would include which of the following?
  a. Energy conservation
  b. Joint conservation
  c. Review of total hip arthroplasty precautions
  d. All of the above

5. _____ is a rare complication of rheumatoid arthritis resulting in inflammatory disease in small to medium-sized blood vessels and may lead to an ischemic motor or sensory mononeuropathy.
  a. Rheumatoid vasculitis
  b. Rheumatoid nodule
  c. Fibromyalgia
  d. Scleritis

References

1. Chung MP, Yi CA, Lee HY, Han J, Lee KS. Imaging of pulmonary vasculitis. *Radiology.* 2010;255:322–341.
2. Hellmich B. Update on the management of systemic vasculitis: what did we learn in 2009? *Clin Exp Rheumatol.* 2010;28(1 Suppl 57):98–103.
3. Herlyn K, Moosig F, Gross WL. The significance of health-related quality of life in systemic vasculitides. *Z Rheumatol.* 2010;69:220–226.
4. Dantzer R. Cytokine-induced sickness behaviour: a neuroimmune response to activation of innate immunity. *Eur J Pharmacol.* 2004;500:399–411.
5. Dantzer R. Cytokine induced sickness behavior: mechanisms and implications. *Ann N Y Acad Sci.* 2001;933:222–234.
6. Dantzer R. Innate immunity at the forefront of psychoneuroimmunology. *Brain Behav Immun.* 2001;15:7–24.
7. Jacobi C, Lenhard T, Meyding-Lamade U. Vasculitis of the nervous system in infectious diseases. *Nervenarzt.* 2010;81:172–180.
8. Leelavathi M, Aziz SA, Gangaram HB, Hussein SH. Cutaneous vasculitis: a review of aetiology and clinical manifestations in 85 patients in Malaysia. *Med J Malaysia.* 2009;64:210–212.
9. Rowley AH, Shulman ST. Pathogenesis and management of Kawasaki disease. *Expert Rev Anti Infect Ther.* 2010;8:197–203.
10. Holle JU, Laudien M, Gross WL. Clinical manifestations and treatment of Wegener's granulomatosis. *Rheum Dis Clin North Am.* 2010;36:507–526.
11. Agras PI, Guveloglu M, Aydin Y, Yakut A, Kabakus N. Lower brachial plexopathy in a child with Henoch-Schonlein purpura. *Pediatr Neurol.* 2010;42:355–358.
12. Pettersson T, Karjalainen A. Diagnosis and management of small vessel vasculitides. *Duodecim.* 2010;126:1496–1507.
13. Pierrot-Deseilligny Despujol C, Pouchot J, Pagnoux C, Coste J, Guillevin L. Predictors at diagnosis of a first Wegener's granulomatosis relapse after obtaining complete remission. *Rheumatology (Oxford).* 2010;49:2181–2190.
14. Hanly JG. ACR classification criteria for systemic lupus erythematosus: limitations and revisions to neuropsychiatric variables. *Lupus.* 2004;13:861–864.
15. Rao JK, Allen NB, Pincus T. Limitations of the 1990 American College of Rheumatology classification criteria in the diagnosis of vasculitis. *Ann Intern Med.* 1998;129:345–352.
16. Saleh A, Stone JH. Classification and diagnostic criteria in systemic vasculitis. *Best Pract Res Clin Rheumatol.* 2005;19:209–221.
17. Bussone G, La Mantia L, Frediani F, Tredici G, Petruccioli Pizzini MG. Vasculitic neuropathy in panarteritis nodosa: clinical and ultrastructural findings. *Ital J Neurol Sci.* 1986;7:265–269.
18. Fathers E, Fuller GN. Vasculitic neuropathy. *Br J Hosp Med.* 1996;55:643–647.
19. Griffin JW. Vasculitic neuropathies. *Rheum Dis Clin North Am.* 2001;27:751–760.
20. Pagnoux C, Guillevin L. Peripheral neuropathy in systemic vasculitides. *Curr Opin Rheumatol.* 2005;17:41–48.
21. Pender MP, Chalk JB. Connective tissue disease mimicking multiple sclerosis. *Aust N Z J Med.* 1989;19:469–472
22. Agarwal V, Singh R, Wiclaf, et al. A clinical, electrophysiological, and pathological study of neuropathy in rheumatoid arthritis. *Clin Rheumatol.* 2008;27:841–844.
23. Albani G, Ravaglia S, Cavagna L, Caporali R, Montecucco C, Mauro A. Clinical and electrophysiological evaluation of peripheral neuropathy in rheumatoid arthritis. *J Peripher Nerv Syst.* 2006;11:174–175.
24. Gemignani F, Giovanelli M, Vitetta F, et al. Non-length dependent small fiber neuropathy: a prospective case series. *J Peripher Nerv Syst.* 2010;15:57–62.
25. Genc H, Balaban O, Karagoz A, Erdem HR. Femoral neuropathy in a patient with rheumatoid arthritis. *Yonsei Med J.* 2007;48:891–893.
26. Bartels C, Bell C, Rosenthal A, Shinki K, Bridges A. Decline in rheumatoid vasculitis, prevalence among US veterans: a retrospective cross-sectional study. *Arthritis Rheum.* 2009;60:2553–2557.
27. Kerschbaumer F, Kerschbaumer GY. Peripheral nerve entrapment syndrome of the upper extremities in cases of inflammatory, rheumatic joint diseases. *Z Rheumatol.* 2007;66:9–12, 14.

28. Sahatciu-Meka V, Rexhepi S, Manxhuka-Kerliu S, Rexhepi M. Extra-articular manifestations of seronegative and seropositive rheumatoid arthritis. *Bosn J Basic Med Sci.* 2010; 10:26–31.

29. Sugiura F, Kojima T, Oguchi T, et al. A case of peripheral neuropathy and skin ulcer in a patient with rheumatoid arthritis after a single infusion of tocilizumab. *Mod Rheumatol.* 2009;19:199–203.

30. Tatsumura M, Mishima H, Shiina I, et al. Femoral nerve palsy caused by a huge iliopectineal synovitis extending to the iliac fossa in a rheumatoid arthritis case. *Mod Rheumatol.* 2008;18:81–85.

31. Tektonidou MG, Serelis J, Skopouli FN. Peripheral neuropathy in two patients with rheumatoid arthritis receiving infliximab treatment. *Clin Rheumatol.* 2007;26: 258–260.

32. Mikuls TR, Hughes LB, Westfall AO, et al. Cigarette smoking, disease severity and autoantibody expression in African Americans with recent-onset rheumatoid arthritis. *Ann Rheum Dis.* 2008;67:1529–1534.

33. Harel-Meir M, Sherer Y, Shoenfeld Y. Tobacco smoking and autoimmune diseases. *Nat Clin Pract Rheumatol.* 2007;3: 707–715.

34. Carbajal-Rodriguez L, Perea-Martinez A, Loredo-Abdala A, Rodriguez-Herrera R, del Angel-Aguilar A, Reynes-Manzur JN. Neurologic involvement in juvenile rheumatoid arthritis. *Bol Med Hosp Infant Mex.* 1991;48:502–508.

35. El-Sayed ZA, Mostafa GA, Aly GS, El-Shahed GS, El-Aziz MM, El-Emam SM. Cardiovascular autonomic function assessed by autonomic function tests and serum autonomic neuropeptides in Egyptian children and adolescents with rheumatic diseases. *Rheumatology (Oxford).* 2009;48:843–848.

36. Lindehammar H, Lindvall B. Muscle involvement in juvenile idiopathic arthritis. *Rheumatology (Oxford).* 2004;43: 1546–1554.

37. Scola MP, Imagawa T, Boivin GP, Giannini EH, Glass DN, Hirsch R, Grom AA. Expression of angiogenic factors in juvenile rheumatoid arthritis: Correlation with revacularization of human synovium engrafted into SCID mice. Arthritis and Rheumatism. 2001;44:794–801.

38. Quartier P, Taupin P, Bourdeaut F, et al. Efficacy of etanercept for the treatment of juvenile idiopathic arthritis according to the onset type. *Arthritis Rheum.* 2003;48: 1093–1101.

39. Ayaz NA, Ozen S, Bilginer Y, et al. MEFV mutations in systemic onset juvenile idiopathic arthritis. *Rheumatology (Oxford).* 2009;48:23–25.

40. Honczarenko K, Budzianowska A, Ostanek L. Neurological syndromes in systemic lupus erythematosus and their association with antiphospholipid syndrome. *Neurol Neurochir Pol.* 2008;42:513–517.

41. Brown AC. Lupus erythematosus and nutrition: a review of the literature. *J Ren Nutr.* 2000;10:170–183.

42. Ilniczky S, Kamondi A, Aranyi Z, et al. Simultaneous central and peripheral nervous system involvement in systemic lupus erythematosus. *Ideggyogy Sz.* 2007;60:398–402.

43. Bultink IE, Lems WF, Kostense PJ, Dijkmans BA, Voskuyl AE. Prevalence of and risk factors for low bone mineral density and vertebral fractures in patients with systemic lupus erythematosus. *Arthritis Rheum.* 2005;52:2044–2050.

44. Santos MS, de Carvalho JF, Brotto M, Bonfa E, Rocha FA. Peripheral neuropathy in patients with primary antiphospholipid (Hughes') syndrome. *Lupus.* 2010;19: 583–590.

45. Yu KH, Yang CH, Chu CC. Swallowing disturbance due to isolated vagus nerve involvement in systemic lupus erythematosus. *Lupus.* 2007;16:746–749.

46. Brooks WH. Systemic lupus erythematosus and related autoimmune diseases are antigen-driven, epigenetic diseases. *Med Hypotheses.* 2002;59:736–741.

47. Santos MS, de Carvalho JF, Brotto M, Bonfa E, Rocha FA. Peripheral neuropathy in patients with primary antiphospholipid (Hughes') syndrome. *Lupus.* 2010;19: 583–590.

48. Yu KH, Yang CH, Chu CC. Swallowing disturbance due to isolated vagus nerve involvement in systemic lupus erythematosus. *Lupus.* 2007;16:746–749.

49. Maisonobe T, Denys V, Amoura Z. Sensory neuropathy and autoimmune diseases. *Rev Neurol (Paris).* 2009;165(Suppl 3): S70–76.

50. Voulgarelis M, Tzioufas AG. Pathogenetic mechanisms in the initiation and perpetuation of Sjogren's syndrome. *Nat Rev Rheumatol.* 2010;6:529–537.

51. Gemignani F, Giovanelli M, Vitetta F, et al. Non-length dependent small fiber neuropathy: a prospective case series. *J Peripher Nerv Syst.* 2010;15:57–62.

52. Gono T, Kawaguchi Y, Katsumata Y, et al. Clinical manifestations of neurological involvement in primary Sjogren's syndrome. *Clin Rheumatol.* 2011;30:485–490.

53. Chai J, Logigian EL. Neurological manifestations of primary Sjogren's syndrome. *Curr Opin Neurol.* 2010;23:509–513.

54. Sakai K, Hamaguchi T, Yamada M. Multiple cranial nerve enhancement on MRI in primary Sjogren's syndrome. *Intern Med.* 2010;49:857–859.

55. Akbulut L, Gur G, Bodur H, Alli N, Borman P. Peripheral neuropathy in Behcet disease: an electroneurophysiological study. *Clin Rheumatol.* 2007;26:1240–1244.

56. Cho BS, Kim HS, Oh SJ, et al. Comparison of the clinical manifestations, brain MRI and prognosis between neuroBechet's disease and neuropsychiatric lupus. *Korean J Intern Med.* 2007;22:77–86.

57. Siva A, Saip S. The spectrum of nervous system involvement in Behcet's syndrome and its differential diagnosis. *J Neurol.* 2009;256:513–529.

58. Finsterer J. Systemic and non-systemic vasculitis affecting the peripheral nerves. *Acta Neurol Belg.* 2009;109:100–113.

59. Nanke Y, Kotake S, Goto M, Matsubara M, Ujihara H. A Japanese case of Behcet's disease complicated by recurrent optic neuropathy involving both eyes: a third case in the English literature. *Mod Rheumatol.* 2009;19:334–337.

60. Rudwaleit M, van der Heijde D, Landewé R, et al. The development of assessment of Spondyloarthritis International Society classification criteria for axial spondyloarthritis (part II): validation and final selection. *Ann Rheum Dis.* 2009;68:777–783.

61. Olivieri I, Barozzi L, Padula A, De Matteis M, Pavlica P. Clinical manifestations of seronegative spondylarthropathies. *Eur J Radiol.* 1998;27(Suppl 1):S3–6.

62. Barozzi L, Olivieri I, De Matteis M, Padula A, Pavlica P. Seronegative spondylarthropathies: imaging of spondylitis, enthesitis and dactylitis. *Eur J Radiol.* 1998;27(Suppl 1): S12–17.

63. Rehart S, Kerschbaumer F, Braun J, Sieper J. Modern treatment of ankylosing spondylitis. *Orthopade.* 2007;36: 1067–1078.

64. Chan JW, Castellanos A. Infliximab and anterior optic neuropathy: case report and review of the literature. *Graefes Arch Clin Exp Ophthalmol.* 2010;248:283–287.

65. Gunduz OH, Kiralp MZ, Ozcakar L, Cakar E, Yildirim P, Akyuz G. Nerve conduction studies in patients with ankylosing spondylitis. *J Natl Med Assoc.* 2010;102:243–246.

66. Tham VM, Cunningham E Jr. Anterior ischaemic optic neuropathy in a patient with HLA-B27 associated anterior uveitis and ankylosing spondylitis. *Br J Ophthalmol.* 2001; 85:756.

67. Rudwaleit M, Braun J, Sieper J. Treatment of reactive arthritis: a practical guide. *BioDrugs*. 2000;13:21–28.

68. Carter JD, Hudson AP. The evolving story of Chlamydia-induced reactive arthritis. *Curr Opin Rheumatol*. 2010;22: 424–430.

69. Ackerman AB. Reiter syndrome and Hans Reiter: neither legitimate! *J Am Acad Dermatol*. 2009;60:517–518.

70. Aksu K, Gokhan K, Eker D. Reactive arthritis following tetanus and rabies vaccinations. *Rheumatol Int*. 2006;27: 209–210.

71. Chou YS, Horng CT, Huang HS, Hu SC, Chen JT, Tsai ML. Reactive arthritis following *Streptococcus viridans* urinary tract infection. *Ocul Immunol Inflamm*. 2010;18:52–53.

72. van der Helm-van Mil AH. Acute rheumatic fever and poststreptococcal reactive arthritis reconsidered. *Curr Opin Rheumatol*. 2010;22:437–442.

73. Li CW, Ma JJ, Yin J, Liu L, Hu J. Reiter's syndrome in children: a clinical analysis of 22 cases. *Zhonghua Er Ke Za Zhi*. 2010;48:212–215.

74. Miranda S, Vernet M, Heron F, Vittecoq O, Levesque H, Marie I. Acute reactive arthritis after intravesical instillation of bacillus Calmette-Guerin. Two case reports and literature review [in French]. *Rev Med Interne*. 2010;31:558–561.

75. Kim SK, An JY, Park MS, Kim BJ. A case report of Reiter's syndrome with progressive myelopathy. *J Clin Neurol*. 2007;3: 215–218.

76. Candia L, Cuellar ML, Marlowe SM, Marquez J, Iglesias A, Espinoza LR. Charcot-like arthropathy: a newly-recognized subset of psoriatic arthritis. *Clin Exp Rheumatol*. 2006;24: 172–175.

77. Narayanaswami P, Chapman KM, Yang ML, Rutkove SB. Psoriatic arthritis-associated polyneuropathy: a report of three cases. *J Clin Neuromuscul Dis*. 2007;9:248–251.

78. Rothenberg RJ, Sufit RL. Drug-induced peripheral neuropathy in a patient with psoriatic arthritis. *Arthritis Rheum*. 1987;30:221–224.

79. Kane D, Stafford L, Brenihan B, Fitzgerlad O. A prospective, clinical and radiological study of early psoriatic arthritis: an early synovitis clinic experience. *Rheumatology*. 2003;42: 1460–1468.

80. McGonagle D, Gibbon W, O'Connor P, Green M, Pease C, Emery P. Characteristic magnetic resonance imaging entheseal changes of knee synovitis in spondylarthropathy. *Arthritis Rheum*. 1998;41:694–700.

81. Riise OR, Handeland KS, Cvancarova M, et al. Incidence and characteristics of arthritis in Norwegian children: a population-based study. *Pediatrics*. 2008;121:e299–306.

82. Karimi O, Pena AS. Indications and challenges of probiotics, prebiotics, and synbiotics in the management of arthralgias and spondyloarthropathies in inflammatory bowel disease. *J Clin Gastroenterol*. 2008;42(Suppl 3 Pt 1): S136–141.

83. Colombo E, Latiano A, Palmieri O, Bossa F, Andriulli A, Annese V. Enteropathic spondyloarthropathy: a common genetic background with inflammatory bowel disease? *World J Gastroenterol*. 2009;15:2456–2462.

84. Kono M, Oshitani N, Sawa Y, et al. Crohn's disease complicated by adult-onset Still's disease. *J Gastroenterol*. 2003;38:891–895.

85. Zhang JL, Jin JY, Li HX, Zhu J, Huang F. The clinical characters of 30 patients with enteropathic arthritis and literature review. *Zhonghua Nei Ke Za Zhi*. 2010;49: 223–225.

86. Orchard TR, Wordworth BP, Jewell DP. Peripheral arthropathies in inflammatory bowel disease: their articular distribution and natural history. *Gut*. 1998;42:387–391.

87. Smale S, Natt RS, Orchard TR, Russell AS, Bjarnason I. Inflammatory bowel disease and spondylarthropathy. *Arthritis Rheum*. 2001;44:2728–2736.

88. Bergfeldt L. HLA-B27-associated cardiac disease. *Ann Intern Med*. 1997;127(8 Pt 1):621–629.

89. Jones S, D'Souza C, Haboubi NY. Patterns of clinical presentation of adult coeliac disease in a rural setting. *Nutr J*. 2006;5:24.

90. Maki M, Collin P. Coeliac disease. *Lancet*. 1997;349: 1755–1759.

91. Feighery C. Coeliac disease. *BMJ*. 1999;319:236–239.

92. Collin P, Reunala T, Pukkala E, Laippala P, Keyrilainen O, Pasternack A. Coeliac disease—associated disorders and survival. *Gut*. 1994;35:1215–1218.

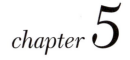

chapter 5

Environmental Toxic Neuropathies

Stephen J. Carp, PT, PhD, GCS

"Poison is in everything, and nothing is without poison. The dosage makes it either a poison or a remedy."

—Paracelsus (1493–1541)

Objectives

On completion of this chapter, the student/practitioner will be able to:

- Identify common environmental toxins and exposure vectors that may lead to peripheral neuropathy.
- Discuss the type of neuropathy associated with each toxin and the common clinical picture including signs and symptoms that may be encountered by rehabilitation therapists.
- Construct treatment intervention schema for each of the common environmental toxic neuropathies presented.

Key Terms

- Alcohol
- Arsenic
- Lead
- Mercury
- Nitrous oxide
- Thallium

Introduction

Knowledge of the neurotoxicity of environmental compounds and elements has a very practical application in the evaluation of patients with signs and symptoms of peripheral neuropathy. Consultation on patients with numerous neurotoxic exposures including environmental compounds and elements; prescribed, over-the-counter, and recreational drugs; and dietary and absorption compromises is common.

Exposure often is occupational or related to a hobby, but occasionally there is exposure by happenstance or, especially in cases of nitrous oxide, **thallium,** and ethylene glycol, purposeful exposure. These compounds and elements produce signs and symptoms common to neuropathies associated with medication, primary or secondary disease processes, and biomechanical forces. An astute clinician is able to identify the etiological agent through careful history-taking, follow-up questioning, laboratory data analysis, and a valid and reliable physical examination.

For example, **nitrous oxide,** a potent etiological agent for peripheral neuropathy, is commonly found in the aerospace, automobile, and food preparation industries. It is also used as a dental anesthetic. Additionally, nitrous oxide is a popular recreational drug. Ethylene glycol is a very common toxin because of its use as a coolant in automobiles. Metal toxicity (thallium, **arsenic,** and **lead**) receives much commentary in neurological and pathophysiology textbooks and is of interest to medical practitioners when investigating the etiology of peripheral neuropathy. The etiology of **alcohol** neuropathy is most likely twofold: (1) a nutritionally based neuropathy primarily owing to thiamine deficiency and (2) the direct toxic effects of alcohol on the peripheral nerve.

In this chapter, we discuss the relationship of the exposure of specific common environmental compounds and elements and the onset and pathogenesis of peripheral neuropathy. Toxins are discussed under specific headings as follows: anesthetic agent, heavy metal toxicities, and chemical toxicities including alcohol-related neuropathy. There are hundreds of environmentally and clinically available toxins that, with exposure, may lead to symptoms of peripheral neuropathy. It is beyond the scope of this book to include all of these toxins. Chapter 11 discusses medication-associated neuropathy.

Anesthetic Agent

Nitrous Oxide

Nitrous oxide (N_2O) is more commonly known to the lay population as "laughing gas." It is a nonflammable, inorganic gas used in medicine, in industry, and as a recreational drug. It is a major source of air pollution as well as a major source of greenhouse emissions.[1]

In industry, N_2O is used as an oxidizer and monopropellant in rocket engines. In the presence of a heated catalyst, N_2O decomposes exothermically into hydrogen and oxygen. Because of the large heat release and its relative lack of toxicity, it is an effective propellant and thruster fuel source. In the automobile industry, nitrous oxide, often referred to simply as "nitrous," allows the engine to burn more fuel and air resulting in a more powerful combustion and a greater horsepower surge. In automobiles, N_2O is stored as a compressed liquid and injected into the intake manifold. In the food industry, N_2O has been approved as a food additive and spray propellant. The stable nature of N_2O makes it an effective aerator for whipped cream canisters (Fig. 5-1). As a food additive, N_2O is known as E942 and has two primary functions: as a propellant for cooking sprays and to displace oxygen in snack food packing that functions to limit bacterial growth on the food.[1]

N_2O has been used as an anesthetic in dentistry for more than 150 years.[2,3] It is now administered during

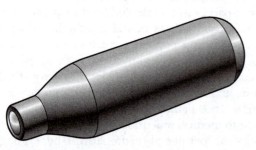

Figure 5-1 Canister of nitrous oxide used as a whipping cream agent. Canisters of nitric oxide used to aerosolize cream into whipped cream are a common source of nitrous oxide used for recreational purposes.

dental procedures via a relative analgesia machine with a demand valve inhaler over the nose. Because the N_2O is minimally metabolized by humans, it retains its potency when exhaled into the room by the patient. When used as an anesthetic, a continuous fresh air ventilation system or N_2O "scavenger system" must be used to protect medical personnel from waste-gas buildup.[2]

Along with the medical benefits as a mild to moderate anesthetic, N_2O may also cause analgesia, depersonalization, hallucinations, dizziness, euphoria, sight and sound distortion, suggestibility, and increased imagination.[4] In 1799, the first documented "laughing gas parties" were held by upper class Englishmen.[3] This recreational usage of N_2O has continued to the present day. The gas is typically obtained illegally via contacts in the medical and food industries. The gas is initially sold by the cylinder to an individual and then individually to recreational users via "nitrous oxide balloons." The N_2O used in rockets and automobiles is typically spiked with sulfur dioxide to prevent recreational drug use and is not used for recreational purposes.

The pharmacological mechanism of action of N_2O in recreational and medical usage is not fully known. However, N_2O has been shown to modulate directly a broad range of ligand-gated ion channels,[5] and this likely plays a major role in many of its therapeutic effects. N_2O moderately blocks N-methyl-D-aspartate (NMDA) receptor and slightly potentiates gamma-aminobutyric acid and glycine receptors.[6] Although N_2O affects numerous ion channels, its anesthetic, euphoric, and hallucinogenic effects are likely caused predominantly via inhibition of NMDA receptor-mediated currents.[5,6] In addition to its effects on ion channels, ingested N_2O may act on the central nervous system (CNS) as well, and this may relate to its anxiolytic and distortion function.[7] N_2O also oxidizes the monovalent core of cobalamin (vitamin B_{12}), affecting the mitochondrial enzyme dependent on the cobalamin-derived cofactors. The net result is a vitamin B_{12}–deficient state exacerbating the N_2O effects.[8]

N_2O is also a strong anxiolytic. Animal studies show that benzodiazepine-tolerant animals are also partially tolerant to N_2O administration.[9] In a human model, persons[10] given N_2O and benzodiazepine receptor antagonists did not have an alteration of motor control skills, whereas persons given N_2O alone did.

The analgesic effects of N_2O are linked to the interaction between the endogenous opioid pathway and the descending noradrenergic pathway. When animals are given morphine, they develop tolerance to the drug after a period of time.[11] Morphine-tolerant animals given N_2O exhibit similar tolerance behaviors. Drugs that inhibit the breakdown of endogenous opioids also potentiate the antinociceptive effects of N_2O.[11]

Similar to other NMDA antagonists such as ketamine, N_2O has been demonstrated to produce central neurotoxicity in the form of Olney's lesions (damage to the posterior cingulate and retrosplenial cortices of the cerebral cortex) in a rodent model.[7] However, it also simultaneously exerts widespread neuroprotective effects via inhibiting glutamate-inducing toxicity, and it has been argued that on account of its very short duration under normal circumstances, N_2O may not share the neurotoxicity of other NMDA antagonists.[6,12] In rodents, short-term exposure results in only mild injury that is rapidly reversible, and permanent neuronal death occurs only after constant and sustained exposure.[10] Exposure to N_2O causes short-term decreases in mental performance, audiovisual ability, and manual dexterity.[10]

Chronic N_2O exposure may also lead to peripheral myeloneuropathy, which was first reported in 1978.[13] Clinically, myeloneuropathy associated with N_2O is similar and potentially related to cobalamin deficiency.[14] Patients with cobalamin deficiency can develop a myeloneuropathy with only one exposure to N_2O (Table 5-1). Researchers have attempted to determine the length of exposure to N_2O required to produce peripheral neurological symptoms. Estimates

range from 3 months to 5 years, but the onset of symptoms is most likely associated with frequency of exposure and gas concentration along with duration of exposure.[15]

Classically, peripheral neuropathy manifests with mild, transient numbness in a stocking-glove distribution.[16] As exposure persists, the large 1a afferent neurons become involved with loss of dynamic ambulatory balance, difficulty walking or standing with eyes closed (Romberg examination), and progression to a motor neuropathy with involvement of the intrinsic and extrinsic muscles of the hands and feet. The neurological examination reveals impaired vibratory, light touch, proprioception, and kinesthetic appreciation; positive Romberg test; impaired Timed Up and Go test; positive upper extremity pronator drift test; and gait dysfunction (wide-based, shortened stride length) similar to ataxia.[17] Deep tendon reflexes are symmetrically decreased distally and normal proximally. Manual muscle testing and dynamometry reveal weakness of the intrinsic and extrinsic muscles of the feet and hands. The onset of upper motor neuron signs including hyperreflexia, positive Babinski sign, and clonus has been reported.[18]

Electroneuromyography studies reveal an axonal neuropathy with reduced amplitude of sensory nerve and motor action potentials. Motor and sensory conduction velocities are typically normal but may be slightly decreased. Needle examination shows denervation potentials in distal leg and arm muscles.[19]

Treatment is symptomatic and directed toward the removal of the exposure toxin. Improvement is typically seen clinically, subjectively, and electrophysiologically in weeks to months after complete removal of the offending toxin.[20–22]

Heavy Metal Toxicities

Lead

Lead intoxication (also known as saturnism, plumbism, colica pictonum, Devon's colic, and painter's colic) is caused by increased plasma and tissue levels of lead. Lead interferes with various body processes and is toxic to tissues in the cardiac, gastrointestinal, neurological, renal, and reproductive systems. Lead interferes with the development of the nervous system and is particularly toxic to fetuses and children, causing potentially permanent cognitive, learning, reasoning, and behavior disorders.[23] Lead has no known physiologically relevant role in the body.[23]

Since first identified by French physician L. Tanqueral des Plances in 1839, the frequency of lead-induced peripheral neuropathy has waxed and waned throughout the years.[24] Humans have been mining and using lead for thousands of years—including its use in goblets, dinner plates, cutlery, and cookware, poisoning

Table 5-1	Clinical Features of Nitrous Oxide Peripheral Myeloneuropathy
Clinical indication	Anesthetic agent for selective invasive procedures, especially dental
Recreational indication	Euphoria, pain control, disassociation
Method of administration	Inhalation
Impairments with chronic use	Stocking-glove distribution of positive sensory signs; large-fiber (proprioception and kinesthetic) sensory loss; symmetrically diminished deep tendon reflexes, positive Babinski sign
Electroneuromyogram studies	Reduced sensory and motor potentials distal > proximal; normal or mildly reduced nerve conduction velocities, distal denervation potentials via electromyography
Nerve biopsy studies	Axonal degeneration and axonal atrophy

Data from Maze M, Fujinaga M. Recent advances in understanding the actions and toxicity of nitrous oxide. *Anaesthesia*. 2000;55:311–314; Dohrn CS, Lichtor JL, Coalson DW, Uitvlugt A, de Wit H, Zacny JP. Reinforcing effects of extended inhalation of nitrous oxide in humans. *Drug Alcohol Depend*. 1993;31:265–280; Wu LT, Schlenger WE, Ringwalt CL. Use of nitrite inhalants ("poppers") among American youth. *J Adolesc Health*. 2005;37:52–60; and Wu LT, Pilowsky DJ, Schlenger WE. Inhalant abuse and dependence among adolescents in the United States. *J Am Acad Child Adolesc Psychiatry*. 2004;43:1206–1214.

themselves in the process. Although lead poisoning is one of the oldest known work and environmental hazards, the modern understanding of the small amount of lead necessary to cause harm did not come about until the latter half of the 20th century. No safe threshold for lead exposure has been discovered—that is, there is no known amount of lead that is too small to cause the body harm.[23]

The waxing and waning of lead intoxication frequency over the past 300 years is due partially to the use of lead in industry during a particular era and the level of exposure as allowed by industry, government, and health regulations.[25] The present time is a period of rare lead intoxication—a large difference from published epidemiological studies from the early and middle industrial age.

Routes of exposure (Box 5-1) to lead include contaminated water, air, soil, and food and the purposeful additives used in consumer products such as crystal and earthenware.[26] Occupational exposure is a common cause of lead poisoning in adults. One of the largest

threats to children is lead in paint, used as a fungicide additive to paint. This tainted paint still exists in many older homes and businesses. The U.S. federal government banned lead as an additive to interior and exterior paint in 1978, but homes built before 1978 may have lead paint underlying newer painted areas. Lead paint can become exposed as the later paint weathers and cracks and with the scraping and sanding of painted surfaces in preparation for repainting. Children who demonstrate pica behavior—the eating of substances that are not food—should be monitored for potential paint chip eating (Fig. 5-2).[27] Authorities such as the American Academy of Pediatrics define lead poisoning requiring medical intervention as blood lead levels (BLLs) greater than 10 mcg/dL.[27,28]

After exposure, lead is stored in blood, soft tissues, and bone. The half-life of lead in these tissues is measured in weeks for blood, months for soft tissues, and years for bone.[29] The estimated half-life of lead in bone is 20 to 30 years, and bone, with ongoing remodeling, can introduce lead into the bloodstream long after the initial exposure is gone.[30] Lead in the teeth, hair, and nails is bound tightly and unavailable to other tissues and is generally thought to be harmless.[31] In adults, 94% of absorbed lead is deposited in the bones and

BOX 5-1

Potential Occupational Sources of Lead Exposure

Battery manufacturing
Battery recycling
Bridge painting
Commercial and institutional refinishing
Demolition
House refinishing
Lead glaze pottery finishing
Lead, copper, or zinc mining
Lead, copper, or zinc smelting
Munitions industry
Plastics industry
Plumbing
Roofing
Rubber industry
Soldering with the use of lead
Stained glass manufacturing
Welding

Data compiled from Guidotti T, Ragain L. Protecting children from toxic exposure: three strategies. *Pediatr Clin North Am.* 2007;54:227–235; Ekong E, Jaar B, Weaver V. Lead-related nephrotoxicity: a review of the epidemiologic evidence. *Kidney Int.* 2006;70:2074–2084; Cleveland LM, Minter ML, Cobb KA, Scott AA, German VF. Lead hazards for pregnant women and children: part 1: immigrants and the poor shoulder most of the burden of lead exposure in this country. Part 1 of a two-part article details how exposure happens, whom it affects, and the harm it can do. *Am J Nurs.* 2008;108:40–49; Payne M. Lead in drinking water. *Can Med Assoc J.* 2008;179: 253–254; Rossi E. Low level environmental lead exposure—a continuing challenge. *Clin Biochem Rev.* 2006;29:63–70; and Hu H, Shih R, Rothenberg S, Schwartz S. The epidemiology of lead toxicity in adults: measuring and consideration for other methodological issues. *Environ Health Persp.* 2007;115:455–462.

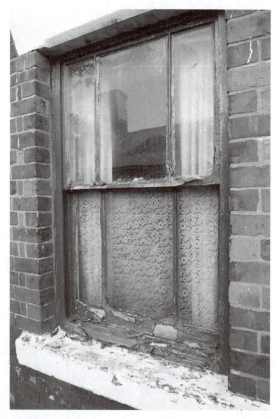

Figure 5-2 Lead was a common additive to house paint before 1978. Lead was added to paint to increase the drying rate, increase durability, maintain a fresh appearance, and resist moisture that causes corrosion.

teeth, but children store only 70% in this manner, a fact that may partially account for the more serious health effects of lead exposure in children.[27] The half-life of lead in the blood in men is about 40 days, but it may be longer in children and pregnant women, whose bones are undergoing accelerated osteoclastic and osteoblastic activity, which allows the lead to be continuously reintroduced into the bloodstream.[27] Many other tissues store lead, and tissues with the highest concentrations (other than blood, bone, and teeth) are the brain, spleen, kidneys, liver, and lungs. Lead is removed from the body very slowly, primarily through renal filtration.[28] Smaller amounts of lead are also eliminated through the feces, and very small amounts are eliminated in hair, nails, and sweat.[28]

Elevated BLLs can cause a variety of signs and symptoms depending on the individual and the duration of lead exposure.[29] Symptoms are nonspecific and may be subtle, and someone with elevated BLLs may have no symptoms.[30] Symptoms usually develop over weeks to months as BLL concentration increases with chronic exposure, but acute symptoms from brief, intense exposures also occur.[31] Symptoms from exposure to organic lead, which is probably more toxic than inorganic lead because of its lipid solubility, occur rapidly.[32] Poisoning by organic lead compounds has symptoms predominantly in the CNS, such as insomnia, delirium, cognitive deficits, hallucinations, and seizures.

Symptoms may be different in adults and children. In adults, symptoms may begin with a BLL of approximately 40 mcg/dL but are more likely to occur at BLLs greater than 50 to 60 mcg/dL.[32] These symptoms include headache; abdominal pain; back pain; lethargy; impotence; and weakness, pain, or tingling in the extremities.[30] The classic signs and symptoms in children, which typically begin to appear at BLLs of 60 mcg/dL, are loss of appetite; pain; vomiting; weight loss; constipation; anemia; kidney failure; irritability; and the behavioral/cognitive grouping of erratic behavior, cognitive impairment, and loss of attention.[30] Children may also experience hearing loss; delayed growth; drowsiness; clumsiness; and loss or delay of developmental milestones such as speech, creeping, and bipedal gait.[33] In adults, abdominal colic, involving episodes of pain, may appear at BLLs greater than 80 mcg/dL.[32] Signs that occur in adults at BLLs exceeding 100 mcg/dL include distal motor paralysis such as wrist drop and footdrop and signs of toxic encephalopathy.[28] In children, signs of encephalopathy such as bizarre behavior, dyscoordination, and apathy occur at BLLs exceeding 70 mcg/dL.[23] For both adults and children, it is rare to be asymptomatic if BLLs exceed 100 mcg/dL.[32]

Lead affects both the male and female reproductive systems. In men, when BLLs exceed 40 mcg/dL, sperm count is reduced, and there are associated

Table 5-2 U.S. Centers for Disease Control and Prevention Management Guidelines for Children with Elevated Blood Lead Levels

Blood Lead Level (mcg/dL)	Treatment
10–14	Education, serial screening
15–19	Repeat screening, multidisciplinary focus to abate sources
20–44	Medical evaluation, case management, multidisciplinary focus to abate sources
45–69	Medical evaluation, chelation, case management
>69	Hospitalization, immediate chelation, case chelation, case management

Data from Jones L, Homa M, Meyer A, et al. Trends in blood lead levels and blood lead testing among US children aged 1 to 5 years, 1988–2004. *Pediatrics.* 2009;123:e376–e385; and Murata K, Iwata T, Dakeishi M, Karita K. Lead toxicity: does the critical level of lead resulting in adverse effects differ between adults and children? *J Occup Health.* 2009;51:1–12.

changes in the sperm motility and morphology.[33] An elevated BLL in a pregnant woman can lead to miscarriage, premature birth, and low birth weight and later problems with motor and cognitive development in the child.[25,33] Lead is able to pass through the placenta impacting the fetus and into breast milk impacting the newborn. BLLs of mothers with lead toxicity and their newborns are usually similar.[33] Even with withdrawal of the acute and chronic causes of lead poisoning, the fetus may still be poisoned in utero if lead from the mother's bones is subsequently mobilized by the changes in metabolism secondary to pregnancy. Increased calcium intake in pregnancy may help mitigate this phenomenon (Table 5-2).[25,34]

Chronic poisoning usually manifests with symptoms affecting multiple systems but is associated with three main types of impairments: gastrointestinal, neuromuscular, and neurological. CNS signs typically result from acute poisoning, whereas gastrointestinal symptoms usually result from exposure over longer periods.[31] Signs of chronic exposure include loss of short-term memory and concentration, depression, nausea, abdominal pain, loss of coordination, and paresthesias in the extremities.[35] Additional manifestations of chronic lead poisoning include fatigue, problems with sleep, headaches, stupor, inattention, slurred speech, and anemia.[31] A gray "lead hue" of the skin with generalized pallor is another common feature of chronic poisoning.[36] A blue line along the gum with bluish black edging to the teeth may also be an indication of chronic lead poisoning.[36]

Elevated lead in the body can be detected by the presence of changes in blood cells visible with a microscope and dense lines in the bones of children seen on x-ray.[37] Anemia accompanied by basophilic stippling is a common characteristic of lead intoxication. BLL is typically measured as micrograms of lead per deciliter of blood (mcg/dL).

Enzymes used in hemoglobin synthesis, δ-aminolevulinic acid dehydratase and coproporphyrinogen, are particularly susceptible to elevated lead concentrations.[38] The urinary metabolites of abnormal hemoglobin synthesis can be identified in the urine of toxic individuals. Inhibition of ferrochelatase, the enzyme responsible for incorporating ferritin into the porphyrin core, results in an elevated blood level of erythrocyte protoporphyrin[28,35]; this is a very sensitive test to determine lead exposure. Serum creatinine (Cr), blood urea nitrogen (BUN), and uric acid levels begin to increase at blood levels of 40 mcg/dL indicating impaired renal function. Chronically elevated Cr and BUN levels by themselves may lead to signs of peripheral neuropathy. Lead poisoning inhibits excretion of the waste product urate and causes a predisposition for gout, in which urate concentration increases and eventually precipitates.[39,40] This condition is known as saturnine gout.

Electroneuromyography studies typically reveal an axonal neuropathy with mildly generally reduced motor nerve conduction studies accompanied by increased amplitude of waveform. Needle examination reveals denervation potentials supporting a diagnosis of an axonal process. Typically, lead concentrations greater than 40 mcg/dL result in electroneuromyography changes with severe abnormalities occurring with BLLs greater than 60 mcg/dL. Autopsy studies support the theory of axonal involvement. Much research interest over the past 3 decades has focused on the correlation between elevated BLL and the onset of motor neuron disease such as amyotrophic lateral sclerosis. To date, the evidence has been insufficient to prompt a correlation between lead and motor neuron disease.[27,34,35]

Along with axonal abnormalities, elevated lead concentrations also affect the renal system. In the kidneys, lead interferes with vitamin D metabolism resulting in renal tubulopathy (Fanconi syndrome) characterized by proteinuria and eventually interstitial fibrosis and tubular atrophy.[35]

Prevention can be divided into individual (measures taken by a family), preventive medicine (identifying and intervening with high-risk individuals), and public health (reducing risk on a population level) strategies.[23] Testing kits are commercially available for detecting lead in consumer items and paint. Swabs, when wiped on a surface, turn pink in the presence of lead[27]; this is an excellent method for identifying lead-based paint in homes. Screening is an important method in preventive medicine strategies.[23,27] Screening programs exist to test the blood of children at high risk for lead exposure, such as children who live near lead-related industries and children living in older homes located in lower income neighborhoods.

Recommended steps by individuals to reduce the risk of elevated BLLs in children include increasing their frequency of hand washing and their intake of calcium and iron; discouraging them from putting their hands to their mouths; vacuuming frequently; and eliminating the child's access to lead-containing objects such as old paint, stained glass, plumbing supplies, nails, ammunition, and lead crystal.[23,27] Lead pipes or lead-based plumbing solder in houses can be replaced.[41] A less permanent but less expensive method of dealing with lead plumbing is running water in the morning to flush out the most contaminated water. Lead testing kits are commercially available for detecting the presence of lead in the household water supply.[32]

Prevention measures also exist on national and municipal levels. Recommendations by health care professionals for decreasing childhood exposures include banning the use of lead where it is not essential and strengthening regulations that limit the amount of lead in soil, water, air, household dust, and products. Regulations exist to limit the amount of lead in paint; for example, a 1978 law in the United States restricted the lead in paint for residences, furniture, and toys to 0.06% or less.[42] In October 2008, the U.S. Environmental Protection Agency (EPA) reduced the allowable lead level by a factor of 10 to 0.15 mcg per cubic meter of air, giving states 5 years to comply with the standards. The Restriction of Hazardous Substances Directive from the European Union limits the use of toxic substances in electronics and electrical equipment. In some places, remediation programs exist to reduce the presence of lead when it is found to be high, for example, in public drinking water.[42,43] As a more radical solution, entire towns located near former lead mines have been "closed" by the government and the population resettled elsewhere, as was the case with Picher, Oklahoma, in 2009.[42]

The mainstays of treatment are removal from the source of lead and, for people who have significantly high BLLs or symptoms of poisoning, chelation therapy.[35] Correction of potential iron, calcium, and zinc deficiencies, which are associated with increased lead absorption, is mandatory.[35] When lead-containing materials are present in the gastrointestinal tract (as evidenced by abdominal x-rays), bowel irrigation, endoscopic procedures, or surgical removal may be used to eliminate the lead from the gut and prevent further exposure.[43] Lead-containing bullets and shrapnel may also present a threat of further exposure and may need to be surgically removed if they are in or near fluid-filled spaces.[43,44] If lead encephalopathy is present, anticonvulsants can be given to control seizures. Treatment of organic lead poisoning involves removing the lead compound from the skin, preventing further exposure, treating seizures, and possibly chelation therapy for people with high BLL concentrations.[30]

Thallium

Thallium (Greek: *thallos*, a green twig or stick) is a chemical element with the symbol TI and atomic number 81. This soft gray metal was accidentally discovered by Sir William Crookes in 1861 by burning the dust from a sulfuric acid industrial plant in England.[45] Approximately 60% to 70% of thallium production is used in the electronics industry, and the remainder is used in the pharmaceutical and pesticide industries and in the production of the green color used in fireworks and glass manufacturing.[46] In the last 20 years, thallium has been used in medical imaging studies (thallium-201 is widely used in myocardial imaging). Thallium is also present in the environment in its natural state. Its use has been decreased or eliminated in many countries because of its nonselective toxicity. Use of thallium as a rodent poison was banned in the United States in 1972.

Thallium is extremely soft and malleable and can be cut with a knife at room temperature. It has a metallic luster, but when exposed to air, it quickly tarnishes with a bluish gray tinge that resembles lead. It may be preserved by keeping it under oil. A heavy layer of oxide builds up on thallium if left in air.

Thallium and its compounds are extremely toxic and should be handled with great care. Contact with skin is dangerous, and adequate ventilation should be provided when melting this metal. Thallium compounds have a high aqueous solubility and are readily absorbed through the skin. Exposure to them should not exceed 0.1 mg per m^2 of skin in an 8-hour time-weighted average (40-hour work week). Thallium is a suspected human carcinogen.[47] For a long time, thallium compounds were easily available commercially as rodent poison. This fact and the fact that it is water soluble and nearly tasteless led to frequent intoxications by accident or by criminal intent.[48] Because of its use for murder, thallium has gained the nicknames "the poisoner's poison" and "inheritance powder."[47] Part of the reason for the high toxicity of thallium is that when present in aqueous solution as the univalent thallium ion (Tl^+), it exhibits some similarities with essential alkali metal cations, particularly potassium (because the atomic radius is almost identical). It can enter the body via potassium uptake pathways. Among the distinctive effects of thallium poisoning are loss of hair (which led to its initial use as a depilatory before its toxicity was properly appreciated) and painful peripheral neuropathy.[49]

Severe symptoms have been reported with purposeful or accidental ingestion of a single dose of 100 mg or more in adults (Table 5-3).[5] Symptoms are specific as to whether the intoxication of thallium is acute (large single dose) or chronic (small multiple doses over

Table 5-3   Clinical Signs and Symptoms of Acute and Chronic Thallium Poisoning

Acute Poisoning	Chronic Poisoning
Gastrointestinal	Gastrointestinal
Retrosternal and abdominal pain	Weight loss
Anorexia	Anorexia
Vomiting	Vomiting
Constipation	Constipation
Neurological	Neurological
Motor and sensory neuropathy	Motor and sensory neuropathy
Insomnia with agitation	Insomnia with agitation
Delirium	Visual loss
Hallucination	Integument
Seizure	Darkening of hair roots
Integument	Alopecia
Darkening of hair roots	Cardiopulmonary
Alopecia	ST-T ECG changes
Mees' lines	Hypotension
Peripheral cyanosis	Arrhythmia
Cardiopulmonary	Genitourinary
ST-T ECG changes	Hematuria
Hypotension	Albuminuria
Arrhythmia	

Data from Gettler A, Weiss L. Thallium poisoning. III. Clinical toxicology of thallium. *Am J Clin Pathol*. 1943;13:422–429; Prick JJG. Thallium poisoning. In: Vinken PJ, Bruyn GW, eds. *Intoxications of the Nervous System. Handbook of Clinical Neurology*. vol 36. New York: Elsevier Science; 1978:239–278; Chamberlain PH, Stavinoha WB, Davis H, Kniker WT, Panos TC. Thallium poisoning. *Pediatrics*. 1958;22:1170–1182; Herrero F, Fernández E, Gómez J, et al. Thallium poisoning presenting with abdominal colic, paresthesia, and irritability. *Clin Toxicol*. 1995;33:261–264; Luckit J, Mir N, Hargreaves M, Costello C, Gazzard B. Thrombocytopenia associated with thallium poisoning. *Hum Exp Toxicol*. 1990;9:47–48; Malbrain ML, Lambrecht GL, Zandijk E, et al. Treatment of severe thallium intoxication. *J Toxicol Clin Toxicol*. 1997;35:97–100; McMillan TM, Jacobson RR, Gross M. Neuropsychology of thallium poisoning. *J Neurol Neurosurg Psychiatry*. 1997; 63:247–250; and Moeschlin S. Thallium poisoning. *Clin Toxicol*. 1980;17:133–146.

a period of time). Exposure routes include oral, dermal, and inhalation. Signs and symptoms of acute intoxication include gastrointestinal symptoms of anorexia, constipation, vomiting, and abdominal pain.[50] Neurological symptoms are generally a mild length-dependent motor and sensory neuropathy—typically initiating with painful paresthesias.[51] Integument changes are darkening of hair, alopecia, and horizontal white lines on nail beds (Mees lines).[52] With lethal dosages, causes of death include gastrointestinal hemorrhage, cardiac arrest, and respiratory failure.[52,53] Signs and symptoms of chronic exposure differ from signs of acute exposure. Signs of chronic exposure include visual loss, weight loss, progressive delirium or psychoses, arrhythmia, hematuria, and albuminuria.[54,55] Nerve biopsy typically shows both axonal degeneration and segmental demyelination.[56,57] To assess the effects of thallium on the conduction velocities of faster and slower nerve fibers, the distribution of conduction velocities in sensory fibers of the median nerve was examined in a patient with acute thallium poisoning 2 months and 11 months after the onset of symptoms. In the first examination, the patient showed evidence of a distal sensorimotor neuropathy and had an elevated urinary thallium concentration (3.5 mg/L); the conduction velocities of faster fibers were below the normal lower limit, whereas the conduction velocities of slower fibers were within normal limits. At the second examination, with the return of normal thallium concentrations, the conduction velocities of all faster and slower fibers were increased and were within normal limits; clinical signs and symptoms of neuropathy almost disappeared. It was concluded that the conduction velocities of faster fibers significantly decrease in an early stage of acute thallium poisoning and recover after recuperation from the poisoning; the conduction velocities of slower fibers are minimally affected and then improve.[58]

Diagnosis is based on the clinical presentation, the history, and the presence of thallium in body fluids.

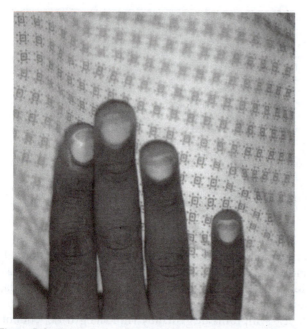

Figure 5-3 The fingers of a young person with a diagnosis of heavy metal intoxication. Note the Mees fingernail lines—dense lines of demarcation. Mees lines, also called Aldrich-Mees lines, are lines of discoloration across the fingernails and toenails often associated with heavy metal poisoning and renal failure.

Typically, a simple urine screen for thallium is sufficient to make the diagnosis. The classic triad of clinical signs of thallium intoxication is gastroenteritis, alopecia, and neuropathy.[47]

Treatment is intravenous potassium chloride, which effectively drives the thallium from body tissues into the plasma where it is excreted through urine and stool. Symptoms and signs often immediately worsen with the onset of treatment, owing to the increase in plasma thallium concentrations.[59] One of the main methods of removing thallium (both radioactive and normal) from humans is the use of Prussian blue, which is a material that absorbs thallium.[60] Up to 20 g per day of Prussian blue is fed by mouth to the person, and it passes through the digestive system and comes out in the stool. Hemodialysis is also used to remove thallium from the blood serum.[60]

Arsenic

Arsenic is primarily known by its use as a homicidal agent from the times of ancient Greece and Rome to the present time.[61] In Frank Capra's film *Arsenic and Old Lace,* two elderly spinsters used arsenic in elderberry wine to murder their male suitors. Most current exposure is through occupational or environmental exposures. Arsenic trioxide (As_2O_3), the inorganic form of arsenic, is used primarily in pesticides and as a wood preservative. Inorganic arsenic is not found naturally; it is the by-product of the copper and lead ore smelting industry. People at risk for exposure to arsenic are individuals who work in the smelting industry (chronic arsenic intoxication that occurs as a result of smelting is called Ronnskar disease—a name derived from the Ronnskar smelting plant in Sweden), individuals who imbibe water from contaminated wells and aquifers near smelting plants and mines, painters, tree sprayers, farmers, leatherworkers, taxidermists, and jewelers.[61] The two areas of the world affected the worst by arsenic aquifer contamination are in Bangladesh and West Bengal, India. In those two areas alone, almost 120 million people are exposed to groundwater arsenic concentrations that are above the maximum permissible limit of 50 mcg/L set by the World Health Organization.[62,63] In the late 19th century and early 20th century, inorganic arsenic was employed in the treatment of trypanosomiasis and syphilis[61]; there are now much more effective agents available. The only current pharmaceutical use of arsenic trioxide is in the treatment of promyelocytic leukemia, based on its mechanism as an inducer of apoptosis (programmed cell death).[64] Arsenic is a key nutritional item in the diet of some animals and is an additive to their food (Box 5-2).[65]

Absorption occurs predominantly from ingestion from the small intestine, although minute absorption occurs from skin contact and inhalation. Peripheral neuropathy is the primary presenting sign with chronic arsenic exposure or after survival from exposure to a

BOX 5-2

Signs and Symptoms of Acute Arsenic Poisoning

- Clinical features manifest in most body systems
- Prominent features are nausea, vomiting, profuse watery diarrhea, abdominal pain, and excessive saliva production
- Acute psychoses and neuroses
- Cardiomyopathy with congestive heart failure and hypotension
- Pulmonary edema
- Peripheral motor and sensory neuropathy
- Metabolic encephalopathy
- Elevated urine arsenic concentration

Data compiled from Balakumar P, Kaur J. Arsenic exposure and cardiovascular disease. *Cardiovasc Toxicol.* 2009;9(4):169; Steinmaus C, Moore L, Hopenhayn-Rich C, Biggs ML, Smith A. Arsenic in drinking water and bladder cancer. *Cancer Invest.* 2000;18:174–182; Buchet JP, Lison D. Clues and uncertainties in the risk assessment of arsenic in drinking water. *Food Chem Toxicol.* 2000;38:S81–85; Campbell JP, Alvarez JA. Acute arsenic intoxication. *Am Fam Physician.* 1989;40:93–97; Schoolmeester WL, White DR. Arsenic poisoning. *South Med J.* 1980;73:198–208; and Goddard MJ, Tanhehco JL, Dau PC. Chronic arsenic poisoning masquerading as Landry-Guillain-Barre syndrome. *Electromyogr Clin Neurophysiol.* 1992;32:419–423.

BOX 5-3

Signs and Symptoms of Chronic Arsenic Poisoning

- Clinical features manifest in most body systems
- Absorbed arsenic accumulates in kidneys, heart, lungs, and liver with smaller concentrations in muscles, tendons, gastrointestinal tract, and spleen
- High concentrations of arsenic are deposited in keratin-rich tissues such as nails, hair, and skin
- Mees lines develop in fingernails and toenails
- Dermatological changes include hyperpigmentation, hyperkeratosis, and sloughing of skin of the palms of the hands and soles of the feet
- There is increased risk of cardiovascular disease, diabetes, peripheral vascular disease, cerebrovascular disease, and neutropenia

Data compiled from Balakumar P, Kaur J. Arsenic exposure and cardiovascular disease. *Cardiovasc Toxicol.* 2009;9(4):169; Steinmaus C, Moore L, Hopenhayn-Rich C, Biggs ML, Smith A. Arsenic in drinking water and bladder cancer. *Cancer Invest.* 2000;18:174–182; Buchet JP, Lison D. Clues and uncertainties in the risk assessment of arsenic in drinking water. *Food Chem Toxicol.* 2000;38:S81–85; Campbell JP, Alvarez JA. Acute arsenic intoxication. *Am Fam Physician.* 1989;40:93–97; Schoolmeester WL, White DR. Arsenic poisoning. *South Med J.* 1980;73:198–208; and Goddard MJ, Tanhehco JL, Dau PC. Chronic arsenic poisoning masquerading as Landry-Guillain-Barre syndrome. *Electromyogr Clin Neurophysiol.* 1992;32:419–423.

large dose. Large doses, used to commit homicide, cause a quick death as a result of vomiting, diarrhea, and vasomotor collapse. A length-dependent sensorimotor neuropathy results from acute and chronic exposure. Although the large myelinated afferents are primarily affected, sensory testing typically reveals loss in all the tactile modalities. Ascending distal motor weakness begins after the sensory component. On examination, along with ascending motor weakness (similar to Guillain-Barré syndrome), deep tendon reflexes are hypoactive or absent. Cranial nerves are rarely involved.[66]

CNS changes are also common and include changes in behavior and mood escalating to psychoses and neuroses. In a study of 8,102 men with chronic arsenic exposure, cognitive changes and an elevated risk for cerebrovascular disease, primarily small vessel vascular disease, were found (Box 5-3).[67]

A primary feature of chronic exposure is the classic integument signs, which include hyperpigmentation, hyperkeratosis, sloughing of skin from the palms and soles of the feet, and Mees lines on the fingernails. Although watery stools are a classic sign of acute arsenic exposure, in chronic toxicity, diarrhea occurs in recurrent bouts and may be associated with vomiting. Exposure should be suspected with complaints of diarrhea in the presence of skin changes and peripheral motor and sensory neuropathy.[67] Recovery after mild chronic exposure is rapid and complete; however, there are often residual neuropathic impairments after significant toxicity.[61]

From a diagnostic standpoint, because arsenic is easily filtered by the kidneys, blood arsenic levels are helpful for only a few days after acute exposure. Urine clearance can often be measured. Low-level chronic exposure is difficult to identify by blood test. Anemia and pancytopenia are typically present. Arsenic binds to the keratin of the nails and hair, and the measured tissue content can be a valid and reliable measure of toxicity. Electroneuromyography studies reveal an axonal neuropathy. Sensory nerve action potential amplitudes are reduced. Needle examination shows denervation with increased insertional activity with fibrillations. In individuals with chronic intoxication, enlarged motor units with polyphasic potentials are seen. Nerve biopsy reveals axonal degeneration.[68]

Treatment with penicillamine or British antilewisite (BAL) has been used in the past with some success. BAL (also known as dimercaprol) displaces the arsenic from the sulfhydryl groups of enzyme proteins to produce an excretable compound. Penicillamine facilitates excretion of arsenic from the kidneys. A regimen of vitamins, mineral supplements, and antioxidant therapy has been advocated more recently. Fully developed neuropathy as a result of arsenic is not affected by arsenic remediation treatment and is often permanent.[69,70]

Mercury

Mercury poisoning, also known as hydrargyria or mercurialism, is a disease caused by exposure to mercury or one of its organic or inorganic compounds.[71] Mercury exists in elemental, inorganic, and organic forms. The population is primarily exposed to organic mercury from fish consumption and mercury vapor from the processing of dental amalgam.[72] The concentration of mercury bioaccumulates up the food chain; large predator species such as tuna, shark, swordfish, whale, and marlin may have very high concentrations of mercury in their tissues. Mercury vapor exposure occurs primarily in dentistry, mining, and the manufacture of electrical equipment and medical instruments.[72,73] Thimerosal, a mercury-containing preservative, has been essentially phased out of the vaccine industry.[74] Elemental mercury exposure can occur through spilling of mercury or improper disposal of fluorescent lamps.[75,76]

The efficiency of absorption of mercury depends on the form of mercury and the route of absorption. Elemental mercury absorption is minimal through an oral route.[75] Mercury vapor is well absorbed through inhalation.[77] Oral absorption of mercury compounds is poor depending on the precise form. Oral absorption of organic mercury is nearly 100%.[75] Once absorbed, mercury is distributed through the vascular system to the kidneys, CNS, and peripheral nervous system.[71] The half-life of organic mercury in the body is about 70 days, and the half-life of inorganic mercury in the body is about 40 days.[78]

The signs and symptoms of mercury poisoning include oral symptoms of gingivitis, stomatitis, excessive salivation, and a strong metallic taste. Neurological manifestations include paresthesias secondary to peripheral sensory neuropathy and central effects such as personality changes, irritability, intention tremor, fatigue, memory loss, difficulty with concentration and learning, and sleep disturbances. Integument signs include desquamation of the hands and feet and pink cheeks, fingers, and toes. Mercury poisoning in a pregnant woman may result in the occurrence of potential neuropsychiatric diagnoses in the child.[79–81]

Diagnosis of mercury poisoning can be made through the measure of mercury concentrations in the blood or urine.[71] With potential organic mercury poisoning, the blood value is the preferred method of assessment. Studies suggest that developing fetuses may be affected by mercury blood levels of 40 mcg/L; in adults, symptoms appear at 100 mcg/L.[81]

Identifying the source of mercury poisoning and removal of the source are imperative. Contaminated clothing must be removed and bagged. For acute oral intoxication, treatment is gastric lavage, charcoal, and chelation therapy including penicillamine.[71,78] Supportive measures may include items such as correcting electrolyte imbalance, hemodialysis for renal failure, and possible surgical intervention for gastrointestinal perforation.[79] Contaminated skin must be scrubbed with soap and water. Eye contact is treated with saline lavage. Many of the toxic effects of mercury are partially or wholly reversible, either through specific therapy or through natural elimination of the metal after exposure has been discontinued.[79] However, large acute or chronic long-term exposure may result in irreversible damage, particularly in fetuses, infants, and young children. Young syndrome, also known as azoospermia sinopulmonary infections, sinusitis-infertility syndrome, and Barry-Perkins-Young syndrome, is a rare condition that encompasses a combination of syndromes such as bronchiectasis, rhinitis, sinusitis, and reduced fertility, and may be a long-term consequence of early childhood mercury poisoning.[82] Common use of mercuric chloride, a chemical previously used in the photography industry and used as an injectable, oral, and topical medication for the treatment of syphilis, has been all but discontinued because of the many potentially dangerous side effects.[83] Methyl mercury (also known as methylmercuy) an environmental toxin, has entered the human food chain resulting in mercury exposure and illness.[84] The EPA has classified mercuric chloride and methyl mercury as possible human carcinogens. Peripheral neuropathy associated with mercury is typically reversible, but this may take considerable time if the neuropathy is axonotmetic.[82–84]

Chemical Toxicities

Ethylene Glycol

Ethylene glycol (ethane-1,2-diol) is an organic compound widely used as an automotive antifreeze, coolant, solvent, and airplane deicer. In its pure form, it is an odorless, colorless, syrupy, sweet-tasting liquid. Ethylene glycol is toxic, and ingestion can result in death. Approximately 60% of ethylene glycol produced is used for antifreeze manufacturing, and the remainder is mainly used as a precursor to polymers. Because this material is cheaply available, there are many niche applications. The primary source of ethylene glycol in the environment is from runoff at airports where it is used in deicing agents for runways and airplanes. Ethylene glycol can also enter the environment through the disposal of products that contain it, such as radiator antifreeze. In air, ethylene glycol degrades in about 10 days; in soil and water, the process takes about 2 weeks (85).

Exposure is typically oral and includes accidental ingestions, suicide attempts, and ingestions by alcoholics. Toxicity levels are greater than 25 mg/dL, and the lethal level is greater than 200 mg/dL. Ethylene glycol is rapidly absorbed from the gastrointestinal tract. Clinical features are usually described in relation to hours after ingestion (Table 5-4).[86]

One of the leading factors for the frequency of accidental ingestion of ethylene glycol is its sweet taste.

Table 5-4	Clinical Phases of Ethylene Glycol Poisoning
30 Minutes to 12 Hours	CNS depression Sleepiness
12–24 Hours	Nausea, vomiting Abdominal pain Noncardiac chest pain Myalgia Confusion Discoordination Renal toxicity
5–20 days	Cranial nerve VII distribution weakness bilaterally Optic neuritis with edema and atrophy Loss of hearing Dysphagia Hoarseness Dysarthria Coma Seizure Diffuse, asymmetric weakness Distal sensory loss of vibration, tactile, and temperature Diminished deep tendon reflexes

Data from Hess R, Bartels MJ, Pottenger LH. Ethylene glycol: an estimate of tolerable levels of exposure based on a review of animal and human data. *Arch Toxicol.* 2004;78:671–680; Tobe TJM, Braam GB, Meulenbelt J, van Dijk GW. Ethylene glycol poisoning mimicking Snow White. *Lancet.* 2002;359:444; Spillane L, Roberts JR, Meyer AE. Multiple cranial nerve deficits after ethylene glycol poisoning. *Ann Emerg Med.* 1991;20:208–210; Hasbani MJ, Sansing LH, Perrone J, Asbury AK, Bird SJ. Encephalopathy and peripheral neuropathy following diethylene glycol ingestion. *Neurology.* 2005;64:1273–1375; Zhou L, Zabad R, Lewis RA. Ethylene glycol intoxication: electrophysiological studies suggest a polyradiculopathy. *Neurology.* 2002;59:1809–1810; and Lewis LD, Smith BW, Mamourian AC. Delayed sequelae after acute overdoses or poisonings: cranial neuropathy related to ethylene glycol ingestion. *Clin Pharmacol Ther.* 1997;61:692–699.

Because of the taste, children and animals are more inclined to consume large quantities of it than they are other poisons. On ingestion, ethylene glycol is oxidized to glycolic acid, which is oxidized to oxalic acid, which is toxic. Oxalic acid and its toxic by-products affect the CNS first, then the heart, and finally the kidneys. Ingestion of sufficient amounts can be fatal if untreated.[87,88]

According to the annual report of the American Association of Poison Control Centers' National Poison Data System in 2007, there were about 1,000 total cases of ethylene glycol ingestions resulting in 16 deaths. The 2008 annual report of the American Association of Poison Control Centers' National Poison Data System listed seven deaths.[89]

The neuropathy associated with ethylene glycol ingestion typically occurs after diagnosis; the CNS, cardiac, and renal symptoms outweigh the severity of the neuropathic symptoms.[85] Cranial nerve involvement, especially the facial nerve; distal motor weakness; and painful distal paresthesias are typically seen. Electroneuromyography studies typically reveal a sensorimotor radiculopathy similar to Guillain-Barré syndrome but with an atypical distribution. If the patient survives the ingestion, there is typically a good recovery from the neuropathic involvement.[90]

Alcohol-Related Neuropathy

Debate has occurred over the past few decades about the etiology of alcohol-related neuropathy. Is the peripheral neuropathy associated with alcoholism a true toxic neuropathy that is due to the direct or indirect impact of alcohol on peripheral nerves, or is it directly related to nutritional—particularly thiamine—deficiency, or is it a combination of the two?[91]

Alcoholism is a disorder characterized by addiction to alcohol that is prevalent worldwide. Individuals with this addiction crave alcoholic beverages and eventually develop tolerance to the intoxicating effects. Alcoholism is defined as recurrent episodes of excessive drinking despite serious economic, social, familial, or medical consequences with symptoms of withdrawal when drinking is stopped.[91] Alcoholism has a large societal cost. Of U.S. hospital admissions, 20% involve medical complications of excessive acute or chronic alcohol ingestion; the socioeconomic cost is greater than $100 billion annually.[91]

Ethanol, the active ingredient in alcoholic beverages, enters the bloodstream within minutes of ingestion and quickly diffuses throughout the vascular system. Virtually all alcohol is detoxified in the liver where alcohol dehydrogenase converts ethanol to acetaldehyde, which is metabolized by aldehyde dehydrogenase to acetate. Excessive accumulation of acetaldehyde results in the typically seen "alcoholic flush" as a result of the vasodilatory response and the associated tachycardia and hypotension.[92]

Ethanol rapidly crosses the blood-brain barrier, and the ethanol concentration in the brain matches that of the peripheral circulation soon after ingestion.[93] Emotionally, alcohol ingestion usually results in euphoria, a loss of social inhibitions, garrulousness, and outgoing behavior. However, some persons react with belligerence, gloominess, tiredness, or depression.[94] Blood alcohol content (BAC) is most commonly used as a metric of intoxication for legal or medical purposes. BAC is usually expressed as a fractional percentage in terms of volume of alcohol per volume of blood in the body. It is a ratio without units that is commonly expressed as a decimal with two to three significant digits followed by a percentage sign (Table 5-5).[95]

Alcoholic tolerance may be acute or chronic. The acute tolerance phenomenon is typically seen with someone who initially appears inebriated, continues to

Table 5-5　Behavioral Changes and Impairments Associated with Progressive Blood Alcohol Concentrations 0.01% to Greater than 4.00% by Volume

Blood Alcohol Concentration (% by vol.)	Behavior Changes	Impairment
0.010–0.029	Average individual appears normal	Subtle effects that can be detected with special tests
0.030–0.059	Mild euphoria Sense of well-being Friendliness Relaxation Joyousness Talkativeness Decreased inhibition Increased libido	Concentration Recall Cognitive/learning ability
0.06–0.10	Blunted feelings Disinhibition Extroversion	Reasoning Depth perception Peripheral vision Glare recovery Fine motor control
0.11–0.20	Overexpression Emotional swings Angriness or sadness Boisterousness Superhuman feeling Decreased libido	Reflexes Reaction time Gross motor control Staggering Slurred speech
0.21–0.29	Stupor Loss of understanding Impaired sensations	Severe motor impairment Loss of consciousness Memory
0.30–0.39	Severe CNS depression Unconsciousness Death possible	Loss of bladder function Breathing Heart rate
0.40 or greater	General lack of behavior Unconsciousness Death	Breathing Heart rate

Data from Lewis LD, Smith BW, Mamourian AC. Delayed sequelae after acute overdoses or poisonings: cranial neuropathy related to ethylene glycol ingestion. *Clin Pharmacol Ther.* 1997;61:692–699; Lieber CS. Interaction of alcohol with other drugs and nutrients: implication for the therapy of alcoholic liver disease. *Drugs.* 1990;40:23–44; Wetterling T, Veltrup C, Driessen M, John U. Drinking pattern and alcohol-related medical disorders. *Alcohol Alcohol.* 1990;34:330–336; Manzo L, Costa LG. Manifestations of neurotoxicity in occupational diseases. In: Costa, LG, Manzo L, eds. *Occupational Neurotoxicology.* Vol 2. Boca Raton, FL: CRC Press; 1998:1–20; Claus D, Egger R, Engelhardt A, Neundorfer B, Warecka K. Ethanol and polyneuropathy. *Acta Neurol Scand.* 1985;72:312–316; Burrit MF, Anderson CF. Laboratory assessment of nutritional status. *Hum Pathol.* 1984;15:130–133; Dyck PJ. Detection, characterization and staging of polyneuropathy assessed in diabetics. *Muscle Nerve.* 1998;11:21–32; and Behese F, Buchtal F. Alcoholic neuropathy: clinical, electrophysiological and biopsy findings. *Ann Neurol.* 1997;2:95.

drink, and appears to become sober even though the BAC is markedly elevated. Chronic tolerance is a characteristic feature of alcoholism. Eventually, the emotional and physical reactions to a given volume of alcohol diminish; however, the BAC continues to increase as ingestion increases.[94]

Peripheral polyneuropathy is the most common neurological complication seen with alcoholism.[94] Presenting symptoms include paresthesias, pain, and intrinsic and extrinsic muscle weakness of the feet. The paresthesias and dysesthesias may be so painful that walking and standing are affected. Physical examination typically reveals a nerve length–dependent relationship of reduced pain, tactile, and proprioceptive and kinesthetic perception. The corporal appearance often mimics a malnourished state. It is frequently difficult to separate muscle atrophy from cachexia. There is often a nerve length–dependent relationship of motor weakness and atrophy; this is more commonly seen in the lower extremities than in the upper extremities. Deep tendon reflexes are often diminished or absent distally compared with proximally. Gait dysfunction is common secondary to either large fiber afferent neuropathy resulting in ataxia or primary cerebellar degeneration or Wernicke syndrome. Distal trophic changes such as hair loss and hypohydrosis suggest a concomitant autonomic neuropathy. Although most of the presenting signs and symptoms are slowly progressive, there have been reported cases of acute presentation similar to that seen with Guillain-Barré syndrome. Patients with alcoholism frequently have compressive or tensile neuropathies associated with abnormal static posturing when inebriated.[94–96]

Prevalence of neuropathy is difficult to determine.[95–97] Studies suggest that 10% to 15% of persons with chronic alcoholism develop signs and symptoms of peripheral neuropathy.[95] If electroneuromyography evidence is used as the criteria of diagnosis, 33% of persons with chronic alcoholism may have peripheral neuropathy.[97] The quantity and frequency of alcoholic ingestion required to develop neuropathy are difficult to determine because of the many individual and extrinsic factors involved.

Laboratory testing generally reveals mild to moderate liver enzyme abnormalities with evidence of malnutrition (diminished serum protein and albumin). Cerebrospinal fluid assessment is typically normal.[95] Electroneuromyography typically reveals reduced sensory nerve action potentials, mildly reduced distal compound motor potentials, and relative preservation of sensory and motor nerve conduction velocities. Needle examination often shows distal denervation.[96–98]

As previously mentioned, even with the extensive body of literature related to alcoholic neuropathy, there is no clear evidence to support a single theory of pathogenesis. The most compelling evidence for a nutritional etiology is the correlation of malnutrition, including low serum thiamine, albumin, and total protein concentrations, with a neuropathy that is very similar in appearance to known nutritional-induced neuropathies. Evidence also suggests that alcohol interferes with the intestinal absorption of thiamine and may increase the metabolic corporal demands for thiamine, further implicating a nutritional etiology.

Other studies appear to support a direct toxic impact of alcohol on the peripheral nervous system. Most persons with alcoholism and neuropathy have no direct laboratory rationale to implicate a nutritional etiology.[95] One large study showed little correlation between thiamine levels in persons with alcoholism with and without neuropathy as diagnosed with electroneuromyography. Behse and Buchthal reported differences in electroneuromyography and biopsy analysis of nerves of persons with alcoholic neuropathy and persons with gastric bypass–induced nutritional neuropathy suggesting a nonnutritional etiology.[99]

The only effective treatment of alcohol-related neuropathy is the complete avoidance of alcohol and nutritional supplementation of thiamine, vitamins, protein, and carbohydrates. Improvement is often indolent with noticeable functional improvement occurring 6 months after risk factor remediation.[91,95,100]

CASE STUDY

Amy is a 3-year-old girl who lives in a house that was built in the late 1800s. Amy was diagnosed as having pica behavior—the eating of nonfood items such as soil, cotton, and paint chips. Because of developmental delay (height, weight, motor milestones), recent weight loss, loss of appetite, poorly healing wounds, and evidence of mild chronic kidney disease, Amy's family physician tested Amy for lead intoxication. The serum lead level was reported as 70 mcg/dL.

Case Study Questions

1. Noting Amy's history, the high levels of lead in her blood most likely are the result of which of the following?
   a. Ingesting lead-based paint
   b. Poor quantity of food intake
   c. Lack of social integration
   d. A medication side effect

2. Which symptom experienced by Amy is not typically associated with lead intoxication in children?
   a. Developmental delay
   b. Weight loss
   c. Kidney failure
   d. Poorly healing wounds

3. Amy's physician, noting the results of Amy's serum lead level, recommended that Amy's mother also undergo serum lead level testing. What is the reason for this recommendation?
   a. Amy's mother may also have lead intoxication and may have passed the high level of lead to Amy while Amy was in utero.
   b. Lead intoxication is contagious.
   c. Amy's mother eats a diet rich in fruit and vegetables.
   d. Amy's mother has a medical history of hypertension.

4. If Amy is not treated for the lead intoxication, her symptoms may progress to which of the following?
   a. Encephalopathy
   b. Bizarre behavior
   c. Abdominal colic
   d. All of the above

5. Additional signs of lead intoxication in children include which of the following?
   a. Changes in the shape of blood cells
   b. Dense lines seen in the bones seen on x-ray
   c. A blue line along the gum line
   d. All of the above

References

1. Maze M, Fujinaga M. Recent advances in understanding the actions and toxicity of nitrous oxide. *Anaesthesia.* 2000;55:311–314.
2. Yamakura T, Harris RA. Effects of gaseous anesthetics nitrous oxide and xenon on ligand-gated ion channels. *J Anesth.* 2000;93(4):1095–1101.
3. Keys TE. The development of anesthesia. *Anesth J.* 1977;2:552–574.
4. Jevtovic-Todorovic V, Beals J, Benshoff N, Olney JW. Prolonged exposure to inhalational anesthetic nitrous oxide kills neurons in adult rat brain. *Neuroscience.* 1997;122:609–616.
5. Yamakura T, Harris RA. Effects of gaseous anesthetics nitrous oxide and xenon on ligand-gated ion channels. *J Anesth.* 2000;93(4):1095–1101.
6. Sawamura S, Kingery WS, Davies MF, et al. Antinociceptive action of nitrous oxide is mediated by stimulation of noradrenergic neurons in the brainstem and activation of adrenoceptors. *J. Neurosci.* 2000;20:9242–9251.
7. Branda EM, Ramza JT, Cahill FJ, Tseng LF, Quock, RM. Role of brain dynorphin in nitrous oxide antinociception in mice. *Pharmacol Biochem Behav.* 1999;65:217–221.
8. Dohrn CS, Lichtor JL, Coalson DW, Uitvlugt A, de Wit H, Zacny JP. Reinforcing effects of extended inhalation of nitrous oxide in humans. *Drug Alcohol Depend.* 1993;31:265–280.
9. David HN, Ansseau M, Lemaire M, Abraini JH. Nitrous oxide and xenon prevent amphetamine-induced carrier-mediated dopamine release in a memantine-like fashion and protect against behavioral sensitization. *Biol Psychiatry.* 2009;60:49–57.
10. Berkoitz BA, Finck AD, Hynes MD, Ngai SH. Tolerance to nitrous oxide analgesia in rats and mice. *J Anesth.* 1979;51:309–312.

11. Benturquia N, Le Guen S, Canestrelli C. Specific blockade of morphine- and cocaine-induced reinforcing effects in conditioned place preference by nitrous oxide in mice. *Neuroscience.* 2009;149:477–486.

12. Jevtovic-Todorovic V, Benshoff N, Olney JW. Ketamine potentiates cerebrocortical damage induced by the common anesthetic nitrous oxide in rats. *Br J Pharm.* 2000;130: 1692–1698.

13. Wu LT, Schlenger WE, Ringwalt CL. Use of nitrite inhalants ("poppers") among American youth. *J Adolesc Health.* 2005;37:52–60.

14. Turner CF, Lessler JT, Gfroerer JC, eds. *Survey measurement of drug use: methodological studies.* DHHS Publication No. ADM 92-1929. Rockville, MD: National Institute on Drug Abuse; 1992.

15. Wu LT, Pilowsky DJ, Schlenger WE. Inhalant abuse and dependence among adolescents in the United States. *J Am Acad Child Adolesc Psychiatry.* 2004;43:1206–1214.

16. Woody GE, Donnell D, Seage GR, et al. Non-injection substance use correlates with risky sex among men having sex with men: data from HIVNET. *Drug Alcohol Depend.* 1999;53:197–205.

17. Schütz CG, Chilcoat HD, Anthony JC. The association between sniffing inhalants and injecting drugs. *Compr Psychiatry.* 1994;35:99–105.

18. Storr CL, Westergaard R, Anthony JC. Early onset inhalant use and risk for opiate initiation by young adulthood. *Drug Alcohol Depend.* 2005;78:253–261.

19. Seage GR 3rd, Mayer KH, Horsburgh CR Jr, Holmberg SD, Moon MW, Lamb GA. The relation between nitrite inhalants, unprotected receptive anal intercourse, and the risk of human immunodeficiency virus infection. *Am J Epidemiol.* 1992;135:1–11.

20. Soderberg LS. Immunomodulation by nitrite inhalants may predispose abusers to AIDS and Kaposi's sarcoma. *J Neuroimmunol.* 1998;83:157–161.

21. Tapia-Conyer R, Cravioto P, De La Rosa B, Velez C. Risk factors for inhalant abuse in juvenile offenders: the case of Mexico. *Addiction.* 1995;90:43–49.

22. Wu LT, Pilowsky DJ, Schlenger WE. High prevalence of substance use disorders among adolescents who use marijuana and inhalants. *Drug Alcohol Depend.* 2005;78: 23–32.

23. Guidotti T, Ragain L. Protecting children from toxic exposure: three strategies. *Pediatr Clin North Am.* 2007;54: 227–235.

24. Ekong E, Jaar B, Weaver V. Lead-related nephrotoxicity: a review of the epidemiologic evidence. *Kidney Int.* 2006;70: 2074–2084.

25. Cleveland LM, Minter ML, Cobb KA, Scott AA, German VF. Lead hazards for pregnant women and children: part 1: immigrants and the poor shoulder most of the burden of lead exposure in this country. Part 1 of a two-part article details how exposure happens, whom it affects, and the harm it can do. *Am J Nurs.* 2008;108:40–49.

26. Payne M. Lead in drinking water. *Can Med Assoc J.* 2008; 179:253–254.

27. Ragan P, Turner T. Working to prevent lead poisoning in children: getting the lead out. *J Am Acad Physician Assist.* 2008;22:40–45.

28. Timbrel JA. Biochemical mechanisms of toxicity: specific examples. In: Timbrell JA, ed. *Principles of Biochemical Toxicology.* 4th ed. London: Informa Healthcare; 2008.

29. Baselt RC. Therapeutic drug monitoring and chemical aspects of toxicology. In: Marshall WJ, Bangert SK, eds. *Clinical Chemistry.* 6th ed. St Louis: Mosby; 2008:366.

30. Sanborn MD, Abelsohn A, Campbell M, Weir E. Identifying and managing adverse environmental health effects: 3. lead exposure. *Can Med Assoc J.* 2002;166: 1287–1292.

31. Needleman H. Lead poisoning. *Ann Rev Med.* 2004;55: 209–222.

32. Brodkin E, Copes R, Mattman A, Kenned J, Kling R, Yassi A. Lead and mercury exposures: interpretation and action. *Can Med Assoc J.* 2006;176:59–63.

33. Bellinger DC. Lead. *Pediatrics.* 2004;113:1016–1022.

34. Goyer RA. Transplacental transport of lead. *Environ Health Perspect.* 2006; 89:101–105.

35. Rossi E. Low level environmental lead exposure—a continuing challenge. *Clin Biochem Rev.* 2006;29:63–70.

36. James W, Berger T, Elston D. *Andrews' Diseases of the Skin: Clinical Dermatology.* 10th ed. Philadelphia: Saunders; 2005.

37. Woolf A, Goldman R, Bellinger D. Update on the clinical management of childhood lead poisoning. *Pediatr Clin North Am.* 2007;54:271–294.

38. Hu H, Shih R, Rothenberg S, Schwartz S. The epidemiology of lead toxicity in adults: measuring and consideration for other methodological issues. *Environ Health Persp.* 2007;115:455–462.

39. Jones L, Homa M, Meyer A, et al. Trends in blood lead levels and blood lead testing among US children aged 1 to 5 years, 1988–2004. *Pediatrics.* 2009;123:e376–e385.

40. Murata K, Iwata T, Dakeishi M, Karita K. Lead toxicity: does the critical level of lead resulting in adverse effects differ between adults and children? *J Occup Health.* 2009;51:1–12.

41. Mañay N, Cousillas AZ, Alvarez C, Heller T. Lead contamination in Uruguay: the "La Teja" neighborhood case. *Rev Environ Contam Toxicol.* 2009;195:93–115.

42. Pokras M, Kneeland M. Lead poisoning: using transdisciplinary approaches to solve an ancient problem. *Ecohealth.* 2008;5:379–385.

43. Schep J, Fountain S, Cox, M, Pesola R. Lead shot in the appendix. *N Engl J Med.* 2006;354:1757.

44. Madsen HH, Skjødt T, Jørgensen PJ, Grandjean P. Blood lead levels in patients with lead shot retained in the appendix. *Acta Radiol.* 1987;29:745–746.

45. Chandler HA, Scott M. A review of thallium toxicology. *J R Nav Med Serv.* 1996;72:75–79.

46. Barroso-Moguel R, Méndez-Armenta M, Villeda-Hernández J, Ríos C, Galván-Arzate S. Experimental neuromyopathy induced by thallium in rats. *J Appl Toxicol.* 1996;16:385–389.

47. Gettler A, Weiss L. Thallium poisoning. III. Clinical toxicology of thallium. *Am J Clin Pathol.* 1943;13:422–429.

48. Prick JJG. Thallium poisoning. In: Vinken PJ, Bruyn GW, eds. *Intoxications of the Nervous System. Handbook of Clinical Neurology.* vol 36. New York: Elsevier Science; 1978:239–278.

49. Chamberlain PH, Stavinoha WB, Davis H, Kniker WT, Panos TC. Thallium poisoning. *Pediatrics.* 1958;22:1170–1182.

50. Herrero F, Fernández E, Gómez J, et al. Thallium poisoning presenting with abdominal colic, paresthesia, and irritability. *Clin Toxicol.* 1995;33:261–264.

51. Luckit J, Mir N, Hargreaves M, Costello C, Gazzard B. Thrombocytopenia associated with thallium poisoning. *Hum Exp Toxicol.* 1990;9:47–48.

52. Malbrain ML, Lambrecht GL, Zandijk E, et al. Treatment of severe thallium intoxication. *J Toxicol Clin Toxicol.* 1997;35:97–100.

53. McMillan TM, Jacobson RR, Gross M. Neuropsychology of thallium poisoning. *J Neurol Neurosurg Psychiatry.* 1997;63: 247–250.

54. Moeschlin S. Thallium poisoning. *Clin Toxicol.* 1980;17: 133–146.

55. Mulkey JP, Oehme FW. A review of thallium toxicity. *Vet Hum Toxicol.* 1993;35:445–453.

56. Dumitru D, Kalantri A. Electrophysiological investigation of thallium poisoning. *Muscle Nerve.* 1990;13:433–437.

57. Limos CL, Ohnishi A, Suzuki N, et al. Axonal degeneration and focal muscle fiber necrosis in human thallotoxicosis: histopathological studies of nerve and muscle. *Muscle Nerve.* 1982;5:598–706.

58. de Groot G, van Heijst ANP, van Kesteren RG, Maes RAA. An evaluation of the efficacy of charcoal haemoperfusion in the treatment of three cases of acute thallium poisoning. *Arch Toxicol.* 1985;57:61–66.

59. Kamerbeek HH, Rauws AG, Ten Ham M, van Heijst ANP. Prussian blue in therapy of thallotoxicosis: an experimental and clinical investigation. *Acta Med Scand.* 1971;189:321–324.

60. Kravzov J, Ríos C, Altagracia M, Monroy-Noyola A, López F. Relationship between physicochemical properties of Prussian blue and its efficacy as antidote against thallium poisoning. *J Appl Toxicol.* 1993;13(3):213–216.

61. Balakumar P, Kaur J. Arsenic exposure and cardiovascular disease. *Cardiovasc Toxicol.* 2009;9(4):169.

62. Steinmaus C, Moore L, Hopenhayn-Rich C, Biggs ML, Smith A. Arsenic in drinking water and bladder cancer. *Cancer Invest.* 2000;18:174–182.

63. Buchet JP, Lison D. Clues and uncertainties in the risk assessment of arsenic in drinking water. *Food Chem Toxicol.* 2000;38:S81–85.

64. Campbell JP, Alvarez JA. Acute arsenic intoxication. *Am Fam Physician.* 1989;40:93–97.

65. Schoolmeester WL, White DR. Arsenic poisoning. *South Med J.* 1980;73:198–208.

66. Goddard MJ, Tanhehco JL, Dau PC. Chronic arsenic poisoning masquerading as Landry-Guillain-Barre syndrome. *Electromyogr Clin Neurophysiol.* 1992;32:419–423.

67. Quatrehomme G, Ricq O, Lapolus P. Acute arsenic intoxication: forensic and toxicologic aspects. *J Forensic Sci.* 1992;37:1163–1171.

68. Mazumder DN, Das-Gupta J, Santra A, Pal A, Ghose A, Sarkar S. Chronic arsenic toxicity in West Bengal—the worst calamity in the world. *J Indian Med Assoc.* 1998;96: 4–7, 18.

69. Axelson O, Dahlgren E, Jansson CD, et al. Arsenic exposure and mortality: a case-referent study from a Swedish copper smelter. *Br J Ind Med.* 1978;35:8–15.

70. Fincher RM, Koerker RM. Long term survival in acute arsenic encephalopathy: follow up using newer measures of electrophysiologic parameters. *Am J Med.* 1987;82:549–552.

71. Clarkson TW, Magos L. The toxicology of mercury and its chemical compounds. *Crit Rev Toxicol.* 2006;36:609–662.

72. Cursh JB, Clarkson TW, Miles E, Goldsmith LA. Percutaneous absorption of mercury vapour by man. *Arch Environ Health.* 1989;44:120–127.

73. Mozaffarian D, Rimm EB. Fish intake, contaminants, and human health: evaluating risks and benefits. *JAMA.* 2006;296:1885–1899.

74. Thompson WW, Price C, Goodson B. Early thimersol exposure and neuropsychological outcomes at 7 to 10 years. *N Engl J Med.* 2007; 357:1281–1292.

75. Aucott M, McLinden M, Winka M. Release of mercury from broken fluorescent bulbs. *J Air Waste Manag Assoc.* 2003;53:143–151.

76. Tunnessen WW Jr, McMahon KJ, Baser M. Acrodynia: exposure to mercury from fluorescent light bulbs. *Pediatrics.* 1987;79:786–789.

77. Liang YX, Sun RK, Chen ZQ, Li LH. Psychological effects of low exposure to mercury vapor: application of computer-administered neurobehavioral evaluation system. *Environ Res.* 1993;60:320–327.

78. Langford NJ, Ferner RE. Toxicity of mercury. *J Hum Hypertens.* 1999;13:651–656.

79. Cherian MG, Hursh JG, Clarkson TW. Radioactive mercury distribution in biological fluids and excretion in human subjects after inhalation of mercury vapor. *Arch Environ Health.* 1978;33:190–214.

80. Risher JF, Amler SN. Mercury exposure: evaluation and intervention in the inappropriate use of chelating agents in the diagnosis and treatment of putative mercury poisoning. *Neurotoxicology.* 2005;26:691–699.

81. Ngim CH, Foo SC, Boey KW, Keyaratnam J. Chronic neurobehavioral effects of elemental mercury in dentists. *Br J Ind Med.* 1992;49:782–790.

82. Hendry WF, A'Hern FPA, Cole PJ. Was Young's syndrome caused by mercury exposure in childhood? *BMJ.* 1993;307: 1579–1582.

83. Mutter J, Naumann J, Schneider R, Walach H, Haley B. Mercury and autism: accelerating evidence? *Neuro Endocrinol Lett.* 2005;26:439–446.

84. Ibrahim D, Froberg B, Wolf A, Rusyniak DE. Heavy metal poisoning: clinical presentations and pathophysiology. *Clin Lab Med.* 2006;26:67–97.

85. Hess R, Bartels MJ, Pottenger LH. Ethylene glycol: an estimate of tolerable levels of exposure based on a review of animal and human data. *Arch Toxicol.* 2004;78:671–680.

86. Tobe TJM, Braam GB, Meulenbelt J, van Dijk GW. Ethylene glycol poisoning mimicking Snow White. *Lancet.* 2002;359:444.

87. Spillane L, Roberts JR, Meyer AE. Multiple cranial nerve deficits after ethylene glycol poisoning. *Ann Emerg Med.* 1991;20:208–210.

88. Hasbani MJ, Sansing LH, Perrone J, Asbury AK, Bird SJ. Encephalopathy and peripheral neuropathy following diethylene glycol ingestion. *Neurology.* 2005;64:1273–1275.

89. Zhou L, Zabad R, Lewis RA. Ethylene glycol intoxication: electrophysiological studies suggest a polyradiculopathy. *Neurology.* 2002;59:1809–1810.

90. Lewis LD, Smith BW, Mamourian AC. Delayed sequelae after acute overdoses or poisonings: cranial neuropathy related to ethylene glycol ingestion. *Clin Pharmacol Ther.* 1997;61:692–699.

91. Lieber CS. Interaction of alcohol with other drugs and nutrients: implication for the therapy of alcoholic liver disease. *Drugs.* 1990;40:23–44.

92. Wetterling T, Veltrup C, Driessen M, John U. Drinking pattern and alcohol-related medical disorders. *Alcohol Alcohol.* 1990;34:330–336.

93. Manzo L, Costa LG. Manifestations of neurotoxicity in occupational diseases. In: Costa, LG, Manzo L, eds. *Occupational Neurotoxicology.* Vol 2. Boca Raton, FL: CRC Press; 1998:1–20.

94. Claus D, Egger R, Engelhardt A, Neundorfer B, Warecka K. Ethanol and polyneuropathy. *Acta Neurol Scand.* 1985;72: 312–316.

95. Burrit MF, Anderson CF. Laboratory assessment of nutritional status. *Hum Pathol.* 1984;15:130–133.

96. Dyck PJ. Detection, characterization and staging of polyneuropathy assessed in diabetics. *Muscle Nerve.* 1998; 11:21–32.

97. Behese F, Buchtal F. Alcoholic neuropathy: clinical, electrophysiological and biopsy findings. *Ann Neurol.* 1997; 2:95.

98. Bosch EP, Pelham RW, Rasool CG, Chattorjee A, Lasch RW, Brown L. Animal models of alcoholic neuropathy: morphological, electrophysiological and biochemical findings. *Muscle Nerve.* 1979;2:133–144.

99. Behse F, Buchthal F. Alcoholic neuropathy: Clinical, electrophysiological, and biopsy finds. *Ann of Neurology.* 1977;2:95–110.

100. Palliyath S, Schwartz BD. Peripheral nerve functions improve in chronic alcoholic patients on abstinence. *J Stud Alcohol.* 1993;54:684–686.

Chapter 6

Critical Illness Polyneuropathy

Stephen J. Carp, PT, PhD, GCS

"It is in moments of illness that we are compelled to recognize that we live not alone but chained to a creature of a different kingdom, whole worlds apart, who has no knowledge of us and by whom it is impossible to make ourselves understood: our body."

—Marcel Proust

Objectives

On completion of this chapter, the student/practitioner will be able to:

- Define critical illness and its two subsets: critical illness polyneuropathy and critical illness myopathy.
- Demonstrate an understanding of the relationship between critical illness and critical illness polyneuropathy and critical illness myopathy.
- Apply knowledge of critical illness polyneuropathy and critical illness myopathy to the development of a valid rehabilitation assessment and goal-oriented intervention schema.

Key Terms

- Critical illness
- Critical illness myopathy (CIM)
- Critical illness polyneuropathy (CIP)

Introduction

Critical illness polyneuropathy (CIP) and **critical illness myopathy (CIM)** are two major complications of **critical illness.** CIP and CIM affect many aspects of the therapeutic intervention spectra of critical illness. These include the progression and success of ventilator weaning; the initiation and progression of physical, emotional, and vocational rehabilitation; and the risk of idiopathic and iatrogenic complications of long-term bedrest. Etiological factors for CIP and CIM include sepsis, acute respiratory failure, systemic inflammatory response syndrome (SIRS), and multiple organ failure. This chapter focuses on the epidemiology, diagnostics, pathophysiology, risk factors, clinical consequences, and potential therapeutic interventions to reduce the incidence and severity of CIP and CIM. This chapter is written for the rehabilitative clinician but may also benefit residents, interns, primary care physicians, nurse practitioners, hospital-based nurses, and critical care physicians.

CIP and CIM were first described by Bolton et al. in 1984[1] and further elucidated by Bolton et al. in 1986.[2] Five patients admitted to an acute care hospital in London, Ontario, Canada, with multiple primary diagnoses all complicated by multisystem organ failure and sepsis were described as having difficulties in weaning from the ventilator when the primary illness had subsided and development of flaccid and areflexic limbs. Early electroneurodiagnostic studies, especially the needle examination, provided definitive evidence of an acute, systemic motor neuropathy. Bolton et al.[1] described the symptoms as "a primary axonal polyneuropathy with sparing of the central nervous system." These investigators believed that nutritional issues may have provided the etiology of the motor loss because, as they noted, symptoms appeared to have improved with the addition of total parenteral nutrition. Williams et al.[3] reported similar findings in children.

CIM and CIP have similar symptoms, signs are often difficult to differentiate, and they frequently co-occur. Combined electroneurophysiological testing and histological studies often show the overlap.[4] From an interventional standpoint, these illnesses are often treated together—hence the often used diagnostic interpretation of CIM/CIP. Because the relationship of CIP and CIM is so intertwined in the literature dealing with etiology, pathogenesis, and treatment of critical illness and many researchers believe the two components are part of the same disease process, the collective term CIP/CIM is used in the remainder of this chapter.

Clinical Signs and Symptoms

CIP/CIM is a manifestation of a critical illness in the peripheral nervous and skeletal muscle systems. For this reason, the signs and symptoms of CIP/CIM are of lower motor neuron origin or muscle origin. Elevated tone and tendon reflexes, the presence of clonus and Babinski sign, and encephalopathy-induced changes in mental status are possible symptoms of the impact of severe illness on the central nervous system—symptoms associated with involvement of upper motor neurons and higher centers—but are not part of CIP/CIM complications. Patients with CIP/CIM exhibit the major clinical signs of flaccid symmetrical paralysis or symmetrical weakness; absent or diminished deep tendon reflexes; myopathic pain; and a distal loss of sensitivity to pain, temperature, and vibration. Facial muscles tend to be spared but may be involved in rare instances. Ventilator weaning issues are typically due to diaphragm paralysis or weakness secondary to phrenic and intercostal nerve involvement resulting from the CIP/CIM.[5]

The Medical Research Council (MRC) sum score is a screening tool for CIP/CIM.[6] In individuals with critical illness, manual muscle tests of six muscle groups bilaterally are assessed on a scale of 0 to 5. The maximum score is 60. CIP/CIM is arbitrarily diagnosed if the MRC sum score is less than 48. Two conditions affect the reliability of the MRC sum score: (1) there can be no confounding cause of muscle weakness (e.g., isolated nerve compression or Guillain-Barré syndrome) affecting the manual muscle tests of the tested muscles, and (2) the patient must be sufficiently awake, cooperative, and alert to be tested.

Laboratory and electroneuromyography testing can assist with pinpointing the diagnosis of CIM/CIP. Electroneuromyography evidence is often the first indication of CIM/CIP before manifestation of clinical symptoms. At 2 to 5 days after the onset of a critical illness, there is a reduction in amplitude of nerve conduction potentials or sensory nerve action potentials, or both, with preserved conduction velocities. One study cited data showing most patients admitted to one hospital for sepsis demonstrated reduced nerve conduction amplitudes within 3 days of admission and that change of baseline nerve conduction response amplitude at 1 week was predictive of the development of acquired lower motor neuron impairment.[7] At 2 to 3 weeks after onset of critical illness, fibrillation potentials and positive sharp waves appeared on the needle examination.[8] One study reported that electrophysiological screening using peroneal compound muscle action potential reduction greater than 2 standard deviations below the normal value is reliable in determining a diagnosis of CIM/CIP.[9]

Serum creatine kinase (CK) concentrations are diagnostically helpful if they are normal, but often elevated CK concentrations may be secondary to trauma, long-term bedrest, or surgical intervention. CK may be more beneficial as related to the specificity rather than the sensitivity for this particular diagnosis. Muscle biopsy is also an effective diagnostic tool. Three subtypes of acute myopathy found in intensive care units (ICUs) have been reported and are often noted as "acute quadriplegic myopathy."[10] These subtypes are diffuse nonnecrotizing cachectic myopathy, thick-filament myopathy or myopathy with selective loss of thick myosin filaments, and acute necrotizing myopathy. Nonnecrotizing myopathy is accompanied by abnormal variation of muscle fiber size, atrophy of predominantly type II fibers, angulated fibers, internalized nuclei, rimmed vacuoles, fatty degeneration of muscle fibers, and fibrosis. In thick filament myopathy, there is a selective loss of myosin filaments. Acute necrotizing myopathy of critical illness is characterized by prominent myonecrosis with vasculization and phagocytosis of the muscle fibers. In a few of these patients, the myopathy may progress to rhabdomyolysis.[5]

Incidence is related to the particular ICU case mix being studied. Of patients with sepsis or SIRS, 70% may develop CIM/CIP.[5] With the addition of a diagnosis of multiple organ failure, the incidence may increase to 100%.[11] Patients with a diagnosis of acute respiratory distress syndrome have a 60% chance of developing CIM/CIP.[11] Among all patients with diagnoses requiring mechanical ventilation for at least 4 days, the incidence is 25%[12] on clinical evaluation, and this number increases to 58% on electroneurodiagnostic evaluation.[13]

Pathophysiology

Similar to the etiology, the pathophysiology of CIM/CIP is unclear. The appearance of CIM/CIP in patients with multiple organ system failure may raise the possibility that the presenting signs and symptoms are evidence of failure of additional systems such as musculoskeletal and peripheral neurological.[14] Bolton et al.[1] hypothesized that the failure of the microcirculation secondary to cardiopulmonary collapse resulted in impaired circulation to muscles, tendons, and peripheral nerves, which may result in CIM/CIP.[1] Fenzi et al.[15] added to this argument by hypothesizing that the microvascular collapse may be secondary to the systemic effects of the proinflammatory cytokines expressed by macrophages/monocytes at the site of the inflammation. The impact of the proinflammatory cytokine messengers may be increased vascular permeability resulting in endoneural edema inducing hypoxemia and energy depletion. This "bioenergetic failure" as discussed by Bolton[16] may also be exacerbated by rapid swings in blood sugar concentration and the passage of neurotoxic factors into the endoneurium in the critically ill patient leading to neuropathy.

The pathophysiology of the myopathy component of CIM/CIP is equally complex. Muscle biopsies in these patients reveal a decrease in total amino acid concentration and glutamine levels. Glutamine is known to stimulate protein synthesis and inhibit protein breakdown.[17] There appears to be a relative deficiency of glutamine secondary to the increased physiological demands in critical illness.

Diaphragmatic studies using animal models[18,19] elucidated how even a relatively short immobilization period may lead to diminished diaphragm function. Diaphragm immobilization under mechanical ventilation for only 18 hours induced a significant decrease in diaphragmatic force coupled with muscle atrophy and an increase in muscle markers of oxidative stress and calpain and ubiquitin-proteasome activity. Preliminary data in humans suggest that the combination of short-term diaphragmatic inactivity and mechanical ventilation results in marked atrophy of human diaphragm myofibers and loss of sarcomeres.[20]

Prevention and Intervention

The primary functional problem associated with a diagnosis of CIM/CIP in a patient who is dependent on a ventilator is ventilator weaning. In addition, the diagnosis of CIM/CIP increases the risk of complications of long-term bedrest, including hospital-acquired pneumonia, deep vein thrombosis and pulmonary embolism, the development of pressure neuropathies, and skin breakdown. In addition, length of stay is increased, inpatient rehabilitation is often delayed, and patient costs are increased.

A review of preventive and interventional therapies reveals numerous attempts to affect the development and pathogenesis of CIM/CIP. These include nutritional schemas and interventions; supplemental therapies; antioxidant therapy; and the use of testosterone derivatives, human growth hormone, and immunoglobulins.[5] None of these interventions has shown a beneficial result in preventing or improving functional outcome associated with CIM/CIP.

More recently, studies have been published examining the relationship between intensive insulin therapy in mechanically ventilated patients and the prevention of CIM/CIP. These studies were prompted by a finding by Witt et al. in 1991[21] noting a relationship between hyperglycemia and CIM/CIP. The authors concluded that avoidance of prolonged hyperglycemic concentrations during the critical illness periods intuitively may affect the development of CIM/CIP. Insulin, along with the blood sugar concentration control function, also provides endothelial protection[22] and anti-inflammatory effects[23] and has been shown to have neuroprotective effects in animals.[24] Two trials compared the use of intensive therapy (proactively prescribing insulin to maintain blood sugar concentrations of 80 to 110 mg/dL and conventional insulin therapy—prescribing insulin only when blood sugar values exceeded 220 mg/dL) in patients with ventilator-dependent critical illnesses.[25,26] In the subanalyses,[27,28] intensive insulin therapy aiming to maintain blood sugar concentrate of 80 to 110 mg/dL offered to ventilator-dependent patients with critical illnesses in medical and surgical ICUs decreased the incidence of CIM/CIP from 49% to 25% in the surgical ICU and from 51% to 39% in the medical ICU as measured via electroneurodiagnostic studies. In addition, the requirement for mechanical ventilation of 2 weeks or longer decreased from 42% to 32% in the surgical ICU and from 47% to 35% in the medical ICU. A relationship was noted between the tightness of glucose control and lower incidence of CIM/CIP and ventilator dependency of greater than 2 weeks.

The effectiveness of corticosteroids in the prevention or treatment of CIM/CIP remains speculative. Corticosteroids are an effective intervention in certain classes of patients with septic shock, acute respiratory distress syndrome, acute asthma, and multiple organ failure—all of which have been linked to CIM/CIP. In two studies, corticosteroids showed a beneficial impact on the prevention of CIM/CIP.[27,28] However, three additional studies concluded that prescriptive use of corticosteroids in ventilator-dependent patients with critical illness is a risk factor for the development of CIM/CIP.[13,29]

The impact to persons performing rehabilitation services is related to prevention and intervention. Knowledge of specific predictor criteria for the development of CIM/CIP allows the therapist to act proactively to prevent complications related to neuropathy, myopathy, prolonged ventilator dependence, and longer lengths of stays in the acute and rehabilitation settings.

Early identification of patients with diagnoses of acute respiratory distress syndrome, multiple organ failure, or sepsis in combination with ventilator dependency is important because these patients should be strictly monitored with serial assessments of skin

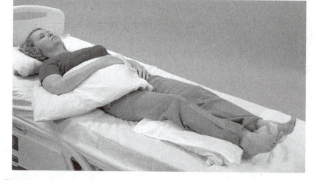

Figure 6-1 Proper bed positioning for patients on long-term bedrest assists with preventing integumentary and musculoskeletal complications. Examples of proper bedrest positioning techniques include frequent positional changes, avoidance of long-term flexion at all joints, pressure relief over superficial bony prominences such as the calcaneus and sacrum, and positioning to prevent loss of range of motion of two-joint muscle.

BOX 6-1

High-Risk Locations for Pressure-Related Skin Ulcers

Occiput
Acromion
Lateral epicondyle of the elbow
Sacrum
Greater trochanter
Fibular head
Lateral malleolus
Calcaneus

BOX 6-2

Locations for Possible Tensile and Compressive Neuropathies in Patients on Long-Term Bedrest

Brachial plexus
Axillary nerve at the humerus
Radial nerve at the elbow
Ulnar nerve at the elbow
Median nerve at the wrist
Lumbar nerve roots in the low back
Common peroneal nerve at the level of the fibular head

---

integrity, muscle weakness, sensory neuropathy, myalgias, and neuropathic pain along with the common complications of long-term bedrest, including pneumonia, atelectasis, and deep vein thrombosis. Preventive integument measures include every-2-hour changes in bed positioning—supine, left side lying, right side lying—to assist with unweighting bony prominences for the prevention of pressure-induced peripheral neuropathies. The use of an outcome measure such as the Braden Scale[30] is often helpful in identifying patients at risk for skin breakdown. The judicious use of pillows, towel rolls, specialty beds and coverlets, and over-the-counter braces and supports may assist with pressure ulcer prevention (Fig. 6-1). Common areas of breakdown include the skin over the calcaneus, lateral malleolus, fibular head, greater trochanter, sacrum, acromion, elbow, scapula, and occiput. Common nerves associated with pressure-related and tensile-related neuropathies include the common peroneal nerve at the level of the fibular head, the ulnar nerve posterior to the elbow, the axillary nerve at the shoulder, the brachial plexus, and the median nerve at the wrist (Boxes 6-1 and Box 6-2).

Musculoskeletal complications are very common and reflect the prolonged abnormal positional stresses and lack of muscular activity associated with enforced bedrest. Abnormalities include fixed flexion deformities, especially at the shoulders, hips, knees, cervical spine, and ankles; progressive instability of joints, most notably at the glenohumeral joint; osteoporosis; and fractures. Cervical and lumbar radiculopathy is common and may manifest as neck and back pain often with variable radicular sensory symptoms and rarely motor signs. Radiculopathy is typically related to bed positioning. Goals of intervention should include the maintenance of articular, axial, muscular, and neurological ranges of motion and the prevention of adaption shortening of tissues; normalizing muscle strength; and early mobilization including weight-bearing activities. The two-joint muscles that are typically adaptively shortened with prolonged bedrest are the biceps, rectus femoris, gastrocnemius, and hamstrings. The maintenance of range of motion is accomplished through daily passive, active-assistive, and active range-of-motion exercises supervised by the therapist.

Deep vein thrombosis prophylaxis should also be instituted early in the hospitalization course. Effective intervention along with pharmaceuticals includes anti-embolism stockings, pneumatic antithrombotic stockings, ankle exercises, and frequent shifting of position in bed (Fig. 6-2). To assist with the prevention of hospital-acquired pneumonia, patients should be instructed in coughing and deep breathing, frequent positional changes, and the use of incentive spirometry. An early mobilization functional plan should be instituted progressing the patient from bed mobility activities to sitting upright to sitting upright over the edge of the bed to out of bed to chair, and so forth.

Martin et al.,[31] Aldrich and Karpel,[32] Sprague and Hopkins,[33] and Martin et al.[34] have published well-constructed research studies on the effectiveness of inspiratory muscle strength training (IMST) on weaning of failure-to-wean patients. In most of the studies, IMST was performed 5 days per week with a

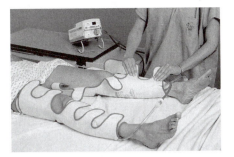

Figure 6-2 Pneumatic antiembolism stockings along with other forms of deep vein thrombosis prophylaxis may lessen the risk of leg clots that can delay mobilization.

threshold inspiratory muscle trainer that provided a threshold inspiratory pressure load between -4 cm H_2O and -20 cm H_2O. The IMST device was attached to the tracheotomy tube, and the cuff remained inflated. Subjects used room air during the intervention and were asked to perform multiple sets of 4 to 10 breaths per day with 2 minutes of rest and ventilator support between each set. Subjects were asked to inhale and exhale as forcibly as possible during the training. Evidence suggests that IMST intervention provided improved maximum inspiratory pressure and weaning outcome compared with conventional and sham treatment.[32–34]

CASE STUDY

John is a 70-year-old man admitted to the ICU with acute respiratory distress secondary to a very aggressive bacterial pneumonia. He was placed on the ventilator and prescribed antibiotics. John's medical history is significant for a 40 pack-year history of cigarette smoking, moderate chronic obstructive pulmonary disease, and hypertension. After 3 days in the ICU, his white blood cell count and temperature are trending downward, and his lungs are clearing as per the chest x-ray. However, weaning has become problematic.

The therapist treating John has been performing daily active-assistive range of motion to prevent loss of articular range of motion, daily strengthening exercises, and a functional progression including bed mobility and supine-to-sit transfers. John has been in a chair for up to 2 hours per day.

Case Study Questions

1. On day 3 of the hospital stay, the physical therapist notes a progression in muscle weakness and loss of deep tendon reflexes. Differential diagnoses include all of the following except:
   a. CIM/CIP
   b. Guillain-Barré syndrome
   c. Metabolic encephalopathy
   d. Urinary tract infection

2. Clinical signs of CIM/CIP include which of the following?
   a. Distal loss of vibration and pain
   b. Symmetrical paralysis
   c. Myalgias
   d. All of the above

3. Often _____ is/are the first diagnostic sign of CIM/CIP.
   a. Electrodiagnostic studies
   b. Elevated blood urea nitrogen
   c. Weakness
   d. Elevated muscle enzymes

4. Extended time on a ventilator may lead to which of the following complications?
   a. Deep vein thrombosis
   b. Skin breakdown
   c. Longer length of stay
   d. All of the above

5. The Braden Scale is a useful assessment tool to assist the therapist with identifying ventilator-dependent patients at risk for which of the following complications?
   a. Deep vein thrombosis
   b. Pneumonia
   c. Skin breakdown
   d. Fall risk

References

1. Bolton CF, Gilbert JJ, Hahn AF, Sibbald WJ. Polyneuropathy in critically ill patients. *J Neurol Neurosurg Psychiatry*. 1984; 47(11):1223–1231.
2. Bolton CF, Laverty DA, Brown JD, Witt NJ, Hahn AF, Sibbald WJ. Critically ill polyneuropathy: electrophysiological studies and differential from Guillain Barre syndrome. *J Neurol Neurosurg Psychiatry*. 1986;49(5):563–573.
3. Williams S, Horrocks IA, Ouvrier RA, Gillis J, Ryan MM. Critical illness polyneuropathy and myopathy in pediatric intensive care: a review. *Pediatr Crit Care Med*. 2007;8:18–22.
4. Latronico N, Fenzi F, Recupero D, et al. Critical illness myopathy and neuropathy. *Lancet*. 1996;347:1579–1582.
5. Hermans G, De Jonghe B, Bruyninckx F, Van den Berghe G. Critical illness polyneuropathy and myopathy. *Crit Care*. 2008;12:238–253.
6. De Jonghe B, Sharshar T, Lefaucheur JP, et al; Groupe de Réflexion et d'Etude des Neuromyopathies en Réanimation. Paresis acquired in the intensive care unit: a prospective multicenter study. *JAMA*. 2002;288:2859–2867.
7. Khan J, Harrison TB, Rich MM, Moss M. Early development of critical illness myopathy and neuropathy in patients with severe sepsis. *Neurology*. 2006;67:1421–1425.
8. Tennila A, Salmi T, Pettila V, Roine RO, Varpula T, Takkunen O. Early signs of critical illness polyneuropathy in ICU patients with systemic inflammatory response syndrome or sepsis. *Intensive Care Med*. 2000;26:1360–1363.
9. Coakley JH, Nagendran K, Yarwood GD, Honavar M, Hinds CJ. Patterns of neurophysiological abnormality in prolonged critical illness. *Intensive Care Med*. 1998;24:801–807.
10. Hund E. Myopathy in critically ill patients. *Crit Care Med*. 1999;27:2544–2547.

11. Tennila A, Salmi T, Pettila V, Roine RO, Varpula T, Takkunen O. Early signs of critical illness polyneuropathy in ICU patients with systemic inflammatory response syndrome or sepsis. *Intensive Care Med.* 2000;26:1360–1363.
12. Bercker S, Weber-Carstens S, Deja M, et al. Critical illness polyneuropathy and myopathy in patients with acute respiratory distress syndrome. *Crit Care Med.* 2005;33: 711–715.
13. Douglass JA, Tuxen DV, Horne M, et al. Myopathy in severe asthma. *Am Rev Respir Dis.* 1992;146:517–519.
14. Leijten FS, de Weerd AW, Poortvliet DC, De Ridder VA, Ulrich C, Harink-De Weerd JE. Critical illness polyneuropathy in multiple organ dysfunction syndrome and weaning from the ventilator. *Intensive Care Med.* 1996;22: 856–861.
15. Fenzi F, Latronico N, Refatti N, Rizzuto N. Enhanced expression of E-selectin on the vascular endothelium of peripheral nerve in critically ill patients with neuromuscular disorders. *Acta Neuropathol.* 2003;106:75–82.
16. Bolton CF. Neuromuscular manifestations of critical illness. *Muscle Nerve.* 2005;32:140–163.
17. Gamrin L, Andersson K, Hultman E, Nilsson E, Essen P, Wernerman J. Longitudinal changes of biochemical parameters in muscle during critical illness. *Metabolism.* 1997;46:756–762.
18. Shanely RA, Zergeroglu MA, Lennon SL, et al. Mechanical ventilation-induced diaphragmatic atrophy is associated with oxidative injury and increased proteolytic activity. *Am J Respir Crit Care Med.* 2002;166:1369–1374.
19. Testelmans D, Maes K, Wouters P, Powers SK, Decramer M, Gayan-Ramirez G. Infusions of rocuronium and cisatracurium exert different effects on rat diaphragm function. *Intensive Care Med.* 2007;33:872–879.
20. Levine S, Nguyen T, Taylor N, et al. Rapid disuse atrophy of diaphragm fibers in mechanically ventilated humans. *N Engl J Med.* 2008;358:1327–1335.
21. Witt NJ, Zochodne DW, Bolton CF, et al. Peripheral nerve function in sepsis and multiple organ failure. *Chest.* 1991;99: 176–184.
22. Langouche L, Vanhorebeek I, Vlasselaers D, et al. Intensive insulin therapy protects the endothelium of critically ill patients. *J Clin Invest.* 2005;115:2277–2286.
23. Hansen TK, Thiel S, Wouters PJ, Christiansen JS, Van den Berghe G. Intensive insulin therapy exerts anti-inflammatory effects in critically ill patients and counteracts the adverse effect of low mannose-binding lectin levels. *J Clin Endocrinol Metab.* 2003;88:1082–1088.
24. Ishii DN, Lupien SB. Insulin-like growth factors protect against diabetic neuropathy: effects on sensory nerve regeneration in rats. *J Neurosci Res.* 1995;40:138–144.
25. Van den Berghe G, Wouters P, Weekers F, et al. Intensive insulin therapy in the critically ill patients. *N Engl J Med.* 2001;345:1359–1367.
26. Van den Berghe G, Wilmer A, Hermans G, et al. Intensive insulin therapy in the medical ICU. *N Engl J Med.* 2006;354: 449–461.
27. Van den Berghe G, Schoonheydt K, Becx P, Bruyninckx F, Wouters PJ. Insulin therapy protects the central and peripheral nervous system of intensive care patients. *Neurology.* 2005;64:1348–1353.
28. Hermans G, Wilmer A, Meersseman W, et al. Impact of intensive insulin therapy on neuromuscular complications and ventilator-dependency in MICU. *Am J Respir Crit Care Med.* 2007;175:480–489.
29. Vespa P. Deep venous thrombosis prophylaxis. *Neurocrit Care.* 2011;15(2):295–297.
30. Kozier B, Erb G, Snyder S, Berman B. *Fundamentals of Nursing: Concepts, Process, and Practice.* 8th ed. Upper Saddle River, NJ: Pearson Education; 2008:905–907.
31. Martin AD, Davenport PD, Franceschi AC, Harman E. Use of inspiratory muscle strength training to facilitate ventilator weaning: a series of 10 consecutive patients. *Chest.* 2002;122: 192–196.
32. Aldrich TK, Karpel JP. Inspiratory muscle resistive training in respiratory failure. *Am Rev Respir Dis.* 1985;131:461–462.
33. Sprague SS, Hopkins PD. Use of inspiratory strength training to wean six patients who were ventilator-dependent. *Phys Ther.* 2003;83:171–181.
34. Martin AD, Smith BK, Davenport PD, et al. Inspiratory muscle strength training improves weaning outcome in failure to wean patients: a randomized trial. *Crit Care.* 2011;15: 96–108.

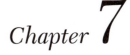

Chapter 7

Diabetes Mellitus and Peripheral Neuropathy

Stephen J. Carp, PT, PhD, GCS

"Someone once told me that God figured that I was a pretty good juggler. I could keep a lot of balls in the air at one time. So He said, 'Let's see if you can juggle another one.'"

—Arthur Ashe (1943–1993)

Objectives

On completion of this chapter, the student/practitioner will be able to:

- Discuss the signs and symptoms of diabetes and diabetic neuropathy.
- Discuss the possible etiologies of diabetic neuropathy.
- Explain the difference between the three classic subgroups of diabetic neuropathy.
- Discuss, compare, and contrast the common presentations of diabetic neuropathy.
- Discuss physical therapy intervention for diabetic neuropathy.

Key Terms

- Diabetes
- Gestational diabetes
- Insulin

Introduction

Diabetes mellitus (DM), or simply **diabetes,** is a chronic health condition in which the body either fails to produce a sufficient amount of **insulin** or responds abnormally to insulin production.[1] DM as a disease entity has been known for centuries. DM takes its name from the Greek for "passing through" because of one of its main symptoms—excessive urine production. During the 15th century, the word "mellitus" was added from the Latin for "honey" when it was noted that many patients with diabetes had high levels of sugar in their blood and urine.[2,3] Classically, diabetes is divided into three broad subcategories: type 1 diabetes, type 2 diabetes, and **gestational diabetes.** The primary impairment of all three types of diabetes is a high blood glucose level, or hyperglycemia. The pathophysiology of DM is very complex because the disease is characterized by different etiologies that share similar signs, symptoms, and complications. The etiology may be primary or secondary as the result of tumor, trauma, obesity, or medication.

Pathophysiology of Diabetes Mellitus

The pathophysiology of the different types of DM is related to the hormone insulin, which is secreted by the beta cells of the pancreas. This hormone is responsible for maintaining a homeostatic glucose level in the blood. Insulin allows cells to use glucose as a main energy source. However, in a person with DM, because of abnormal insulin metabolism, the body cells and tissues do not make use of glucose from the blood. This situation results in an elevated level of glucose outside the cell and a high blood glucose concentration. Over time, a high glucose level in the bloodstream may lead

75

to severe complications, such as ocular disorders, cardiovascular diseases, renal insufficiency, cerebral blood insufficiency, peripheral vascular disease, and neuropathy.[4]

In type 1 DM, the pancreas cannot synthesize a sufficient amount of insulin hormone as required by the metabolic demands of the body. The pathophysiology of type 1 DM suggests that it is an autoimmune disease affecting the beta cells of the pancreas. Consequently, the pancreas secretes little or no insulin. Type 1 diabetes is more common in children and young adults than in older adults. Because it is common among young individuals and insulin hormone is used for treatment, type 1 diabetes is also referred to by its older nomenclature: insulin-dependent diabetes mellitus or, when affecting children, juvenile diabetes.[5]

In type 2 DM, there is normal production of insulin hormone, but cells are resistant to insulin resulting in an elevated blood concentration of glucose. Type 2 DM commonly manifests in middle-aged adults (older than 40 years). Because insulin is often not necessary for treatment of type 2 diabetes and adults are mostly affected, it is also known as non–insulin-dependent diabetes mellitus or adult-onset diabetes.[5]

Pregnant women who have never been diagnosed with diabetes before pregnancy but who have high blood glucose levels during pregnancy have gestational diabetes. Gestational diabetes affects about 4% of all pregnant women. There are approximately 135,000 new cases of gestational diabetes in the United States each year. The placenta provides nutritional and protective support to the fetus as it grows. Gestational diabetes develops when the mother's body is unable to make and use all the insulin it needs for pregnancy. Without enough insulin, glucose cannot exit the blood and pass through the cell walls. Glucose concentration increases in the blood. Gestational diabetes affects the mother during the later stages of pregnancy. Because of this, gestational diabetes does not cause the kinds of complications sometimes seen in babies whose mothers had diabetes before pregnancy. However, untreated or poorly controlled gestational diabetes can injure the fetus. High blood glucose passes through the placenta, resulting in the fetus having high blood glucose levels. The relative hyperglycemia stimulates the fetus's pancreas to produce extra insulin to normalize the blood glucose levels. Because the fetus is often receiving more glucose than it needs to grow and develop, the extra glucose is stored as fat; this can lead to macrosomia, or "fat baby syndrome." Babies with macrosomia who are delivered vaginally face potential complications, including structural damage to the shoulders and brachial plexus lesions. Because of the extra insulin made by the fetal pancreas during gestation, newborns may have very low blood glucose levels at birth and are at higher risk for respiratory issues during the neonatal period. Babies with excess insulin grow up to be

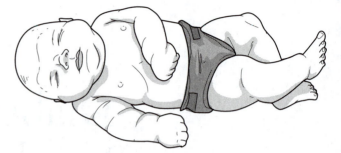

Figure 7-1 Newborn with macrosomia secondary to gestational diabetes. Elevated blood glucose levels in a pregnant woman with gestational diabetes also occur in the growing fetus resulting in higher-than-expected body weight at birth. Excessive weight may result in injury to the infant at birth and potential long-term health concerns.

children who are at risk for obesity and adults who are at risk for type 2 diabetes (Fig. 7-1).[2,6]

In "borderline" or "prediabetes," fasting blood glucose concentration is impaired. In this condition, the fasting blood glucose concentration is elevated above what is considered to be normal. However, these levels are not sufficiently elevated to be diagnostic of DM. The "prediabetic state," for want of a better term, is associated with insulin resistance and an increased risk of cardiovascular pathologies. According to the World Health Organization,[7] fasting plasma glucose levels between 110 mg/dL and 125 mg/dL are diagnostic for prediabetes.

Complications of Diabetes

The quantity and severity of the complications of diabetes are directly related to the duration of the disease and the quality of short-term and long-term blood sugar control. Short-term blood sugar control is best measured by frequent finger-stick assessments, and long-term control is best measured via the hemoglobin A_{1c} blood test. Complications typically affect the visual, integument, cardiovascular, neurological, renal, immune, and reproductive systems.

The most common visual complication of diabetes is diabetic retinopathy. Diabetic retinopathy affects 80% of all patients who have diabetes for 10 years or more.[6] However, research indicates that at least 90% of these new cases could be eliminated if there were proper and vigilant treatment and monitoring of the eye and improved glycemic control.[8]

Diabetic retinopathy often has no early warning signs. Even macular edema, which may enhance the rate of visual loss, may not have any warning signs for some time. In general, a person with macular edema is likely to have blurred vision prompting complaints of difficulty with driving, reading, and performing fine motor tasks. In some cases, the quality of vision may change throughout the day, often relative to the blood glucose concentration.

As new blood vessels form at the back of the eye as a part of proliferative diabetic retinopathy, bleeding may occur with resultant loss of visual acuity. Symptoms following the initial bleed may be minor or not noticeable to the patient. In many cases, funduscopic examination identifies blood specks floating in the visual field, although the spots often disappear after a few hours or days. These specks are often followed within a few days or weeks by a much greater leakage of blood, which blurs vision. In extreme cases, with recurrent bleeds or a major bleed, the patient is able to determine only light from dark in that eye. Clearance of blood may take a few days to months or years to clear from the inside of the eye, and in some cases the blood does not completely clear. These types of large hemorrhages tend to occur more than once, often during sleep.[8]

Elevation of blood glucose levels can also cause edema (swelling) of the crystalline lens (hyperphaco-sorbitomyopicosis) as a result of osmotic changes associated with sorbitol accumulating in the lens. This edema often causes transient myopia, whereas near vision remains constant. The lens edema, as a result of the hyperglycemia, is often symptomatic via decreased visual acuity.

Individuals with diabetes are more likely to have length-dependent integument concerns because of the length-dependent nerve-related and blood vessel–related damage. The further from the heart, the greater the risk of neural and vessel damage and the greater the associated risk of skin complications. Large-fiber and small-fiber neuropathy may lead to insensate skin areas increasing the risk for pressure and traumatic ulcerations (Fig. 7-2). Motor neuropathy may lead to focal or patterned muscle weakness, which leads to gait dysfunction and a heightened risk for ulceration because of improper weight-bearing vectors through the lower extremity. Vascular complications include a length-dependent stenosis of the vasculature leading to intermittent claudication and possibly ischemia (Fig. 7-3). Both neuropathy and vasculopathy may result in slow healing of or an inability to heal skin wounds and a greater than expected risk of infection. Small sores or breaks in the skin may turn into deep skin ulcers if not treated properly. If these skin ulcers do not improve or progress in size and depth, amputation of the affected limb may be needed.

Skin care is an effective preventive measure of the loss of skin integrity in patients with diabetes. Patients with diabetes should be encouraged to learn proper skin care and precautions. Although tedious and time-consuming, frequent skin checks are of utmost importance in preventing limb injury or loss. Examples of

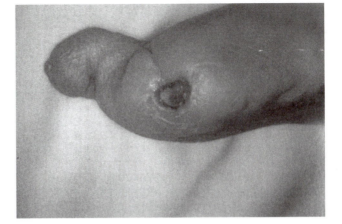

Figure 7-2 Ulcerations associated with diabetes mellitus may be due to many factors, including microvascular and macrovascular disease, afferent neuropathy, autonomic neuropathy, and abnormal foot mechanics. Ulcerations may become infected potentially leading to limb loss.

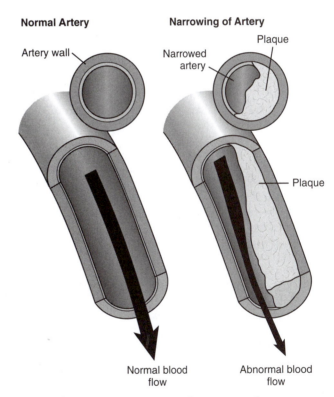

Figure 7-3 Progressive stenosis of an artery subject to prolonged hyperglycemia. Elevated hemoglobin A_{1c} has been correlated with worsening microvascular and macrovascular disease, often the result of atherosclerotic plaque formation. Many of the impairments associated with diabetes—retinopathy, renal disease, cerebrovascular disease, peripheral vascular disease, and heart disease—are associated with diminished blood flow or blood vessel pathology.

BOX 7-1

Diabetic Skin Care

- **Monitor and work toward a healthy blood glucose level.** Perform frequent blood glucose monitoring. Ask your physician about a home testing kit. Ask your physician about routine hemoglobin A_{1c} testing. Work with your health care team to keep your blood glucose in your target range. Maintain your prescribed diet. Exercise. Take your medication.
- **Monitor the skin on your legs and feet daily.** Check your bare feet and legs for red spots, cuts, swelling, and blisters. If you cannot see the bottoms of your feet, use a mirror or ask someone for help.
- **Exercise daily.** Ask your physician for a referral to a physical therapist for an exercise prescription.
- **Wash your feet every day with a mild soap and warm water.** Dry them carefully, especially between the toes.
- **Keep your skin soft and smooth.** Rub a thin coat of skin lotion over the tops and bottoms of your feet but not between your toes.
- **If you can see and reach your toenails, trim them when needed.** Trim your toenails straight across and file the edges with an emery board or nail file. Have your nails trimmed by a podiatrist if you cannot see your toenails clearly, if you have trouble reaching them, or if you have ever had a wound related to your diabetes on your feet.
- **Wear shoes and socks at all times.** Never walk barefoot. Wear comfortable shoes that fit well and protect your feet. Check inside your shoes before wearing them. Make sure the lining is smooth and there are no objects inside.
- **Protect your feet from hot and cold.** Wear shoes at the beach or on hot pavement. Do not put your feet into hot water. Test water before putting your feet in it just as you would before bathing a baby.
- **Keep the blood flowing to your feet.** Put your feet up when sitting. Wiggle your toes and move your ankles up and down for 5 minutes two or three times a day. Do not cross your legs for long periods of time.
- **Do not smoke.** Smoking is detrimental to circulation.
- **Visit your eye doctor regularly.** Diabetes may result in severe eye complications.
- **Visit your dentist regularly.** Diabetes can hasten gum and tooth diseases.
- **Get started now.** Begin taking good care of your feet today. Set a time every day to check your feet.

diabetic skin care include skin checks such as daily examination of the feet and legs with a mirror for signs of ulceration, redness, edema, or infection; clipping of toenails by a podiatrist; and avoidance of walking in socks or barefoot (Box 7-1). Monofilament examinations should be performed routinely every 3 months to assess for insensate skin areas (Fig. 7-4). An individual with a suspected skin lesion should be referred to a health care practitioner for evaluation.

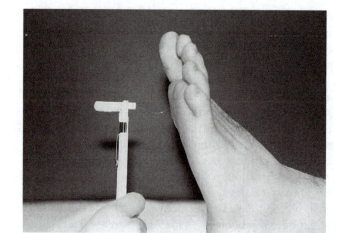

Figure 7-4 Use of Semmes Weinstein monofilaments to assess tactile and protective sensation. Ongoing filament analysis of tactile perception related to dermatomal geography is an excellent method of predicting the risk of developing insensate foot ulcers related to trauma. Filaments of various sizes are pressed to the dermal areas, and the patient is asked to vocalize when he or she feels the filament touch the skin. The greater the diameter of the filament, the greater the pressure needed to excite the dermal pressure receptors—and a greater risk of developing foot ulcers because of insensate skin.

Cardiovascular and cerebrovascular complications are common and include vascular cardiomyopathy, myocardial infarction, arrhythmia, stroke, and renal disease. Untreated hypertension, hyperlipidemia, and hypercholesterolemia may increase the risk of an adverse event. Other complications of diabetes include a greater than expected risk of infections of the female genitourinary tract, chronic kidney disease, polyuria, polydipsia, polyphagia, weight loss, confusion, and impotence in men (Fig. 7-5).

Early and correct detection of the specific type of diabetes affecting the patient is necessary to prevent severe downstream health effects. After diagnosis, a physician may prescribe appropriate medications and lifestyle changes to assist with glycemic control. Examples of lifestyle modifications include dietary restrictions and an exercise prescription for regular aerobic exercise.[9,10] Glycemic control is directly related to three variables: caloric intake of food, activity, and medication.

Diabetic neuropathies—neuropathies associated with prediabetes, type 1 diabetes, type 2 diabetes, and gestational diabetes—are heterogeneous; affect different parts of the nervous system; and result in the presentation of diverse clinical symptoms and impairments secondary to involvement of the sensory, motor, and autonomic nervous systems. Diabetic neuropathies are characterized by a progressive loss of nerve fibers, which can be assessed noninvasively by several tests of

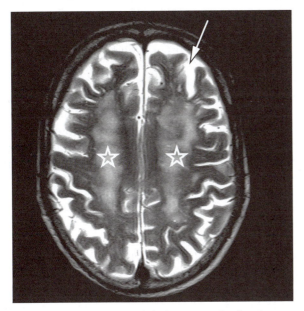

Figure 7-5 Poorly controlled diabetes may lead to lacunar (small, deep) brain infarcts as a result of cerebrovascular disease. As the number of infarcts increases, functional and cognitive impairments similarly increase.

Table 7-1	Classification of Diabetic Neuropathy
Symmetrical Polyneuropathies	Distal symmetrical sensorimotor polyneuropathy
	Small-fiber neuropathy
	Diabetic autonomic neuropathy
	Diabetic neuropathic cachexia
Asymmetrical Neuropathies	Cranial mononeuropathy
	Somatic mononeuropathies
	Diabetic thoracic radiculoneuropathy
	Diabetic radiculoplexus neuropathy
	Charcot neuropathy

nerve function, including nerve conduction studies and electromyography, quantitative sensory testing, and autonomic function tests.[11]

A widely accepted definition of diabetic peripheral neuropathy is "the presence of symptoms and/or signs of peripheral nerve dysfunction in people with diabetes after exclusion of other causes."[12] Diabetic neuropathy is classified into several syndromes, each with a distinct pattern of involvement of peripheral nerves. Patients often have multiple or overlapping syndromes (Table 7-1).

Peripheral neuropathies have been described in patients with primary (types 1 and 2) and secondary diabetes of diverse causes suggesting a common etiologic mechanism based on chronic hyperglycemia. The contribution of hyperglycemia has received strong support from the Diabetes Control and Complications Trial (DCCT).[9] An association between impaired glucose tolerance and peripheral neuropathy has been construed as further evidence of a dose-dependent effect of hyperglycemia on nerves, although this relationship remains controversial for type 2 diabetes and prediabetes.[12–14] Pathologically, numerous changes have been demonstrated in both myelinated and unmyelinated fibers.[15]

The etiology of diabetic neuropathy is unclear; many conflicting hypotheses exist. The diabetic neuropathies may be focal or diffuse. Most common among the neuropathies are chronic sensorimotor distal symmetrical polyneuropathy and autonomic neuropathies.[16] The early recognition and appropriate management of neuropathy in a patient with diabetes is important for the following reasons: (1) Of diabetic neuropathies, 50% may be subclinical or asymptomatic and early, medically supervised risk factor modification may elicit downstream benefits[17]; (2) nondiabetic neuropathies may be present in patients with diabetes[18]; (3) an increasing number of treatment options exist for symptomatic diabetic neuropathy; (4) patients with diabetic neuropathy are at risk for insensate injury to their feet, and provision of education and appropriate foot care may result in a reduced incidence of ulceration and consequently amputation[19]; and (5) autonomic neuropathy, if unrecognized and untreated, may cause substantial morbidity and increased mortality, particularly if cardiovascular autonomic neuropathy is present.[20]

Demographics

Among all persons with a diagnosis of diabetes, regardless of the duration of the disease, the incidence of neuropathy was noted to be 5% to 100%[18] depending on the diagnostic criteria, and 7.5% of persons with a new diagnosis of diabetes have objective evidence of neuropathy.[20] These results are similar for studies outside the United States. More than half of patients with a new diagnosis of diabetes have distal symmetrical polyneuropathy. Focal syndromes such as carpal tunnel syndrome (14% to 30%),[20] radiculopathies/plexopathies, and cranial neuropathies account for the rest of neuropathies. Solid prevalence data for the common syndromes are lacking. A Belgian study reported that after 25 years of having diabetes, the incidence of neuropathy increased to 45%.[21]

Patients with poorly controlled diabetes as measured by daily blood glucose levels and hemoglobin A_{1c} titers have significantly higher rates of neuropathy and higher rates of neuropathic complications.[21] There does not appear to be varying incidences of neuropathy associated with race.[22] Men with type 2 diabetes often develop neuropathy earlier than women when duration and severity of disease are controlled.[22] Diabetic neuropathy accounts for more hospitalizations than all other diabetic complications combined and are responsible for 50% to 75% of nontraumatic amputations. Older adults with diabetic neuropathy, owing to generalized system decline with age, are especially at risk for falls because of neuropathic effects on stability, gait, balance, muscle strength, pain, and sensorimotor function.[23,24]

Pathophysiology of Diabetic Neuropathy

Seminal discussions regarding the etiology of diabetic neuropathy continue to evolve; there is not yet a consensus. Possible etiologies can be classified into one of three groups: the polyol pathway theory, the microvascular theory, and the glycosylation end-product theory.

Polyol Pathway

The polyol pathway is a two-step metabolic pathway in which glucose is reduced to sorbitol, which is converted to fructose.[25] It is one of the most attractive candidate mechanisms to explain, at least in part, the cellular toxicity of diabetic hyperglycemia because

- the pathway becomes active when intracellular glucose concentrations are elevated above normal[26];
- the two enzymes required for pathway completion are present in human tissues and organs that are sites of common diabetic complications, such as eye, kidney, and nerve[27]; and
- the products of the pathway and the altered balance of cofactors generate the types of cellular stress that occur at the sites of diabetic complications.[28]

The polyol pathway is so named because polyol is the general term for sugar alcohols, of which glucose is one.[29] Glucose uptake in the peripheral nerve, in contrast to most corporal tissues, is not insulin-dependent.[30] Elevated blood glucose levels always lead to elevated intracellular nerve glucose concentrations. High intracellular concentrations of nerve glucose lead to conversion of glucose to sorbitol via the polyol pathway using the enzyme aldose reductase.[31] This conversion also occurs in the renal glomerulus, lens, and retina.[32] In a rat model, high sorbitol concentration leads to cataract formation.[33]

There is also evidence that increased sorbitol concentration in peripheral nerve leads to decreased *myo*-inositol levels in the peripheral nerve.[33] *Myo*-inositol is a sugar that is very similar molecularly to glucose. Intracellular *myo*-inositol levels are decreased in the diabetic rat model.[34] *Myo*-inositol supplementation prevents nerve conduction abnormalities in the rat model

without changing the level of hyperglycemia or the sorbitol or fructose levels, suggesting that *myo*-inositol itself may be an important polyol.[34] The mechanism for decreased intracellular *myo*-inositol concentrations causing decreased nerve conduction velocity is unclear. Evidence suggests that decreased *myo*-inositol concentrations may lead to decreased phosphoinositides.[34] Phosphoinositides are labile phospholipids, important structural components of the nerve membrane. Aberrant membrane structure may affect the sodium-potassium pump resulting in increased intracellular sodium, as evidenced by osmotic-induced paranodal nerve swelling in rats with diabetes.[33]

Microvascular Theory

The microvascular theory, also known as the microvascular ischemic theory of diabetic neuropathy, is well known and well represented in the literature.[35–45] Diabetes of long duration has been correlated with microvascular changes in the kidney, retina, and nerve.[37] These changes include capillary basement membrane thickening and endothelial cell hypertrophy.[38] Evidence suggests that these alterations could result in changes in oxygen and nutrient distribution and uptake by the peripheral nerve.[38,39] In addition to the capillary wall changes, findings of erythrocyte and platelet abnormalities have been found.[39] These abnormalities are characterized by decreased red cell deformability and an increase in red cell and platelet aggregation. These findings may result in decreased oxygen delivery to perineural tissues. These protein aggregates permanently bind to the blood vessel walls via attachments to collagen and may be the locus of attachment for monocyte/macrophage complexes.[40–42] The monocytes/macrophages produce proinflammatory cytokines such as tumor necrosis factor-α and interleukin-1β leading to the local inflammatory changes of angiogenesis, scarring, and alterations in vascular permeability combining to result in accelerated atherosclerosis and progressive tissue ischemia.[42–45]

Nonenzymatic Glycosylation Theory

The nonenzymatic glycosylation theory expands on the notion that glucose attaches to proteins at a rate proportional to glucose concentration.[46] The resultant protein:glucose structures are called "nonenzymatic glycosylation products" and can bind to proteins of the erythrocyte membrane, basement membrane, intraneural tubulin, or other exposed proteins. The glycosylation products accumulate over time hastening in correlation with above-average blood glucose levels.[47]

Inhibition or ablation of aldose reductase, the first and rate-limiting enzyme in the pathway, prevents diabetic retinopathy in diabetic rodent models, but the results of a major clinical trial have been disappointing.[48] It has become evident that truly informative indicators of polyol pathway activity or inhibition are elusive but are likely to be other than sorbitol levels if meant to predict tissue consequences accurately. The spectrum of abnormalities known to occur in human diabetic retinopathy has enlarged to include glial and neuronal abnormalities, which in experimental animals are mediated by the polyol pathway. The endothelial cells of human retinal vessels have been noted to have aldose reductase. Specific polymorphisms in the promoter region of the aldose reductase gene have been found associated with susceptibility or progression of diabetic retinopathy.[49] This new knowledge has rekindled interest in a possible role of the polyol pathway in diabetic retinopathy and in methodological investigation that may prepare new clinical trials. Only new drugs that inhibit aldose reductase with higher efficacy and safety will make it possible to learn if the resilience of the polyol pathway means that it has a role in human diabetic retinopathy.[50]

Classification and Clinical Characteristics of Diabetic Neuropathies

Diabetic neuropathy is not a homogeneous disorder. Rather, diabetic neuropathy comprises a group of syndromes with various clinical presentations and impairments often associated with different types of diabetes and with varying prognoses. A generally accepted classification of diabetic neuropathies divides them broadly into symmetrical and asymmetrical neuropathies. Development of symptoms depends on many risk factors, such as total hyperglycemic exposure; elevated lipids; blood pressure; smoking; increased height; and high exposure to other potentially neurotoxic agents such as ethanol, lead, and neurotoxic medications. Genetic factors may also play a role. Establishing the diagnosis requires careful evaluation because patients with diabetes may have neuropathy from another cause.

Symmetrical Neuropathies

Distal Symmetrical Sensorimotor Polyneuropathy
Distal symmetrical sensorimotor polyneuropathy is the most common presentation of diabetic neuropathy.[51] For proper diagnosis, the patient must have DM as determined by the definitions outlined by the American Diabetes Association or World Health Organization.[51] Additionally, the severity of the polyneuropathy should parallel the duration and severity of the disease, and other differential diagnoses should have been excluded. Sensory, motor, and autonomic impairments are present in varying degrees with the sensory impairments most apparent. There is a length-dependent, symmetrical pattern of nerve involvement.[6] Symptoms begin as painful paresthesias and numbness in the toes

and ascend proximally in a stockinglike distribution.[52] Similar symptoms in the upper extremity (glovelike distribution) may occur.[53] Clinicians often combine the two terms and refer to distal symmetrical sensory polyneuropathy as being a "stocking-glove sensorimotor neuropathy."[53] Mild intrinsic muscle foot weakness may be present bilaterally, and there may be a loss of or diminishment of the Achilles reflex bilaterally. Vibratory sense is typically diminished in the feet and hands. Foot ulcerations or slow-healing wounds may be present. There may be evidence of loss of proprioception in the lower extremities as noted by a diminished Romberg, Berg, and other balance examination tools.[54]

Small-Fiber Neuropathy
Small-fiber neuropathy involves primarily the small-diameter, unmyelinated sensory fibers such as the A delta and C fibers.[52] Symptoms include painful paresthesias that patients characterize as "burning," "fiery," "achy," and "cramping."[54] Similar to distal symmetrical sensorimotor polyneuropathy, symptoms of small-fiber neuropathy tend to be length-dependent and begin in a stocking-glove distribution with the feet and legs often experiencing the worst symptoms. Symptoms are often improved during the day and worsened at night. Typically, there is no motor weakness, and reflexes are preserved. Tactile sensation is also typically intact. There are no balance issues unrelated to pain.

Diabetic Autonomic Neuropathy
Pure autonomic diabetic neuropathy is extremely rare.[55] Some degree of autonomic involvement is present in most patients with distal symmetrical diabetic polyneuropathy, but patients may not notice or appreciate the presence of the autonomic symptoms.[55] Common autonomic signs include labile blood pressure and heart rate (especially with postural change and severe effort), an absent ability to sweat, orthostatic hypotension, resting tachycardia, anhydrosis of the extremities, bowel or bladder dysfunction, pupils sluggishly reacting to light and accommodation, and impotence.[20,55-57] Often autonomic symptoms are the predominant complaint early on in the course of type 1 diabetes.[57]

Diabetic Neuropathic Cachexia
The hallmark of diabetic neuropathic cachexia is a precipitous and profound weight loss followed by severe and unremitting cutaneous pain, small-fiber neuropathy, and autonomic dysfunction. Diabetic neuropathic cachexia appears most commonly in older men.[51,55] Concomitant impotence is common, although muscle weakness is uncommon. Weight loss symptoms improve with improved glycemic control; however, the cutaneous pain symptoms do not.[2]

Asymmetrical Neuropathies

Cranial Mononeuropathy
Cranial mononeuropathies typically affect cranial nerves (cranial nerve [CN] II, CN III, CN IV, CN VI,

and CN VII). Involvement of CN III, CN IV, and CN VI is typically manifested as acute or subacute periorbital pain or headache with diplopia.[56] Muscle weakness is not generalized; it is limited to the myotome of the involved nerve.[57] Pupillary light reflexes are spared. Complete spontaneous recovery occurs within 3 to 6 months.[58] Facial neuropathy, simulating idiopathic Bell's palsy, can be recurrent and bilateral. Most facial neuropathies recover spontaneously in 3 to 6 months. Anterior ischemic optic neuropathy manifests as acute visual loss or visual field cuts. The optic disc often appears pale and edematous. Hemorrhages may be present.[59]

Somatic Mononeuropathies

Somatic mononeuropathies are focal sensory and motor neuropathies occurring in the extremities that are caused by entrapment, compression, ischemia, or epineural or endoneural fibrosis.[20] Entrapments typically occur at common entrapment sites similar to sites found in persons without diabetes.[60] Treatment, along with risk factor modification, includes interventions such as release and neurolysis—similar procedures used for nondiabetic neuropathies. Neuropathy secondary to nerve infarction, a rare occurrence resulting from the frequent extraneural and intraneural blood vessel anastomoses, manifests acutely, usually with focal pain, associated with weakness and variable sensory loss in the distribution of the affected nerve. Multiple nerves may be affected (mononeuritis multiplex).[60]

Diabetic Thoracic Radiculoneuropathy

The hallmark of diabetic thoracic radiculoneuropathy is burning, stabbing, and aching pain at, just below, or just above the beltline.[61] Allodynia and dermatomal numbness may occur in the distribution of the intercostal nerves or thoracic spinal nerves. Multiple nerves may be involved.[62] Truncal weakness from either the anterior or the posterior divisions of the thoracic nerve root may occur. Anterior division weakness may lead to trunk instability and bulging abdomen. Posterior division weakness may lead to overuse backache, scoliosis, and truncal weakness. Except for the pain, intercostal weakness rarely results in a functional impairment. Men older than age 50 are most affected.[61] This syndrome often coexists with distal symmetrical polyneuropathy. Recovery is often spontaneous over a period of months.

Diabetic Radiculoplexus Neuropathy

Synonyms for diabetic radiculoplexus neuropathy often found in the literature include diabetic amyotrophy, Bruns-Garland syndrome, and diabetic plexopathy.[62] The initial complaint is a sudden onset of unilateral neck, low back, or hip pain quickly followed by allodynia, paresthesias, and sensory loss. Weakness typically follows within a few weeks or months. Symmetrical attacks may occur. Reflexes in the affected limbs become diminished or absent. The syndrome is associated with significant weight loss, elevated hemoglobin A_{1c}, and labile finger-stick blood sugar values.[62] The

course is typically self-limiting with some degree of improvement over many months.[11] Residual weakness or sensory losses often remain. When occurring in the hip, this syndrome is often confused with an acute femoral neuropathy. However, careful examination reveals weakness in the obturator nerve distribution along with the femoral nerve distribution muscles, and electromyography needle examination reveals widespread spontaneous activity in all muscle groups.[15]

Charcot Neuropathy

Charcot neuropathy is a progressive malady associated with diabetes and neuropathy of long duration and characterized by joint pain, dislocation/subluxation, pathological fracture, and functional impairment.[63] The most common location of Charcot neuropathy is in the ankle, subtalar, or midtarsal joints.[9] The current theory regarding the articular changes is that diabetes-induced autonomic neuropathy increases blood flow to the affected joint resulting in bone resorption and osteopenia. Concomitant motor neuropathy results in muscle imbalance leading to abnormal biomechanics and eventually joint dislocation and fracture. Tendon shortening may be caused by the abnormal precipitation of glycation end products.[63] Sensory abnormalities lead to a decreased perception of pain resulting in further joint degradation and abnormal biomechanics secondary to large-fiber (proprioceptive) feedback (Fig. 7-6).

Intervention

The most effective treatment to prevent and to slow the progression of diabetic neuropathy is optimal glycemic control as reported by the Diabetes Control and Complications Trial (DCCT) (Box 7-2).[9] With the benefits

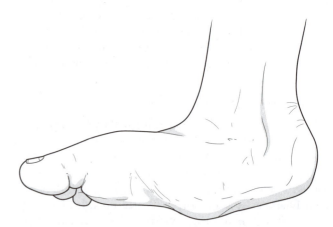

Figure 7-6 Charcot arthropathy: collapse of midfoot arch secondary to diabetic neuropathy. Charcot arthropathy, also called diabetic neuropathic arthropathy, leads to biomechanical changes in the feet. The combination of Charcot arthropathy, abnormal perception of tactile and pain sense, and microvascular and macrovascular pathology puts the patient at great risk for developing pressure ulcers on the feet that may be slow to heal and prone to infection.

BOX 7-2

Benefits of Improved Glycemic Control from the Diabetes Control and Complications Trial (DCCT) and Epidemiology of Diabetes Interventions and Complications (EDIC)

DCCT Study Findings
Intensive blood glucose control reduces risk of:

Eye disease: 76% reduced risk
Kidney disease: 50% reduced risk
Nerve disease: 60% reduced risk

EDIC Study Findings
Intensive blood glucose control reduces risk of:

Any cardiovascular disease event: 42% reduced risk
Nonfatal heart attack, stroke, or death from
  cardiovascular causes: 57% reduced risk

Data from The effect of intensive treatment of diabetes on the development and progression of long-term complications in insulin-dependent diabetes mellitus. The Diabetes Control and Complications Trial Research Group. *N Engl J Med.* 1993;329(14):977–986; and Nathan DM, Cleary PA, Backlund JY, et al; Diabetes Control and Complications Trial/Epidemiology of Diabetes Interventions and Complications (DCCT/EDIC) Study Research Group. Intensive diabetes treatment and cardiovascular disease in patients with type 1 diabetes. *N Engl J Med* 353(25):2643–2653, 2005.

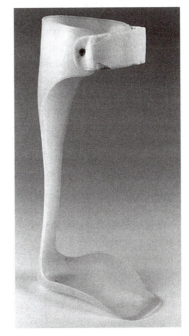

Figure 7-7 Plastic footplate on posterior leaf spring to assist with ankle dorsiflexion in a patient with diabetes mellitus with secondary common peroneal neuropathy. Focal motor neuropathy is a common complication of diabetes. To prevent knee collapse during heel strike and stance, a brace with a locked knee has been prescribed.

of improved glycemic control from DCCT and Epidemiology of Diabetes Interventions and Complications (EDIC) as methods of blood sugar monitoring and the development and administration venues of insulin and noninsulin medications improve, there is real hope that the incidence and severity of diabetic neuropathy will be reduced. Eventually, therapies will move from controlling to curing this complicated disease. The initial reports of halting the progression of diabetic neuropathy in patients with type 1 diabetes with pancreatic transplantation are highly encouraging.[64]

Most aspects of current treatment for diabetic neuropathy involve the use of patient education, modalities to control nerve pain, and physical therapy for therapeutic exercise and bracing related to weakened muscles.[65] Many insurance companies now provide coverage for diabetes education programs for persons with a new diagnosis of diabetes.[66] Along with discussions related to the types of diabetes, medications, pathophysiology, terminology, and diabetic technology, certified diabetic educators also teach patients skin monitoring and checks to assist with early detection of ulcerations.[66] Serial Semmes Weinstein filament testing can identify the existence or progression of dermatomal areas with diminished or absent perception of pain.[67]

The science of pharmacology as related to the treatment of nerve pain is evolving. To date, all medications appear to be symptom related; there is of yet no proven pharmaceutical agents that halt or diminish diabetic neuropathy. It is hoped that ongoing studies of aldose reductase inhibitors, aspirin, nerve growth factors, and insulin-like growth factors will produce positive results.[68–71]

For symptomatic relief of diabetic neuropathic pain, tricyclic antidepressants such as amitriptyline are sometimes successful.[72] Gabapentin (Neurontin), phenytoin, and carbamazepine appear to be less successful.[73] Capsaicin-containing creams and topical lidocaine have reported moderate success.[74] Physical therapy modalities including transcutaneous electrical nerve stimulation, ultrasound, and thermal modalities have shown little effectiveness.[75,76] Bed cradles can be used to lift sheets and blankets off sensitive legs.[77]

Ongoing daily exercise, along with diet and medication, is one of the hallmarks of improved glycemic control.[78] Because of the common comorbidities of diabetes that may have a potential impact on exercise tolerance, physical therapists are often asked to develop exercise programs for patients with diabetes.[79] Other potential physical therapy and medicine interventions are determined by whether large-fiber or small-fiber neuropathy is present. Interventions related to large-fiber neuropathies include strength, gait, and balance training; fall prevention initiatives; pain management; orthoses fitted with specialty shoes; tendon stretching to prevent deformity; bisphosphonates for the treatment of osteopenia; and total contact casting for the treatment of insensate ulcerations (Fig. 7-7).[80,81] Interventions related to small-fiber neuropathies include foot protection such as orthoses, specialty shoes, and white padded socks; twice-daily self-foot inspection with a mirror (many patients are too obese to see the bottoms of their feet); monthly visits with a podiatrist for nail and skin care; serial Semmes Weinstein filament examination by a health professional; and education regarding the prevention of thermal injury (e.g., from hot bathwater or winter weather) and the use of emollient creams to maintain skin moisture.[81]

CASE STUDY

Harold is a 44-year-old man who presents to his primary care practitioner with a 4-week history of an unexplained 20-pound weight loss, polyuria, polydipsia, increased appetite, gait dysfunction, and impotence. Routine blood testing was normal except for a fasting blood glucose of 242 mg/dL (normal, 70 to 110 mg/dL) and a hemoglobin A_{1c} of 8.2% (normal, 4% to 5.9%). Type 2 diabetes was diagnosed, and Harold was immediately begun on oral antihyperglycemic agents. He was referred to a urologist for the impotence and to a physical therapist for gait dysfunction.

After taking the history of the present illness, medical history, and social/vocational history, the therapist began her physical evaluation. The results were as follows:

Cardiovascular: 118/66, 76, 24, 98% oxygen saturation, 0/10 pain scale at rest and with activity. The lungs were clear to auscultation.

Musculoskeletal: Tone was normal. Upper extremity and lower extremity strength testing revealed symmetrical strength at 5/5 with focal weakness of right anterior tibialis, extensor hallucis longus, and peroneal muscle group of 2/5. Range of motion was functional throughout except for a 10-degree plantar flexion contracture at the right ankle.

Integument: Distal lower extremity and upper extremity pulses were +2. No skin openings, rashes, or contusions were noted. Calves were without edema, nontender, and without palpable cords.

Neurological: Cranial nerves II through XII were intact. Vision was 20/20 in each eye with adaptive eyewear. Sensory examination revealed loss of tactile (light touch, pin), vibration, proprioception, and kinesthesia in both lower extremities from the knees to the toes. Monofilament testing revealed large areas on the plantar surface of both feet that exhibited loss of protective sensation. Bowel and bladder were intact. Mini-mental state examination revealed no cognitive disability. Bowel and bladder were intact. Berg Balance Scale was 49; Romberg test eyes open was 15 seconds, eyes closed 8 seconds; and unilateral leg stance was 9 seconds on the left and 7 seconds on the right—all indicative of a potential fall risk.

Problems identified by the physical therapist included loss of protective sensation in both feet; loss of tactile sensation; decreased proprioceptive and kinesthetic sensation; a heightened fall risk; weakness of the right anterior tibialis, peroneal, and extensor hallucis longus muscles; and lack of patient knowledge about diabetes and the complications of diabetes.

The therapist's treatment plan included ongoing diabetes-related education using multimedia, including oral discussion, Internet sites, handouts, and referral to a diabetes educator. Fall prevention guidelines were provided including a home-safety checklist, education, and the use of a cane. To assist the therapist with clinical decision making regarding whether or not to order an ankle brace to compensate for the extrinsic weakness, the therapist referred the patient for an electroneurodiagnostic examination. The needle examination revealed an axonal injury consistent with diabetic neuropathy. With that information, the therapist recommended and ordered a custom-molded ankle-foot orthosis. With the addition of the orthosis, balance testing scores improved to the point where the therapist advised the patient he no longer needed the cane. Lastly, the therapist prescribed a long-term exercise program comprising aerobic, anaerobic, flexibility, and balance exercises for Harold to assist with maintaining good glycemic control.

Case Study Questions

1. Which of the following testing methods is the best method to use for identifying whether a patient with diabetes has protective sensation over a particular dermatomal area?
   a. Electroneurodiagnostic testing
   b. Monofilament testing
   c. Berg Balance Scale
   d. Vibrometer

2. Which blood test is best for determining long-term (3 months) blood glucose control?
   a. Blood urea nitrogen
   b. Hemoglobin
   c. Finger-stick blood sugar
   d. Hemoglobin A_{1c}

3. Which of the following is a symptom of diabetic autonomic neuropathy?
   a. Elevated fall risk
   b. Weakness of the gastrocnemius muscle
   c. Inability to sweat
   d. Renal failure

4. Small-fiber neuropathy is typically associated with which symptom of diabetes?
   a. Painful paresthesias
   b. Motor weakness
   c. Kidney failure
   d. Stroke

5. Charcot neuropathy is associated with which body part?
   a. Head and neck
   b. Shoulder
   c. Knee
   d. Ankle

References

1. Zochodne DW. Diabetic polyneuropathy: an update. *Curr Opin Neurol.* 2008;21(5):527–533.

2. Knuiman M, Welborn T, McCann V, Stanton K, Constable I. Prevalence of diabetic complications in relation to risk factors. *Diabetes.* 1986;35:1332–1339.

3. Vinik AI, Mitchell BD, Leichter SB, Wagner AL, O'Brian JT, Georges LP. Epidemiology of the complications of diabetes. In: Leslie RDG, Robbins DC, eds. *Diabetes: Clinical Science in Practice.* Cambridge: Cambridge University Press; 1995:221–287.

4. Vinik AI, Pittenger GL, Milicevic Z, Cuca J. Autoimmune mechanisms in the pathogenesis of diabetic neuropathy. In: Eisenbarth RG, ed. *Molecular Mechanisms of Endocrine and Organ Specific Autoimmunity.* Georgetown, TX: Landes Company; 1998:217–251.

5. Pirart J. Diabetes mellitus and its degenerative complications: a prospective study of 4,400 patients observed between 1947 and 1973. *Diabetes Care.* 1978;1:252–263.

6. Caputo GM, Cavanagh PR, Ulbrecht JS, Gibbons GW, Karchmer AW. Assessment and management of foot disease in patients with diabetes. *N Engl J Med.* 1994;331:854–860.

7. World Health Organization. Definition, Diagnosis and Classification of Diabetes Mellitus and its Complications. http://whqlibdoc.who.int/hq/1999/who_ncd_ncs_99.2.pdf. 1999. Accessed October 30, 2014.

8. Costa LA, Canani LH, Lisboa HR, Tres GS, Gross JL. Aggregation of features of the metabolic syndrome is associated with increased prevalence of chronic complications in type 2 diabetes. *Diabet Med.* 2004;21:252–255.

9. The effect of intensive treatment of diabetes on the development and progression of long-term complications in insulin-dependent diabetes mellitus. The Diabetes Control and Complication Trial Research Group. *N Engl J Med.* 1993;329:977–986.

10. Nathan DM, Cleary PA, Backlund JY, et al. Diabetes Control and Complications Trial/Epidemiology of Diabetes Interventions and Complications (DCCT/EDIC) Study Research Group. Intensive diabetes treatment and cardiovascular disease in patients with type 1 diabetes. *N Engl J Med.* 2005;353(25):2643–2653.

11. Boulton AJ, Malik RA. Diabetic neuropathy. *Med Clin North Am.* 1998;82(4):909–929.

12. Harati Y. Diabetes and the nervous system. *Endocrinol Metab Clin North Am.* 1996;25(2):325–359.

13. Young MJ, Boulton AJ, MacLeod AF, Williams DR, Sonksen PH. A multicentre study of the prevalence of diabetic peripheral neuropathy in the United Kingdom hospital clinic population. *Diabetologia.* 1993;36(2):150–154.

14. Pirart J. Diabetes mellitus and its degenerative complication: a prospective study of 4,400 patient observed between 1947 and 1973. *Diabetes Care.* 1978;1:168–188.

15. Dyck PJ, Kratz KM, Karnes JL, Litchy WJ, Klein R, Pach JM, et al. The prevalence by staged severity of various types of diabetic neuropathy, retinopathy, and nephropathy in a population-based cohort: the Rochester Diabetic Neuropathy Study. *Neurology.* 1993;43(4):817–824.

16. Lozeron P, Nahum L, Lacroix C, Ropert A, Guglielmi JM, Said G. Symptomatic diabetic and non-diabetic neuropathies in a series of 100 diabetic patients. *J Neurol.* 2002;249(5):569–575.

17. Ziegler D. Treatment of diabetic neuropathy and neuropathic pain: how far have we come? *Diabetes Care.* 2008;31(Suppl 2):S255–261.

18. Apfel SC. Neurotrophic factors in the therapy of diabetic neuropathy. *Am J Med.* 1999;107(2B):34S–42S.

19. Bromberg MB. Peripheral neurotoxic disorders. *Neurol Clin.* 2000;18(3):681–694.

20. Vinik A, Mehrabyan A. Diagnosis and management of diabetic autonomic neuropathy. *Compr Ther.* 2003;29(23):130–145.

21. Vinik AI, Holland MT, LeBeau JM, Liuzzi FJ, Stansberry KB, Colen LB. Diabetic neuropathies. *Diabetes Care.* 1992;15:1926–1975.

22. Llewelyn JG, Tomlinson DR, Thomas PK. Diabetic neuropathies. In: Dyck PJ, Thomas PK, eds. *Peripheral Neuropathies.* 4th ed. Philadelphia: Saunders; 2005:1951–1991.

23. Inzitari M, Carlo A, Baldereschi M, et al. Risk and predictors of motor-performance decline in a normally functioning population-based sample of elderly subjects: the Italian Longitudinal Study on Aging. *J Am Geriatr Soc.* 2006;54:318–324.

24. Schwartz AV, Hillier TA, Sellmeyer DE, et al. Older women with diabetes have a higher risk of falls: a prospective study. *Diabetes Care.* 2002;25:1749–1754.

25. Lorenzi M. The polyol pathway as mechanism for diabetic retinopathy; attractive, elusive and resilient. *Exp Diab Res.* 2007:22(15):32–42.

26. Szwergold BS, Kappler F, Brown TR. Identification of fructose 3-phosphate in the lens of diabetic rats. *Science.* 1990;247(4941):451–454.

27. González RG, Miglior S, Von Saltza I, Buckley L, Neuringer LJ, Cheng H-M. ^{31}P NMR studies of the diabetic lens. *Magn Reson Med.* 1988;6(4):435–444.

28. Barnett PA, González RG, Chylack LT Jr, Cheng H-M. The effect of oxidation on sorbitol pathway kinetics. *Diabetes.* 1986;35(4):426–432.

29. Williamson JR, Chang K, Frangos M, et al. Hyperglycemic pseudohypoxia and diabetic complications. *Diabetes.* 1993;42(6):801–813.

30. Lassègue B, Clempus RE. Vascular NAD(P)H oxidases: specific features, expression, and regulation. *Am J Physiol Regul Integr Comp Physiol.* 2003;285(2):R277–R297.

31. Dagher Z, Park YS, Asnaghi V, Hoehn T, Gerhardinger C, Lorenzi M. Studies of rat and human retinas predict a role for the polyol pathway in human diabetic retinopathy. *Diabetes.* 2004;53(9):2404–2411.

32. Lorenzi M, Gerhardinger C. Early cellular and molecular changes induced by diabetes in the retina. *Diabetologia.* 2001;44(7):791–804.

33. Obrosova IG, Minchenko AG, Vasupuram R, et al. Aldose reductase inhibitor fidarestat prevents retinal oxidative stress and vascular endothelial growth factor overexpression in streptozotocin-diabetic rats. *Diabetes.* 2003;52(3):864–871.

34. Obrosova IG, Pacher P, Szabó C, et al. Aldose reductase inhibition counteracts oxidative-nitrosative stress and poly(ADP-ribose) polymerase activation in tissue sites for diabetes complications. *Diabetes.* 2005;54(1):234–242.

35. Kassab E, McFarlane SI, Sowers JR. Vascular complications in diabetes and their prevention. *Vasc Med.* 2001;6:249–255.

36. American Diabetes Association. Economic costs of diabetes in the U.S. in 2002. *Diabetes Care.* 2003;26:917–932.

37. Skyler JS. Microvascular complications—retinopathy and nephropathy. *Endocrinol Metab Clin North Am.* 2001;30: 833–855.
38. Nathan DM. Long-term complications of diabetes mellitus. *N Engl J Med.* 1993;328:1676–1685.
39. Hanefeld M, Fischer S, Julius U, et al. Risk factors for myocardial infarction and death in newly detected NIDDM: The Diabetes Intervention Study, 11-year follow-up. *Diabetologia.* 1996;39:1577–1583.
40. Cummings M, Browne D. Endothelial dysfunction—from research to clinical practice. *Practical Diabetes International.* 2001;18(6):184–185.
41. Ishii H, Koya D, King GL. Protein kinase C activation and its role in the development of vascular complications in diabetes mellitus. *J Mol Med.* 1998;76:21–31.
42. American Diabetes Association. Standards of medical care for patients with diabetes mellitus. *Diabetes Care.* 2000; 23(Suppl 1):S32–S42.
43. UK Prospective Diabetes Study Group. Tight blood pressure control and risk of macrovascular and microvascular complications in type 2 diabetes (UKPDS 38). *BMJ.* 1998; 317:703–713.
44. Ohkubo Y, Kishikawa H, Araki E, et al. Intensive insulin therapy prevents the progression of diabetic microvascular complications in Japanese patients with non–insulin-dependent diabetes mellitus: a randomized prospective 6-year study. *Diabetes Res Clin Pract.* 1995;28:103–117.
45. Swidan SZ, Montgomery PA. Effect of blood glucose concentrations on the development of chronic complications of diabetes mellitus. *Pharmacotherapy.* 1998;18:961–972.
46. Koenig RJ, Cerami A. Synthesis of hemoglobin A_{1c} in normal and diabetic mice: potential model of basement membrane thickening. *Proc Natl Acad Sci U S A.* 1975;72:3687–3691.
47. Bunn HF, Haney DN, Kamin S, et al. The biosynthesis of human hemoglobin A_{1c}: slow glycosylation of hemoglobin in vivo. *J Clin Invest.* 1976;57:1652–1659.
48. Koenig, Peterson, Jones, et al. The correlation of glucose regulation and hemoglobin A_{1c} in diabetes mellitus. *N Engl J Med.* 1976;295:417–420.
49. Fluckiger R, Winterhalter KH. In vitro synthesis of hemoglobin A_{1c}. *FEBS Lett.* 1976;71:356–360.
50. Cole RA, Bunn HF, Soeldner JS. New rapid assay method for hemoglobin (hemoglobin A_{1c}) and total fast Hb. *Diabetes.* 1977;26(Suppl 1):392.
51. O'Brien SP, Schwedler M, Kerstein MD. Peripheral neuropathies in diabetes. *Surg Clin North Am.* 1998;78(3): 393–408.
52. Galer BS, Gianas A, Jensen MP. Painful diabetic polyneuropathy: epidemiology, pain description, and quality of life. *Diabetes Res Clin Pract.* 2000;47(2):123–128.
53. Boulton AJ, Malik RA. Neuropathy of impaired glucose tolerance and its measurement. *Diabetes Care.* 2010;33(1): 207–209.
54. Vinik AI, Erbas T. Recognizing and treating diabetic autonomic neuropathy. *Cleve Clin J Med.* 2001;68(11): 928–944.
55. Baumgartner RN. Body composition in healthy aging. *Ann N Y Acad Sci.* 2000;904:437–448.
56. Young MJ, Boulton AJM, MacLeod AF, Williams DRR, Sonksen PH. A multicenter study of the prevalence of diabetic peripheral neuropathy in the United Kingdom hospital clinic population. *Diabetologia.* 1993;36:1–5.
57. Goetz CG, Pappert EJ. *Textbook of Clinical Neurology.* Philadelphia: Saunders; 1999.
58. Martin CL, Albers J, Herman WH, et al. Neuropathy among the diabetes control and complications trial cohort 8 years after trial completion. *Diabetes Care.* 2006;29(2): 340–344.
59. Vinik AI, Park TS, Stansberry KB, Pittenger GL. Diabetic neuropathies. *Diabetologia.* 2000;43(8):957–973.
60. Wilbourn AJ. Diabetic entrapment and compression neuropathies. In: Dyck PJ, Thomas PK, eds. *Diabetic Neuropathy.* Philadelphia: Saunders; 1999:481–508.
61. Skyler JS. Diabetic complications. The importance of glucose control. *Endocrinol Metab Clin North Am.* 1996;25(2): 243–254.
62. Krendel DA, Costigan DA, Hopkins LC. Successful treatment of neuropathies in patients with diabetes mellitus. *Arch Neurol.* 1995;52:1053–1061.
63. Young MJ, Marshall M, Adams JE, Selby P, Boulton AJM. Osteopenia, neurological dysfunction, and the development of Charcot neuroarthropathy. *Diabetes Care.* 1995;18:34–38.
64. Ruhnau KJ, Meissner HP, Finn R, et al. Effects of 3-week oral treatment with the antioxidant thioctic acid (alpha-lipoic acid) in symptomatic diabetic polyneuropathy. *Diabet Med.* 1999;16(12):1040–1043.
65. Valensi P, Le DC, Richard JL, Farez C, et al. A multicenter, double-blind, safety study of QR-333 for the treatment of symptomatic diabetic peripheral neuropathy. A preliminary report. *J Diabetes Complications.* 2005;19:247–253.
66. Gruessner AC, Sutherland DE. Pancreas transplant outcomes for United States (US) and non-US cases as reported to the United Network for Organ Sharing (UNOS) and the International Pancreas Transplant Registry (IPTR) as of June 2004. *Clin Transplant.* 2005;19(4):433–455.
67. Feng Y, Schlosser FJ, Sumpio BE. The Semmes Weinstein monofilament examination as a screening tool for diabetic peripheral neuropathy. *J Vasc Surg.* 2009;50(3):675–682.
68. Forst T, Nguyen M, Forst S, Disselhoff B, Pohlmann T, Pfutzner A. Impact of low frequency transcutaneous electrical nerve stimulation on symptomatic diabetic neuropathy using the new Salutaris device. *Diabetes Nutr Metab.* 2004;17(3): 163–168.
69. Jin DM, Xu Y, Geng DF, Yan TB. Effect of transcutaneous electrical nerve stimulation on symptomatic diabetic peripheral neuropathy: a meta-analysis of randomized controlled trials. *Diabetes Res Clin Pract.* 2010;89(1):10–15.
70. Pieber K, Herceg M, Paternostro-Sluga T. Electrotherapy for the treatment of painful diabetic peripheral neuropathy: a review. *J Rehabil Med.* 2010;42(4):289–295.
71. Veves A, Backonja M, Malik RA. Painful diabetic neuropathy: epidemiology, natural history, early diagnosis, and treatment options. *Pain Med.* 2008;9(6):660–674.
72. Morello CM, Leckband SG, Stoner CP, Moorhouse DF, Sahagian GA. Randomized double-blind study comparing the efficacy of gabapentin with amitriptyline on diabetic peripheral neuropathy pain. *Arch Intern Med.* 1999;159: 1931–1937.
73. Dworkin RH, Backonja M, Rowbotham MC, et al. Advances in neuropathic pain: diagnosis, mechanisms, and treatment recommendations. *Arch Neurol.* 2003;60:1524–1534.
74. LaRoche SM, Helmers SL. The new antiepileptic drugs: scientific review. *JAMA.* 2004;291:605–614.
75. Rosenstock J, Tuchman M, LaMoreaux L, Sharma U. Pregabalin for the treatment of painful diabetic peripheral neuropathy: a double-blind, placebo-controlled trial. *Pain.* 2004;110:628–638.
76. Andersen H, Gjerstad MD, Jakobsen J. Atrophy of foot muscles: a measure of diabetic neuropathy. *Diabetes Care.* 2004;27:2382–2385.
77. Bus SA, Yang QX, Wang JH, Smith MB, Wunderling R, Cavanag PR. Intrinsic muscle atrophy and toe deformity in the diabetic neuropathic foot. *Diabetes Care.* 2002;V25: 1444–1450.
78. Cavanagh PR, Derr JA, Ulbrecht JS, Maser RE, Orchard TJ. Problems with gait and posture in neuropathic patients with

insulin-dependent diabetes mellitus. *Diabet Med.* 1992;9: 469–474.

79. Nelson ME, Fiatarone MA, Morganti CM, Trice I, Greenberg RA, Evans WJ. Effects of high-intensity strength training on multiple risk factors for osteoporotic fractures. A randomized controlled trial. *JAMA.* 1994;272:1909–1914.

80. Liu-Ambrose T, Khan KM, Eng JJ, Janssen PA, Lord SR, McKay HA. Resistance and agility training reduce fall risk in women aged 75 to 85 with low bone mass: a 6-month randomized, controlled trial. *J Am Geriatr Soc.* 2004;52: 657–665.

81. Murray H, Veves A, Young M, Richie D, Boulton A. Role of experimental socks in the care of the high risk diabetic foot. A multi-center patient evaluation study. American Group for the Study of Experimental Hosiery in the Diabetic Foot. *Diabetes Care.* 1993;16:1190–1192.

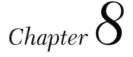

Chapter 8

Peripheral Neuropathy and Infection

STEPHEN J. CARP, PT, PHD, GCS

"Tut, man, one fire burns out while another's burning. One pain is lessen'd by another's anguish; turn giddy and behold by backward turning; one's desperate grief is cured by another's languish: take thou to some new infection of thine eye and the rank of poison of."

—WILLIAM SHAKESPEARE (1564–1616)

Objectives

On completion of this chapter, the student/practitioner will be able to:

- Define the common infection diagnoses that may lead to peripheral neuropathy.
- Develop a clinical understanding of the typical neurological signs and symptoms associated with specific infections that may lead to peripheral neuropathy.
- Apply knowledge of the common infection diagnoses into "clinical scripts" used in the development of the differential diagnoses list.
- Choose the appropriate assessment tools that will "map back" to the potential diagnosis.

Key Terms

- Hepatitis
- Infection
- Lyme disease
- Parasite

Introduction

When comparing the prevalence of etiologies of suspected peripheral nerve disease, infectious causes are much less frequent than traumatic, overuse, metabolic, environmental, and degenerative etiologies. However, many of the infectious etiologies described in this chapter, such as tuberculosis (TB), **hepatitis,** HIV, **Lyme disease,** and leprosy, have prevalence rates in the United States and worldwide that are either staying consistent or increasing. One would expect peripheral nerve injuries resulting from the aforementioned infectious diseases to, at best, remain at their current levels or, at worst, increase in prevalence. HIV-related neuropathy is discussed in detail in Chapter 27.

The clinician attempting to identify the etiology of suspected peripheral nerve injury must be aware of the potential of **infection** to cause neuropathy. This statement is true for several reasons. Correct diagnosis is a requirement for correct intervention. With many infectious etiologies, time from onset to treatment may have a great impact on potential recovery. Lastly, many of the diseases described in this chapter are contagious. Early diagnosis may prevent further dissemination of the offending agent. As with all peripheral nerve injury etiologies, exhaustive history taking, review of the clinical data set, and performance of valid and reliable tests and measures are required for the diagnostician to reach the correct diagnosis.

Lyme Disease

A large amount of knowledge has been acquired since the original descriptions of Lyme borreliosis (LB) and of its causative agent, *Borrelia burgdorferi*. The complexity of the organism, the variations in the clinical manifestations of LB caused by the different *B. burgdorferi* species, and the difficulty in obtaining an evidence-based treatment regimen were not originally anticipated. Considerable improvement in reliability and validity of the detection of *B. burgdorferi* by laboratory and physical assessment as well as in the effectiveness of therapy has occurred since the early stage of disease presentation.[1-3]

The etiologic agent, *B. burgdorferi*, was recovered in 1982 from the vector tick *Ixodes dammini* (now *Ixodes scapularis*) and subsequently, from skin biopsy, cerebrospinal fluid (CSF), and blood specimens of patients with LB in the United States[4] and Europe.[5] In the United States, the Centers for Disease Control and Prevention (CDC) initiated surveillance for LB in 1982,[2] and the Council of State and Territorial Epidemiologists adopted a resolution making LB a nationally notifiable disease in 1990.[3] LB is the most common vector-borne disease in North America and represents a major public health challenge.[1] Since 1982, more than 200,000 LB cases in the United States have been reported to the CDC, with about 17,000 cases reported yearly between 1998 and 2001. In 2002, the number of cases of LB in the United States increased to 23,763, with a national incidence of 8.2 cases per 100,000 persons. Approximately 95% of the cases occurred in 12 states located in the northeastern, mid-Atlantic, and north-central regions: Connecticut, Delaware, Maine, Maryland, Massachusetts, Minnesota, New Hampshire, New Jersey, New York, Pennsylvania, Rhode Island, and Wisconsin. LB is widely distributed in European countries and occurs in Far Eastern Russia and in some Asian countries.[6]

Infection with *B. burgdorferi* can result in dermatological, neurological, cardiac, and musculoskeletal impairments. The basic clinical spectra of the disease are similar worldwide, although differences in clinical manifestations between LB occurring in Europe and North America are well documented. Such differences are attributed to differences in *B. burgdorferi* species causing LB on the two continents.[5-7] In addition, differences in clinical presentations exist among geographic regions of Europe, presumably secondary to differences in the rates of occurrence of infection caused by distinct *B. burgdorferi* subspecies.[5]

Patients with *B. burgdorferi* infection may experience one or more clinical syndromes of early or late

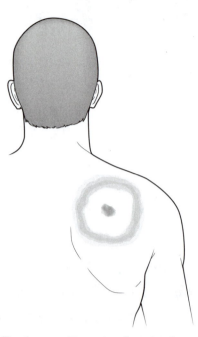

Figure 8-1 Erythema migrans is often the first objective sign of *B. burgdorferi* infection. Note the central macule with the expanding circular patch of erythema with central clearing. Erythema migrans occurs in approximately 70% to 80% of infected persons and begins at the site of the tick bite after a delay of 3 to 30 days (mean, 7 days).

LB. In approximately 80% of patients, the first clinical sign of early infection is a localized erythema migrans (EM) at the site of the tick bite, which may be followed within days or weeks by clinical evidence of disseminated infection that may affect the skin, nervous system, heart, or joints (Fig. 8-1).[8] Arthritis appears to be more frequent in patients in North America, whereas lymphocytoma, chronic atrophic acrodermatitis (also known as acrodermatitis chronica atrophicans), and encephalomyelitis have been seen primarily in patients in Europe.[5-7]

The EM rash begins as a red macule or papule at the site of the tick bite, rapidly enlarges, and sometimes develops central clearing.[8] The clinical diagnosis of early LB with EM relies on recognition of the characteristic appearance of a skin lesion at least 5 cm in diameter.[9] At this stage, patients may be asymptomatic or, more commonly in the United States, experience flu-like symptoms such as headache, myalgias, arthralgias, or fever.[8-10] The presence of constitutional signs and symptoms in a patient with EM has been considered evidence of dissemination by some investigators, but this declaration is not evidence-based.[9]

Hematogenous dissemination of *B. burgdorferi* to the nervous system, joints, heart, or other skin areas as well as occasionally to other organs may give rise to a wide spectrum of clinical manifestations in early LB.[11,12] Usually, patients with objective evidence of dissemination experience one or more of the following syndromes: multiple EM lesions, atrioventricular conduction defects (primarily heart block), myopericarditis, arthritis, facial palsy, meningitis, and meningoradiculoneuritis (Bannwarth syndrome).[12] Lyme arthritis begins as intermittent attacks of joint pain, loss of range of motion, inflammation, and effusion involving primarily the appendicular skeleton. In 10% of patients, the typically seen monarticular or pauciarticular arthritis, especially of large joints, may persist for months or years despite treatment with antimicrobials. Treatment-resistant arthritis is seen more frequently in patients with the certain HLA DRB alleles. Autoimmunity has been suggested to play a role in this clinical entity.[6,7]

Late LB may develop in some untreated patients months to a few years after tick-transmitted infection. The major manifestations of late LB include worsening arthritis, progressive heart block, and neuroborreliosis (peripheral neuropathy or encephalomyelitis).[7,8,10,11,13,14] The peripheral neuropathy seen with late LB is typically large and small fiber afferent, primarily in a stocking-glove distribution neuropathy, but motor symptoms have also been reported.[7,8]

Poliomyelitis

Poliomyelitis originally appeared in epidemic form, became endemic on a global scale, and has been reduced to near-elimination, all within the span of medical history. The earliest references to the disease include an ancient Egyptian frieze from 1580 B.C.E. showing an adult with a crutch and an atrophied leg quite similar to more modern photographic images of patients with monoplegic poliomyelitis. Sir Walter Scott wrote about an attack of "infantile paralysis" in 1773 that left him with a permanent limp and withered leg.[15] By 1880, there were numerous reports of paralysis epidemics. The epidemic phase eventually was replaced by annual seasonal outbreaks during the first half of the 20th century, and by the latter second half of the 20th century, there was a near elimination of the disease.[16] A striking aspect of poliomyelitis infection is the seasonality of infections in temperate zones. This seasonality was most marked in the colder climates and is gradually decreased toward the equator. The disease was almost totally absent in the tropics. The wild poliovirus was eliminated in the United States by 2000. The annual prevalence of 600,000 new cases per year in the United States alone in 1940 dwindled to less than 1,000 new cases worldwide in 2000. Localized circulation of poliovirus types 1 and 3 in Asia and Africa continue to be intermittently problematic preventing total disease eradication.[17]

Polioviruses are enteroviruses that are transmitted from person to person following improper handling of feces and pharyngeal virus excretion via a hand-to-mouth route.[17] The virus has been identified only in humans and a few subhuman primate species; there is no known nonhuman reservoir for the virus.[17] After infection, the virus replicates in the gastrointestinal tract and may cause a viremia with symptoms of malaise, fever, loss of appetite, and gastrointestinal symptoms. Occasionally (about 1 in 150 cases), the virus invades the anterior horn cells of the spinal cord producing a clinically distinctive motor loss with only rare sensory involvement.[18]

In the anterior horn cell, the poliovirus spreads along nerve fiber pathways, preferentially replicating in and destroying motor neurons within the spinal cord or peripheral nerve leading to a lower motor neuron paralysis. The various forms of paralytic poliomyelitis (spinal, bulbar, and bulbospinal) vary only with the amount of neuronal damage and inflammation that occurs and the regions of the central nervous system (CNS) or peripheral nervous system (PNS) that are affected.[17]

The destruction of neuronal cells produces lesions within the spinal ganglia; these may also occur in the reticular formation, vestibular nuclei, and cerebellar vermis, and deep cerebellar nuclei.[18] Macroscopically, inflammation associated with nerve cell destruction often alters the color and appearance of the gray matter in the spinal column, causing it to appear reddish and swollen. Early symptoms of paralytic polio include high fever, headache, stiffness in the back, nuchal rigidity, asymmetrical weakness of various muscles, sensitivity to touch, dysphagia, myalgia, loss of superficial and deep reflexes, paresthesia, irritability, constipation, and difficulty with initiation of urinating.[19] Paralysis generally develops 1 to 10 days after early symptoms begin, progresses for 2 to 3 days, and is usually complete within 7 to 10 days, coinciding with the return to being afebrile.[17–19]

The likelihood of developing paralytic polio increases with age, as does the extent of paralysis.[19] In children, nonparalytic meningitis is the most likely consequence of CNS involvement, and paralysis occurs in only 1 in 1,000 cases. In adults, paralysis occurs in 1 in 75 cases.[20] In children younger than 5 years old, paralysis of one leg is most common; in adults, extensive paralysis of the chest and abdomen and paraplegia and quadriplegia are more common than a monoplegia. Paralysis rates also vary depending on the serotype of the infecting poliovirus; the highest rates of paralysis (1 in 200) are associated with poliovirus type 1, the lowest rates (1 in 2,000) are associated with type 2.[19,20]

The extent of spinal paralysis depends on the region of the cord affected, which may result in any combination of cranial, cervical, thoracic, or lumbar dorsal and ventral root myotomal weakness. Weakness may be unilateral or bilateral but is often in an asymmetrical distribution. Proximal motor nerves are often more affected than distal motor nerves.[20,21]

Bulbar polio, which accounts for about 2% of cases of paralytic polio, occurs when poliovirus invades and destroys nerves within the bulbar region of the spinal cord—the white matter pathway connecting the cortex to the brainstem.[16] The destruction of these nerves weakens the muscles supplied by the cranial nerves, inducing symptoms of encephalitis, and causes respiratory difficulties, dysarthria, and dysphagia. Critical nerves affected are the glossopharyngeal, vagus, accessory, and trigeminal nerves.[16,17]

Approximately 19% of patients with paralytic polio have both bulbar and spinal symptoms; this subtype of polio is called respiratory polio or bulbospinal polio.[16] The virus, along with the extremity and truncal impact, also affects the midcervical roots (C3 through C5), and paralysis of the diaphragm occurs. The critical nerves affected are the two phrenic nerves that drive the diaphragm to inflate the lungs and the nerves that drive the muscles needed for swallowing. By injuring these nerves, this form of polio affects breathing, making it difficult or impossible for the patient to breathe without the support of an assistive device and to swallow. Along with the appendicular and axial weakness, this form of polio is especially devastating.

The polio vaccine was introduced into the United States in 1955[16] with the oral version arriving in 1961.[17] Both versions were designed to protect immunized recipients. The annual incidence of polio declined exponentially beginning in 1955 as more and more Americans were immunized. The last U.S. outbreak occurred in 1979 in an underimmunized Amish population and was caused by a wild poliovirus traced back to a visitor from Turkey via The Netherlands and Canada.[22,23]

HIV Infection

The story of the AIDS virus began with numerous clinical articles published in the early 1980s describing an increased incidence of heretofore uncommon medical illnesses such as Kaposi's sarcoma and *Pneumocystis carinii* pneumonia in certain populations, most noticeably homosexual men, intravenous drug users, and patients receiving blood transfusions.[24] Subsequent reports found that the causative agent was a microscopic agent transmitted from person to person via blood or body fluid contact, primarily through sexual contact, intravenous drug use, or the receiving of blood and blood products. This agent was found to impact T-cell immunity resulting in a global immunodeficiency syndrome.[25]

Since the onset of the AIDS pandemic in 1981, infection with HIV has spread exponentially throughout the world; at the present time, 60 million children and adults are affected.[24] There are approximately 16,000 new infections per day.[25] More than 8,000 deaths occur daily as a result of AIDS.[26] In the United States alone, reports indicate that there are more than 1 million infections; almost 1 in 300 persons harbors HIV.[25] In some African countries, the infection rate approaches 30% of the population.[25] Since the introduction of highly active antiretroviral therapy (HAART) in communities where this treatment is available and affordable, AIDS is becoming a chronic illness with dramatic reductions in morbidity and mortality. However, in most of the world, where HAART therapy is either not available or not affordable, AIDS remains an acute illness with a high morbidity rate.

HIV is a neuroinvasive and neurovirulent (resulting in myopathy, myelopathy, radiculopathy, and dementia) disease with neurological signs, along with fever, often being among the earliest signs and symptoms of the disease (Table 8-1).[26] Classification, incidence, prevalence, and etiological agent of peripheral neuropathy associated with HIV infection is quite complex. The immunosuppression associated with HIV may lead to secondary infections such as TB, herpes zoster, and Guillain-Barré syndrome (GBS) that may themselves,

Table 8-1 HIV-Related Peripheral Neuropathies	
Occurring During Early-Stage HIV Infections	Inflammatory demyelinating polyradiculoneuropathy Cranial nerve VII palsy Large-fiber–induced sensory gait ataxia
Occurring During Intermediate-Stage HIV Infections	Multiple mononeuropathy (sensory and motor)
Occurring During Late-Stage HIV Infections	Distal symmetrical polyneuropathy Lumbosacral polyradiculopathy/cauda equina syndrome Brachial plexopathy Autonomic neuropathy Diffuse infiltrative lymphocytosis syndrome
Occurring at Any Time of Infection	Herpes zoster radiculitis (sensory) Mononeuropathy (motor and sensory)

Data from CDC. HIV AIDS resources: prevention in the United States at a critical crossroads. http://cdc.gov/hiv/resources/reports/hiv_prev_us.htm; Time from HIV-1 seroconversion to AIDS and death before widespread use of highly active antiretroviral therapy: a collaborative re-analysis. Collaborative Group on AIDS Incubation and HIV Survival including the CASCADE EU Concerted Action. Concerted Action on SeroConversion to AIDS and Death in Europe. *Lancet.* 2000;355(9210):1131–1137; Schneider MF, Gange SJ, Williams CM, et al. Patterns of the hazard of death after AIDS through the evolution of antiretroviral therapy: 1984–2004. *AIDS.* 2005;19(17):2009–2018; Reeves JD, Doms RW. Human immunodeficiency virus type 2. *J Gen Virol.* 2002;83(Pt 6):1253–1265; Agnello V, Chung RT, Kaplan LM. A role for hepatitis C virus infection in type II cryoglobulinemia. *N Engl J Med.* 1992;327:1490–1495; and Agnello V, Abel G. Localization of hepatitis C virus in cutaneous vasculitic lesions in patients with type II cryoglobulinemia. *Arthritis Rheum.* 1997;40:2007–2015.

along with the AIDS virus, elicit neuropathic symptoms. Noninfection comorbidities possibly associated with HIV, such as diabetes mellitus, vitamin B$_{12}$ deficiency, malnutrition, anorexia, cachectic syndrome, alcohol abuse, and recreational drug use, all may predispose HIV-infected persons to peripheral neuropathy. Lastly, many antiretroviral medications used to treat HIV may themselves cause neuropathy.[27,28]

Peripheral neuropathy rates in patients with symptomatic HIV infection range from 0% to 95%.[24,27] The variance is most likely due to the manner of diagnostics; researchers who used solely a physical examination to document neuropathy had lower incidences, whereas researchers who used electroneurodiagnostics had middle percentages, and researchers who used postmortem sural biopsies had the highest percentages. In all instances, the duration of HIV infection in symptomatic individuals was directly correlated with CD4+ T-cell count and with the prevalence of symptoms of peripheral neuropathy. In asymptomatic patients with HIV infection, the incidence of neuropathy was generally less than in individuals with symptomatic HIV. As with the studies of patients with symptomatic HIV infection, the assessment technique influenced prevalence. Independent of the technique, the prevalence rates ranged from 5% to 25%.[24]

The most frequently encountered peripheral nerve disorder induced by HIV is length-dependent distal sensory peripheral neuropathy (DSPN), also referred to in the literature as distal symmetrical polyneuropathy and distal symmetrical sensory polyneuropathy (Table 8-2). The prevalence rate without HAART has been estimated to be about 35% as diagnosed using physical examination and 95% at autopsy using sural nerve biopsy.[24] Risk factors for the development of DSPN include high HIV viral load; low CD4+ T-cell count; length of duration of having HIV; and comorbidities such as diabetes mellitus, alcohol intake, and recreational drug use.[29] Presenting symptoms are the classic "painful and numb feet and ankles," worse with ambulation and better with rest and elevation. The impairment is typically a large- and small-fiber sensory neuropathy with little, if any, motor or autonomic involvement.[27] Physical examination is noted for depressed or absent Achilles deep tendon reflex, a decreased appreciation of tactile and joint position sensation, mild gait ataxia, and lower than expected fall risk assessment (Romberg test, Timed Up and Go test, Berg Balance Scale).[28] Intervention therapy is primarily designed to control risk factors, such as maintaining adequate blood sugar control if the patient has diabetes, correcting vitamin B$_{12}$ levels if required, and eliminating alcohol and recreational drug use.

The nucleoside reverse transcriptase inhibitors used to treat HIV infection such as stavudine and zalcitabine have also been shown to create a dose-dependent, length-dependent peripheral neuropathy with ongoing use. Although the clinical presentations of neuropathies associated with antiretroviral medications and DSPN are similar, the drug-related neuropathies are more likely to be painful and to have an abrupt onset. Medication combinations such isoniazid or hydroxyurea with antiretrovirals may exacerbate the onset and severity of DSPN.[30]

Inflammatory demyelinating neuropathy is a common complication of HIV. GBS and chronic inflammatory demyelinating polyradiculoneuropathy (CIDP) are the two most common variations noted in persons with HIV infection. Most cases of GBS and CIDP arise in HIV-infected patients at or near the time of seroconversion or in HIV-positive patients without evidence of immune compromise or evidence

Table 8-2 HIV-Related Distal Sensory Peripheral Neuropathy

Clinical Findings	• Length-dependent lower > upper limb paresthesias and dysesthesias • Distal weakness • Stocking-glove distribution large- and small-fiber sensory loss • Distal areflexia • Gait ataxia • Decreased performance on balance testing
Laboratory Examination	Electroneuromyography studies show: • Reduced amplitudes of sensory nerve action potential and compound muscle action potentials • Prolongation of distal latencies and possible slowing of conduction velocities • Needle examination shows distal denervation
Symptom Staging	Early- to intermediate-stage infection
Treatment	Risk factor modification: • Check vitamin B$_{12}$ levels • Regulate blood sugar levels of patients with diabetes • Investigate possible medication etiology
Prognosis	If risk factor modification is ineffective, poor, with no spontaneous remission

Data from Time from HIV-1 seroconversion to AIDS and death before widespread use of highly active antiretroviral therapy: a collaborative re-analysis. Collaborative Group on AIDS Incubation and HIV Survival including the CASCADE EU Concerted Action. Concerted Action on SeroConversion to AIDS and Death in Europe. *Lancet.* 2000;355(9210):1131–1137; Schneider MF, Gange SJ, Williams CM, et al. Patterns of the hazard of death after AIDS through the evolution of antiretroviral therapy: 1984–2004. *AIDS.* 2005;19(17):2009–2018; Reeves JD, Doms RW. Human immunodeficiency virus type 2. *J Gen Virol.* 2002;83(Pt 6):1253–1265; Agnello V, Chung RT, Kaplan LM. A role for hepatitis C virus infection in type II cryoglobulinemia. *N Engl J Med.* 1992;327:1490–1495; and Agnello V, Abel G. Localization of hepatitis C virus in cutaneous vasculitic lesions in patients with type II cryoglobulinemia. *Arthritis Rheum.* 1997;40:2007–2015.

of opportunistic infections such as *P. carinii* pneumonia.[28] The early timing of the inflammatory demyelinating neuropathy during the HIV infection course coupled with the evidence of spontaneous improvement tends to suggest that the HIV infection does not directly cause the complication, but rather the etiology may be autoimmune mediated as seen in individuals without HIV infection. However, there are case reports indicating the onset of GBS and CIDP in patients with late-stage HIV infection.[28]

HIV-associated GBS and CIDP have similar clinical pictures as GBS and CIDP occurring in individuals without HIV infection. Areflexia with often ascending proximal and distal limb weakness and variable sensory loss are the typical presenting signs. Myalgias, arthralgias, and neuropathic pain are rare. Facial weakness is more common in GBS than CIDP. Respiratory failure may develop in some individuals. In GBS, the evolution of the ascending weakness develops over days to weeks; a diagnosis of CIDP requires that weakness progress over a period of at least 2 months.[26–29]

Laboratory and electroneuromyography results are similar to the results found in individuals without HIV infection.[30] CSF protein is typically elevated. One distinguishing feature of CSF seen in HIV-positive patients with GBS or CIDP compared with patients with GBS or CIDP without HIV infection is the presence of CSF pleocytosis.[25] The presence of pleocytosis in patients with GBS or CIDP who do not have a diagnosis of HIV should indicate the need for HIV testing. Electroneuromyography assessment typically reveals slowed nerve conduction velocities, delayed F-wave responses, prolonged distal latencies, and conduction block. Needle examination reveals reduced motor unit potential recruitment with denervation potentials.[28]

Treatment of HIV-associated GBS or CIDP is intravenous immune globulin and physical therapy to regain functional status. Corticosteroids and plasma exchange should be used carefully because of the greater risks of this therapy in immunocompromised patients.[26]

Hepatitis C Virus

Hepatitis C virus (HCV) is a parenterally transmitted, hepatotropic and lymphotropic RNA virus. Approximately 170 million people are infected worldwide, and HCV is a primary cause of chronic hepatitis, cirrhosis, and hepatocellular carcinoma. Along with peripheral neuropathy, HCV may be associated with cryoglobulinemia; lymphoproliferation; and various extrahepatic manifestations including sicca syndrome, inflammation of the thyroid, and porphyria cutanea tarda.[31]

In contrast to HIV-related peripheral neuropathy, neuropathy associated with HCV is related to virus-triggered immune-mediated mechanisms rather than direct nerve infection and in situ replication.[32] Neuropathy typically associated with HCV infections is a subacute, distal sensorimotor polyneuropathy but mononeuropathy and multiple mononeuritis have also been reported.[33]

Santoro and Manganelli[34] published the first large prospective survey of randomly selected consecutive series of unrelated patients with HCV infection who underwent systematic clinical and electrophysiological studies to assess the prevalence and characteristics of peripheral neuropathy in the HCV population. In their sample, using a clinical examination assessment model, peripheral neuropathy was found in 10.6% of the subjects. The electrophysiological examination revealed subclinical neuropathy in an additional 4.7% of subjects indicating that a purely clinical assessment tends to underestimate PNS involvement in patients with HCV. A strong correlation was found between the patient's age and the existence of peripheral neuropathy, and a much weaker correlation was found between the duration from first positive diagnostic laboratory test for HCV and neuropathy. This weaker correlation may be partially explained by the timing of the diagnostic workup and the time of the infection by the hepatitis virus.

Tuberculosis

The current TB epidemic is sustained by three important factors: (1) HIV and its association with new active TB cases, (2) recidivism of patients with TB in completing the prescribed course of antibiotics, and (3) increasing resistance of the tubercular strains to most effective first-line anti-TB drugs.[36] Other contributing factors include population expansion, emigration from rural areas to crowded cities, poor case detection and cure rates in impoverished countries, wars, famines, increased prevalence of diabetes mellitus, social decay, and homelessness.[37] Although exposure to *Mycobacterium tuberculosis* leads to active disease in approximately 10% of people exposed, there were a reported 9 million new active disease cases and 2 million deaths reported worldwide in 2008.[37] Nearly one third of the world's population is latently infected with *M. tuberculosis,* and 5% to 10% of infected individuals develop active disease during their lifetime. Coinfection with HIV exacerbates the risk of transitioning from latent to active infection by 5% to 15% per year and by approximately 50% over a lifetime[38]; this is illustrated by the incidence rates of TB and HIV being the highest in sub-Saharan Africa. Although active transmission of the bacterium is the primary route to active infection worldwide, researchers are seeing an increased number of active cases precipitated by coinfection with HIV).[39]

TB is a communicable infection and disease spread by inhalation of droplet nuclei (1- to 5-μm particles) containing *M. tuberculosis* expectorated by patients with active pulmonary or laryngeal TB, typically with a cough or sneeze.[37] Transmission is facilitated in small households, crowded places, and repetitive close contact. The chance of acquisition is higher in immunocompromised and older patients compared with younger and healthier individuals.

Immediately after entry of the *M. tuberculosis*, alveolar macrophages and monocytes produce proinflammatory cytokines and chemokines that serve to signal infection. Monocytes, macrophages, neutrophils, and lymphocytes migrate to the infection site but often are unable to kill the invading bacteria efficiently because *M. tuberculosis* resists the phagosome-lysosome fusion. The bacteria multiply in the phagosome and eventually escape. The released bacteria multiply extracellularly developing a new inflammatory cascade reaction. Bacteria continue to escape developing distant metastasis. The accumulation of macrophages, T cells, and other host cells (dendritic cells, fibroblasts, endothelial cells, and stromal cells) leads to the formation of granuloma at the site of infection.[38]

Diabetes mellitus and TB have a strong clinical relationship. Besides resulting in multiple complications including vascular disease, neuropathy, and increased susceptibility to infection, poorly controlled diabetes mellitus may also lead to increased susceptibility to disease caused by *M. tuberculosis* via multiple mechanisms. These mechanisms include those directly related to hyperglycemia and cellular insulinopenia as well as indirect effects on macrophage and lymphocyte function leading to diminished ability to contain the tubercular organism. The most important effector cells for containment of TB are phagocytes (alveolar macrophages and their precursor monocytes) and lymphocytes. Diabetes is known to affect chemotaxis, phagocytosis, activation, and antigen presentation by phagocytes in response to *M. tuberculosis*. In patients with diabetes, chemotaxis of monocytes is impaired, and this defect does not improve with insulin. In mice with streptozotocin-induced persistent diabetes mellitus (streptozotocin is an islet-cell toxin), macrophages had one tenth of the phagocytic activity of control mice but similar intracellular killing. In these experiments, 90% of mice died after challenge with TB compared with 10% of normal mice.[39]

Studies of diabetes mellitus and TB generally focus on active TB disease. However, in one study in a general medicine clinic in Spain, 69 (42%) of 163 patients with diabetes mellitus had a positive tuberculin skin test, suggesting a high rate of latent TB in patients with diabetes mellitus, although this could have been confounded by age, geographic location, and lack of a control group. Several case-control studies have shown that the relative odds of developing TB in patients with diabetes range from 2.44% to 8.33%. Several large-scale longitudinal cohort studies have shown similar findings.[40]

Infections, including TB, often worsen glycemic control in patients with diabetes mellitus, and poorly controlled diabetes mellitus may augment the severity of infections. Some studies suggest that TB can precipitate diabetes in persons not previously known to be diabetic.[39] Many studies have used oral glucose tolerance testing to show that patients with TB have higher rates of glucose intolerance than community controls.[39]

Nutritional status is significantly lower in patients with active pulmonary TB compared with healthy control subjects in different studies in Indonesia, England, India, and Japan.[41] The TB abscess usually resolves with antituberculous drug therapy. However, failure of improvement or deterioration in neurological status on antituberculous drug therapy is an indication of surgical decompression.[42] Cauda equina syndrome has been reported to be caused by TB. Cauda equina syndrome is a surgical emergency, and in cases related to TB, early drainage is important for early recovery of bladder and bowel control. Kallmann and Resiner studied several factors responsible for a successful outcome in cauda equina syndrome and believed that early diagnosis and early decompression are the most important predictors of a successful outcome.[43]

The standard treatment for TB in the United States and Canada is daily self-administered therapy with isoniazid (INH) for 9 months, but this regimen can often be reduced to 6 months in patients with seronegative HIV testing. The overall efficacy of INH therapy is greater than 90% in individuals who successfully complete the course of prescribed therapy. However, completion rates with ongoing clinical monitoring are only 30% to 64% and in nonclinical settings only 10%. Although INH is tolerated relatively well, there is a risk of hepatotoxicity in selected patients, especially patients with high levels of alcohol ingestion. INH can result in peripheral neuropathy, primarily a length-dependent, large-fiber and small-fiber afferent sensory impairment. The risk of INH-induced peripheral neuropathy can be decreased with adjuvant vitamin B$_6$.[42]

Varicella-Zoster Virus Infections

The varicella-zoster virus (VZV) is a human neurotropic alpha-herpesvirus. Primary infection causes varicella (chickenpox), after which the virus becomes latent in cranial nerve ganglia, dorsal root ganglia, and autonomic ganglia. Years later, most likely as a result of diminished cell-mediated immunity in elderly and immunocompromised individuals, VZV reactivates initiating a wide spectrum of neurological diagnoses, including herpes zoster, postherpetic neuralgia (PHN), vasculopathy, myelopathy, retinopathy, cerebellitis, and zoster sine herpete (ZSH).[44]

Initial VZV infection results in varicella, which is typically seen in children 1 to 9 years old but may also occur in adults.[45] Adult infections tend to be more severe than infections in children with accompanying high fever and interstitial pneumonia.[46] Infection in immunocompromised individuals causes widespread disseminated disease.[47] Varicella infection is characterized by fever and a self-limiting rash on the skin and mucosa. Headache, malaise, loss of appetite, and fever are often seen. The rash begins as macules, rapidly progressing to papules, vascularization, and eventually slough. Slough occurs 1 to 3 weeks after infection (Figs. 8-2 and 8-3).[48] Spread is via direct contact with the skin lesions or by respiratory aerosols from cough

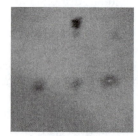

Figure 8-2 Varicella macules. Varicella is an extremely contagious disease and appears most commonly in children younger than 8 years old. The typical skin rash appears 1 or 2 days after the onset of flu-like symptoms. Skin lesions pass through four distinct stages: (1) A small area of redness appears, (2) the area of redness evolves into a papule, (3) the papule becomes a serum-filled blister, and (4) the papules dry and crust.

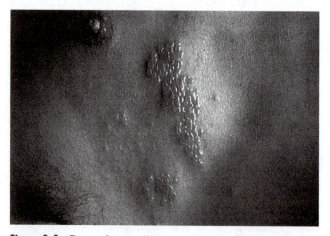

Figure 8-3 Crusted varicella-zoster lesions. Blisters associated with zoster infections typically form in one and occasionally two or three adjacent dermatomes. As with chickenpox, the blisters begin as red spots, become raised, fill with fluid, and eventually crust.

or sneeze. The diagnosis is made by the atypical vesicular rash. Treatment is symptomatic. Antiviral medications may be given to immunocompromised individuals and newborns exposed to VZV during the perinatal period.

VZV reactivation may lead to numerous peripheral neuropathic diagnoses.[49,50] Herpes zoster (zoster), the most common of the reactivation manifestations, affects 1 million individuals per year in the United States.[49] Most patients are older than age 60 or have a diagnosis leading to concomitant immune compromise.[47] The annual incidence of zoster is approximately 5 to 6.5 per 1,000 individuals at age 60 and increasing to 8 to 11 per 1,000 individuals at age 70.[49] Zoster begins with a prodromal phase characterized by pain, itching, paresthesias, dysesthesias, and allodynia in one to three dermatomes. All dermatomal segments may be affected by zoster, but most infections are found in the dorsal roots of the cervical, thoracic, and lumbar nerve roots followed by the face, typically in the ophthalmic distribution of the trigeminal nerve.

Herpes zoster ophthalmicus is often accompanied by keratitis, which can lead to blindness if unrecognized and untreated.[57] Involvement of the optic nerves with subsequent optic neuritis has occurred rarely in association with zoster ophthalmicus and other zoster eruptions.[52] Ophthalmoplegia after zoster most frequently involves cranial nerve (CN) III, CN VI, and CN VII and less frequently CN VI.[53] Zoster involving the CN VII ganglion may cause weakness or paralysis of the ipsilateral muscles of facial expression with rash in the ear canal (zoster oticus) or on the ipsilateral anterior two thirds of the tongue and hard palate.[54] Ramsay Hunt syndrome is traditionally defined as a lower motor neuron facial palsy with zoster oticus. Many patients also have hearing loss, vomiting, nausea, vertigo, and nystagmus.[55]

Cervical, thoracic, and lumbar distribution zoster may be followed by lower motor neuron weakness or paralysis in the muscles of the segmental nerve distribution. Rare cases of thoracic zoster may cause abdominal weakness leading to hernia, and there have been case reports of diaphragm weakness secondary to zoster involving CN III through CN V.[56]

Approximately 40% of patients older than age 60 with zoster develop PHN.[57] PHN is characterized by constant, severe, stabbing or burning dysesthetic pain in the segmental distribution of the involved nerve or nerves that persists months to years after infection. The etiology of PHN is unknown. Management is a challenge. Treatments including tricyclic antidepressants, neuroleptic drugs, analgesics, antivirals, and opiates have been attempted.[48]

ZSH (pain without rash) is caused by reactivation of VZV, a concept supported by patient descriptions of dermatomal distribution radicular pain in areas distinct from pain with rash in patients with zoster.

Historically, most clinicians regard ZSH as a rare occurrence of chronic radicular pain without rash with virologic confirmation. However, in recent years, the detection of VZV DNA and anti-VZV antibody in patients with meningoencephalitis, vasculopathy, myelitis, cerebral ataxia, and cranial polyneuritis, all without rash, has expanded the spectrum of ZSH. Prevalence estimates of VZV-induced pathology without rash require additional studies. ZSH should be considered in the differential diagnosis for patients with unexplained radicular pain or the above-listed diagnoses who are immunocompromised.[48]

Parasitic Infections

Parasitic infections of the nervous system can produce various signs and symptoms. Because many of the neurological symptoms produced by **parasites** are minimal or nonspecific, diagnosis can be difficult. Familiarity with the basic epidemiological characteristics, laboratory findings, and imaging studies can increase the likelihood of detection and proper treatment of parasitic infections affecting the PNS and CNS.

Cestodes, trematodes, and protozoans can infect the CNS or PNS, producing various clinical signs and symptoms.[58-61] Cestodes and trematodes are members of Platyhelminthes, a phylum characterized by an inability to live outside the host. Cestodes are often referred to as "tapeworms" and may exist in either adult or larva forms. Anatomically, cestodes are ribbon-shaped, segmentally differentiated worms with a scolex in the anterior portion used to attach to the host. In general, larval forms are more pathogenic to the human nervous system because adult forms rarely spread outside the gastrointestinal tract. Neurocysticercosis, caused by the cestode *Taenia solium,* is perhaps the most common cause of epilepsy in the world (Fig. 8-4).[59] The most common cestode is *Echinococcus,* also known as hydatid disease, and is endemic in the Mediterranean, the Middle East, Latin America, and the Arctic.[60] Epidemiological data support transmission from dogs, cats, foxes, and rodents to humans. *Echinococcus* resides in the intestinal tract of dogs and other canids. It quickly transits to the liver, blood, lymph, lung, pericardium, and brain. Humans and sheep are intermediate hosts and acquire infection by ingesting eggs eliminated by infected animals. Human infection results in the formation of hydatid cysts that contain serous fluid. Most of the cysts occur in the liver. Hydatid infections often remain undetected until the cyst becomes problematic, which usually occurs when the cyst bursts spreading infection and resulting in the development of space-occupying lesions primarily in the CNS. Clinical signs and symptoms include motor and sensory neuropathy; upper motor signs such as spasticity, clonus, and Babinski sign; and clinical signs

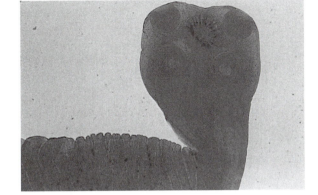

Figure 8-4 Taeniasis in humans is a parasitic infection caused by the tapeworm species *T. saginata* (beef tapeworm), *T. solium* (pork tapeworm), and *T. asiatica* (Asian tapeworm). Humans can become infected with these tapeworms by eating raw and undercooked beef (*T. saginata*) or pork (*T. solium* and *T. asiatica*). People with taeniasis may not know they have a tapeworm infection because symptoms are usually mild or nonexistent. Parasitic flatworms (tapeworms) tend to occur in areas that lack adequate sanitation. Eggs are generally ingested through food, water, or soil contaminated with host feces.

of increasing intracranial pressure. Cyst removal is the most effective treatment.[61]

Sparganosis is an infection caused by the larval form of tapeworms from the genus *Spirometra*. *Spirometra* are parasites of cats, dogs, birds, and humans that eat raw and undercooked fish. Sparganosis is common in the Gulf states of the United States. Clinically, infected patients develop a discrete subcutaneous nodule that migrates locally. Metastasis to the brain is common with seizures, slowly progressing motor and sensory hemiparesis, and headache. Diagnosis is made based on eosinophilia and biopsy.[62]

Trematodes, also referred to as "flukes," can invade the nervous system secondarily after a primary infection occurring in the blood, liver, intestinal mucosa, or lung. Most species are hermaphroditic and are capable of reproduction within the host. Trematodes have two anterior suckers used to attach to the host (Fig. 8-5). *Paragonimus* is the only mammalian lung fluke capable of infecting humans. An estimated 20 million people are infected worldwide. Human infection is almost always acquired through incorrectly cooked freshwater crab or crayfish. Domesticated cats, dogs, and pigs can harbor the fluke and transmit it to humans. Initial infections produce intestinal symptoms. There are often migratory subcutaneous masses typically located in the abdominal region. With time, migration to the lung parenchyma occurs. Adult worms may live 20 or more years. Long-standing infection typically results in worm transmission to brain tissue. CNS infection can produce meningoencephalitis, headache, weakness

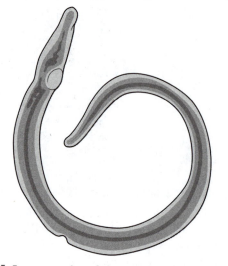

Figure 8-5 Long-standing fluke parasites are a type of parasitic flatworm or trematode that can migrate from host tissue (primarily digestive) to the central nervous system resulting in upper motor neuron and sensory impairment.

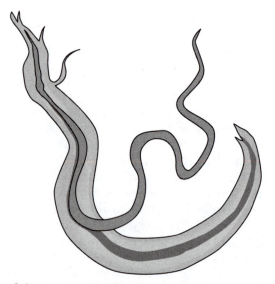

Figure 8-6 *S. mansoni* is a human trematode parasite that is the major disease agent for schistosomiasis. Early symptoms may mimic scabies. Diagnosis is confirmed via eggs in the stool.

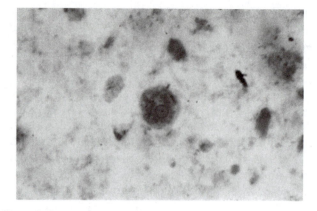

Figure 8-7 Numerous species of parasitic protozoa using various vectors can infect the human body. Often the intestine is the site of initial infection, but infection may also begin in capillaries, skin, stomach, and blood. Neurological symptoms often depend on the site of migration.

(general or focal), nausea, and seizures. Diagnosis is based on serum and CSF eosinophilia, biopsy specimen showing egg material, and serum antibody detection testing.[63]

Schistosomiasis, also known as bilharziasis, is an extremely common parasite, infecting more than 300 million people worldwide per year. CNS and PNS involvement has been reported in three of the species: *Schistosoma mansoni*, *Schistosoma haematobium*, and *Schistosoma japonicum*. Humans and at least 30 other mammals are possible hosts (Fig. 8-6).[63] Infection is spread through contaminated water sources including drinking, bathing, washing clothes, washing dishes, and walking barefoot. Initial infection occurs when the forked tail penetrates the skin. The tail is then shed, and the larva migrates into the venous system. Clinical symptoms depend on which species infects; each species has a different corporal locus. *S. mansoni* infects the inferior mesenteric vein, *S. haematobium* infects the peri-bladder veins, and *S. japonicum* infects the superior mesenteric veins. Eggs from *S. japonicum* tend to metastasize to the brain, whereas the larger eggs of *S. mansoni* and *S. haematobium* typically metastasize to the spinal cord. The metastasized eggs do not develop into worms; rather, their presence initiates an inflammatory cascade reaction culminating in a granulomatous response as tissues attempt to wall off the invading parasite.[65] After a period of time, the granulomas become exudative, invasive, and necrotic, damaging local upper motor neuron and lower motor neuron tissue beginning weeks after the acute infection. Lower motor neuron involvement often mimics cauda equina syndrome or conus medullaris syndrome.[66] Diagnosis is made by biopsy or detection of eggs in stool or urine. For patients with spinal cord infection, CSF enzyme-linked immunosorbent assay for immunoglobulin G against egg antigens is recommended. Praziquantel is effective against all *Schistosoma* species and is curative in 90% of patients.[67]

Protozoans are classified by mode of locomotion and can be either free-living or obligate parasites. The spectrum of clinical symptoms and signs of protozoa infections is diverse, and nervous system infection may occur secondary to distant infection. Because of their large size, protozoan infections are easily identified via light microscopy (Fig. 8-7). American trypanosomiasis, also known as Chagas disease, is endemic to South and Central American countries. With increased emigration and urbanization, infection is becoming more common in the United States. Infection is spread by the reduviid bug (*Triatoma infestans*) or by ingesting meat of the guinea pig.[68] Infection may also be spread via blood transfusion or organ transplantation. The protozoa may pass through the placenta to the fetus. Primary infection occurs when the reduviid bug takes a blood meal from the host and leaves fecal material behind containing *Trypanosoma cruzi* eggs. The eggs remain on the skin until embedded through itching of the bug bite. The cells migrate quickly via binary fusion and metastasize to distant sites through venous and arterial blood circulation.[69] Protozoa reproduce within host cells, and when the host cell ruptures, additional vectors are created.

Acute infections result in malaise, myalgia, headache, asthenia, and anorexia. Romaña's sign (unilateral or bilateral palpebral edema) is pathognomonic for Chagas disease. Cardiac failure and intestinal symptoms are the major cause of morbidity and mortality. In Brazil, the primary cause of acute congestive heart failure is Chagas disease. Only 5% of infected persons develop severe complications. Neurological symptoms are limited to meningitis with headache, malaise, and photophobia. Only acute Chagas disease can be eradicated by treatment. Chronic infections can be treated symptomatically only. Benznidazole is the treatment of choice.[70]

African trypanosomiasis, also known as human African trypanosomiasis and sleeping sickness, is endemic to sub-Saharan Africa—primarily in the Democratic Republic of the Congo and Uganda. Widespread political unrest and poor reporting procedures most likely diminish the actual number of cases. Officially, the World Health Organization reports approximately 300,000 new cases in Africa each year.[71] The tsetse fly is the vector for infection. The prevalence of infection is directly related to the concentration of tsetse flies in a particular region. Only a few dozen cases have been reported in the United States over the past few years with most of these occurring in persons with recent travel to the African subcontinent. Following the fly bite, a superficial chancre develops at the site of the bite. Larvae within the chancre migrate through blood and lymphatic vessels to the CNS, maturing and reproducing during the migratory process. When the infection reaches the CNS, an immune response is created with a severe inflammatory response. Peri-infection edema causes the clinical findings of behavioral abnormalities, a reversal in sleep patterns (sleep during the day and insomnia at night), hypothermia or hyperthermia, ataxia, hypertonus, and akinesia. Fatal arrhythmia secondary to parasitic invasion of the heart is the most common cause of death. Definitive diagnosis is made through blood, CSF, or chancre sampling. Drug regimens are fairly effective, although drug resistance is emerging.[71]

Chronic Fatigue Syndrome

Chronic fatigue syndrome (CFS) is the most common name given to a variably debilitating disorder or disorders generally defined by persistent fatigue unrelated to exertion, not substantially relieved by rest, and accompanied by the presence of other specific symptoms for a minimum of 6 months.[72] The disorder may also be referred to as postviral fatigue syndrome (when the condition arises after a flu-like illness) or myalgic encephalomyelitis.[73] The disease process in CFS displays a range of neurological, immunological, and endocrine system abnormalities. Although classified by the World Health Organization under diseases of the nervous system, the etiology of CFS is unknown, and there is no diagnostic laboratory test or biomarker to confirm the presence or absence of the disorder.[74]

Intermittent fatigue is a common symptom in many illnesses, but CFS is a multisystemic disease and is rare by comparison. Symptoms of CFS include postexertional malaise; unrefreshing sleep; widespread myalgia and arthralgia affecting the axial and appendicular skeletons; cognitive deficits; chronic, often severe mental and physical exhaustion; and other characteristic symptoms in a previously healthy and active person. Patients with CFS may report additional symptoms, including patterned or unpatterned muscle weakness, hypersensitivity to sensory stimuli, and orthostatic hypotension with positional changes. Vague symptoms of depression, cardiopulmonary symptoms, a depressed immune system, and respiratory problems have been reported. It is unclear if these additional symptoms represent comorbid or reactive symptoms to CFS or the medication used to treat the disorder or conditions produced by an underlying etiology of CFS.[75]

The prevalence of CFS varies widely, ranging from 7 to 3,000 cases of CFS for every 100,000 adults, but national health organizations have estimated more than 1 million Americans and approximately a quarter of a million people in the United Kingdom have CFS. CFS occurs most often in people in their 40s and 50s, more often in women than men, and is less prevalent among children and adolescents. A prognosis study review calculated a median full recovery rate of 5% among untreated patients and median improvement rate of approximately 40% compared with premorbid status.[76]

There is agreement on the genuine threat to health, happiness, and productivity posed by CFS, but various physicians' groups, researchers, and patient advocates promote different nomenclature, diagnostic criteria, etiologic hypotheses, and treatments, resulting in marked controversy of the disorder.[76] The name CFS itself is controversial; many patients and advocacy groups as well as some experts want the name changed because they believe that it stigmatizes by not conveying the seriousness of the illness.[77]

There are no characteristic laboratory, clinical, or imaging abnormalities to diagnose CFS, and testing is used to rule out other potential causes for symptoms. When symptoms are attributable to certain other conditions, the diagnosis of CFS is excluded.[78] Rehabilitation therapists should be aware of the existence of this diagnosis and the possibility that symptoms may be related to PNS impairment.

Parsonage-Turner Syndrome

Parsonage-Turner syndrome is a term used to describe a neuritis involving the brachial plexus. It was first described by Feiburg in 1897, who reported a case of unilateral brachial plexopathy associated with an influenza infection. In 1948, Parsonage and Turner described 136 cases of plexopathy and gave it the name "shoulder girdle syndrome." They described a typical presentation of sudden onset of shoulder pain without trauma followed by flaccid paralysis of the shoulder girdle, arm, forearm, and hand at which time the pain subsided. Associated sensory symptoms may or may not be present. Complete recovery of strength occurred in 90% of patients within 3 years. The remaining cohort had residual weakness. More recent research indicates the incidence as 1.64 cases per 100,000 population with men being affected more than women. Peak incidence occurs in the third and seventh decades of life. There is no relationship between hand dominance. The condition occurs bilaterally in 3% of the cases.[80]

Treatment is supportive. In their review of 99 patients, Tsairis et al.[81] found no significant benefit of oral corticosteroids. There was no substantial support of physical therapy modalities such as ultrasound or electrical stimulation. Surgery is indicated only for the small cohort of patients showing no improvement. Surgical intervention includes tendon transfers and shoulder stabilization procedures. A few patients may experience relapse of symptoms, but these tend to be less severe than the original symptoms and of much shorter duration.[85,86] Rehabilitative treatment is directed at maintaining articular passive range of motion, strengthening of the existing and reinnervated musculature, and prevention of glenohumeral subluxation.

Leprosy

The best way to understand the clinical and functional impact of leprosy (Hansen's disease) is to consider it as two conjoined diseases. The first is a chronic mycobacterial infection that may elicit an extraordinary range of cellular immunity responses in humans. The second

is a peripheral neuropathy that is not mediated by the infectious agent, but rather by the immune response. Leprosy, common throughout all of written history, remains a problematic disease in many parts of the world. The number of new cases reported each year (500,000 to 700,000 worldwide) has remained constant for the past decade.[87]

The precise mechanism of transmission of *Mycobacterium leprae* is unknown.[88] No highly effective vaccine has yet been developed.[89] No clinical tests for early diagnosis have been found for a clinically unapparent disease.[87] Leprosy manifests with a wide range of clinical, histopathological, and functional manifestations. This great diversity puzzled and frustrated clinicians and researchers until it was found that this diversity was based on the ability of the host to develop an individualized cellular immune response to *M. leprae*.

The five-part Ridley-Jopling classification of patients with leprosy identifies patients based on the degree of cell-mediated immunity. At one extreme are patients with a high degree of cell-mediated immunity and delayed hypersensitivity presenting with a single, well-demarcated lesion with central hypopigmentation and hypoesthesia. At the other extreme are patients who appear to have no resistance at all to *M. leprae*. These patients present with numerous, poorly demarcated raised or nodular lesions on all parts of the body. Biopsy specimens of the lesions reveal a large number of macrophages and dermis containing numerous individual bacilli and grouped microcolonies of bacilli called globi. This highly nonresistant form of leprosy is called polar lepromatous leprosy.[87]

In contrast to TB and other acquired infections, leprosy has not been observed to have an increased prevalence in individuals with a diagnosis of HIV in areas where both diseases are endemic. Suggestions for this phenomenon include the relatively low virulence of *M. leprae* or that patients with HIV often die before leprosy—with its long incubation period—becomes apparent (Fig. 8-8).[88]

The diagnosis of leprosy is made by a full-thickness skin biopsy specimen obtained from the advancing margin of active lesion, fixed in neutral buffered formalin, embedded in paraffin, and examined microscopically. The primary characteristics of a positive biopsy specimen include the classic histological patterns of the host response in hematoxylin and eosin–stained sections, the involvement of the cutaneous afferent nerves, and the identification of non–acid-fast bacilli within the nerves using the Fite stain. No serological tests are available for the routine laboratory diagnosis of leprosy. An enzyme-linked immunosorbent assay and related immunoassay has been developed to detect antibodies to *M. leprae*, and these have been used in epidemiological studies, but the sensitivity and specificity of the test are below satisfactory levels to enable the test to be used as a diagnostic tool (Table 8-3).[89]

Type 1 leprosy reactions occur in patients in the borderline (less severe) portion of the Ridley-Jopling scale. These are often called "reversible reactions" because early observations suggested that after the reaction has subsided, clinical and histopathological evidence indicated that the immunity in the lesions had increased. Type 1 reactions manifest as indurated and erythematous lesions with edema and progressive sensory greater than motor peripheral neuropathy. These reactions develop gradually and may last for weeks. Patients with type 2 lesions experience an abrupt onset of crops of tender, erythematous nodules that develop throughout the body.[90] Along with the

neuropathy, these patients often experience iridocyclitis, episcleritis, orchitis, myalgias, arthralgias, and myositis.[91]

The neuropathic process of leprosy is directly related to the *M. leprae* infection, and this effect is unique among bacterial pathogens.[87] With infection, there is a strong predilection of the *M. leprae* bacillus to migrate to peripheral nerves.[91] The infection aggregates in the epineural lymphatics and blood vessels and enters the endoneural compartment via the vasa nervorum. If there is no or limited effective immune response, the bacilli proliferate within macrophages and Schwann cells. The resultant perineural and endoneural inflammation and thickening, angiogenesis, and laying down of aberrant connective tissue over time lead to a decrease in nerve conduction velocity and eventually neurapraxic, axontometic, and neurotometic lesions. Infection tends to begin distally and move proximally with the fingers and toes most often infected. There also seems to be a predilection for the facial nerve.[87] Typical pathogenesis in untreated or antibiotic-resistant disease is a progression of lesions with concomitant ascending sensory loss and motor loss.

Treatment is antibiotics. Dapsone, introduced in the 1950s, quickly became the standard treatment, but poor compliance in many areas quickly led to dapsone-resistant leprosy. Rifampin and clofazimine were later introduced, but antibiotic-resistant strains again began to appear. More recently, multidrug cocktails have proved to be an effective intervention, but even with the newer therapies, the number of new cases reported per year has remained relatively constant. Relapse, with a rate of 20 per 1,000 persons, has been reported in patients treated with a 2-year course of multidrug therapy.[92,93]

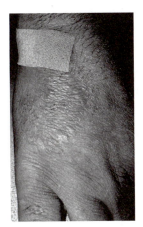

Figure 8-8 Leprous hands. Contrary to folklore, leprosy (Hansen's disease) does not result in body parts "falling off." Rather, secondary infections may result in interventional amputations. Fingers and toes may become shortened and deformed secondary to absorption of cartilage, bone, and connective tissue.

Table 8-3	**Comparison of Clinical Features of Types 1 and 2 Immunological Leprosy Reactions**	
Parameter	Type 1	Type 2
Onset of reaction	Gradual, over weeks to months	Abrupt
Cutaneous lesions	Increased erythema and induration of previously existing lesions	Widespread and numerous erythematous, tender nodules on face, extremities, or trunk, without relationship to prior lesions
Neuritis	Primarily sensory, frequent, often severe	Primarily sensory, frequent, often severe
Systemic symptoms	Malaise	Fever, malaise, chills, loss of appetite
Histopathological features	No specific findings	Polymorphonuclear cell infiltrates in lesions <24 hours old
Course (untreated)	Weeks or months	Days to weeks
Treatment	Corticosteroids	Thalidomide, corticosteroids

Data from Ridley DS, Jopling WH. Classification of leprosy according to immunity. A five-group system. *Int J Lepr Other Mycobact Dis* 1996;34(3):255–273; Modlin RL. Th1-Th2 paradigm: insights from leprosy. *J Invest Dermatol.* 1994;102(6):828–832; James WD, Berger TG. *Andrews' Diseases of the Skin: Clinical Dermatology.* Philadelphia: Saunders; 2006; Jardim MR, Antunes SL, Santos AR. Criteria for diagnosis of pure neural leprosy. *J Neurol.* 2003;250(7):806–809; and Mendiratta V, Khan A, Jain A. Primary neuritic leprosy: a reappraisal at a tertiary care hospital. *Indian J Lepr.* 2006;78(3):261–267.

CASE STUDY

JB, a 46-year-old man, arrived in the physical therapy clinic with a chief complaint of bilateral knee swelling and pain that he believed was due to a long weekend of walking through the woods while hunting. On physical examination, the therapist noted synovitis and tenderness at both knees with a corresponding antalgic gait pattern. The pain was most severe with sit-to-stand transfers and stair climbing. Past medical history was unremarkable. The therapist found no other joint involvement. Neurological examination was unremarkable. Integument examination revealed a red macule that enlarged into a large round circular patch with some central clearing on the patient's right shoulder.

Case Study Questions

1. Considering the history of walking in the woods and the red macule, the therapist should consider which of the following diagnoses?
   a. Poliomyositis
   b. Lyme disease
   c. HIV
   d. Protozoan infection

2. The description of the integument may be labeled as which of the following?
   a. Erythema migrans
   b. Kaposi sarcoma
   c. Varicella
   d. Varicella slough

3. Which of the following is the bacterium that causes Lyme disease?
   a. *Proteus mirabilis*
   b. *Borrelia burgdorferi*
   c. *Escherichia coli*
   d. *Salmonella*

4. Lyme disease may result in impairments to which of the following systems?
   a. Integument
   b. Neurological
   c. Cardiopulmonary
   d. All of the above

5. Treatment for Lyme disease includes which of the following?
   a. Antimicrobials
   b. Radiation
   c. Chemotherapy
   d. Cauterization

References

1. Coyle BS, Strickland GT, Liang YY, Pena C, McCarter R, Israel E. The public health impact of Lyme disease in Maryland. *J Infect Dis.* 1996;173:1260–1262.

2. Wormser GP. Clinical practice. Early Lyme disease. *N Engl J Med.* 2006;354:2794–2801.

3. Tibbles CD, Edlow JA. Does this patient have erythema migrans? *JAMA.* 2007;297:2617–2627.

4. Centers for Disease Control and Prevention. Lyme disease—United States, 2003–2005. *MMWR Morb Mortal Wkly Rep.* 2007;56:573–576.

5. Nowakowski J, McKenna D, Nadelman RB. Failure of treatment with cephalexin for Lyme disease. *Arch Fam Med.* 2000;9:563–567.

6. Sigal LH. Toward a more complete appreciation of the clinical spectrum of *Borrelia burgdorferi* infection: early Lyme disease without erythema migrans. *Am J Med.* 2003;114:74–75.

7. Sigal LH. Summary of the first 100 patients seen at a Lyme disease referral center. *Am J Med.* 1990;88:577–581.

8. Centers for Disease Control and Prevention. Recommendations for test performance and interpretation from the Second National Conference on Serologic Diagnosis of Lyme Disease. *MMWR Morb Mortal Wkly Rep.* 1995;44:590–591.

9. Aguero-Rosenfeld ME, Wang G, Schwartz I, Wormser GP. Diagnosis of Lyme borreliosis. *Clin Microbiol Rev.* 2005;18:484–509.

10. Shapiro ED, Dattwyler R, Nadelman RB, Wormser GP. Response to meta-analysis of Lyme borreliosis symptoms. *Int J Epidemiol.* 2005;34:1437–1439.

11. Cairns V, Godwin J. Post-Lyme borreliosis syndrome: a meta-analysis of reported symptoms. *Int J Epidemiol.* 2005;34:1340–1345.

12. Shadick NA, Phillips CB, Sangha O. Musculoskeletal and neurologic outcomes in patients with previously treated Lyme disease. *Ann Intern Med.* 1999;131:919–926.

13. Kalish RA, Kaplan RF, Taylor E, Jones-Woodward L, Workman K, Steere AC. Evaluation of study patients with Lyme disease, 10–20-year follow-up. *J Infect Dis.* 2001;183:453–460.

14. Klempner MS. Controlled trials of antibiotic treatment in patients with post-treatment chronic Lyme disease. *Vector Borne Zoonotic Dis.* 2002;2:255–263.

15. Heymann DL, Aylward RB. Eradicating polio. *N Engl J Med.* 2004;351:1275–1277.

16. Kidd D, Williams A, Howard RS. Classical diseases revisited—poliomyelitis. *Postgrad Med J.* 1996;72:641–647.

17. Fine PE. Poliomyelitis: very small risks and very large risks. *Lancet Neurol.* 2004;3:703–710.

18. Dalakas MC, Elder G, Hallett M, et al. A long-term follow-up study of patients with post-poliomyelitis neuromuscular symptoms. *N Engl J Med.* 1986;314:959–963.

19. Kidd D, Howard RS, Williams AJ, Heatley FW, Panayiotopoulos CP, Spencer GT. Late functional deterioration following paralytic poliomyelitis. *QJM.* 1997;90:189–196.

20. Sejvar JJ. West Nile virus and poliomyelitis. *Neurology.* 2004;63:206–207.

21. Howard RS. Late post-polio functional deterioration. *Pract Neurol.* 2003;3:66–77.

22. Kilpatrick DR, Nottay B, Yang CF, Yang SJ, Mulders MN, Holloway BP. Group specific identification of poliovirus by PCR using primers containing mixed-base or deoxyinosine residues at positions of codon degeneracy. *J Clin Microbiol.* 1996;34:2990–2996.

23. Alexander LN, Seward JF, Santibanez TA, et al. Vaccine policy changes and epidemiology of poliomyelitis in the United States. *JAMA.* 2004;292:1696–1701.

24. Weiss RA. How does HIV cause AIDS? *Science.* 1993;260(5112):1273–1279.

25. Douek DC, Roederer M, Koup RA. Emerging concepts in the immunopathogenesis of AIDS. *Annu Rev Med.* 2009;60: 471–484.

26. CDC. HIV AIDS resources: prevention in the United States at a critical crossroads. http://cdc.gov/hiv/resources/reports/hiv_prev_us.htm.

27. Time from HIV-1 seroconversion to AIDS and death before widespread use of highly active antiretroviral therapy: a collaborative re-analysis. Collaborative Group on AIDS Incubation and HIV Survival including the CASCADE EU Concerted Action. Concerted Action on SeroConversion to AIDS and Death in Europe. *Lancet.* 2000;355(9210): 1131–1137.

28. Schneider MF, Gange SJ, Williams CM, et al. Patterns of the hazard of death after AIDS through the evolution of antiretroviral therapy: 1984–2004. *AIDS.* 2005;19(17): 2009–2018.

29. Reeves JD, Doms RW. Human immunodeficiency virus type 2. *J Gen Virol.* 2002;83(Pt 6):1253–1265.

30. Agnello V, Chung RT, Kaplan LM. A role for hepatitis C virus infection in type II cryoglobulinemia. *N Engl J Med.* 1992;327:1490–1495.

31. Agnello V, Abel G. Localization of hepatitis C virus in cutaneous vasculitic lesions in patients with type II cryoglobulinemia. *Arthritis Rheum.* 1997;40:2007–2015.

32. Bonetti B, Scardoni M, Monaco S. Hepatitis C virus infection of peripheral nerves in type II cryoglobulinaemia. *Virchows Arch.* 1999;434:533–535.

33. Smith DK, Grohskopf LA, Black RJ, et al; U.S. Department of Health and Human Services. Antiretroviral postexposure prophylaxis after sexual, injection-drug use or other non-occupational exposure to HIV. *MMWR Recomm Rep.* 2005; 54(RR-2):1–20.

34. Santoro L, Manganelli C. Prevalence and characteristics of peripheral neuropathy in hepatitis C virus population. *J Neurol Neurosurg Psychiatry.* 2006;77(5):626–629.

35. Caruntu FA, Benea L. Acute hepatitis C virus infection. *J Gastrointest Liver Dis.* 2006;15(3):249–256.

36. Kamal SM. Acute hepatitis C: a systematic review. *Am J Gastroenterol.* 2008;103(5):1283–1297.

37. Villano SA, Vlahov D, Nelson KE, Cohn S, Thomas DL. Persistence of viremia and the importance of long-term follow-up after acute hepatitis C infection. *Hepatology.* 1999; 29(3):908–914.

38. Parish T, Stoker N. Mycobacteria: bugs and bugbears (two steps forward and one step back). *Mol Biotechnol.* 1999;13(3): 191–200.

39. van Soolingen D, Hoogenboezem T, de Haas PE. A novel pathogenic taxon of the *Mycobacterium tuberculosis* complex. *Int J Syst Bacteriol.* 1997;47(4):1236–1245.

40. Restrepo BI. Convergence of the tuberculosis and diabetes epidemics: renewal of old acquaintances. *Clin Infect Dis.* 1997;45(4):436–438.

41. Nijland HM, Ruslami R, Stalenhoef JE, et al. Exposure to rifampicin is strongly reduced in patients with tuberculosis and type 2 diabetes. *Clin Infect Dis.* 2006; 43(7):848–854.

42. Nnoaham KE, Clarke A. Low serum vitamin D levels and tuberculosis: a systematic review and meta-analysis. *Int J Epidemiol.* 2008;37(1):113–119.

43. Kallmann FJ, Reisner D. Twin studies on the significance of genetic factors in tuberculosis. *Am Rev Tuberc.* 1942;16: 593–617.

44. Kaufmann S. Protection against tuberculosis: cytokines, T cells and macrophages. *Ann Rheum Dis.* 1996;61(Suppl 2): ii54–58.

45. Skeiky YA, Sadoff JC. Advances in tuberculosis vaccine strategies. *Nat Rev Microbiol.* 2006;4(6):469–476.

46. Ibanga H, Brookes R, Hill P, et al. Early clinical trials with a new tuberculosis vaccine, MVA85A, in tuberculosis-endemic countries: issues in study design. *Lancet Infect Dis.* 2006;6(8): 522–528.

47. Steiner I, Kennedy PG, Pachner AR. The neurotropic herpes viruses: herpes simplex and varicella-zoster. *Lancet Neurol.* 2007;6(11):1015–1028.

48. Johnson RW, Dworkin RH. Treatment of herpes zoster and postherpetic neuralgia. *BMJ.* 2003;326(7392):748–750.

49. Kennedy PG. Varicella-zoster virus latency in human ganglia. *Rev Med Virol.* 2002;12(5):327–334.

50. Peterslund NA. Herpesvirus infection: an overview of the clinical manifestations. *Scand J Infect Dis Suppl.* 1991;80: 15–20.

51. Jones AD. Infection. *Viral Immunol.* 2003;16(3):243–258.

52. Dworkin RH, Johnson RW, Breuer J. Recommendations for the management of herpes zoster. *Clin Infect Dis.* 2006; 44(Suppl 1):S1–26.

53. Donahue JG, Choo PW, Manson JE, Platt R. The incidence of herpes zoster. *Arch Intern Med.* 2005;155(15):1605–1609.

54. Araújo LQ, Macintyre CR, Vujacich C. Epidemiology and burden of herpes zoster and post-herpetic neuralgia in Australia, Asia and South America. *Herpes.* 1997;14(Suppl 2): 40A–44A.

55. Cunningham AL, Breuer J, Dwyer DE, et al. The prevention and management of herpes zoster. *Med J Aust.* 2008;188(3): 171–176.

56. Holmes G, Kaplan J, Gantz N, et al. Chronic fatigue syndrome: a working case definition. *Ann Intern Med.* 1998;108(3):387–389.

57. Helgason S, Sigurdsson JA, Gudmundsson S. The clinical course of herpes zoster: a prospective study in primary care. *Eur J Gen Pract.* 1996;2(1):12–16.

58. World Health Organization (WHO). Prevention and control of schistosomiasis and soil transmitted helminthiasis: report of WHO Expert Committee. *WHO Technical Report Series, No. 912.* Geneva: WHO; 2002.

59. UNAIDS/WHO. AIDS epidemic update 2006. http://www.un-ngls.org/spip.php?page=article_s&id_article=186.

60. Grossman Z, Meier-Schellersheim M, Sousa AE, Victorino RM, Paul WE. CD4+ T-cell depletion in HIV infection: are we closer to understanding the cause. *Nat Med.* 2002;8: 319–323.

61. Borkow G, Bentwich Z. Chronic immune activation associated with chronic helminthic and human immunodeficiency virus infections: role of hypo-responsiveness and energy. *Clin Microbiol Rev.* 2004;17(4): 1012–1030.

62. MacDonald AS, Araujo MI, Pearce EJ. Immunology of parasite helminth infections. *Infect Immun.* 2002;70: 427–433.

63. Secor WE, Shah A, Mwinzi PM, Ndenga BA, Watta CO, Karanja DM. Increased density of human immunodeficiency virus type 1 co-receptors CCR5 and CXCR4 on the surfaces of CD4+ T cells and monocytes of patients with *Schistosoma mansoni* infection. *Infect Immun.* 2003;71: 6668–6671.

64. Kalinkovich A, Borkow G, Weisman Z, Tsimanis A, Stein M, Bentwich Z. Increased CCR5 and CXCR4 expression in Ethiopians living in Israel: environmental and constitutive factors. *Clin Immunol.* 2001;100(1):107–117.

65. Shapira-Nahor O, Kalinkovich A, Weisman Z, et al. Increased susceptibility to HIV-1 infection of peripheral blood mononuclear cells from chronically immune activated individuals. *AIDS.* 1998;12:1731–1733.

66. Fincham JE, Markus MB, Adams VJ. Could control of soil-transmitted helminthic infection influence the HIV/AIDS pandemic? *Acta Trop.* 2003;86(2–3):315–333.

67. Gupta S, Narang S, Nunavath V, Singh S. Chronic diarrhea in HIV patients: prevalence of coccidian parasites. *Indian J Med Microbiol.* 2008;26:172–175.

68. Kelly P, Todd J, Sianongo S, et al. Susceptibility to intestinal infection and diarrhea in Zambian adults in relation to HIV status and CD4 count. *BMC Gastroenterol.* 2009;9:7.

69. Habtamu B, Kloos H. Intestinal parasitism. In: Berhane Y, Hailemariam D, Kloos H, eds. *Epidemiology and Ecology of Health and Diseases in Ethiopia.* Addis Ababa: Shama Books; 2006:519–538.

70. Cheesbrough M. *District Laboratory Practice in Tropical Countries, Part 1.* Cambridge: Cambridge University Press; 2000.

71. Awole M, Gebre-Selassie S, Kassa T, Kibru G. Prevalence of intestinal parasites in HIV-infected adult patients in southwestern Ethiopia. *Ethiop J Health Dev.* 2003;17:71–78.

72. Sharpe M, Archard L, Banatvala J, et al. A report—chronic fatigue syndrome: guidelines for research. *J R Soc Med.* 2006; 84(2):118–121.

73. Carruthers BM, Jain AK, De Meirleir KL, et al. Myalgic encephalomyelitis/chronic fatigue syndrome: clinical working definition, diagnostic and treatment protocols. *Journal of Chronic Fatigue Syndrome.* 2006;11(1):7–97.

74. Reeves WC, Lloyd A, Vernon SD, et al. Identification of ambiguities in the 1994 chronic fatigue syndrome research case definition and recommendations for resolution. *BMC Health Serv Res.* 2006;3(1):25.

75. Jason LA, Corradi K, Torres-Harding S, Taylor RR, King C. Chronic fatigue syndrome: the need for subtypes. *Neuropsychol Rev.* 2005;15(1):29–58.

76. Whistler T, Unger ER, Nisenbaum R, Vernon SD. Integration of gene expression, clinical, and epidemiological data to characterize chronic fatigue syndrome. *J Transl Med.* 2006;1(1):10.

77. Kennedy G, Abbot NC, Spence V, Underwood C, Belch JJ. The specificity of the CDC-1994 criteria for chronic fatigue syndrome: comparison of health status in three groups of patients who fulfill the criteria. *Ann Epidemiol.* 2004;14(2): 95–100.

78. Whiting P, Bagnall AM, Sowden AJ, Cornell JE, Mulrow CD, Ramirez G. Interventions for the treatment and management of chronic fatigue syndrome: a systematic review. *JAMA.* 2006;286(11):1360–1368.

79. Parsonage MJ, Turner JW. Neuralgic amyotrophy; the shoulder-girdle syndrome. *Lancet* 1948;1(6513):973–978.

80. Magee KR, DeJong RN. Paralytic brachial neuritis. *JAMA.* 1960;174:1258–1262.

81. Tsairis P, Dyck PJ, Mulder DW. Natural history of brachial plexus neuropathy. Report of 99 patients. *Arch Neurol.* 1972; 27:109–117.

82. McCarty EC, Tsairis P, Warren RF. Brachial neuritis. *Clin Orthop.* 1999;368:37–43.

83. Misamore GW, Lehman DE. Parsonage-Turner syndrome (acute brachial neuritis). *J Bone Joint Surg Am.* 1996;78: 1405–1408.

84. Sarikaya S, Sumer M, Ozdolap S, Erdem CZ. Magnetic resonance neurography diagnosed brachial neuritis: a case report. *Arch Phys Med Rehabil.* 2005;86:1058–1059.

85. Sasaki S, Takeshita F, Okuda K, Ishii N. Mycobacterium leprae and leprosy: a compendium. *Microbiol Immunol.* 2006; 45(11):729–736.

86. Leprosy disabilities: magnitude of the problem. *Wkly Epidemiol Rec.* 1995;70(38):269–275.

87. Smith DS. Leprosy overview. *eMedicine Infectious Diseases.* http://emedicine.medscape.com/article/220455-overview.

88. Singh N, Manucha V, Bhattacharya SN, Arora VK, Bhatia A. Pitfalls in the cytological classification of borderline leprosy in the Ridley-Jopling scale. *Diagn Cytopathol.* 2004;30(6): 386–388.

89. Ridley DS, Jopling WH. Classification of leprosy according to immunity. A five-group system. *Int J Lepr Other Mycobact Dis* 1996;34(3):255–273.

90. Modlin RL. Th1-Th2 paradigm: insights from leprosy. *J Invest Dermatol.* 1994;102(6):828–832.

91. James WD, Berger TG. *Andrews' Diseases of the Skin: Clinical Dermatology.* Philadelphia: Saunders; 2006.

92. Jardim MR, Antunes SL, Santos AR. Criteria for diagnosis of pure neural leprosy. *J Neurol.* 2003;250(7): 806–809.

93. Mendiratta V, Khan A, Jain A. Primary neuritic leprosy: a reappraisal at a tertiary care hospital. *Indian J Lepr.* 2006; 78(3):261–267.

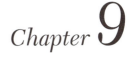

Chapter **9**

Peripheral Neuropathy Associated With Nutritional Deficiency

Joseph I. Boullata, PharmD, RPh, BCNSP

"He that takes medicine and neglects diet wastes the skills of the physician."
—Ancient Chinese Proverb

Objectives

On completion of this chapter, the student/practitioner will be able to:

- List the common presenting signs and symptoms of nutrition-related peripheral nerve injury.
- Describe the etiologies of alcohol-related neuropathy.
- Discuss the role of "balanced" nutrients in homeostasis.
- List and describe diagnostic neuropathic patterns related to common nutritional deficiencies.
- Explain the complex roles of vitamins and nutrients in peripheral nerve health.

Key Terms

- Macronutrient
- Mineral
- Neuropathies
- Nutrient
- Nutritional deficiency
- Vitamin

Introduction

Localization of lesions in neurology is paramount to identification and management of disease. In clinical practice, the primary site and cause of a peripheral neuropathy may not be easy to determine. Peripheral nerve disorders may reflect damage to a neuronal cell body, its axon, the myelin sheath, supporting tissue, and the vascular supply. Nerve conduction studies and specific neurological physical examinations can be useful. Otherwise, the clinical presentation and past medical history provide the etiological clues. The influence of **nutritional deficiency** always needs to be considered.

The cells of the peripheral nervous system (PNS) and central nervous system (CNS) require a steady supply of **nutrients** to maintain optimal function. Similarly, other tissues within the body require an assortment of nutrients for maintaining metabolic processes at the cellular and molecular levels. Manifestations of nutrient deficits throughout the body continue to be characterized; the focus in this chapter is on currently recognized signs and symptoms associated with the nervous system, their clinical cause, and their pathological description.

Nutrients, Nutritional Status, and the Nervous System

Nutrients and Nutritional Status

Human metabolism requires substrate materials that cannot be synthesized by the body or are detected in quantities insufficient to meet the body's needs. These essential substrates are the nutrients that are consumed daily through a healthy diet. The nutrients have been reasonably well classified as either **macronutrients** or micronutrients.

Macronutrients are required in gram quantities daily, whereas micronutrients are generally required in milligram or microgram quantities. Macronutrients include proteins, carbohydrates, fats, and water. The three carbon-based nutrients flow through common routes of intermediary metabolism and contribute to the energy needs of the body, with most reactions occurring in environments containing water. Besides roles in energy metabolism, macronutrients play important structural and transport roles within the body. The fundamental units of any protein are amino acids, which are obtained daily via nutrient consumption. Proteins serve a structural role in all cells of the body and function as enzymes, hormones, and membrane transporters. Individual amino acids and fatty acids have specific physiological roles at cellular targets.[1]

Although micronutrients do not provide calories toward energy needs, this group of nutrients, which includes **vitamins** and **minerals,** is physiologically important in regulating metabolism through roles as coenzymes and cofactors, in free radical scavenging, in intracellular signaling, and in gene expression. If any one of these compounds is lacking in the diet, biochemical alterations lead to changes in tissue or organ structure or function that subsequently result in clinical manifestations known as deficiency diseases. Minerals are further differentiated as macrominerals (i.e., electrolytes) and microminerals (i.e., trace elements). It is important to consider not only the amount of a single micronutrient but also the balance among all required vitamins and minerals because of the significant nutrient-nutrient interactions among them. Given the role of agricultural and industrial technology in the food supply that provides dietary sources of the micronutrients, environmental science and environmental toxicology are becoming more tied in with nutritional and clinical status.[1]

An individual's nutritional status is considered optimal when nutrient requirements are balanced by nutrient intake, while maintaining a healthy body composition and function. Nutritional status is regularly evaluated by health care providers to identify risk factors for deficits and toxicities. Malnutrition ("poor nutritional status") refers generally to nutrient intake out of balance with nutrient requirements. It is more common than appreciated and includes conditions of underweight, overweight, and obesity as well as specific nutrient imbalances and altered states of metabolism.[1] Patient-related factors, as elicited from clinical history, can indicate patients at risk for malnutrition. An appreciation of the complex absorption and subsequent disposition of each nutrient—requiring transporters and enzymes that are each susceptible to the influence of gene polymorphism and environmental exposures—provides an explanation for the many ways that deficits may occur short of a classic nutrient deficiency. Such nutrient deficits can adversely influence clinical presentations and patient outcomes (Table 9-1).

Nutrition and the Nervous System

Central Nervous System

The brain depends on the delivery of glucose for energy needs. A steady supply of amino acids is also necessary

Table 9-1 Patient-Related Factors Indicative of Malnutrition Risk	
Mechanism for Risk	Examples of Patient-Related Factors
Reduced food consumption	Impaired appetite, gastrointestinal disease, traumatic neurological disorders interfering with self-feeding, neuropsychiatric disorders, disease of soft or hard oral tissue, alcoholism, pregnancy, anorexia and vomiting, food hypersensitivity, adverse drug effects, and disease requiring a restricted diet
Altered nutrient absorption	Absence of normal digestive secretions, intestinal hypermotility, reduction of effective absorbing surface, impairment of intrinsic mechanism of absorption, and drugs preventing absorption
Altered utilization or storage	Impaired liver function, hypothyroidism, neoplasm of the gastrointestinal tract, and drug therapy or radiation
Increased tissue destruction	Severe trauma, achlorhydria in the gastrointestinal tract, heavy metals, and other metabolic antagonists
Increased nutrient excretion	Lactation, burns, glycosuria and albuminuria, acute or chronic blood loss, and drug interaction/side effect
Increased nutrient requirements	Increased physical activity, periods of rapid growth, pregnancy and lactation, fever, hyperthyroidism, drug therapy, poor status, homeless status, substance addiction, and unconventional dietary habits

From Boullata JI. Nutrients and associated substances. In: Loyd A, ed. *Remington: The Science and Practice of Pharmacy.* 22nd ed. Philadelphia: Pharmaceutical Press & Philadelphia College of Pharmacy; 2012.

for protein and neurotransmitter synthesis. Additionally, numerous fatty acids are required by myelin and nonmyelin cell membranes to maintain neuronal and supporting cell structure and associated function.[2] Notwithstanding influences on brain maturation (e.g., neurogenesis) that may continue beyond early development, deficits of these nutrients may influence cognitive performance. Micronutrient deficits can also influence the CNS. In particular, cognitive function is known to be influenced by deficits in iodine, iron, selenium, and possibly zinc.[2] For example, zinc colocalizes with the neurotransmitter glutamate in some glutamatergic neurons and may possibly act as a neuromodulator.[3]

Peripheral Nervous System

Peripheral nerves also require ongoing sources of energy and substrate for structural support and function. Much more is known about the influence of nutrient status on the PNS. Numerous nutritional **neuropathies** and myeloneuropathies are recognized. Appreciating a patient's complete medical history can be informative. For example, many familiar neuropathies attributed to chronic alcoholism are nutritional in origin, especially as energy from ethanol displaces nutrient-dense food. An individual with a history of malabsorption—whether functional (e.g., inflammatory bowel disease) or anatomical (e.g., after bariatric surgery)—is likely to exhibit many nutrient deficits over time. Many of these manifest as neurological complications.[4-6] Although neurological manifestations of gastrointestinal disease often have a nutritional explanation, they sometimes may be independent.[7,8] In less common situations, individuals with many inborn errors of metabolism (e.g., abetalipoproteinemia) may present with neurological manifestations that can be managed with nutritional treatment as well. It can be difficult to disentangle PNS from CNS effects because they may manifest together in a patient with nutrient deficits.

Neuropathy by Presentation

Clinical presentation depends on both the primary site of the disorder and the most likely cause and can include encephalopathy, myelopathy, optic neuropathy, myopathy, and polyneuropathy. Patient presentations may include cognitive dysfunction and gait abnormalities related to the CNS and deafness, blindness, and sensory and motor deficits related to the PNS.[2]

Although the axon fiber type affected may vary, nutritionally related peripheral neuropathy generally affects all cell bodies to a similar extent, resulting in a symmetrical presentation. Sensory or motor deficits can be observed on clinical examination; however, most known lesions secondary to nutrient deficiency affect the sensory side. Sensory complaints include heaviness, numbness, paresthesia, pain, and dysesthesia. As a result, tactile discrimination, vibration, and position sense are diminished. Residual impact on pain and temperature sensation may also occur. With a peripheral neuropathy, patients complain of burning feet, dysesthesia of the soles and palms, numbness, and paresthesia. Patients may also report decreased distal sensation to light touch, pinprick, and vibration. Cell body lesions on the motor side can manifest as muscle weakness with wasting and possible diminution of deep tendon reflexes. Dorsolateral myelopathy can manifest as difficulty walking with leg weakness and brisk knee reflexes in the presence of slow ankle reflexes. Except for absent ankle reflexes, patients rarely present asymptomatically. Complaints with a myeloneuropathy include distal sensory neuropathy in combination with ataxia, brisk knee and slow ankle reflexes, and sphincter instability.

Distal sensory and motor deficits are usually symmetrical, which is often a result of axonal degeneration. Neuronal damage implicates deficits of essential nutrients and nutrients (e.g., antioxidants) that otherwise protect neurons from injury. Initial effects on the neuron affect the most distal aspect of the axon as metabolic needs are interrupted. The process of "dying back" (degeneration) toward the cell body can occur if the damage is not addressed in a timely fashion. This phenomenon may also explain why lower extremities with their longer afferent fibers are the site of initial presentation compared with the upper extremities. A demyelinating lesion may be present secondary to axonal degeneration but could also be primary as the nutritive functions of the highly metabolic Schwann cells are interrupted. The initial damage can occur to the most metabolically active neurons (i.e., cochlea, retina, dorsal root, distal axons). For example, the large myelinated distal axons depend on active transport systems to maintain their functional and structural integrity whereby deficits of substrate, including needs for adenosine triphosphate (ATP) production, initiate disruptions that manifest as neuropathy—"glove-and-stocking" symptoms.

Burning mouth syndrome is a neurosensory disorder that may include nutrient deficits (e.g., vitamin B_{12}, iron) in the differential diagnosis.[8] Most complaints involve the anterior tongue, hard palate, and lower lip and may be accompanied by dysgeusia. The effect may be attributed to medications (e.g., angiotensin-converting enzyme inhibitors) that cause a nutrient deficit (e.g., zinc) leading to the oral symptoms.

Visual impairment following optic neuropathy may have a nutritional etiology.[10,11] Patients with optic neuropathy complain of blurred vision, photophobia, decreased visual acuity, and possible changes in color vision. Hearing impairment, although correlated with peripheral neuropathy (e.g., in diabetes), has not yet been linked with any nutrient imbalance.[12]

Neuropathies and myeloneuropathies in tropical settings described in numerous historical reports may have nutritional roots. Many individuals with weight loss and chronic fatigue from a poor diet associated with economic sanctions in Cuba subsequently developed neurological symptoms that were at least partly attributable to nutrient deficits.[13] Originating as an optic neuropathy with progressive bilateral loss of visual acuity, sensorineural deafness and myeloneuropathy were eventually observed as well.[14] This neuropathy is also reported in other tropical regions[15] Deficits of several of the so-called B vitamins, particularly cyanocobalamin (vitamin B_{12}), along with deficits of sulfur-containing amino acids (e.g., methionine), minerals (e.g., selenium), and carotenoids (e.g., lycopene) seemed to be the major factors in this epidemic neuropathy.[14,16,17]

There is complexity in the etiology of malnutrition-related epidemics.[16] For example, an interaction between a host's nutrient deficiency and a symbiotic viral genome causes conversion to greater virulence and associated neuropathy.[17] Peripheral neuropathy attributed to chronic alcoholism is due partly to direct neurotoxicity of ethanol, but some features are also due to the associated nutrient (e.g., thiamine) deficits in patients with poor nutritional status.[18] It can be difficult to attribute a clinical finding to the deficiency of a single nutrient because multiple nutrient deficits may be concurrent. Clinical heterogeneity in presentation may also be the result of genetic variability in nutrient-associated pathways or accompanying etiologies.

The following sections describe reports of specific nutrient deficits causing neuropathy and their pathophysiological mechanisms and potential for reversibility when known. Manifestations of most nutrient deficiencies affect multiple systems, and it is not the intent of this chapter to provide a broad description of all signs and symptoms.

Neuropathy by Specific Nutrient

Macronutrients

When protein-calorie malnutrition is recognized in adults who are underweight or in children with stunted growth, micronutrient deficiencies may be observed as well. Altogether an individual is placed at risk for morbidity and mortality. The influence on the nervous system, which in some cases may take time to develop, is less often appreciated. Chronic malnutrition, as in the setting of anorexia nervosa, has been associated with the development of peripheral neuropathy.[19] This condition appears to be a distal sensorimotor disorder. Decreased amplitudes on sensory evoked potentials with less reduction in conduction velocities would suggest axonal degeneration. Nonspecific

proximal muscle weakness also accompanies protein-calorie malnutrition.[20] Aside from classic dermatological manifestations, deficits of essential fatty acids may result in peripheral neuropathy and abnormal visual function.[21] Dietary deficiencies of specific amino acids have also been implicated in optic neuropathy.[11] Any additive or synergistic role played by micronutrients in these presentations remains unclear.

Vitamins

Retinol (Vitamin A)

A patient may develop vitamin A deficiency as a result of reduced intake, malabsorption, or a metabolic defect such as abetalipoproteinemia. Because this nutrient is required for the synthesis of glycoproteins in the cornea and conjunctiva and the aldehyde form is needed to produce rhodopsin for phototransduction, patients present with corneal and conjunctival xerosis, retinopathy, and night blindness.[22] A functional retinoid cycle is required at the rod and cone cells in the retina, which serve as the peripheral receptors for vision. Night blindness occurs early and responds well to repletion in the presence of adequate protein and zinc status.

Given multiple sources of vitamin A, such as dietary supplements, total intake may exceed the recommended dietary allowance (i.e., 700 mcg for women, 900 mcg daily for men). It is important to note total intake of vitamin A because vitamin A toxicity can also manifest neurologically. Signs and symptoms include insomnia, irritability, headache with increased intracranial pressure, papilledema without focal neurological signs, and myalgias.

Thiamine (Vitamin B_1)

Thiamine has a coenzyme role in energy production of all cells, including neurons, which is necessary for fuel oxidation and ATP production. Aside from energy production, thiamine is important to neuronal membrane ion gating, axonal membrane transport, and neurotransmitter synthesis.[23] Given limited capacity for body stores of thiamine, deficiency may develop within 2 weeks of poor dietary intake, reduced absorption, or increased needs. Clinically, thiamine deficiency can affect the cardiovascular system, the CNS, and the PNS. Neurotoxicity associated with thiamine deficits can begin to occur within days.[23] Manifestations include a symmetrical, distal sensorimotor peripheral neuropathy, referred to as dry beriberi, which may or may not be accompanied by edema and congestive heart failure (i.e., wet beriberi). Dry beriberi is more often associated with a chronic marginal deficiency. Patients initially may complain of anorexia, headache, lethargy, fatigue, and irritability. The neuropathy may start with tingling and numbness at the toes before progressing to burning/stabbing pain of the feet. This neuropathy may cause an unsteady gait and can interfere with sleep. Beriberi neuropathy is motor dominant, influencing superficial and deep sensation.[18] Patients complain of a burning sensation in the soles of the feet, calf muscle tenderness, muscle cramps, and general muscular weakness with possible areflexia; loss of sensation, muscle weakness, and paralysis may occur in upper extremities as well over time. Leg weakness and numbness are followed by the loss of the ankle jerk reflex and footdrop. Glove-stocking hyperesthesia, and surface anesthesia with deep skeletal muscle pain can occur.

When manifesting as acute denervation (i.e., rapidly progressive weakness), beriberi can imitate Guillain-Barré syndrome.[24,25] Normal sensory-nerve (and motor-nerve) conduction velocities coexist with reduced compound sensory action potentials. Segmental demyelination can occur along with axonal degeneration, but small myelinated and unmyelinated axons are preserved.[26] Axonal degeneration has been identified particularly with large myelinated fibers.[27] This degeneration includes disruption of neurotubules, neurofilaments, and myelin sheaths. Glutamate-mediated excitotoxicity, decreased synaptic transmission, mitochondrial dysfunction, and apoptosis are possible mechanisms of damage.[23]

Thiamine deficiency may also be present in the CNS as Wernicke-Korsakoff syndrome, most commonly in the setting of alcoholism. Numerous factors are likely to predispose to the development of this syndrome.[23] Patients with Wernicke encephalopathy present acutely with nystagmus, gaze palsies, gait ataxia, apathy, disorientation, and confusion. Chronic manifestations include Korsakoff psychosis, amnesia, confusion, and dementia. Most of these patients also experience peripheral neuropathy, which is a consequence of ongoing thiamine deficiency. Generally, alcoholism causes a chronic symmetrical sensory peripheral neuropathy, whereas beriberi is associated with an acute form of neuropathy with weakness (distal greater than proximal), paresthesias, and neuropathic pain (burning discomfort with ache, occasional sharp pains).

The administration of 100 mg of thiamine intravenously, followed by daily oral supplementation, corrects the neuropathy and confusion, whereas ataxia and memory impairment may remain. Neuropathic recovery is better for motor than sensory findings.[24] The distal sensory (burning feet) neuropathy may also respond to several other B vitamins (e.g., niacin, folic acid, pantothenic acid), highlighting the interplay among many of the B vitamins and supporting the caution to avoid large repletion doses of one B vitamin without the others.

Riboflavin (Vitamin B₂)

Riboflavin deficits have been associated with neuropathy, and repletion of this vitamin has been effective in its treatment (28, 29). Deficiencies of B vitamins generally result in an axonal polyneuropathy. Despite some commonalities between B-vitamin deficiency and clinical presentations, it is difficult to discern the specific effect of riboflavin deficits. Based on animal models, riboflavin deficiency manifests with demyelination and Schwann cell hypertrophy with initial sparing of the axons.[30]

Niacin (Vitamin B₃)

Niacin (nicotinic acid and nicotinamide) is essential for the proper functioning of several coenzymes. Deficiency may develop in people who use corn as their main dietary carbohydrate and people with alcoholism and malabsorption. Niacin deficiency may be secondary to other nutrient deficits (e.g., pyridoxine) and other disorders (e.g., Hartnup syndrome).[2] Deficiency of niacin is characterized by dermatitis, diarrhea, and dementia. CNS deficits and lesions are well described, but a peripheral neuropathy is also recognized, although it is difficult to distinguish clearly from thiamine deficiency.[23] Patients may complain of burning sensations of the tongue and oral cavity. On neuropathological examination, chromatinolysis can be identified in niacin deficiency. It has been suggested that nicotinamide riboside may be a more specific substrate for peripheral neuron function.[31]

The administration of nicotinamide initially at 100 mg every 6 hours and then 25 to 50 mg once or twice daily encourages the reversal of diarrhea and dermatitis. Higher doses may be necessary for neurological impairment, and other B vitamins are often indicated as well.

Pyridoxine (Vitamin B₆)

Deficiency of pyridoxine has numerous manifestations, including seizures and peripheral neuropathy. Symmetrical distal neuropathy may progress to a sensory ataxia and limb weakness.[2] Degeneration and regeneration of axons on both myelinated and unmyelinated fibers has been observed. Although biochemical abnormalities are corrected with 25 mg of pyridoxine, the neuropathy is also reversible with oral replacement of the vitamin at doses of 50 to 100 mg daily.

There may be an etiological role of pyridoxine overuse in chronic idiopathic axonal polyneuropathy. Pyridoxine is considered to have a narrow therapeutic index in that larger doses (greater than 200 mg daily) may precipitate a sensory neuropathy and ataxia in the absence of weakness.[32] In a group of patients dependent on parenteral nutrition, peripheral neuropathy was associated with elevated pyridoxine concentrations but not with any B-vitamin deficits.[33] The mechanism for neuronal degeneration as a result of excess pyridoxine is unclear.

Biotin (Vitamin B₇)

Paresthesias of the extremities may accompany depression and lethargy in individuals with biotin deficits. Biotin deficiency may decrease pyruvate carboxylase activity, allowing for lactic acid accumulation as a contributing factor. This condition is expected to be reversible within 2 weeks of supplementation.

Folic Acid (Vitamin B₉)

Deficiency of folic acid may occur within months of the onset of malnutrition. This deficiency may be observed in patients with gastrointestinal disease or be a result of drug effects such as ethanol. This nutrient is important in one-carbon metabolism, as is vitamin B_{12}, but less commonly causes neurological manifestations. When present, deficits may be manifest as an affective disorder and mental status changes.[23] However, peripheral neuropathy including subacute combined degeneration and myelopathy is rarely observed.[34] Optic neuropathies leading to bilateral visual loss also have been attributed to folic acid deficiency in the absence of alcohol abuse or other deficits of B vitamins.[35] A hypothesized mechanism involves the accumulation of formic acid, normally cleared in the presence of adequate tetrahydrofolate, with subsequent mitochondrial impairment and neuronal damage.

Cyanocobalamin (Vitamin B₁₂)

Deficits of vitamin B_{12} are often seen in elderly individuals, individuals with natural or iatrogenic gastric achlorhydria, and individuals with malabsorption syndromes. Given significant body stores of this nutrient, the deficits may take at least 1 to 2 years to develop. The metabolic conversion of methylmalonyl CoA to succinyl CoA is impaired with deficiency, resulting in reduced availability of activated methyl groups necessary for synthesis of myelin and neurotransmitters.[2] The brain, spinal cord, optic nerves, and peripheral nerves all are affected by vitamin B_{12} deficiency. Vitamin B_{12} deficiency with neuropsychiatric findings may exist in the absence of anemia, macrocytosis, or markedly low serum cobalamin concentrations.[36] Deficiency of this vitamin should be included in the differential diagnosis of any patient with peripheral nerve and neuropsychiatric manifestations.[37]

Neurological manifestations of vitamin B_{12} deficiency include a myelopathy that may be accompanied by a neuropathy, paresthesias, optic neuropathy, and cognitive impairment.[23] The neuropathy is characterized by a spastic paraparesis, extensor plantar response, and impaired perception of both vibration and position. Patients complain of tingling, paresthesias, and pins-and-needles sensations in the feet, but it can also occur in the hands.[38] Although some patients have axonal neuropathy and demyelination, this glove-stocking distribution may reflect dorsal column lesions more than alterations in peripheral nerves. Symptoms occur secondary to a decrease in the universal methyl donor (S-adenosylmethionine). Particularly vulnerable are the long tracts of white matter in the posterior and lateral spinal columns that are responsible for conducting vibration and position sense. Posterior spinal columns are more adversely affected than lateral columns; anterior column involvement is rare. Nerve conduction studies suggest a somatosensory and motor axonopathy, with abnormalities also present on visual evoked potentials. Vitamin B_{12} deficits have been associated with optic neuropathy and loss of visual acuity.[10,39] The myelopathy is referred to as "subacute combined degeneration."

Subacute combined degeneration manifests as sensory ataxia, spasticity, and lower extremity weakness. It is due to posterior and lateral column degeneration in the spinal cord.[37] As these manifestations become chronic, they can be quite disabling leading to an unsteady gait from the loss of proprioception and postural sense. Leg weakness and stiffness become progressive as brisk knee reflexes and a positive Babinski sign are present. Without intervention, patients may develop ataxic paraplegia with spasticity and contractures. Abnormal production of the neurotrophic factors (e.g., epidermal growth factor) in vitamin B_{12} deficiency also contributes to neural damage.

Pathology initially reveals separation of myelin lamellae, vacuolization, and axonal damage in the dorsal columns of the upper spinal cord. Later, the lesions are more scattered in a characteristic "honeycomb" pattern. Spongy degeneration of the optic nerve leads to the visual loss. Neuronal demyelination appears in both the PNS and the CNS.

Although oral repletion with crystalline vitamin B_{12} is considered appropriate in patients with adequate absorptive area, parenteral dosing may be considered initially for patients with severe symptoms or for patients with insufficient gastrointestinal surface area. The degree of reversibility with vitamin B_{12} repletion depends largely on the duration of deficits, and deficits are less responsive after 1 year. Myeloneuropathy, exhibited as muscle weakness of less than 3 months' duration, is reversible a few weeks from the onset of repletion. Paresthesias are more likely to respond to cobalamin repletion than ataxia.[37] Sensory deficits may take much longer. Repletion is more likely to improve impaired sense of touch, pain, and position than impaired vibration sense. Most patients have a residual abnormality of tibial somatosensory evoked potentials after treatment.[37]

Pantothenic Acid (Vitamin B₁₅)

Vitamin B_{15} is important in carbohydrate and fatty acid metabolism throughout the body—particularly within the nervous system. Deficits can result in numbness and burning sensations of the feet that can be reversed only by pantothenic acid regardless of other concurrent deficits.[40] Peripheral nerve lesions can be accompanied by cramping of the legs and impaired motor coordination.

α-Tocopherol (Vitamin E)

Vitamin E represents a number of compounds: α-, β-, γ-, and δ-tocopherol (each of which can exist in various stereoisomers) and α-, β-, γ-, and δ-tocotrienol. Clinically, the term vitamin E refers to the tocopherols with the biological activity of α-tocopherol. One function of vitamin E is to serve as an antioxidant to prevent peroxidative damage to cell membranes. With a deficit of vitamin E, membrane lipid peroxidation is more likely, which may interfere with neuronal function.[41] Although the peripheral nerves contain more vitamin E than the brain, they still degenerate in the face of deficits.[41] The neurological role of vitamin E was first recognized in deficient animals in the early years after its discovery in the 1920s. More recently, neurological findings in humans have been attributed to deficiency of the vitamin, although it rarely manifests as an isolated neuropathy.[23] These are most often secondary to malabsorption or to genetic abnormalities in vitamin E disposition rather than dietary insufficiency.

Vitamin E deficits may occur in patients with chronic malabsorption (e.g., cystic fibrosis, short bowel syndrome) or defects in vitamin E disposition (e.g., hypolipoproteinemia or abetalipoproteinemia, α-tocopherol transport protein mutation). With chronic malabsorption, vitamin E deficiency may take years to emerge. A rare, autosomal recessive syndrome produces vitamin E deficiency with neurological manifestations (e.g., hyporeflexia, tremor, gait ataxia, loss of proprioception and vibratory sensation) and has been referred to as "ataxia with vitamin E deficiency" (AVED).[42] AVED is characterized in young adults by a progressive peripheral neuropathy of the large-caliber myelinated axons of sensory neurons.[43] Patients may present with areflexia, gait and limb ataxia, sensory impairment, muscle weakness, amyotrophy, decreased vibration sense, and bilateral Babinski sign.[44] With ongoing vitamin E deficiency, besides a loss of deep tendon reflexes, truncal and limb ataxia, and reduced vibrational and positional sense, ophthalmoplegia and muscle weakness can occur.[41] On pathological examination, damage is to large-fiber axons and dorsal root ganglia. Lipofuscin may accumulate in the Schwann cell cytoplasm and in dorsal root sensory neurons.[41] Peripheral sensory nerves exhibit neuroaxonal dystrophy (dystrophic degeneration with secondary demyelination).[41] Motor neuron demyelination has been reported in patients complaining of impaired sensation in the feet and feeling unsteady when walking,[45] but the usual presentation is of significantly reduced sensory nerve action potentials without abnormalities in motor conduction. Sensory nerve conduction studies reveal low-amplitude action potentials and limited delays in conduction velocities.[43] Although basophilic deposits throughout the muscle fiber may play a role, muscle weakness may also be the result of a denervation-reinnervation process with a variation of muscle fiber size.[41] In vitamin E–deficient patients with peripheral neuropathy, α-tocopherol content in the sural nerve is significantly lower.[46] The low levels and accompanying biochemical alterations appear to precede histological degeneration.

Reversibility of these lesions with oral or parenteral vitamin E supplementation is not guaranteed and may require 6 months to 4 years of therapy. The most dramatic recovery occurs if the condition is diagnosed and treated early. Best results occur in patients with AVED, but larger daily doses may be necessary for patients with abetaliporoteinemia.[44,47] There may be only partial recovery of efferent nerve conduction after vitamin E supplementation despite recovery of sensory conduction.[45]

Calciferol (Vitamin D)

Deficits of vitamin D are common because of reduced sun exposure, minimal dietary intake, or malabsorption. Aside from bone-related consequences, vitamin D deficits may cause a proximal myopathy of lower and upper extremities and hyperesthesia unresponsive to opioid analgesics.[48,49] The association between vitamin D deficits and multiple sclerosis requires further study.[2]

Electrolytes

Magnesium

Magnesium is an abundant intracellular mineral essential for regulation of numerous cellular functions. Neuronal injury is enhanced by magnesium deficiency.[50] This enhanced injury may occur partly as the result of substance P release from C fibers after N-methyl-D-aspartate receptor activation.[51]

Trace Elements

Copper

As a critical cofactor for many enzymes, copper deficiency affects physiological function in numerous systems. A deficiency of copper is uncommon except in cases of malabsorption after gastric surgery (i.e., gastrectomy, bypass) or inadequate copper intake in the presence of excess zinc intake with which it competes for absorption. Adverse neurological consequences of copper deficits influence both the CNS and the PNS. The neuropathy attributed to copper deficiency in particular may reflect a relative deficiency compared with zinc excess and the combined effect on the stability of the neuronal cell membrane.[52] Peripheral neuropathy may precede anemia or pancytopenia often associated with copper deficiency.[52] Patients can present with a myelopathy or a neuropathy that can mimic those seen with vitamin B_{12} deficiency.[53,54] Reduced mobility and an unsteady spastic gait may be combined with sensory loss at the soles of the feet and vibration sensation to the knees.[53] A positive Romberg test may be present indicating a proprioceptive lesion. Sensory symptoms may also occur in the hands.[53] The sensory ataxia is caused by dysfunction in the dorsal column.[23] Footdrop may be present, and optic neuritis with peripheral neuropathy has also been reported. Optic neuropathy with diminished peripheral vision and posterolateral myelopathy is a rare presentation in patients with copper deficiency.[54] A cessation of neurological deterioration is more likely to accompany copper repletion than an outright improvement in neurological symptoms.[23]

In patients presenting with a peripheral nerve disorder, the influence of nutrient deficits should be considered. A thorough history and physical examination and appropriate diagnostic tests are valuable in identifying peripheral neuropathy associated with nutritional deficiency and in optimizing patient outcome.

CASE STUDY

WM has chronic alcoholism. He resides alone in a small apartment that does not have a kitchen. He estimates his alcohol intake per day at 12 to 18 cans of beer. He is employed part-time as a dishwasher in an Asian restaurant. The owner of the restaurant allows her employees to take home leftover food; this is primarily rice of some sort. WM often skips breakfast and lunch and eats the leftover rice as his dinner.

Over a period of 1 month, WM's supervisor at the restaurant has become concerned about WM's loss of memory, confabulation, and, on one occasion, an auditory hallucination. She also noted that WM has been dragging his foot when walking. After many unsuccessful attempts to have WM see his family physician, she eventually drove him to the hospital.

On examination, the physician suspected thiamine deficiency, which was corroborated with a blood test. Intravenous thiamine was ordered followed by daily oral dosages.

Case Study Questions

1. Thiamine deficiency is also known as which of the following?
   a. Beriberi
   b. Scurvy
   c. Rhabdomyolysis
   d. Dysphagia

2. Common symptoms of thiamine deficiency include all of the following *except*:
   a. Insomnia owing to foot pain
   b. Gait dysfunction
   c. Fatigue
   d. Skin rash

3. "Dry" thiamine deficiency involves primarily the peripheral nerves. Symptoms of "wet" thiamine deficiency include which of the following?
   a. Hair loss (alopecia)
   b. Loss of central vision
   c. Peripheral edema and congestive heart failure
   d. Constipation

4. Rapidly evolving thiamine deficiency characterized by acute motor neuropathy may mimic which of the following diseases?
   a. Multiple sclerosis
   b. Guillain-Barré syndrome
   c. Muscular dystrophy
   d. Parkinson's disease

5. WM's memory loss, confabulation, and auditory hallucinations may be related to which of the following complications of alcoholism?
   a. Wernicke-Korsakoff syndrome
   b. Elevated liver enzymes
   c. Weight loss
   d. Osteoporosis

References

1. Boullata JI. Nutrients and associated substances. In: Loyd A, ed. *Remington: The Science and Practice of Pharmacy*. 22nd ed. Philadelphia: Pharmaceutical Press & Philadelphia College of Pharmacy; 2012.
2. Román GC. Nutritional disorders of the nervous system. In: Shils ME, Shike M, Ross AC, Caballero B, Cousins RJ, eds. *Modern Nutrition in Health and Disease*. 10th ed. Philadelphia: Lippincott Williams & Wilkins; 2006:1362–1380.
3. Tóth K. Zinc in neurotransmission. *Annu Rev Nutr*. 2011;31:139–153.
4. Freeman HJ. Neurologic disorders in adult celiac disease. *Can J Gastroenterol*. 2008;22:909–911.
5. Chang CG, Adams-Huet B, Provost DA. Acute post-gastric reduction surgery (APGARS) neuropathy. *Obes Surg*. 2004;14:182–189.
6. Juhasz-Pocsine K, Rudnicki SA, Archer RL, Harik SI. Neurologic complications of gastric bypass surgery for morbid obesity. *Neurology*. 2007;68:1843–1850.
7. Ghezzi A, Zaffaroni M. Neurologic manifestations of gastrointestinal disorders, with particular reference to the differential diagnosis of multiple sclerosis. *Neurol Sci*. 2001;22: S117–122.
8. Vaknin A, Eliakim R, Ackerman Z, Steiner I. Neurological abnormalities associated with celiac disease. *J Neurol*. 2004; 251:1393–1397.
9. Brown RS, Farquharson AA, Sam FE, Reid E. A retrospective evaluation of 56 patients with oral burning and limited clinical findings. *Gen Dentist*. 2006;Jul-Aug:267–271.
10. Stambolian D, Behrens M. Optic neuropathy associated with vitamin B12 deficiency. *Am J Ophthalmol*. 1977;83:465–468.
11. Sadun AA. Metabolic optic neuropathies. *Semin Ophthalmol*. 2002;17:29–32.
12. Bainbridge KE, Hoffman HJ, Cowie CC. Risk factors for hearing impairment among U.S. adults with diabetes. *Diabetes Care*. 2011;34:1540–1545.
13. Menéndez AR-O, Matos CM, Acosta SJ, et al. Evaluación del estado nutricional de enfermos con neuropatía epidémica al año de evolución: indicadores bioquímicos. *Rev Cuban Med Trop*. 1998;50:254–258.
14. Román GC. An epidemic in Cuba of optic neuropathy, sensorineural deafness, peripheral sensory neuropathy and dorsolateral myeloneuropathy. *J Neurol Sci*. 1994;127:11–28.
15. Madhusudanan M, Menon MK, Ummer K, Radhakrishnanan K. Clinical and etiological profile of tropical ataxic neuropathy in Kerala, South India. *Eur Neurol*. 2008;60: 21–26.

16. Bowman BA, Bern C, Philen RM. Nothing's simple about malnutrition: complexities raised by epidemic neuropathy in Cuba. *Am J Clin Nutr.* 1996;64:383–384.

17. Beck MA, Levander OA, Handy J. Selenium deficiency and viral infection. *J Nutr.* 2003;133:1463S–1467S.

18. Koike H, Sobue G. Alcoholic neuropathy. *Curr Opin Neurol.* 2006;19:481–486.

19. MacKenzie JR, LaBan MM, Sackeyfio AH. The prevalence of peripheral neuropathy in patients with anorexia nervosa. *Arch Phys Med Rehabil.* 1989;70:827–830.

20. Wade AN, Dolan JM, Cambor CL, Boullata JI, Rickels MR. Fatal malnutrition 6 years after gastric bypass surgery. *Arch Intern Med.* 2010;170:993–995.

21. Uauy R, Dangour AD. Nutrition in brain development and aging: role of essential fatty acids. *Nutr Rev.* 2006;64: S24–S33.

22. Smith J, Steinemann TL. Vitamin A deficiency and the eye. *Int Ophthalmol Clin.* 2000;40(4):83–91.

23. Kumar N. Neurologic presentations of nutritional deficiencies. *Neurol Clin.* 2010;28:107–170.

24. Koike H, Misu K, Hattori N, et al. Postgastrectomy polyneuropathy with thiamine deficiency. *J Neurol Neurosurg Psychiatry.* 2001;71:357–362.

25. Murphy C, Bangash IH, Varma A. Dry beriberi mimicking the Guillain-Barré syndrome. *Pract Neurol.* 2009;9:221–224.

26. Kril JJ. Neuropathology of thiamine deficiency disorders. *Metab Brain Dis.* 1996;11:9–17.

27. Koike H, Iijima M, Mori K, et al. Postgastrectomy polyneuropathy with thiamine deficiency is identical to beriberi neuropathy. *Nutrition.* 2004;20:961–966.

28. Osuntakun B, Aladetoyinbo A, Bademosi O. Vitamin B nutrition in the Nigerian tropical ataxic neuropathy. *J Neurol Neurosurg Psychiatry.* 1985;48:154–156.

29. Mashima Y, Kigasawa K, Wakakura M, Oguchi Y. Do idebenone and vitamin therapy shorten the time to achieve visual recovery in Leber hereditary optic neuropathy? *J Neuroophthal.* 2000;20:166–170.

30. Cai Z, Blumbergs PC, Finnie JW, Manavis J, Thompson PD. Selective vulnerability of peripheral nerves in avian riboflavin deficiency demyelinating polyneuropathy. *Vet Pathol.* 2009;46: 88–96.

31. Bogan KL, Brenner C. Nicotinic acid, nicotinamide, and nicotinamide riboside: a molecular evaluation of NAD+ precursor vitamins in human nutrition. *Annu Rev Nutr.* 2008; 28:115–130.

32. Parry GJ, Bredesen DE. Sensory neuropathy with low-dose pyridoxine. *Neurology.* 1985;35:1466–1468.

33. Mikalunas V, Fitzgerald K, Rubin H, McCarthy R, Craig RM. Abnormal vitamin levels in patients receiving home total parenteral nutrition. *J Clin Gastroenterol.* 2001;33: 393–396.

34. Parry TE. Folate-responsive neuropathy. *Presse Med.* 1994;23: 131–137.

35. Hsu CT, Miller NR, Wray ML. Optic neuropathy from folic acid deficiency without alcohol use. *Ophthalmology.* 2002;216: 65–67.

36. Stabler SP, Allen RH, Savage DG, Lindenbaum J. Clinical spectrum and diagnosis of cobalamin deficiency. *Blood.* 1990; 76:871–881.

37. Hemmer B, Glocker FX, Schumacher M, Deuschl G, Lücking CH. Subacute combined degeneration: clinical, electrophysiological, and magnetic resonance imaging findings. *J Neurol Neurosurg Psychiatry.* 1998;65:822–827.

38. Healton EB, Savage DG, Brust JCM, et al. Neurologic aspects of cobalamin deficiency. *Medicine.* 1991;70:229–245.

39. Moschos M. Optic neuropathy in vitamin B12 deficiency (correspondence). *Lancet.* 1998; 352:146–147.

40. Glusman M. The syndrome of "burning feet" as a manifestation of nutritional deficiency. *Am J Med.* 1947;3(2): 211–223.

41. Sokol RJ. Vitamin E and neurologic function in man. *Free Rad Biol Med.* 1989;6:189–207.

42. Traber MG. Vitamin E. In: Zempleni J, Rucker RB, McCormick DB, Suttie JW (eds). *Handbook of Vitamins.* 4th ed. Boca Raton, FL:CRC Press; 2007:153–174.

43. Sokol RJ, Kayden HJ, Bettis DB, et al. Isolated vitamin E deficiency in the absence of fat malabsorption—familial and sporadic cases: characterization and investigation of causes. *J Lab Clin Med.* 1988;111:548–559.

44. Benomar A, Yahyaoui M, Marzouki N, et al. Vitamin E deficiency ataxia associated with adenoma. *J Neurol Sci.* 1999; 162:97–101.

45. Puri V, Chaudhry N, Tatke M, Prakash V. Isolated vitamin E deficiency with demyelinating neuropathy. *Muscle Nerve.* 2005;32:230–235.

46. Traber MG, Sokol RJ, Ringel SP, et al. Lack of tocopherol on peripheral nerves of vitamin E-deficient patients with peripheral neuropathy. *N Engl J Med.* 1987;317:262–265.

47. Kayden HJ. The neurologic syndrome of vitamin E deficiency: a significant cause of ataxia. *Neurology.* 1993;43:2167–2169.

48. Russell JA. Osteomalacic myopathy. *Muscle Nerve.* 1994;17: 578–580.

49. Gloth FM, Lindsay JM, Zelesnick LB, et al. Can vitamin D deficiency produce an unusual pain syndrome? *Arch Intern Med.* 1991;151:1662–1664.

50. Oyanagi K, Kawakami E, Kikuchi-Horie K, et al. Magnesium deficiency over generations in rats with special references to the pathogenesis of the parkinsonism-dementia complex and amyotrophic lateral sclerosis of Guam. *Neuropathology.* 2006; 26:115–128.

51. Weglicki WB. Hypomagnesemia and inflammation: clinical and basic aspects. *Annu Rev Nutr.* 2012;32:4.1–4.17.

52. Imataki O, Ohnishi H, Kitanaka A, et al. Pancytopenia complicated with peripheral neuropathy due to copper deficiency: clinical diagnostic review. *Intern Med.* 2008;47: 2063–2065.

53. Bertfield DL, Jumma O, Pitceathly RDS, Sussman JD. Copper deficiency: an unusual case of myelopathy with neuropathy. *Ann Clin Biochem.* 2008;45:434–435.

54. Pineles SL, Wilson CA, Balcer LJ, Slater R, Galetta SL. Combined optic neuropathy and myelopathy secondary to copper deficiency. *Surv Ophthalmol.* 2010;55:386–392.

Chapter 10

Peripheral Neuropathy and Chronic Kidney Disease

Susan Bray, MD

"Happiness is nothing more than good health and a bad memory."
—Albert Schweitzer

Objectives

On completion of this chapter, the student/practitioner will be able to:

- Discuss renal physiology and the function of the kidneys.
- Define the possible etiologies and clinical characteristics of chronic kidney disease.
- Compare the various methods of dialysis.
- Describe the various peripheral neuropathies associated with chronic kidney disease.

Key Terms

- Capillary filtration coefficient
- Chronic kidney disease
- Glomerular filtration rate
- Hemodialysis
- Renal blood flow

Introduction

Following a brief overview of renal physiology and **chronic kidney disease** (CKD), this chapter discusses the interaction between kidney disease and peripheral neuropathy. With increasing life expectancy and the increased prevalence of diabetes mellitus and hypertension, CKD, also known as chronic renal failure, chronic renal insufficiency, and chronic kidney failure, now affects 26 million Americans.[1]

The primary function of the kidney is to remove metabolic waste products and excess water from the body. In early stages of CKD, symptoms rarely occur. Symptoms may not appear until kidney function is less than one tenth of normal. The final stage of CKD is called end-stage renal disease (ESRD). The two most common causes of CKD are diabetes and uncontrolled high blood pressure. Less common etiologies include renal artery atherosclerotic disease, genetic diseases such as polycystic kidney disease, drug interaction, autoimmune disorders such as systemic lupus erythematosus and scleroderma, glomerulonephritis, renal calculi, and reflux nephropathy.[2-4] Culturally, African Americans, Hispanics, Pacific Islanders, American Indians, and adults older than age 60 are at greater risk for the development of CKD compared with Caucasians and northern Asian groups.[2,3]

Presenting symptoms include anorexia, malaise, pruritus, dry skin, and weight loss. Later symptoms include drowsiness and confusion, changes in skin pigmentation, excessive thirst, insomnia, edema, and peripheral neuropathy.[2,3] A wide variety of neuropathies are associated with CKD because of the strong correlation of diabetes and CKD and the large amount of downstream corporal system impairment associated with CKD.

Functions of the Kidney

The kidneys serve multiple functions. The first is to rid the body of waste materials and products that are either

---

Box 10-1

Functions of the Kidney

Excretion of metabolic waste products and foreign chemicals
Gluconeogenesis
Regulation of acid-base balance
Regulation of water and electrolyte balances
Regulation of arterial blood pressure
Secretion, metabolism, and excretion of hormones
Regulation of body fluid osmolality and electrolyte concentration

---

ingested or produced by metabolism. A second function is to control the volume and composition of the body fluids. For water and virtually all electrolytes in the body, balance between intake (secondary to oral or parenteral ingestion or metabolic production) and output (secondary to excretion or metabolic consumption) is maintained largely by the kidneys. The regulatory function of the kidney allows cells to function in an optimally stable metabolic environment (Box 10-1).

The kidneys are the primary means for the body to excrete metabolic wastes. These products include urea (from the metabolism of amino acids), creatinine (from muscle creatine), uric acid (from nucleic acids), the end products of hemoglobin breakdown (bilirubin), and metabolites of various hormones. The kidneys also work to eliminate toxins that are either produced by the body or ingested, such as pesticides, recreational and prescribed drugs, and food additives.

For cells to function efficiently, water and electrolyte homeostasis must be maintained. The kidneys match excretion to intake. If excretion is greater than intake, electrolyte concentrations decrease; if excretion is less than intake, electrolyte concentrations increase. Electrolyte concentrations controlled by the kidney include sodium, potassium, hydrogen, chloride, calcium, magnesium, and phosphate. Failure to control electrolyte concentrations affects many corporal systems.

The kidneys also play a dominant role in the long-term and short-term maintenance of arterial blood pressure. Long-term control is accomplished by excreting variable quantities of sodium and water. Short-term control is performed by the secretion of vasoactive factors or substances, such as renin, which either directly or indirectly assist with the excretion of vasoactive products such as angiotensin II. Many blood pressure–controlling medications exert their actions directly on the kidney.

Along with the lungs and various body fluid buffers, the kidneys contribute to regulation of acid-base balance by regulating the body fluid buffer stores. The

kidneys are the only means for eliminating from the body certain types of acids generated by metabolic processes such as sulfuric and phosphoric acid.

The quantity of red blood cells is an important homeostatic element for cellular function. The kidneys secrete erythropoietin, which stimulates the production of red blood cells. The stimulus for secretion is the relative oxygen content in the circulating blood. In a healthy person, the kidneys have the sole responsibility for erythropoietin secretion and regulation. In patients with severe CKD, anemia develops secondary to decreased erythropoietin production and secretion.

Vitamin D is an important adjunct to many chemical processes within the body. The kidneys produce the active form of vitamin D, 1,25-dihydroxyvitamin D_3 (calcitriol) by hydroxylating this vitamin at the number "1" position. Calcitriol is essential for normal calcium deposition in osteogenesis and for reabsorption by the gastrointestinal tract.

The kidneys also assist with glucose synthesis from amino acids and other precursors during prolonged fasting. This process is called gluconeogenesis. The ability of the kidneys to add glucose to the bloodstream during fasting rivals that of the liver.

CKD or acute kidney failure disrupts all these homeostatic functions resulting in severe abnormalities of fluid volume, electrolyte concentration, red blood concentration, acid-base balance, calcitonin concentration, and aberrant glucose levels during fasting. Intervention, such as **hemodialysis,** is an attempt to restore these balances.

Kidney Physiology

Urine formation begins with filtration of large amounts of fluid through the glomerular capillaries into Bowman's capsule. Similar to most capillaries, the glomerular capillaries are relatively impermeable to proteins, so that the filtered fluid is essentially protein-free and devoid of cellular elements including blood products. Concentrations of the other constituents of the glomerular filtrate are similar to those of plasma.

The **glomerular filtration rate** (GFR) is determined by the balance of colloid osmotic forces and hydrostatic pressure acting across the capillary membrane. A key determinant is also the **capillary filtration coefficient** (K_f), the product of the permeability and filtering surface areas of the capillaries.[5] The high glomerular hydrostatic pressure and large K_f allow for a much higher rate of filtration within the glomerular capillaries than with other capillaries throughout the body.[6] In a typical adult, the GFR is about 125 mL/min or 180 L/day.[5] The fraction of the renal plasma flow that is filtered, known as the filtration fraction, averages about 20%[5] indicating that on average about 20% of plasma flowing through the kidney at a given time is filtered through the glomerular capillaries. The formula for filtration fraction is as follows:[7]

Filtration fraction = GFR/Renal plasma flow

Determinants of GFR that are most variable and subject to physiological control include the glomerular hydrostatic pressure and the glomerular capillary colloid osmotic pressure. Factors that may influence these particular variables include activity of the sympathetic nervous system, hormones and autacoids (vasoactive substances that are released by the kidneys and act locally), and other feedback controls that are particular to kidney function. Essentially all blood vessels within the kidney have rich sympathetic and parasympathetic innervation. Sympathetic stimulation may constrict the renal arterioles and decrease **renal blood flow,** decreasing GFR. Hormones that constrict afferent and efferent arterioles, such as norepinephrine and epinephrine released from the adrenal medulla, may also cause a reduction in GFR.[3]

The effectiveness of renal blood flow volume may also affect GFR. In an average 70-kg man, the combined blood flow through both kidneys averages 1,100 mL/min, or about 20% of the cardiac output. Because both kidneys combined constitute only about 0.4% of total body weight, one can easily see that the kidneys receive a disproportionate amount of blood flow compared with other organs or tissues. A small percentage of this volume is used to nourish the kidney with oxygen, sugars, proteins, and fats, but the large percentage of the volume is used for filtration.[4] Renal blood flow is determined by the pressure gradient across the renal vasculature (the calculated difference between renal vein and renal artery hydrostatic pressure) divided by the total renal vascular resistance:[5]

Renal blood flow = (renal artery pressure − renal vein pressure)/total renal vascular resistance

Chronic Kidney Disease

CKD is a huge health problem in the United States affecting 26 million people. In 2007 in the United States, there were about 527,000 individuals with ESRD requiring dialysis or transplantation (Table 10-1). Americans receiving hemodialysis or peritoneal dialysis numbered 368,265 in 2007. The cost to treat Americans with CKD in 2007 was $35.32 billion. As the prevalence of diabetes and hypertension continue to increase, the prevalence of CKD will also increase.[1]

Any pathology that results in permanent loss of nephrons will result in CKD. The nephron is the functional unit of the kidney that filters water, waste, electrolytes, acids, and bases and is also responsible for selective reabsorption and excretion of ions. The permanent loss of nephrons results in a correlative

Table 10-1	Etiology of Chronic Kidney Disease
Etiology	Number in the United States
Diabetes	197,037
Hypertension	127,935
Glomerulonephritis	81,599
Cystic kidney	24,828
Urological disease	13,139
All other	82,745

Data from U.S. Department of Health and Human Services. National Kidney and Urologic Diseases Information Clearinghouse (NKUDIC). http://kidney.niddk.nih.gov/kudiseases/pubs/kustats/#2. Accessed November 12, 2012.

percentile loss in GFR. The progressive inability of the kidney to filter plasma affects all corporal systems. Many disease processes may result in a comorbidity of CKD: uncontrolled hypertension, urinary tract obstruction, urinary tract infection, hereditary defects of the kidneys, glomerular disorders, renal neoplasm, diabetes mellitus, and systemic lupus erythematosus. Chronic and persistent use or overuse of certain medications such as nonsteroidal anti-inflammatory drugs and acetaminophen may result in CKD. There is also a relationship between aging and CKD. Age-related reduced GFR and the increased frequency of concurrent diseases among elderly adults may lead to progressive diminished GFR. Age-related reduced GFR may lead to greater susceptibility to nephrotoxic side effects of certain medications.[2-7]

As a result of the chronic and cumulative loss of nephrons, CKD is marked by the inability of the kidney to remove metabolic waste products from the blood adequately, to regulate fluid and electrolyte homeostasis, and to balance the pH of the extracellular fluids. Normal kidney function is defined as a GFR of 100 mL/min.[3] A diagnostic criterion for CKD is a chronically low GFR for at least 3 months' duration.[4]

CKD, as indicated in Table 10-2, is classified into five stages. The normal GFR is 100 mL/min (mL/min/1.73 m²).[3] The GFR is determined by the patient's serum creatinine value and a prediction equation.[3] Many patients move through the early stages of CKD unaware of the decline in renal function. In early CKD, functioning nephrons may compensate for the damaged or nonfunctional nephrons. Loss of 80% of nephrons may occur without the patient becoming symptomatic. With loss of greater than 90% of the nephrons, the patient experiences multisystem signs and symptoms and requires dialysis or renal transplantation to sustain body viability (Table 10-3).[7]

A patient with ESRD is at risk for developing a wide spectrum of systemic impairments. Although interventions such as dialysis may improve many of

Table 10-2 Stages of Chronic Kidney Disease

Description	GFR (mL/min/1.73 m²)
Normal kidney function	125
At risk for development of CKD	91–124 with CKD risk factors
Stage 1: Kidney damage with normal or increase in kidney function	≥90
Stage 2: Kidney damage with mild loss of kidney function	60–89
Stage 3: Moderate loss of kidney function	30–59
Stage 4: Severe loss of kidney function	15–29
Stage 5: Kidney failure	<15

CKD, Chronic kidney disease; GFR, glomerular filtration rate.
Data compiled from National Kidney Foundation. K/DOQI clinical practice guidelines for chronic kidney disease: evaluation, classification, and stratification. *Am J Kidney Dis.* 2002;39(2 Suppl 1):S1–266; Levey AS, Eckardt KU, Tsukamoto Y, et al. Definition and classification of chronic kidney disease: a position statement from Kidney Disease: Improving Global Outcomes (KDIGO). *Kidney Int.* 2005;67:2089; Fraser CL, Arieff AI. Nervous system complications in uremia. *Ann Intern Med.* 1988;109:143; and Foley RN, Murray AM, Li S, et al. Chronic kidney disease and the risk for cardiovascular disease, renal replacement, and death in the United States Medicare population, 1998 to 1999. *J Am Soc Nephrol.* 2005;16:489.

Table 10-3 Systemic Signs and Symptoms of End-Stage Renal Disease

Corporal System	Clinical Signs and Symptoms
Gastrointestinal	Nausea, vomiting, anorexia, diarrhea, constipation, abdominal pain, stomatitis
Cardiovascular	Hypertension, arrhythmias, uremic pericarditis, congestive heart failure, peripheral edema, shortness of breath
Hematological	Anemia of chronic disease, increased bleeding tendencies, impaired leukocyte function
Musculoskeletal	Soft tissue calcifications, myositis ossificans, bone pain, pathological fractures, osteoporosis, joint pain, joint effusion
Respiratory	Pulmonary edema, pneumonia, pleural effusions, Kussmaul's respiration
Integumentary	Pruritus, dry skin, altered pigmentation, pallor
Neurological	Peripheral neuropathy, headaches, insomnia, altered level of consciousness, weakness, asterixis, coma

these impairments, not all conditions are reversible. Patients with ESRD require lifelong medical intervention to manage the accompanying symptoms.

CKD is associated with a high risk of cardiovascular disease (CVD), and the management of patients with CKD includes management of CVD as well, including active treatment of existing disease and risk factor modification preventing hypertension, hyperlipidemia, congestive heart failure, and coronary artery disease.[6] Some of the medications used in this population include angiotensin-converting enzyme inhibitors, angiotensin receptor blockers, statins, beta blockers, aspirin, nitrates, and niacin. The risk of death from CVD is much higher than the risk of mandatory dialysis therapy. Traditional CVD risk factors, including hypertension, smoking history, diabetes, dyslipidemia, and older age, are very prevalent in patients with CKD.[7] These patients are more likely to have metabolic syndrome, defined as insulin resistance, dyslipidemia, elevated serum glucose, abdominal obesity, and hypertension. Metabolic syndrome is an obvious contributor to CVD risk.[5]

Hemodialysis is the process by which plasma water and chemical solutes are filtered from the patient's blood as the blood passes through a semipermeable membrane. Blood is directed from the patient's vascular access through tubing and a semipermeable membrane. The semipermeable membrane is often referred as an "artificial kidney" or dialyzer. Types of vascular access to the patient's blood are via an arteriovenous fistula, arteriovenous graft, and temporary catheters (Fig. 10-1). An arteriovenous fistula is created by anastomosing an artery to a vein. An arteriovenous fistula is the preferred method of access because of a much lower risk of infection and clotting than the other methods. An arteriovenous graft is created by "bridging" a peripheral artery and vein with a synthetic material. Synthetic material grafts have an increased risk of infection and clotting compared with fistulas. Large-bore catheters, placed in the femoral, subclavian, or jugular veins, may be used for temporary or emergent access. Hemodialysis can be performed in outpatient, inpatient, or home settings.

Common side effects of hemodialysis include hypotension, muscle cramping, bleeding from the access site, and risk of local and systemic infection. Hypotension and muscle cramping often occur as a result of rapid changes in osmolality of the blood. Maintaining graft or fistula competency is another concern. Frequent assessment for a bruit and thrill in the dialysis access is mandatory, and prompt action must be undertaken if the graft or fistula becomes occluded.[8]

Peritoneal dialysis (PD) is a safe and effective alternative to hemodialysis therapy. Approximately 8% of patients undergoing dialysis use PD as their method of choice. PD involves inserting approximately 2 L of dialysis solution into the patient's peritoneal cavity. The

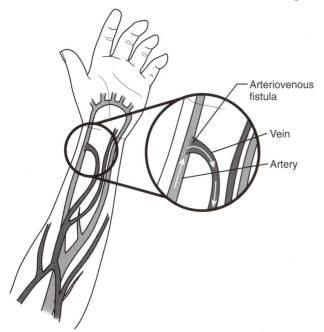

Figure 10-1 An arteriovenous shunt, also known as an arteriovenous fistula, is a connection between an artery and a vein that permits blood to flow between the two bypassing the capillary system. Fistulas can occur congenitally, traumatically, or surgically. Surgical fistulas are often created to facilitate hemodialysis procedures. A surgeon creates an arteriovenous fistula by connecting an artery directly to a vein, frequently in the forearm. Connecting the artery to the vein causes more blood to flow into the vein. As a result, the vein grows larger and stronger. The stronger walled vein facilitates the repeated needle insertions required by ongoing hemodialysis.

unique constituents of the dialysis solution coupled with the principles of osmosis and diffusion allow fluid and solute to pass from the patient's blood into the dialysis solution. Access to the peritoneum is via a catheter through the abdominal wall. Repeated insertion and withdrawal of dialysis fluid allows for proper metabolic exchange. Automated PD systems called "cyclers" allow patients to perform PD at their convenience. The most common complication of PD is peritonitis, or infection of the peritoneum. Peritonitis results from contamination of the dialysis fluid or access catheter. Rarer complications include hyperglycemia, abdominal pain, protein store losses, and hernia.[9]

Continuous renal replacement therapy (CRRT) is the filtration of blood through a hollow semipermeable membrane located outside the body. CRRT is used in patients who are hemodynamically unstable. CRRT is a slow, continuous process. Patients with hemodynamic instability are patients with hypervolemia, hypovolemia, severe uremia, electrolyte imbalance, and acid-base imbalance.[3]

Chronic Kidney Disease–Induced Neuropathy

Among the many goals of treatment of CKD is management of one of the most severe complications, neuropathy, which occurs in 65% of patients with CKD.[10] Uremic neuropathy has several forms, including peripheral mononeuropathy, peripheral polyneuropathy, motor neuropathy, and encephalopathy.[11] Encephalopathy is a change in mental status secondary to the toxic state of uremia, found in untreated stage 5 CKD. Patients with early uremic encephalopathy may present with fatigue or impaired memory or concentration. As the severity of encephalopathy progresses, hallucinations, disorientation, and coma may develop, followed, if untreated, by death.[12]

With metabolic encephalopathy, electroencephalography (EEG) often reveals generalized slowing and bilateral spike and wave complexes even in the absence of clinically obvious seizure activity. EEG measures of sleep are also abnormal in patients with stage 5 CKD. Computed tomography scan or magnetic resonance imaging (MRI) may show cerebral atrophy but do not reveal findings indicative of CKD specifically.[12]

Peripheral neuropathy secondary to CKD may manifest as peripheral polyneuropathy, autonomic dysfunction, restless legs syndrome (RLS), and peripheral mononeuropathy.[12–14] Neuropathic symptoms do not typically occur unless the GFR is consistently less than 20 mL/min.[13] Generally, the occurrence of neuropathy correlates with the severity of the kidney disease and not so much with the actual type or etiology of underlying kidney disease. However, there are diseases that produce kidney damage and cause neuropathy, including amyloidosis, diabetes mellitus, systemic lupus erythematosus, polyarteritis nodosa, and end-stage liver failure.[15] For this reason, the spectrum of neuropathies occurring with CKD is quite extensive.

Normally, kidneys, along with removal of the by-products of metabolism and respiration, filter and remove excess small proteins from the blood. With advanced CKD, especially in patients receiving dialysis, the concentration of one type of small protein called beta-2-microglobulin, increases in the blood. When this increase occurs, beta-2-microglobulin molecules may join together, similar to the links of a chain, forming a few very large molecules from many smaller ones. These large molecules can deposit onto and eventually damage the surrounding tissues and cause great discomfort. This condition is called dialysis-related amyloidosis (DRA).[16]

DRA is common in patients, especially older adults, who have been on hemodialysis for more than 5 years.[16] Older hemodialysis membranes do not effectively remove the large, complex beta-2-microglobulin proteins from the bloodstream. Newer hemodialysis membranes as well as PD remove beta-2-microglobulin more effectively but not enough to keep blood concentrations normal. As a result, blood levels remain elevated, and deposits form in bone, joints, and tendons.[14] DRA may result in pain, stiffness, and chronic appendicular joint synovitis. Patients with DRA may also develop cysts in some of their bones, and these cysts may lead to pathological bone fractures. Amyloid deposits may cause tears in ligaments and tendons.[14] Most patients with these problems can be helped by surgical intervention. From a neuropathy viewpoint, the amyloid deposits on peripheral nerves result in epineural fibrosis resulting in passive insufficiency of the peripheral nerve. Peripheral nerves stretch to accommodate various axial and appendicular positioning, and the fibrosis limits this extensibility. If patients with CKD and amyloid neural deposits stretch beyond the capability of the peripheral nerve, the supporting structures of the nerve are injured, an inflammatory cascade develops, and more scarring is laid down. Eventually, the fibrosis becomes so thickened the action potential cannot propagate resulting in denervation.

Approximately 50% of patients with DRA also develop carpal tunnel syndrome, which results from the unusual buildup of amyloid at the level of the wrists.[13] If detected before significant motor neuron loss, the condition may be reversible with surgical release. No effective treatment exists for DRA, although a successful kidney transplant may stop the disease from progressing. However, DRA has caught the attention of dialysis engineers, who are attempting to develop new dialysis membranes that can remove larger amounts of beta-2-microglobulin from the blood.[15]

In addition to the compressive and traction neuropathies caused by deposits of amyloid, distal mononeuropathies may occur in an extremity during and after the construction of arteriovenous fistulas. The surgical procedure itself or later trauma to the perifistular tissue may lead to a diminished loss of distal blood flow and ultimately tissue and nerve ischemia. Local weakness, sensory loss, and positive Tinel sign at the site of ischemia are often present.

Common risk factors, along with CKD, for development of distal sensory or motor neuropathy include diabetes, alcoholism, nonalcoholic liver disease, malignancy, and HIV. The neuropathy is distal, symmetrical, and mixed sensorimotor and is seen more commonly in male patients. The symptoms, because of the long axons being more severely damaged, are worse in the lower extremities. Sensory symptoms, such as paresthesias, burning sensations, and pain, occur before the motor symptoms. Findings on physical examination commonly include impaired vibratory perception and absent deep tendon reflexes. Paradoxical heat sensation in the feet can be found in 40% of patients with CKD.[17] Cranial nerve involvement is rare and when present may include transient nystagmus, miosis, impaired extraocular movement, and facial asymmetry.

Autonomic neuropathy (dysautonomia or autonomic dysfunction) is a common problem in patients with CKD.[18] In patients with autonomic neuropathy, clinical findings include abnormal tilt test, orthostatic hypotension, and abnormal heart and respiratory rates at rest and when challenged by exercise and are present in about 50% of patients with stage 5 CKD.[19] Autonomic neuropathy may be a causal factor in the frequent hypotensive episodes seen during dialysis.[19] Some tests that evaluate different aspects of this neuropathy include the Valsalva maneuver, which probes the integrity of the low-pressure and high-pressure baroreceptors in the cardiopulmonary circulation, the afferent and efferent limbs of these pathways, and both sympathetic and parasympathetic function.[18] It is a useful test to detect the existence of autonomic neuropathy but not to identify the site of the abnormality. The amyl nitrate inhalation test evaluates the low-pressure baroreceptors and the resultant efferent sympathetic outflow, which is the expected result when blood pressure decreases.[18] The cold pressor test reflects efferent sympathetic function in response to cold-induced vasoconstriction.[19] The most common autonomic defect in patients undergoing dialysis is in the baroreceptor/afferent side of the autonomic loop.[18,19] This particular dysfunction minimizes the reflex increase in circulating catecholamines that should increase when hypotension occurs during hemodialysis.

Autonomic dysfunction can impair the ability to maintain systolic blood pressure after significant ultrafiltration because of an inability to increase systemic vascular resistance. The decrease in blood pressure occurring secondary to a decrease in intravascular volume cannot be remediated, leading to orthostatic symptoms. There is as yet no effective therapy for autonomic dysfunction in patients undergoing dialysis. There are two possibly helpful drugs that improve symptomatic orthostatic hypotension: midodrine, a selective alpha-1-adrenergic agonist, and sertraline, a central nervous system serotonin reuptake inhibitor. The benefit may be due to an attenuation of sympathetic withdrawal.[20]

Primary sensory dysfunction, along with the classic symptoms of hypothesia and hyperthesia, may also manifest in a patient with CKD as RLS, burning foot syndrome, or paradoxical heat sensation.[21] RLS is a persistent, uncomfortable sensation in the lower extremities that is relieved only by movement of the legs. The symptoms are much more bothersome at night and are quite common in end-stage renal failure (patients on long-term dialysis).[22] Studies of patients with RLS describe a decreased quality of life, and strong correlations exist with concomitant iron deficiency, smoking history, and duration of ESRD.[23] RLS can often be treated by correcting iron deficiency or administering levodopa or dopamine agonists.[22] Burning foot syndrome involves severe pain and a burning sensation distally in the lower extremities. Its presence may be associated with thiamine deficiency (formerly common in dialysis patients).[22] Paradoxical heat sensation, in which low-temperature stimuli above or below the noxious threshold trigger perceived sensations typically seen with high-temperature stimuli, is found in approximately 10% of patients with stage 5 CKD. The perceived sensations may range from warmth to intense burning.[23]

The pathophysiology of uremic neuropathy is not well understood.[12,13] The most sensitive test for detection of neuropathy is the nerve conduction velocity test, which shows slowed sensory nerve conduction velocity. There is also evidence of axonal degeneration and secondary demyelination of peripheral nerves. These conditions may be due to neurotoxic compounds of uremia, which deplete energy supplies via inhibition of nerve fiber enzymes necessary for maintenance of energy production. The long axons degenerate earliest because they have a greater metabolic load for the perikaryon to bear. The "dying back" of axons is more severe in the distal aspect of the neuron, possibly owing to metabolic failure of the perikaryon. The axonal degeneration may initiate the process, and this then leads to secondary segmental demyelination. CKD-associated polyneuropathy is a specific term referring to a generalized homogeneous process affecting many peripheral nerves, with the distal nerves usually being affected most prominently.[11]

Interference with the axon membrane function and inhibition of Na+/K+-activated ATPase by uremic toxins has been theorized as a possible etiology for CKD-induced neuropathy.[12] Potassium (K+), often elevated in uremia, may contribute to the development of neuropathy. Peripheral nerve dysfunction may be related to an interference with the nerve axon membrane function and inhibition of Na+/K+-activated ATPase by toxic factors in uremic serum.[13] Bolton and Young[12] postulated that membrane dysfunction was occurring at the perineurium, which functioned as a diffusion barrier between interstitial fluid and nerve, or within the endoneurium, which acted as a barrier between blood and nerve. As a result, uremic toxins may enter the endoneural space at either site and cause direct nerve damage and water and electrolyte shifts with expansion or retraction of the space.

Other theories for the development of uremic neuropathy include thiamine deficiency; decreased transketolase activity; and reduced concentrations of other compounds or enzymes necessary for proper nerve function, including decreased levels of biotin and zinc and increased concentrations of phenols and myo-inositol. Secondary hyperparathyroidism is also associated with the presence of polyneuropathy.[13]

In addition, the accumulation of uremic toxins of medium molecular weight ("middle molecules") has been a widely held theory explaining the development of uremic polyneuropathy.[3] The nature of the toxic substances in uremia is not clearly defined. Myo-inositol, a precursor of phosphoinositide, is metabolized rapidly in neural membranes. It is elevated abnormally in CKD, poorly eliminated by hemodialysis, but excreted by the renal cortex of successfully transplanted kidneys. Substances of moderate molecular weight (i.e., 500 to 2,000 daltons) can be toxic agents in uremia. Advanced glycosylated end products and parathyroid hormone generally are recognized as major uremic toxins (Box 10-2).[3-5]

The clinical presentation of uremic polyneuropathy usually begins with lower extremity symptoms because

---

Box 10-2

Uremic Toxins Possibly Associated With Uremic Neuropathy

3-Carboxy-4-methyl-5-propyl-2-furanpropionic acid
Advanced glycosylated end products
Asymmetrical dimethylarginine
Beta-2-microglobulin
Complement factor D
Creatinine
Guanidines
Hippuric acid
Homocysteine
Indoles
Indoxyl sulfate
Medium-size to large molecules (500–2,000 daltons)
Oxalate
Oxidation products
Parathyroid hormone
P-cresol polyamines
Peptides (beta-endorphin, methionine-enkephalin, beta-lipotropin, granulocyte inhibiting proteins I and II, degranulation-inhibiting protein, adrenomedullin)
Phosphorus
Protein-bound compounds
Purines
Small water-soluble compounds
Urea

Data compiled from National Kidney Foundation. K/DOQI clinical practice guidelines for chronic kidney disease: evaluation, classification, and stratification. Am J Kidney Dis. 2002;39(2 Suppl 1):S1–266; Levey AS, Eckardt KU, Tsukamoto Y, et al. Definition and classification of chronic kidney disease: a position statement from Kidney Disease: Improving Global Outcomes (KDIGO). Kidney Int. 2005;67:2089; Fraser CL, Arieff AI. Nervous system complications in uremia. Ann Intern Med. 1988;109:143; Foley RN, Murray AM, Li S, et al. Chronic kidney disease and the risk for cardiovascular disease, renal replacement, and death in the United States Medicare population, 1998 to 1999. J Am Soc Nephrol. 2005;16:489; Foley RN, Wang C, Collins AJ. Cardiovascular risk factor profiles and kidney function stage in the US general population: the NHANES III study. Mayo Clin Proc. 2005;80:1270; and Shishehbor MH, Oliveira LP, Lauer MS, et al. Emerging cardiovascular risk factors that account for a significant portion of attributable mortality risk in chronic kidney disease. Am J Cardiol. 2008;101:1741.

the longer axons are affected earliest. Motor symptoms follow the onset of sensory symptoms. Patients typically present with slowly progressive sensory loss and dysesthesias such as numbness, burning sensation in feet, and mild gait abnormalities; this is followed by weakness in the legs and then in the hands. Typical symptoms are insidious in onset and consist of a tingling and prickling sensation in the lower extremities. Paresthesia is the most common and earliest symptom. Additionally, increase in pain sensation is a prominent symptom. Many patients experience RLS and muscle cramping even if they are not yet experiencing neuropathic symptoms. If patients remain untreated, sensory symptoms are followed by motor symptoms (weakness in lower extremities and muscle atrophy.) Later, the symptoms progress to involve the upper extremities.[12]

Obtaining "clinical scripts" from the history followed by a hypothesis-oriented physical evaluation is very important in helping to discern the type of neuropathy with which the patient is presenting. Abnormalities in the physical examination are determined by the type of neuropathy. In patients with uremic axonal polyneuropathy, there may be wasting of the intrinsic muscles of the feet and hands. Distal loss of sensation to pinprick, light touch, vibration, cold, and proprioception may occur as well. Reflexes become hypoactive distally.

The most sensitive ways to detect neuropathy in renal disease are electrophysiological studies (even in clinically asymptomatic patients). Of these, the more commonly used is motor nerve conduction velocity, usually measured in the peroneal nerve. Slowing of the motor nerve conduction velocity worsens with further decline in renal function. Greater than 50% of patients have abnormal studies when the creatinine clearance decreases to 10 mL/min.[24] At this advanced stage of CKD, patients may also experience paradoxical heat sensation.[7]

Polyneuropathy of kidney disease needs to be distinguished from other diseases of the peripheral nervous system, including mononeuropathies and mononeuropathy multiplex. Mononeuropathy refers to focal involvement of a single nerve usually secondary to a local cause, including trauma, compression, or entrapment. An example is carpal tunnel syndrome. Mononeuropathy multiplex refers to simultaneous or sequential involvement of noncontiguous nerve trunks; this usually includes multiple nerve infarcts resulting from a systemic vasculitis process affecting the vasa nervorum.

The later development of motor symptoms can lead to muscle atrophy, myoclonus, and, rarely, paralysis. Complete recovery of this stage of peripheral polyneuropathy is unlikely even with the initiation of dialysis therapy. Untreated, uremic polyneuropathy progresses and becomes less likely to reverse even when kidney transplantation, the only treatment for later stage uremic neuropathy, is performed. After transplantation, clinical recovery occurs over 3 to 6 months and may continue over the next 2 years. Thorough adequate thrice-weekly hemodialysis or daily peritoneal dialysis may halt the progression of neuropathy. Dialysis rarely results in significant and substantial clinical improvement. If neuropathy worsens despite dialysis, this may be an important indicator of insufficient dialysis. Some studies indicate an improved prognosis in neuropathy with daily or nightly hemodialysis compared with thrice-weekly sessions.[25]

Patients with painful neuropathy can benefit from treatment with tricyclic antidepressants such as amitriptyline or with anticonvulsant medications such as sodium valproate or gabapentin. These medications may provide symptomatic or palliative relief from painful symptoms. Vitamin supplements including water-soluble B vitamins, pyridoxine, and methylcobalamin have been shown to help improve neuropathic pain in CKD.[26] Dietary restriction of potassium intake may also be helpful in preventing progression of neuropathy.[27]

CASE STUDY

JG is a 24-year-old woman with a 5-year history of chronic kidney disease secondary to chronic overuse of over-the-counter nonsteroidal anti-inflammatory drugs. Past medical history is significant for chronic alcohol abuse and breast cancer. For the past 2 years, she has received hemodialysis three times weekly at a local dialysis center via a fistula located in her right forearm. She presents to physical therapy with numbness in the palmar surface of both hands and complaints of dropping objects. She has noted atrophy of the muscles at the bases of her thumbs. Complaints include difficulty turning doorknobs and holding utensils when she is cutting food. Sensory examination reveals a loss of tactile sense over the palmar surface of her thumbs and first three fingers bilaterally. There is no overt weakness via manual muscle testing. JG does not complain of any lower extremity symptoms. JG has recently received a diagnosis of type 2 diabetes mellitus.

Case Study Questions

1. Important laboratory values for the outpatient therapist to review before initiating therapy include which of the following?
   a. Thiamine
   b. Hemoglobin A_{1c}
   c. Parathyroid hormone
   d. All of the above

2. For this case study, what is the most important adjunct diagnostic test to determine the severity of the neuropathy?
  a. MRI of the brain
  b. MRI of the cervical spine
  c. Electroneuromyography of both upper extremities
  d. Tinel sign at the level of the median nerve

3. A key clinical script that may lead the therapist to believe the symptoms are not the result of uremic polyneuropathy is which of the following?
  a. Lack of lower extremity symptoms
  b. No focal motor weakness via manual muscle test
  c. Symmetrical presentation of symptoms
  d. Loss of tactile sensation

4. Common risk factors, along with the chronic kidney disease, for development of distal sensory/motor neuropathy in this patient include which of the following?
  a. Diabetes
  b. Alcoholism
  c. Malignancy
  d. All of the above

5. During the integument examination, the therapist should inspect the fistula. "Red flags" include which of the following?
  a. Tenderness
  b. Lack of audible bruit
  c. Rubor
  d. All of the above

References

1. U.S. Department of Health and Human Services. National Kidney and Urologic Diseases Information Clearinghouse (NKUDIC). http://kidney.niddk.nih.gov/kudiseases/pubs/kustats/#2. Accessed November 12, 2012.
2. National Kidney Foundation. K/DOQI clinical practice guidelines for chronic kidney disease: evaluation, classification, and stratification. *Am J Kidney Dis.* 2002; 39(2 Suppl 1):S1–266.
3. Levey AS, Eckardt KU, Tsukamoto Y, et al. Definition and classification of chronic kidney disease: a position statement from Kidney Disease: Improving Global Outcomes (KDIGO). *Kidney Int.* 2005;67:2089.
4. Fraser CL, Arieff AI. Nervous system complications in uremia. *Ann Intern Med.* 1988;109:143.
5. Foley RN, Murray AM, Li S, et al. Chronic kidney disease and the risk for cardiovascular disease, renal replacement, and death in the United States Medicare population, 1998 to 1999. *J Am Soc Nephrol.* 2005;16:489.
6. Foley RN, Wang C, Collins AJ. Cardiovascular risk factor profiles and kidney function stage in the US general population: the NHANES III study. *Mayo Clin Proc.* 2005; 80:1270.
7. Shishehbor MH, Oliveira LP, Lauer MS, et al. Emerging cardiovascular risk factors that account for a significant portion of attributable mortality risk in chronic kidney disease. *Am J Cardiol.* 2008;101:1741.
8. Murphy E, Byrne G. The role of the nurse in the management of acute kidney injury. *Br J Nurs.* 2010;36: 146–152.
9. Prowant B. Peritoneal dialysis nursing. *Nephr Nurs J.* 2009:36; 197–227.
10. Krishnan AV, Kiernan MC. Uremic neuropathy: clinical features and new pathophysiological insights. *Muscle Nerve.* 2007;35:273.
11. Makkar RK, Kochar DK. Somatosensory evoked potentials (SSEPs): sensory nerve conduction velocity (SNCV) and motor nerve conduction velocity (MNCV) in chronic renal failure. *Electromyogr Clin Neurophysiol.* 1994;34:295.
12. Bolton CF, Young GB. Uremic neuropathy. In: *Neurological Complications of Renal Disease.* Boston: Butterworth; 1990: 76–107.
13. Bazzi C, Pagani C, Sorgato G, et al. Uremic polyneuropathy: a clinical and electrophysiological study in 135 short- and long-term hemodialyzed patients. *Clin Nephrol.* 1991;35:176.
14. Benson MD, Kincaid JC. The molecular biology and clinical features of amyloid neuropathy. *Muscle Nerve.* 2007; 36:411.
15. Hafer-Macko C, Hsieh ST, Li CY, et al. Acute motor axonal neuropathy: An antibody-mediated attack on axolemma. *Ann Neurol.* 1996;40:635.
16. Dyck PJ, Dyck JB, Grant IA, Fealey RD. Ten steps in characterizing and diagnosing patients with peripheral neuropathy. *Neurology.* 1996;47:10.
17. England JD, Gronseth GS, Franklin G, et al. Practice parameter: evaluation of distal symmetric polyneuropathy: role of autonomic testing, nerve biopsy, and skin biopsy (an evidence-based review). Report of the American Academy of Neurology, American Association of Neuromuscular and Electrodiagnostic Medicine, and American Academy of Physical Medicine and Rehabilitation. *Neurology.* 2009; 72:177.
18. Ewing DJ, Winney R. Autonomic function in patients with chronic renal failure on intermittent hemodialysis. *Nephron.* 1975;15:424.
19. Henrich WL. Autonomic insufficiency. *Arch Intern Med.* 1982;142:339.
20. Converse RL Jr, Jacobsen TN, Jost CM, et al. Paradoxical withdrawal of reflex vasoconstriction as a cause of hemodialysis-induced hypotension. *J Clin Invest.* 1992; 90:1657.
21. Kavanagh D, Siddiqui S, Geddes CC. Restless legs syndrome in patients on dialysis. *Am J Kidney Dis.* 2004;43:763.
22. Unruh ML, Levey AS, D'Ambrosio C, et al. Restless legs symptoms among incident dialysis patients: association with lower quality of life and shorter survival. *Am J Kidney Dis.* 2004;43:900.
23. Thorp ML. Restless legs syndrome. *Int J Artif Organs.* 2001; 24:755.
24. Nardin R, Chapman KM, Raynor EM. Prevalence of ulnar neuropathy in patients receiving hemodialysis. *Arch Neurol.* 2005;62:271.
25. Rocco M, Lockridge R, Beck G, et al. The effects of frequent nocturnal home hemodialysis: the Frequent Hemodialysis Network Trial. *Kidney Int.* 2011;80:1080–1091.
26. Guay DR. Update on gabapentin therapy of neuropathic pain. *Consult Pharm.* 2003;18:158–170.
27. Dheenan S, Venkatesan J, Grubb BP, Henrich WL. Effect of sertraline hydrochloride on dialysis hypotension. *Am J Kidney Dis.* 1998;31:624.

Chapter 11

Medication-Induced Neuropathy

ROBERT B. RAFFA, PhD

"Awareness of the potential of medications to cause peripheral neuropathy is key to preventing significant nerve damage in treated patients."

—PELTIER AND RUSSELL

Objectives

On completion of this chapter, the student/practitioner will be able to:

- Understand the common classes of medications that can induce neuropathy and the major pathophysiological mechanisms that are likely involved.

Key Terms

- Apoptosis
- Demyelination
- Paresthesia
- Peripheral neuropathy

Introduction

There are about 100 known causes of neuropathy.[1] Medication-induced neuropathy accounts for about 4% of outpatient neurology cases.[2] A representative list of drugs that can have neurotoxic effects is provided in Table 11-1.[3] This chapter concentrates on chemotherapeutic agents (platinum drugs, taxanes, vinca alkaloids, thalidomide, bortezomib, suramin), leflunomide, statins, highly active antiretroviral therapy (HAART), antitumor necrosis factor alpha (anti-TNFα) drugs, and amiodarone.

Mechanisms of Medication-Induced Neuropathy

Neuropathy may be considered medication induced if it meets generally established criteria for associations, such as a temporal association (the onset of neuropathy coincides with the onset of medication use, stabilization or improvement of neuropathy when the drug is temporarily discontinued, and neuropathy resumes when medication is resumed), biological plausibility, absence of likely alternative explanations, and analogy (similar adverse effects occur with similar medications).[56]

The underlying neuropathology typically involves three main processes that damage or destroy nerves: axonal degeneration, segmental **demyelination,** and neuronopathy.[1] Medication-induced neuropathies often involve axonal degeneration, but any or all processes can occur concurrently.[57] Symptoms can give insight into the type of nerve damage causing the neuropathy.[58]

Spinal cord neurons are generally protected by the blood-brain barrier, whereas sensory, autonomic, and peripheral neurons are more vulnerable.[3] The latter are supplied by capillaries with fenestrated walls, allowing relatively free exchange of small molecules with the circulatory system and extracellular fluid within ganglia.[22] Medications can interfere with axonal

Table 11-1 Selected Drugs Associated With Medication-Induced Neuropathy

Drug	Rate of Occurrence	Comments
Amiodarone	3%–30%[4–6]	Duration of treatment affects neurotoxicity[7]
Bortezomib	12%[8] or 31%–45%[9–17]	Dose dependent[13,18]
Carboplatin	4%–6%[19]	>400 mg/m² dose[20]
Cisplatin	12%–60% at conventional doses[3,19,21,22] and 70%–100% at higher doses (>540 mg/m²)[3]	90% of patients who receive cumulative doses of >300 mg/m² experience peripheral neuropathy[23,24]
Docetaxol	17.9%[25]	>600 mg/m² dose[26,27]
Highly active antiretroviral therapy (HAART)	36%–48%[28] overall, 9% severe[29]	HIV can cause neuropathy so rates are unclear; advanced age is associated with higher rates of neuropathy[28]
Leflunomide	1%–10%,[30–32] but one study showed 54%[33]	Unclear if dose dependent
Oxaliplatin—acute neuropathy	60%–98%[22,34–37]	Occurs at onset of therapy; no cumulative effect
Oxaliplatin—chronic neuropathy	~50%[19]	≥540–800 mg/m² dose[20,38,39]
Paclitaxel	4%–20%[22,40,41]	>175–200 mg/m² dose[20,42]; >175 mg/m² any single dose[43]
Suramin	30%–55%[44,45]	Dose dependent[46]
Thalidomide	20%–50%[22,47]	>20 g dose[48]; appears to be cumulative and dose dependent[49,50]
Vincristine	10.5%[51]	>4 mg/m² dose[20]
Vinflunine	<10%–12%[52,53]	Dose dependent, reversible[53]
Zalcitabine	30%–60%[55]	

transport (disrupting cell processes) or can damage the axon and the myelin sheath (Schwann cells). Anticancer agents that interfere with the increased mitochondrial activity that is typical of cancer cells likewise can interfere with mitochondrial activity of neurons and may lead to neuronopathy or death of the nerve cell.[22] Ganglionopathy occurs when ganglia are damaged or die and results in sensory or autonomic symptoms.[59]

Chemotherapeutic Agents

Although chemotherapy-induced **peripheral neuropathy** can give rise to several commonly used antineoplastic agents, the pathophysiology of nerve damage is related to drug class. The resulting symptoms may be sensory, motor, or autonomic and may be dose limiting.[60]

Platinum Drugs

Three major platinum chemotherapeutic agents are cisplatin, carboplatin, and oxaliplatin.[19] Platinum-induced neuropathies are common, are cumulative, and may involve "coasting" (neuropathic symptoms persist in the initial weeks and months after drug discontinuation).[19]

The antineoplastic effect of platinum drugs includes their effect on tumor vasculature.[61] Platinum compounds also bind avidly to plasma proteins[20] and neuronal DNA.[62,63] The number of DNA cross-links in the neurons of the dorsal root ganglia (DRG) has been associated with the drug's degree of neurotoxicity.[64] The resulting DNA repair arrests cell division.[65] The platinum concentration in peripheral nervous tissue is similar to that in tumor tissue in patients treated with platinum agents.[66]

Taxanes

Taxane drugs, including paclitaxel and docetaxel, are associated with dose-dependent drug-induced neuropathy.[20] Taxanes disrupt microtubular dynamics and polymerization within cells, and interrupted axonal transport may be involved in taxane-induced neuropathy.[3] Taxanes appear to have a direct effect on Schwann cells, cause axonal loss, and disturb the cytoplasmic flow in the affected neurons.[67,68]

In a randomized clinical trial comparing paclitaxel with a control group (single-agent gemcitabine or vinorelbine) in chemotherapy-naïve patients, neuropathy occurred significantly more often in patients receiving paclitaxel than control subjects (30% vs. 5%, $P < 0.001$).[40] Although paclitaxel is associated with more severe forms of medication-induced neuropathy than docetaxel,[69] severe docetaxel-induced neuropathy has also been reported.[70]

Risk factors for taxane-induced neuropathy include cumulative dose, high single doses, rapid infusion times, previous or simultaneous administration of other chemotherapeutic agents,[20] and a large number of chemotherapy cycles.[71]

Vinca Alkaloids

Vinca alkaloids inhibit the assembly of microtubules and promote their disassembly, which interferes with cytoskeletal axonal transport within the cell.[22,72] By inhibiting tubulin polymerization into microtubules, vinca alkaloids destabilize the mitotic spindle.[18] Microscopy of sensory neurons reveals cytoskeletal structural changes in the large sensory neurons and myelinated axons as well as an accumulation of neurofilaments in sensory DRG.[73] Vinflunine, a newer vinca alkaloid drug, has less affinity for tubulin-binding sites and appears to be less neurotoxic than vincristine.[74]

Thalidomide

Despite its association with birth defects, thalidomide has reemerged as an approved drug for certain cancers.[47] Thalidomide is thought to modulate cytokines, particularly by decreasing the production of TNFα in monocytes and macrophages and by increasing the elimination of TNFα messenger RNA, which leads to a decrease in the signaling that induces TNFα production.[75,76] Thalidomide also possesses antiangiogenic properties, which appear to function independently of its TNFα-inhibiting effects.[47]

Thalidomide-induced neuropathy is possibly related to neurotrophin dysregulation, leading to inhibition of nuclear factor-κβ, which sensory neurons need to survive.[77,78] Multiple mechanisms may be involved because of the observed "glove-and-stocking" effect (sensory neuropathy in the hands and feet, distributed in a pattern similar to gloves and stockings), suggesting axonal degeneration[79] and poor recovery rates (suggesting permanent damage to the DRG).[80]

Thalidomide neurotoxicity appears to be dose dependent and cumulative,[48,50,80] and it has been recommended that therapy be restricted to courses less than 6 months[81] under careful neurological monitoring.[82]

Bortezomib

Bortezomib, a proteasome inhibitor and boronic acid dipeptide, is a newer agent used in the treatment of multiple myeloma.[9] Bortezomib is thought to treat cancer by inducing **apoptosis,** arresting tumor growth, and reversing chemoresistance in myeloma cells.[83] The mechanisms underlying bortezomib-induced neuropathy remain unclear, but an accumulation of the agent in DRG cells has been observed.[12] Metabolic changes caused by bortezomib accumulation in the DRG and mitochondrial-mediated dysregulation of Ca^{2+} homeostasis and disruption of neurotrophins have been implicated as mechanisms of bortezomib-induced neuropathy.[11] It may also cause demyelination.[11] Because certain neuropathies persist or develop after bortezomib is discontinued, it has been suggested that immune-mediated mechanisms may also play a role.[84]

Preexisting neuropathy has been reported to be a risk factor for the development of a more severe bortezomib-induced neuropathy.[85] Other risk factors for bortezomib-induced neuropathy are cumulative dose,[16] no concurrent dexamethasone administration, male sex,[71] lack of neurological monitoring,[86] and prior use of thalidomide[12,87] or vincristine.[86] Advancing age is likely a risk factor with a suggested 6% increase in risk for every year of age.[88] Diabetes has been explored as a potential risk factor with conflicting results.[13,87]

Suramin

Suramin is an experimental antineoplastic agent[89] and reverse transcriptase inhibitor[90] used in chemotherapeutic applications.[91] Suramin-induced neuropathy has been described as an axonal neuropathy with acute Guillain-Barré–type symptoms, elevated cerebrospinal fluid protein levels, and variable response to plasma exchange.[44,45,92] Rats administered suramin develop axonal degeneration and lysosomal inclusion bodies in the DRG and Schwann cells, but demyelination is rare.[46]

Suramin has numerous cellular effects. It inhibits enzyme function, blocks mitogenic growth factors,[93] blocks nerve growth factor (NGF) binding,[94] and activates and induces phosphorylation and downstream signaling of the NGF receptor.[95–97] Based on results using animal tissue cultures, the mechanism underlying suramin-induced neuropathy may involve glycolipid imbalance, which would lead to neuronal degradation and subsequent cell death.[46]

Leflunomide

Leflunomide is a disease-modifying drug used in the treatment of rheumatoid arthritis. Leflunomide is the prodrug of the active metabolite A77 1726 [N-(4-Trifluoromethylphenyl)-2-cyano-3-hydroxycrotonamide], which has immunosuppressive effects. New and exacerbated peripheral neuropathy, including **paresthesia,** has been reported with leflunomide use[31,98–101] but is relatively rare[30,31,33] and may be reversible.[102]

It has been suggested that the mechanism underlying leflunomide-induced neuropathy involves a neurological vasculitis affecting the peripheral nervous system.[99] Vasculitis may be triggered by a leflunomide-induced immune system response. Nerve biopsy specimens from three patients receiving leflunomide revealed epineurial perivascular inflammation around the large and small myelinated nerve fibers, suggesting a type of axonopathy with features of vasculitis.[31] Electrophysiological study results from 37 patients with leflunomide-induced neuropathy were consistent with distal axonal, sensory, or sensorimotor polyneuropathies.[102]

Risk factors for the development of leflunomide-induced neuropathy include advanced age, diabetes, and the concurrent use of other neurotoxic agents.[32]

Statins

Statins are taken by millions of people around the world to reduce serum cholesterol.[103] Statins interfere with cholesterol synthesis by inhibiting two distinct processes: HMG CoA (3-hydroxy-3-methylglutaryl coenzyme A) reductase and ubiquinone (a mitochondrial respiratory chain enzyme).[104,105] Although statins are generally well tolerated, these inhibitory effects have been suggested to disrupt the energy use patterns of neurons, leading to neuropathic symptoms in some patients.[104]

Statin drugs have been extensively studied in numerous landmark clinical trials, none of which found evidence of statin-induced neuropathy.[106] However, an epidemiological 5-year study found the odds ratio linking idiopathic polyneuropathy with statin use to be 3.7 (95% confidence interval, 1.8 to 7.6) for all cases and 14.2 (95% confidence interval, 5.3 to 38.0) for patients with a diagnosis of "definite" rather than "probable" or "possible" polyneuropathy.[104] Other reports in the literature link long-term statin use to neuropathic symptoms.[107–112] In contrast, in a cross-sectional arm of the Fremantle Diabetes Study (n = 531), patients treated with statins had a significantly *decreased risk* of diabetic neuropathy.[113] The possible neuroprotective mechanisms behind this finding remain to be elucidated. Although statins may confer neuroprotective benefits to diabetic patients, this does not rule out the simultaneous existence of a statin-induced form of neuropathy.[58] The controversy over the existence or extent of statin-induced neuropathy is unresolved.

Highly Active Antiretroviral Therapy

HAART combines at least one nucleoside analog reverse transcriptase inhibitor (NRTI) with at least one protease inhibitor and may include one or more non-nucleoside analog reverse transcriptase inhibitors. Only NRTIs have been associated with neuropathy.[114] When phosphorylated, NRTIs, such as zidovudine, stavudine, fialuridine, didanosine, zalcitabine, and lamivudine, compete with nucleotides for reverse transcriptase binding, which helps prevent the DNA elongation

caused by HIV.[114] These drugs appear to be toxic to mitochondria.[115]

The mechanisms underlying HAART-induced neuropathy are unclear, but viral infections may alter peripheral nerve antigens, which may result in a form of autoimmune response.[116] The presence of antiviral and autoantibodies could promote immunological cross reaction. NRTIs are phosphorylated by thymidine kinase isoforms, allowing them to compete with the substrates for HIV reverse transcriptase, which terminates DNA chains.[114,117] NRTIs also selectively affect γ-DNA polymerase, decreasing mitochondrial DNA replication. Zalcitabine, didanosine, and stavudine preferentially affect axons and Schwann cells, whereas zidovudine affects the mitochondria of skeletal muscles.[118]

Increased longevity conferred by HAART[119,120] makes neurological adverse events increasingly important to address, particularly those that might occur with prolonged use of HAART drugs.[121] Risk factors for HAART-induced neuropathy include advanced age.[122]

Anti–Tumor Necrosis Factor Alpha Drugs

TNFα is an immune-regulatory cytokine with pro-inflammatory properties. Infliximab, etanercept, and adalimumab are TNFα antagonists that are used for treating rheumatoid arthritis and other conditions. These agents launch a T-cell and immune system attack on peripheral nerve myelin, provoke a vasculitis-induced ischemia, and inhibit axonal signaling systems.[123] Anti-TNFα therapy may be associated with an immune-modulated form of neuropathy, although the mechanism is unclear.[18] Anti-TNFα drugs may not have a class effect in terms of neuropathy, in that adalimumab has no clear association with neuropathy.[58]

Infliximab-induced neuropathy appears to be either an axonal sensory polyneuropathy or a multifocal motor neuropathy.[124] Discontinuation of the TNFα blocker is not necessarily required for symptom resolution.[125]

Amiodarone

Amiodarone is a class III antiarrhythmic agent and benzofuran derivative with known dermatological, hepatic, ocular, pulmonary, and thyroid adverse events. Amiodarone neurotoxicity is possibly underreported.[126] Mixed sensory and motor neuropathies have been observed within 6 to 36 months of onset of amiodarone therapy.[5] Nerve biopsy specimens in patients with amiodarone-induced neuropathy may show lamellar inclusions in Schwann cells, possibly a consequence of inactivation of lysosomal enzymes.[72]

Case reports suggest that amiodarone-induced neuropathic symptoms become markedly reduced within days or weeks of discontinuation of the drug.[4,126,127] The primary risk factor for amiodarone-induced neuropathy may be duration of treatment.[63]

Additive and Synergistic Considerations

The literature contains few reports of the additive or synergistic neurotoxicities of specific drug combinations. Combination therapy is typical in chemotherapy, but the combinations have not been reported to be associated with notably higher rates of neurotoxicity than monotherapeutic use of the same drugs.[22,128] The combination of paclitaxel and cisplatin is an exception, in that it may provoke a rapidly progressing medication-induced neuropathy at rates exceeding that of paclitaxel or cisplatin alone.[68,129] Thalidomide and bortezomib may have additive neurotoxicity.[8,15,87,130–132]

Medication-induced neuropathy can be both treatment limiting and treatable. The mechanisms behind medication-induced neuropathies are not thoroughly understood and may be specific to drug class. Although axonal degeneration, disruption of axonal transport, and demyelination have been described, apoptosis increasingly emerges as an important pathway.[3] Conduction block can mimic immune-mediated neuropathy, whereas genuine immune-mediated neuropathies are thought to occur with anti-TNFα agents.

The risk factors for medication-induced neuropathy include the specific drug, acute dose, cumulative dose, frequency of administration, duration of therapy, patient age, and presence of preexisting neuropathy. In many cases, medication-induced neuropathies can be effectively treated by discontinuing the drug, but the damage is permanent in some instances. Many treatment modalities have been proposed apart from drug discontinuation, including the use of neuroprotective agents.[133] Further study is warranted on the additive and synergistic neurotoxic effects of medication combinations.

CASE STUDY

Severe bortezomib-induced neuropathy developed in a 69-year-old man with a 39-month history of multiple myeloma. His previous medications included melphalan, cyclophosphamide, dexamethasone, and thalidomide (which had been discontinued because a stable partial response had been attained, with no neuropathic symptoms). Bortezomib was added as third-line treatment. After two cycles of bortezomib, the man began to complain of paresthesia, numbness, and "lightning-like" pains in both hands, which did not resolve despite reduction of the dose by half for the third cycle. He developed an extremely painful peripheral neuropathy 1 month later, primarily in his lower limbs in a "stocking" distribution. His hand symptoms remained mild and unchanged. The predominant feature was severe burning, which gave rise to sleep disturbance, high levels of distress, and reduced general function. Symptoms progressed to the point that he was virtually bed-bound. The bortezomib was discontinued.

Case Study Questions

1. Which of the following statements about medication-induced peripheral neuropathy is true?
    a. Medication-induced neuropathy is extremely rare and is typically associated with medications for cancer treatment.
    b. Medication-induced neuropathy is relatively common, but the symptoms tend to be mild and do not affect quality of life.
    c. Medication-induced neuropathy is extremely common but is easily treated with medication.
    d. Medication-induced neuropathy is a common side effect of pharmaceutical intervention, the symptoms may have a great impact on the quality of life of the patient, and effective treatment may be difficult to attain.

2. The pathology underlying medication-induced neuropathy typically involves which of the following?
    a. Axonal degeneration
    b. Neuronopathy
    c. Segmented demyelination
    d. All of the above

3. Which of the following is the most susceptible to medication-induced neuropathy?
    a. Central (brain and spinal cord) neurons
    b. Peripheral neurons
    c. Interneurons associated with the basal ganglia
    d. Cutaneous receptors

4. Risk factors for medication-induced neuropathy include which of the following?
    a. Specific drug
    b. Dose
    c. Patient's age
    d. All of the above

5. The primary neuropathic complication of thalidomide is a "stocking-glove" neuropathy. Which of the following best defines "stocking-glove" neuropathy?
    a. A tactile sensory neuropathy involving the hands and feet
    b. A motor neuropathy involving the hands and feet
    c. Loss of proprioception and kinesthesia in the hands and feet but preservation of tactile sense
    d. A tactile sensory and motor neuropathy involving the hands and feet

References

1. McLeod J. Investigation of peripheral neuropathy. *J Neurol Neurosurg Psychiatry.* 1995;58:274–283.
2. Jain KK. Drug-induced peripheral neuropathies. In: Jain KK, ed. *Drug-Induced Neurological Disorders.* 2nd ed. Seattle, WA: Hogrefe & Huber; 2001:237–261.
3. Weimer L. Medication-induced peripheral neuropathy. *Curr Neurol Neurosci Rep.* 2003;3:86–92.
4. Kang H, Kang Y, Kim S, et al. Amiodarone-induced hepatitis and polyneuropathy. *Korean J Intern Med.* 2007;22:225–229.
5. Martinez-Arizala A, Sobol S, McCarty G, Nichols B, Rakita L. Amiodarone neuropathy. *Neurology.* 1983;33(5):643–645.
6. Zimetbaum P. Amiodarone for atrial fibrillation. *N Engl J Med.* 2007;356:935–941.
7. Orr C, Ahlskog E. Frequency, characteristics, and risk factors for amiodarone neurotoxicity. *Arch Neurol.* 2009;66(7):865–869.
8. Richardson P, Barlogie B, Berenson J, et al. A phase 2 study of bortezomib in relapsed, refractory myeloma. *N Engl J Med.* 2003;348(26):2609–2617.
9. Jagannath S, Durie B, Wolf J, et al. Bortezomib therapy alone and in combination with dexamethasone for previously untreated symptomatic multiple myeloma. *Br J Haematol.* 2005;129(6):776–783.
10. Richardson P, Briemberg H, Jagannath S, et al. Frequency, characteristics, and reversibility of peripheral neuropathy during treatment of advanced multiple myeloma with bortezomib. *J Clin Oncol.* 2006;25(19):3113–3120.
11. Argyriou A, Iconomou G, Kalofonos H. Bortezomib-induced peripheral neuropathy in multiple myeloma: a comprehensive review of the literature. *Blood.* 2008;112:1593–1599.
12. El-Cheikh J, Stoppa A, Bouabdallah R, et al. Features and risk factors of peripheral neuropathy during treatment with bortezomib for advanced multiple myeloma. *Clin Lymphoma Myeloma.* 2008;8(3):146–152.
13. Richardson P, Sonneveld P, Schuster M, et al. Reversibility of symptomatic peripheral neuropathy with bortezomib in the phase III APEX trial in relapsed multiple myeloma: impact of a dose-modification guideline. *Br J Haematol.* 2009;144:895–903.
14. Chen SL, Jiang B, Qiu LG, Yu L, Zhong YP, Gao W. Bortezomib plus thalidomide for newly diagnosed multiple myeloma in China. *Anat Rec (Hoboken).* 2010;293:1679–1684.
15. Bang S, Lee J, Yoon S, et al. A multicenter retrospective analysis of adverse events in Korean patients using bortezomib for multiple myeloma. *Int J Hematol.* 2006;83(4):309–313.
16. Cavaletti G, Jakubowiak A. Peripheral neuropathy during bortezomib treatment of multiple myeloma: a review of recent studies. *Leuk Lymphoma.* 2010;51(7):1178–1187.
17. Kaufman J, Nooka A, Vrana M, Gleason C, Heffner L, Lonial S. Bortezomib, thalidomide, and dexamethasone as induction therapy for patients with symptomatic multiple myeloma. *Cancer.* 2010;116:3143–3151.
18. Toyooka K, Fujimura H. Iatrogenic neuropathies. *Curr Opin Neurol.* 2009;22:475–479.
19. McWhinney S, Goldberg R, McLeod H. Platinum neurotoxicity pharmacogenetics. *Mol Cancer Ther.* 2009;8(1):10–16.
20. Quasthoff S, Hartung H. Chemotherapy-induced peripheral neuropathy. *J Neurol* 2002;249:9–17.
21. Strumberg D, Brügge S, Korn M, et al. Evaluation of long-term toxicity in patients after cisplatin-based chemotherapy for non-seminomatous testicular cancer. *Ann Oncol.* 2002;13(2):229–236.
22. Windebank A, Grisold W. Chemotherapy-induced neuropathy. *J Peripher Nerv Syst.* 2008;13:27–46.
23. Hamers F, Gispen W, Neijt J. Neurotoxic side effects of cisplatin. *Eur J Cancer.* 1991;27:372–376.
24. Pace A, Giannarelli D, Galiè E, et al. Vitamin E neuroprotection for cisplatin neuropathy: a randomized, placebo-controlled trial. *Neurology.* 2010;74(9):762–766.
25. Kaya A, Coskun U, Buyukberber S, et al. Efficacy and toxicity of preoperative chemotherapy with docetaxel and epirubicin in locally advanced invasive breast cancer. *J BUON.* 2010;15(2):248–252.
26. Hilkens P, Verweij J, Stoter G, Vecht C, van Putten WL, van den Bent MJ. Peripheral neurotoxicity induced by docetaxel. *Neurology.* 1996;46(1):104–108.
27. Pronk L, Stoter G, Verweij J. Docetaxol (Taxotere): single agent activity, development of combination treatment and reducing side-effects. *Cancer Treat Rev.* 1995;21(5):463–478.
28. Shurie J, Deribew A. Assessment of the prevalence of distal symmetrical polyneuropathy and its risk factors among HAART-treated and untreated HIV infected individuals. *Ethiop Med J.* 2010;48(2):85–93.
29. Forna F, Liechty C, Solberg P, et al. Clinical toxicity of highly active antiretroviral therapy in a home-based AIDS care program in rural Uganda. *J Acquir Immune Defic Syndr.* 2007;44:456–462.
30. Metzler C, Arlt A, Gross W, Brandt J. Peripheral neuropathy in patients with systemic rheumatic disease treated with leflunomide. *Ann Rheum Dis.* 2005;64:1798–1800.
31. Bharadwaj A, Haroon N. Peripheral neuropathy in patients on leflunomide. *Rheumatology.* 2004;43:934.
32. Martin K, Bentaberry F, Dumoulin C, et al. Peripheral neuropathy associated with leflunomide: is there a risk patient profile? *Pharmcoepidemiol Drug Saf.* 2007;16(1):74–78.
33. Richards BL, Spies J, McGill N, et al. Effect of leflunomide on the peripheral nerves in rheumatoid arthritis. *Intern Med J.* 2007;37:101–107.
34. Becouarn Y, Ychou M, Ducreux M, et al. Phase II trial of oxaliplatin as first-line chemotherapy in metastatic colorectal cancer patients. Digestive Group of French Federation of Cancer Centers. *J Clin Oncol.* 1998;16(8):2739–2744.
35. Diaz-Rubio E, Sastre J, Zaniboni A, et al. Oxaliplatin as single agent in previously untreated colorectal carcinoma patients: a phase II multicentric study. *Ann Oncol.* 1998;9(1):105–108.
36. Machover D, Diaz-Rubio E, DeGramont A, et al. Two consecutive phase II studies of oxaliplatin (L-OHP) for treatment of patients with advanced colorectal carcinoma who were resistant to previous treatment with fluoropyrimidines. *Ann Oncol.* 1996;7(1):95–98.
37. Ta L, Low P, Windebank A. Mice with cisplatin and oxaliplatin-induced painful neuropathy develop distinct early responses to thermal stimuli. *Mol Pain.* 2009;5:9–20.
38. Cersosimo C. Oxaliplatin-associated neuropathy: a review. *Ann Pharmacother.* 2005;39:128–135.
39. Peltier A, Russell J. Advances in understanding drug-induced neuropathies. *Drug Saf.* 2006;29(1):23–30.
40. O'Brien M, Socinski M, Popovich A, et al. Randomized phase III trial comparing single-agent paclitaxel polglumex (CT-2103, PPX) with single-agent gemcitabine or vinorelbine for the treatment of PS 2 patients with chemotherapy-naive advanced non-small cell lung cancer. *J Thorac Oncol.* 2009;3:728–734.
41. Chon H, Rha S, Im C, et al. Docetaxel versus paclitaxel combined with 5-FU and leucovorin in advanced gastric

cancer: combined analysis of two phase II trials. *Cancer Res Treat.* 2009;41(4):196–204.

42. Makino H. Treatment and care of neurotoxicity from taxane anticancer agents. *Breast Cancer.* 2004;11(1):100–104.

43. Kannarkat G, Lasher E, Schiff D. Neurologic complications of chemotherapy agents. *Curr Opin Neurol.* 2007;20: 719–725.

44. Soliven B, Dhand U, Kobayashi K, et al. Evaluation of neuropathy in patients on suramin treatment. *Muscle Nerve.* 1997;20(1):83–91.

45. Chaudhry V, Eisenberger M, Sinibaldi V, Sheikh K, Griffin J, Cornblath D. A prospective study of suramin-induced peripheral neuropathy. *Brain.* 1996;119(Pt 6):2039–2052.

46. Russell J, Gill J, Sorenson E, Schultz D, Windebank A. Suramin-induced neuropathy in an animal model. *J Neurol Sci.* 2001;192(1–2):71–80.

47. Matthews S, McCoy C. Thalidomide: a review of approved and investigational uses. *Clin Ther.* 2003;25:342–395.

48. Cavaletti G, Beronio A, Reni L, et al. Thalidomide sensory neurotoxicity: a clinical and neurophysiologic study. *Neurology.* 2004;62(12):2291–2293.

49. Cavaletti G, Marmiroli P. Chemotherapy-induced peripheral neurotoxicity. *Expert Opin Drug Saf.* 2004;3(6):535–546.

50. Lagueny A, Rommel A, Vignolly B, et al. Thalidomide neuropathy: an electrophysiologic study. *Muscle Nerve.* 1986;9(9):837–844.

51. Othieno-Abinya N, Nyabola L. Experience with vincristine-associated neurotoxicity. *East Afr Med J.* 2001;78(7): 376–378.

52. Yun-San Yip A, Yuen-Yuen Ong E, Chow LW. Vinflunine: clinical perspectives of an emerging anticancer agent. *Expert Opin Investig Drugs.* 2008;17(4):583–591.

53. Ng J. Vinflunine: review of a new vinca alkaloid and its potential role in oncology. *J Oncol Pharm Pract.* 2011;17(3): 209–224.

54. Dalakas M, Semino-Mora C, Leon-Monzon M. Mitochrondrial alterations with mitochondrial DNA depletion in the nerves of AIDS patients with peripheral neuropathy induced by 2′,3′-dideoxycytidine (ddC). *Lab Invest.* 2001;81:1537–1544.

55. Maschke M, Kastrup O, Esser S, Ross B, Hengge U, Hufnagel A. Incidence and prevalence of neurological disorders associated with HIV since the introduction of highly active antiretroviral therapy (HAART). *J Neurol Neurosurg Psychiatry.* 2000;69(3):376–380.

56. Miller F, Hess E, Clauw D, et al. Approaches for identifying and defining environmentally associated rheumatic disorders. *Arthritis Rheum.* 2000;43(2):243–249.

57. Pratt R, Weimer L. Medication- and toxin-induced peripheral neuropathy. *Semin Neurol.* 2005;25(2):204–216.

58. Weimer L, Schdev N. Update on medication-induced peripheral neuropathy. *Curr Neurol Neurosci Rep.* 2009;9: 69–75.

59. Giannini F, Volpi N, Rossi S, Passero S, Fimiani M, Cerase A. Thalidomide-induced neuropathy: a ganglionopathy? *Neurology.* 2003;60(5):877–878.

60. Rosson G. Chemotherapy-induced neuropathy. *Clin Podiatr Med Surg.* 2006;23:637–649.

61. Kirchmair R, Walter D, Ii M, et al. Antiangiogenesis mediates cisplatin-induced peripheral neuropathy: attenuation or reversal by local vascular endothelial growth factor gene therapy without augmenting tumor growth. *Circulation.* 2005;111(20):2662–2670.

62. McDonald E, Randon K, Knight A, Windebank A. Cisplatin preferentially binds to DNA in dorsal root ganglion neurons in vitro and in vivo: a potential mechanism for neurotoxicity. *Neurobiol Dis.* 2005;18: 305–313.

63. Ta L, Espeset L, Podratz J, Windebank A. Neurotoxicity of oxaliplatin and cisplatin for dorsal root ganglion neurons correlates with platinum-DNA binding. *Neurotoxicology.* 2006;27:992–1002.

64. Dzagnidze A, Katsarava Z, Makhalova J, et al. Repair capacity for platinum-DNA adducts determines the severity of cisplatin-induced peripheral neuropathy. *J Neurosci.* 2007;27(35):9451–9457.

65. Gill J, Windebank A. Cisplatin-induced apoptosis in rat dorsal root ganglia neurons is associated with attempted entry in the cell cycle. *J Clin Invest.* 1998;101:2842–2850.

66. Screnci D, McKeage M, Galettis P, Hambley T, Palmer B, Baguley B. Relationships between hydrophobicity, reactivity, accumulation and peripheral nerve toxicity of a series of platinum drugs. *Br J Cancer.* 2000;82:966–972.

67. Cavaletti G, Tredici G, Braga M, Tazzari S. Experimental peripheral neuropathy induced in adult rats by repeated intraperitoneal administration of taxol. *Exp Neurol.* 1995; 133:64–72.

68. Sahenk Z, Barohn R, New P, Mendell J. Taxol neuropathy. Electrodiagnostic and sural nerve biopsy findings. *Arch Neurol.* 1994;51(7):726–729.

69. Bhagra A, Rao R. Chemotherapy-induced neuropathy. *Curr Oncol Rep.* 2007;9:290–299.

70. Hilkens PH, Verweij J, Vecht CJ, Stoter G, van den Bent MJ. Clinical characteristics of severe peripheral neuropathy induced by docetaxel (Taxotere). *Ann Oncol.* 1997;8: 187–190.

71. Kanbayashi Y, Hosokawa T, Okamoto K, et al. Statistical identification of predictors for peripheral neuropathy associated with administration of bortezomib, taxanes, oxaliplatin or vincristine while using ordered logistic regression analysis. *Anticancer Drugs.* 2010;21(9):877–881.

72. Saleh F, Seidman R. Drug-induced myopathy and neuropathy. *J Clin Neuromuscul Dis.* 2003;5(2):81–92.

73. Topp K, Tanner K, Levine J. Damage to the cytoskeleton of large diameter sensory neurons and myelinated axons in vincristine-induced painful peripheral neuropathy in the rat. *J Comp Neurol.* 2000;424:563–576.

74. Bennouna J, Delord J, Campone M, Nguyen L. Vinflunine: a new microtubule inhibitor agent. *Clin Cancer Res.* 2008; 14(6):1625–1632.

75. Sampaio E, Sarno E, Galilly R, Cohn Z, Kaplan G. Thalidomide selectively inhibits tumor necrosis factor alpha production by stimulated human monocytes. *J Exp Med.* 1991;173(3):699–703.

76. Moreira A, Sampaio E, Zmuidzinas Z, Frindt P, Smith K, Kaplan G. Thalidomide exerts its inhibitory action on tumor necrosis factor alpha by enhancing mRNA degradation. *J Exp Med.* 1993;177(6):1675–1680.

77. Briani C, Zara G, Rondinone R, et al. Thalidomide neurotoxicity: prospective study in patients with lupus erythematosus. *Neurology.* 2004;62(12):2288–2290.

78. Hamanoue M, Middleton G, Wyatt S, Jaffray E, Hay R, Davies A. p75-mediated NF-kappaB activation enhances the survival response of developing sensory neurons to nerve growth factor. *Mol Cell Neurosci.* 1999;14(1):28–40.

79. Isoardo G, Bergui M, Durelli L, et al. Thalidomide neuropathy: clinical, electrophysiological and neuroradiological features. *Acta Neurol Scand.* 2004; 109(3):188–193.

80. Molloy F, Floeter M, Syed N, et al. Thalidomide neuropathy in patients treated for metastatic prostate cancer. *Muscle Nerve.* 2001;24(8):1050–1057.

81. Reddy G, Mughal T, Lonial S. Optimizing the management of treatment-related peripheral neuropathy in patients with multiple myeloma. *Support Cancer Ther.* 2006;4:19–22.

82. Mateos MV. Management of treatment-related adverse events in patients with multiple myeloma. *Cancer Treat Rev.* 2010;36(Suppl 2):S24–S32.

83. Orlowski R. Bortezomib and its role in the management of patients with multiple myeloma. *Exp Rev Anticancer Ther.* 2004;4:171–179.

84. Ravaglia S, Corso A, Piccolo G, et al. Immune-mediated neuropathies in myeloma patients treated with bortezomib. *Clin Neurophys.* 2008;119:2507–2512.

85. Lanzani F, Mattavelli L, Frigeni B, et al. Role of a pre-existing neuropathy on the course of bortezomib-induced peripheral neurotoxicity. *J Peripher Nerv Syst.* 2008;13:267–274.

86. Velasco R, Petit J, Clapes V, Verdu E, Navarro X, Bruna J. Neurological monitoring replaces the incidence of bortezomib-induced peripheral neuropathy in multiple myeloma patients. *J Peripher Nerv Syst.* 2010;15:17–25.

87. Badros A, Goloubeva O, Dalal J, et al. Neurotoxicity of bortezomib therapy in multiple myeloma: a single-center experience and review of the literature. *Cancer.* 2007;110(5):1042–1049.

88. Corso A, Mangiacavalli S, Varettoni M, Pascutto C, Zappasodi P, Lazzarino M. Bortezomib-induced peripheral neuropathy in multiple myeloma: a comparison between previously treated and untreated patients. *Leuk Res.* 2010;34:471–474.

89. Eisenberger M, Reyno L, Jodrell D, et al. Suramin, an active drug for prostate cancer: interim observations in a phase I trial. *J Natl Cancer Inst.* 1993;85(8):611–621.

90. DeClerq E. Suramin: a potent inhibitor of the reverse transcriptase of RNA tumor viruses. *Cancer Lett.* 1979;8:9–22.

91. Broder S, Yarchoan R, Collins J, et al. Effects of suramin on HTLV-III/LAV infection presenting as Kaposi's sarcoma or AIDS-related complex: clinical pharmacology and suppression of virus replication in vivo. *Lancet.* 1985;2(8456):627–630.

92. LaRocca R, Meer J, Gilliatt R, et al. Suramin-induced polyneuropathy. *Neurology.* 1990;40(6):954–960.

93. Coffey R, Leof E, Shipley G, Moses H. Suramin inhibition of growth factor receptor binding and mitogenicity in AKR-2B cells. *J Cell Physiol.* 1987;132:143–148.

94. Russell J, Windebank A, Podratz J. Role of nerve growth factor in suramin neurotoxicity studied in vitro. *Ann Neurol.* 1994;36:221–228.

95. Gill J, Connolly D, McManus M, Maihle N, Windebank A. Suramin induces phosphorylation of the high-affinity nerve growth factor receptor in PC12 cells and dorsal root ganglion neurons. *J Neurochem.* 1996;66:963–972.

96. Gill J, Windebank A. Direct activation of the high-affinity nerve growth factor receptor by a non-peptide symmetrical polyanion. *Neuroscience.* 1998;87:855–860.

97. Cardinali M, Sartor O, Robbins K. Suramin, an experimental chemotherapeutic drug, activates the receptor for epidermal growth factor and promotes growth of certain malignant cells. *J Clin Invest.* 1992;89:1242–1247.

98. Martin K, Bentaberry F, Dumoulin C, et al. Neuropathy associated with leflunomide: a case series. *Ann Rheum Dis.* 2005;64(4):649–650.

99. Carulli M, Davies U. Peripheral neuropathy: an unwanted effect of leflunomide? *Rheumatology.* 2002;41:952–953.

100. Hill C. Leflunomide-induced peripheral neuropathy: rapid resolution with cholestyramine wash-out. *Rheumatology.* 2004;43:809.

101. Kho L, Kermode A. Leflunomide-induced peripheral neuropathy. *J Clin Neurosci.* 2007;14:179–181.

102. Bonnel R, Graham D. Peripheral neuropathy in patients reated with leflunomide. *Clin Pharmacol Ther.* 2004;75:580–585.

103. Herper M. How many people take cholesterol drugs? Forbes 2008. http://www.forbes.com/2008/10/29/cholesterol-pharmacuticals-statins-biz-cx_mh_1030cholesterol.html. Accessed October 3, 2010.

104. Gaist D, Jeppesen U, Andersen M, Garcia-Rodriguez L, Hallas J, Sindrup S. Statins and risk of polyneuropathy: a case-control study. *Neurology.* 2002;58(9):1333–1337.

105. Walravens P, Greene C, Seerman E. Lovastatin, isoprenes, and myopathy. *Lancet.* 1989;2:1097–1098.

106. Chong P, Boskovich A, Stevkovic N, Bartt R. Statin-associated peripheral neuropathy: review of the literature. *Pharmacotherapy.* 2004;24:1194–1203.

107. Gaist D, Rodriguez LG, Huerta C, Hallas J, Sindrup S. Are users of lipid-lowering drugs at increased risk of peripheral neuropathy? *Eur J Clin Pharmacol.* 2001;56:931–933.

108. Lovastatin 5-year safety and efficacy study. Lovastatin Study Groups I through IV. *Arch Intern Med.* 1993;153:1079–1087.

109. Jeppesen U, Gaist D, Smith T, Sindrup S. Statins and peripheral neuropathy. *Eur J Clin Pharmacol.* 1999;54:835–838.

110. Ahmad S. Lovastatin and peripheral neuropathy. *Am Heart J.* 1995;130:1321.

111. Ziajka P, Wehmeier T. Peripheral neuropathy and lipid-lowering therapy. *South Med J.* 1998;91(7):667–668.

112. Phan T, McLeod J, Pollard J, Peiris O, Rohan A, Halpern J. Peripheral neuropathy associated with simvastin. *J Neurol Neurosurg Psychiatry.* 1995;58:625–628.

113. Davis T, Yeap B, Davis W, Bruce D. Lipid-lowering therapy and peripheral sensory neuropathy in type 2 diabetes: the Fremantle Diabetes Study. *Diabetologia.* 2008;51(4):562–566.

114. Dalakas M. Peripheral neuropathy and antiretroviral drugs. *J Peripher Nerv Syst.* 2001;6(1):14–20.

115. Lewis W, Dalakas M. Mitochondrial toxicity of antiviral drugs. *Nat Med.* 1995;1:417–422.

116. Miller R. Neuromuscular complications of human immunodeficiency virus infection and antiretroviral therapy. *West J Med.* 1994;160:447–452.

117. White A. Mitochondrial toxicity and HIV therapy. *Sex Transm Infect.* 2001;77:158–173.

118. Peltier A, Russel J. Recent advances in drug-induced neuropathies. *Curr Opin Neurol.* 2002;15:633–638.

119. Palella FJ Jr, Delaney KM, Moorman AC, et al. Declining morbidity and mortality among patients with advanced human immunodeficiency virus infection. HIV Outpatient Study Investigators. *N Engl J Med.* 1998;338(13):853–860.

120. Hogg R, Yip B, Kully C, et al. Improved survival among HIV-infected patients after initiation of triple-drug antiretroviral regimens. *Can Med Assoc J.* 1999;160(5):659–665.

121. Kaul M. HIV-1 associated dementia: update on pathological mechanisms and therapeutic approaches. *Curr Opin Neurol.* 2009;22(3):315–320.

122. Lichtenstein KA, Armon C, Baron A, Moorman AC, Wood KC, Holmberg SD; HIV Outpatient Study Investigators. Modification of the incidence of drug-associated symmetrical peripheral neuropathy by host and disease factors in the HIV outpatient study cohort. *Clin Infect Dis.* 2005;40(1):148–157.

123. Stübgen J. Tumor necrosis factor-alpha antagonists and neuropathy. *Muscle Nerve.* 2008;37(3):281–292.

124. Tektonidou M, Serelis J, Skopouli F. Peripheral neuropathy in two patients with rheumatoid arthritis receiving infliximab treatment. *Clin Rheumatol.* 2007;26:258–260.

125. Lozeron P, Denier C, Lacroix C, Adams D. Long-term course of demyelinating neuropathies occurring during tumor necrosis factor-alpha-blocker therapy. *Arch Neurol.* 2009;66(4):490–497.

126. Krauser D, Sega A, Kligfield P. Severe ataxia caused by amiodarone. *Am J Cardiol.* 2005;96:1463–1464.

127. Hindle J, Ibrahim A, Ramaraj R. Ataxia caused by amiodarone in older people. *Age Ageing.* 2008;37: 347–348.

128. Caruba T, Cottu PH, Madelaine-Chambring I, Espie M, Misset JL, Gross-Goupil M. Gemcitabine-oxaliplatin combination in heavily pretreated metastatic breast cancer: a pilot study on 43 patients. *Breast J.* 2007;13(2):165–171.

129. Postma TJ, van Groeningen CJ, Witjes RJ, Weerts JG, Kralendonk JH, Heimans JJ. Neurotoxicity of combination chemotherapy with procarbazine, CCNU and vincristine (PCV) for recurrent glioma. *J Neurooncol.* 1998;38(1): 69–75.

130. Harousseau J, Attal M, Leleu X, et al. Bortezomib plus dexamethasone as induction treatment prior to autologous stem cell transplantation in patients with newly diagnosed multiple myeloma: results of an IFM phase II study. *Heamatologica.* 2006;91(11):1498–1505.

131. Mateos M, Hernandez J, Hernandez M, et al. Bortezomib plus melphalan and prednisone in elderly untreated patients with multiple myeloma: results of a multicenter phase 1/2 study. *Blood.* 2006;108(7):2165–2172.

132. Mateos M, Oriol A, Martinez-Lopez J, et al. Bortezomib, melphalan, and prednisone versus bortezomib, thalidomide, and prednisone as induction therapy followed by maintenance treatment with bortezomib and thalidomide versus bortezomib and prednisone in elderly patients with untreated multiple myeloma: a randomised trial. *Lancet.* 2010;11(10):934–941.

133. Meyer L, Patte-Mensah C, Taleb O, Mensah-Nyagan A. Cellular and functional evidence for a protective action of neurosteroids against vincristine chemotherapy-induced painful neuropathy. *Cell Mol Life Sci.* 2010;67:3017–3034.

Evaluation and Assessment of Peripheral Nerve Injury

Chapter *12*

Electroneurodiagnostic Assessment and Interpretation

Stephen J. Carp, PT, PhD, GCS

"Sometimes the correct questions are more important than the correct answers."
—Nancy Willard (1936–)

Objectives

On completion of this chapter, the student/practitioner will be able to:

- Understand why the electroneurodiagnostic examination is an important diagnostic tool for rehabilitation professionals.
- Define the components of the electroneurodiagnostic examination.
- Discuss the purpose of the electroneurodiagnostic examination.
- Interpret the results of the electroneurodiagnostic examination and translate the results into clinical practice.

Key Terms

- Electromyography
- F wave
- Motor nerve conduction
- Sensory nerve conduction

Introduction

Electroneurodiagnostic studies are the natural physiological extension of the neurological physical examination. They are used to confirm, add to, or remove differential diagnoses suggested by clinical scripts taken from the history, prior diagnostic workup, and physical examination. This chapter is not meant to be a "how to" primer for the performance of the spectrum of electroneurodiagnostic testing; many other well-written texts are available. Rather, the author presents the subject of electroneurodiagnostic testing in a conceptualized state to allow the reader to develop an understanding of the various types of testing available and the clinical and diagnostic implications of normal and aberrant testing results and, for the rehabilitation clinician, to develop an appreciation of the ability of this powerful tool to facilitate diagnostics, goal setting, and interventional planning for patients with peripheral nerve injury.

In the performance of clinical testing, the electroneurodiagnostic clinician works to prove, disprove, or add to the differential diagnosis list via the scientific method. Clinical scripts provide differential diagnoses, and the clinician, through the use of various electroneurodiagnostic tests, collects data, develops the diagnostic hypotheses, collects more data, reworks the diagnostic hypothesis, and confirms or disproves the differential diagnosis. During the testing, the patient is awake and alert and can provide additional historical data if needed to the clinician. In contrast to many diagnostic studies, the electroneuromyogram does not have a strict procedural component; the clinician may perform as many or as few specific tests as needed to isolate a diagnosis. Electroneurodiagnostic testing is a unique test in that the patient by supplying the clinician with information during the study is an active partner in the diagnostic process.

The primary goal of the electroneurodiagnostic evaluation is to determine the site of the lesion; the findings do not identify the process leading to the aberrant findings. To obtain information about the "localization," the following processes are used: motor nerve studies, sensory nerve studies, and needle **electromyography** (EMG). Correlation with aspects of the physical examination and other diagnostic tests is needed to isolate the diagnosis.

Electroneurodiagnostic Process

The complete electroneurodiagnostic process is as follows:

1. History taking: Following the development of the clinician-patient collaborative relationship, the clinician should take a thorough history of the present illness using open-ended questions and follow-up queries. Past medical and surgical histories and current and past medications should be thoroughly documented. Social, nutritional, medication, and vocational histories should be adequately explored with concentration on possible behavioral and chemical influences that may result in peripheral nerve injury.
2. Establishing the agenda of electroneurodiagnostic evaluation: Based on clinical scripts produced during the history-taking process, the clinician develops an agenda of procedures to perform to confirm, disprove, or add to the differential list. The typical study begins with sensory conduction studies and **motor nerve conduction** studies and ends with the needle examination. The agenda may be amended "midstream" based on evidence obtained during the examination. Additional testing such as quantitative sensory testing, autonomic testing, and somatosensory evoked potential testing may be employed.
3. Synthesis and correlation: Following the history taking and electroneurodiagnostic assessment, the clinician begins to define the site of the lesion; the pathological (neurapraxic, axonal, or demyelination) process; possible etiologies of the nerve lesion; and, if possible, the prognosis of healing.

Motor Nerve Conduction Studies

Nerve conduction studies as part of the examination for suspected peripheral nerve injury are an extension of the clinical examination and are important in the management of cranial and peripheral neuromuscular disease as well as contributing to diagnosis of spinal cord lesions. The purpose of nerve conduction testing in suspected peripheral nerve injury is to assess the degree and extent of motor axonal nerve injury, to determine the presence or lack of nerve connectivity (gap), and to identify if the repair process has begun (sprouting, regeneration). Nerve conduction studies can be extremely useful both in localizing lesions and in providing adjuvant data as to the etiologies of the pathological processes responsible. It is vital for the electromyographer to carry out tests accurately and reproducibly and to develop an investigation strategy based on the patient's symptoms and signs rather than a fixed protocol. The investigator should report the results clearly, place them in the context of the clinical situation, and correlate the findings with any supporting diagnostic studies.

Motor conduction studies, also known as motor conduction velocities (MCVs,) are performed by electrically stimulating a nerve and recording the compound muscle action potential (CMAP) from surface electrodes overlying a muscle supplied by that nerve (Table 12-1). The most frequently examined nerves are the peroneal, tibial, ulnar, and median—not coincidentally, all superficial nerves affected by external forces. The primary advantage of motor conduction over sensory conduction studies is that several segments along the course of the nerve are available for motor study. Similar to the sensory examination, side-to-side comparison studies are quite helpful. The active electrode is placed over the muscle belly, and the reference electrode is placed over an electrically inactive site (usually the muscle tendon). A ground electrode is also placed somewhere between the stimulating and recording electrodes providing a zero voltage reference point.

Table 12-1	Common Abbreviations Used in Electroneurodiagnostic Studies
Ach	Acetylcholine
AIDP	Acute inflammatory demyelinating polyneuropathy
AMAN	Acute motor axonal neuropathy
CMAP	Compound muscle action potential
CN	Clinical neurophysiologist
DRG	Dorsal root ganglion
EMG	Electromyography
LEMS	Lambert-Eaton myasthenic syndrome
NAP	Nerve action potential
NCS	Nerve conduction study
NMTD	Neuromuscular transmission disorder
PNE	Peripheral neurophysiological examination
RNS	Repetitive nerve stimulation
SNAP	Sensory nerve action potential
SSEP	Somatosensory evoked potential
TMS	Transcranial magnetic stimulation

For example, the median nerve motor study might involve stimulation at the wrist, the elbow, the axilla (less frequently), and the brachial plexus.

For each motor nerve conduction study, four values are typically obtained and recorded: CMAP amplitude and duration at each stimulation site, latency at each stimulation site, conduction velocity between stimulation sites, and F-wave latencies. The CMAP is a summated voltage response from the individual muscle fiber action potentials. The shortest latency of the CMAP is the time from stimulus artifact to onset of the response and is a biphasic response with an initial upward deflection followed by a smaller downward deflection. The CMAP amplitude is measured from baseline to negative peak (the neurophysiological convention is that negative voltage is demonstrated by an upward deflection) and measured in millivolts (mV).

To record the CMAP, the stimulating current or voltage is gradually increased until a point is reached where an increase in stimulus produces no incremental increase in CMAP amplitude as observed on the oscilloscope. Only at this (supramaximal) point can a reproducible value for CMAP amplitude and the latency between the stimulus and the onset of the CMAP be recorded accurately.

The nerve is stimulated at a more proximal site—in the median nerve examination for carpal tunnel syndrome, this would be the antecubital fossa, close to the biceps tendon. In the normal state, stimulating the median nerve at the wrist and the elbow results in two CMAPs of similar shape and amplitude because the same motor axons innervate the muscle fibers making up the response. However, the latency is greater for elbow stimulation compared with wrist stimulation because of the longer distance between the stimulating and recording electrodes. The difference in latency represents the time taken for the fastest nerve fibers to conduct between the two stimulation points because all other factors involving neuromuscular transmission and muscle activation are common to both stimulation sites. If one measures the distance between the two sites, the fastest motor nerve conduction velocity (FMNCV) can be calculated as follows: FMNCV (m/sec) = distance between stimulation site 1 and site 2 (mm)/[latency site 2 − latency site 1 (msec).

Seddon[1,2] described three major types of traumatic nerve injuries. Neurotmesis implies the nerve cannot regenerate spontaneously because it is either severed completely or disrupted by an obstruction such as internal or external scar tissue. In axonotmesis, regeneration can occur because endoneurial coverings maintain the proper alignment. In neurapraxia, conduction is locally blocked (possibly secondary to focal demyelination), and recovery is relatively rapid—minutes to weeks.

In the first two types nerve injury, wallerian degeneration occurs distal to the lesion, whereas in neurapraxia, no such distal changes take place. In all three types, no response is obtained from stimulation proximal to the lesion. However, with distal stimulation, normal conduction is maintained in neurapraxia and serves to distinguish it from the other states.

The electrical distinction between neurotmesis and axonotmesis may be difficult. If there is some preservation of either voluntary activity or response to electrical stimulation of a nerve, a complete neurotmesis is ruled out. If no such function is preserved, serial studies may be necessary to distinguish between these two processes.

Sensory Nerve Conduction Studies

Sensory nerve conduction studies, often referred to as sensory nerve action potential (SNAP) studies, involve stimulation of a nerve while recording from the skin over the nerve. Sensory nerve studies are extremely useful discriminators regarding the site of the pathology because the presence of a normal sensory action potential implies that large-diameter dorsal root ganglion cells and large myelinated axons are appropriately connected and are likely to be functioning normally. If studies indicate that this component of the peripheral nervous system is normal and if the patient has a large-fiber type of sensory loss, the pathology must be proximal to the dorsal root ganglion.[3]

The SNAP is obtained by electrically stimulating sensory fibers and recording the nerve action potential

Table 12-2 Summary of Electroneurodiagnostic Findings in Various Pathologies

	Anterior Horn Cell Disease	Neuropathy	Myopathy	Neuromuscular Junction Disease	Radiculopathy
Fasciculations at Rest	Present	Rare	Rare	Absent	Rare
Conduction Studies	Normal or slightly slowed	Normal, slightly slowed, or markedly slowed	Normal	Normal	Normal
Repetitive Supramaximal Stimulation	Usually normal	Usually normal	Usually normal	Abnormal	Normal
Motor Unit Potentials Amplitude/Duration	Markedly increased	Increased	Decreased	Occasionally decreased	Increased
Recruitment Pattern	Decreased	Decreased	Increased	Normal	Decreased

From Dyck PJ. Quantitative sensory testing: a consensus report from the Peripheral Neuropathy Association. *Neurology.* 1993;43:1050–1052; and Fisher MA. AAEM Minimonograph #13: H reflexes and F waves: physiology and indications. *Muscle Nerve.* 1992;15:1223–1233.

at a point further along that nerve. Again the stimulus must be supramaximal. Recording the SNAP orthodromically refers to distal nerve stimulation and recording more proximally (the direction in which physiological sensory conduction occurs). Different electroneurodiagnostic testing laboratories prefer antidromic or orthodromic methods for testing different nerves. The sensory latency and the peak-to-peak amplitude of the SNAP are measured. The velocity correlates directly with the sensory latency, and the result may be expressed either as latency over a standard distance or, more commonly, as a velocity (Table 12-2).

Only the 20% largest diameter and fastest conducting sensory fibers are tested using conventional sensory studies functionally supplying fine touch, vibration, and position sense.[4] Predominantly small-fiber neuropathies affecting the other 80% of fibers exist usually with prominent symptoms of pain, and conventional sensory studies may be normal. In such cases, quantitative sensory testing and autonomic testing are required.

F Waves

F waves (F for foot, where they were first described) are a type of late motor response. When a motor nerve axon is electrically stimulated at any point, an action potential is propagated in both directions away from the initial stimulation site. The distally propagated impulse gives rise to the CMAP. However, an impulse also conducts proximally to the anterior horn cell, depolarizing the axon hillock and causing the axon to backfire; this leads to a small additional muscle depolarization (F wave) at a longer latency. Only about 2% of axons backfire with each stimulus. In contrast to the M response, F waves vary in latency and shape because

different populations of neurons normally backfire with each stimulus. The most reliable measure of the F wave is the minimum latency of 10 to 20 firings.[5]

F waves allow testing of proximal segments of nerves that would otherwise be inaccessible to routine nerve conduction studies. F waves test long lengths of nerves, whereas motor studies test shorter segments. F wave abnormalities can be a sensitive indicator of peripheral nerve pathology, particularly if sited proximally. The F wave ratio, which compares the conduction in the proximal half of the total pathway with the distal half, may be used to determine the site of conduction slowing—for example, to distinguish a root lesion from a patient with a distal generalized neuropathy.[6]

Repetitive Nerve Stimulation

Repetitive nerve stimulation (RNS) is used in the evaluation of patients with suspected neuromuscular transmission disorders (NMTDs) such as myasthenia gravis or Lambert-Eaton myasthenic syndrome (LEMS). RNS is a modified motor nerve conduction study in which instead of recording CMAPs with single supramaximal electrical stimuli, a train of 8 to 10 stimuli is applied, and the sequential response amplitudes or areas are measured. This study may be carried out at low-frequency (3 to 4 Hz) or high-frequency (20 to 50 Hz) stimulation. In the latter case, the train is prolonged to allow 2 to 10 seconds of continuous data to be measured. Both distal and proximal muscles and nerves should be studied in every patient suspected to have an NMTD because the sensitivity of the test is greatly increased by this means.[7]

With low-frequency stimulation in normal subjects, the CMAP amplitude or area falls over the first four to five stimuli by a maximum of 10% to 12%. The maximum fall should be between potentials 1 and 2.

Numerous department-specific protocols have been published to study RNS over time both before and after a period of maximum voluntary contraction of the muscle to detect early or late neuromuscular transmission failure.[8]

Electromyography

The electromyograph is a device that amplifies and converts the minute voltages recorded by a needle electrode—typically a fine wire inserted within a 24-gauge hollow needle—inserted into muscle and expresses these currents by speaker or visually by a cathode ray oscilloscope. A permanent record of the examination can be saved and printed. By this means, the electrical potentials of normal, diseased, or denervated muscle can be studied. Normal, healthy muscle has two significant electromyographic characteristics: it emits no detectable impulses at rest, and on insertion of the needle electrode, the electrical activity caused by the mechanical stimulation of insertion is quickly dissipated.

EMG is often performed when patients have unexplained motor weakness. EMG helps to distinguish between muscle conditions in which the problem begins in the muscle and muscle weakness resulting from nerve disorders. EMG can be used to detect true weakness as opposed to weakness from reduced use because of pain or lack of motivation. EMG can also be used to isolate the level of nerve irritation or injury. EMG can detect disease involving the lower motor neuron from the anterior horn cell to the neuromuscular junction, defects in transmission at the neuromuscular junction, and primary muscle disease.

A needle is inserted through the skin into the muscle. Electrical activity—at insertion, at rest, at volitional contraction, and at maximal contraction—is detected by this needle (which serves as an electrode). The activity is displayed visually on an oscilloscope and may be detected audibly with a speaker.

Because skeletal muscles are often large, several needle electrodes may need to be placed at various locations to obtain an informative electromyogram. The presence, size, and shape of the waveform (the action potential) produced on the oscilloscope provide information about the ability of the muscle to respond to nervous stimulation. Each muscle fiber that contracts produces an action potential. The size of the muscle fiber affects the rate (how frequently an action potential occurs) and the size (the amplitude) of the action potential (Figs. 12-1, 12-2, and 12-3).

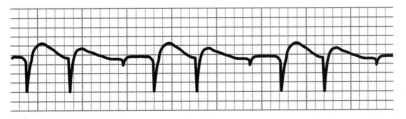

Figure 12-1 Fibrillation potentials and positive sharp waves share many of the same characteristics and have the same clinical importance. Although subtle differences exist, both represent spontaneous muscle activity in association with neural denervation or irritable myopathy. An example of a positive sharp wave is pictured. Positive sharp waves represent spontaneous muscle activity seen on electromyography in association with denervation or irritable myopathy.

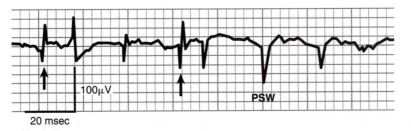

Figure 12-2 Fibrillation potentials, similar to positive sharp waves, are often diagnostic of denervation. In contrast to fasciculations, which may be visibly observed and may be benign, fibrillations cannot visibly observed and are pathological. Fibrillation potentials occur when muscle fibers lose contact with their innervating axon producing a spontaneous action potential that results in muscle contraction of the individual motor unit.

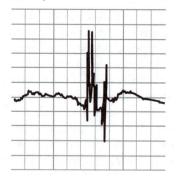

Figure 12-3 Similar to fibrillation potentials and positive sharp waves, giant motor unit potentials are suggestive of denervation. With chronic muscle reinnervation, the amplitude of the motor unit increases, as does its duration, producing the greater size of the new motor unit. A motor unit greater than 5 mV is referred to as a giant motor unit and is consistent with chronic reinnervation.

Normally, some electrical activity occurs when the needle is inserted, but this quickly dissipates. Increased insertional activity, fibrillation potentials, and positive sharp waves[9] can be seen in diseases producing axonal degeneration, blockade of the neuromuscular junction such as often seen with botulinum poisoning[10] or myopathic processes. Repetitive discharges may be seen in myotonia. A relaxed muscle is electrically silent. Fibrillation and fasciculations may be detected in the relaxed denervated muscle. During voluntary contraction, muscle action potentials can be visualized on the oscilloscope. With minimal contraction, often single action potentials may be seen and analyzed. With maximal contraction, an "interference pattern" is visualized on the oscilloscope. The amplitude, duration, number, and configuration of the muscle action potentials are noted in differentiating neurogenic from myogenic involvement. In myogenic weakness, the amplitude of the action potential is decreased with little decrease in the number of action potentials.

Two types of bizarre high-frequency discharges may also be present. In the first, the frequency and amplitude of the action potentials do not wax and wane but are relatively constant. These discharges are usually composed of complex-appearing potentials that tend to stop and start spontaneously. They are not generally provoked by voluntary movement but rather by needle insertion and manipulation or muscle percussion. These have been termed "pseudomyotonic" discharges and are now realized to be a nonspecific finding occurring in lower motor neuron lesions.

The other form of bizarre high-frequency discharges wax and wane to provoke the familiar "dive bomber" sound. These are commonly found in myotonic disorders where needle movement, percussion near the needle insertion, or voluntary motion provokes their appearance. They are the electrical analogy of a clinical myotonia, which is a prominent feature in the genetic diseases myotonia congenita, myotonia dystrophica, and paramyotonia congenita.[11]

Following complete or partial nerve damage, it is essential to know the sequence of changes in the innervated muscle. At first, the only change noted is the absence or decrease of muscle contraction noted on EMG. Fibrillation potentials begin to appear with the insertion or "tweaking" of the recording needle about 1 week after injury. Spontaneous fibrillations begin to appear 2 to 4 weeks after injury. Sequential examinations may reveal additional aberrant tracings or, as reinnervation occurs, the emergence of low-amplitude, often polyphasic, action potentials, which gradually develop normal patterns.

Fasciculation potentials occur in many conditions,[12] including motor neuron disease; cord diseases such as hematomyelia, syringomyelia, and cervical spondylosis; irritative disorders of nerve roots; hypomagnesemia; and pancreatic adenoma with hyperinsulinism. Most commonly, fasciculations are benign and are observed in many individuals especially after severe exercise and concomitant fatigue. Coupled discharges can be seen in latent tetany, induced by hyperventilation or by muscle ischemia.[13]

Activity is also monitored during EMG with volitional contraction of the muscle. When an anterior horn cell is activated, an action potential travels down its axon and terminal nerve fibers to produce an almost synchronous depolarization of the muscle fibers that it innervates. The summated potential generated by these specific muscle fibers is called the motor unit potential. In actuality, the full complement of muscle fibers innervated by one anterior horn cell lie in an area that exceeds the effective pick-up zone of a needle. What is called the motor unit potential is only a fraction of the whole.

The number of active motor units and their frequency of discharge depend on the volitional effort exerted. A small effort recruits a small number of motor units; a large effort recruits much of the muscle. When much of the muscle is recruited, this is called a complete interference pattern. The number of motor units activated can be inferred by monitoring the oscilloscope pattern. The recruitment pattern on maximal exertion reflects the degree of denervation. With complete denervation, no observable motor units are seen. If only a few axons are lost, a complete interference pattern may still be seen. In contrast, myopathies tend to show a complete interference pattern on minimal effort.

The amplitude of the motor unit potential is a function of the number of activated muscle fibers that lie adjacent to the EMG needle. The duration is a variable of the relative degree of asynchronicity between the number of active fibers adjacent to the needle. In addition, because the number of muscle fibers included in a particular motor unit varies, the amplitude and duration vary among normal subjects. Short-duration motor unit potentials are thought to be the result of loss of muscle fibers. The dropout of fibers can account for decreased amplitude or an increased number of phases (polyphasic units). Such motor unit potentials are common in myopathies where random degeneration of muscle fibers develop. BSAPPs is an acronym for brief small abundant polyphasic potentials, and this term has been suggested to describe a recruitment strategy consisting of the aforementioned motor unit potentials. Although BSAPPs are seen in myopathies, they may occur in other pathologies as well. The increased dispersion in conduction along terminal nerve fibers accounts for the long-duration polyphasic motor unit potentials. The greater the disparity of arrival of the action potentials arriving to various muscle fibers, the longer the duration of the motor unit potentials. The long-duration polyphasic potentials as seen during nerve degeneration or regeneration by themselves are not sufficient to diagnose a worsening, static, or improving illness. Giant motor unit potentials are defined as peak-to-peak amplitude greater than 5 mV. These units most likely indicate that reinnervation is occurring or has occurred by the process of collateral sprouting. The appearance of giant motor unit action potentials on EMG indicates a chronic rather than acute process.

Electroneurodiagnostic testing is a vital adjunct to the neurological examination. The qualified examiner, in partnership with the patient, uses the nerve conduction velocity and EMG tests to facilitate the diagnostic process and localize the site or sites of injury and may be able to develop a prognosis for recovery. The electroneuromyogram provides a unique data picture not provided by other methods of diagnostic testing and when correlated with the history and physical examination facilitates the diagnostic process.

CASE STUDY

The patient, DM, developed right wrist and hand pain a few days after painting a ceiling. About the same time, DM noticed that he had begun dropping objects such as pencils and coins. The pain was located in the right lateral four digits and the lateral palm but did not extend proximal to the wrist. The Tinel sign was positive at the wrist. The Phalen sign was present on the right. Medical history was unremarkable.

DM was referred to a neurologist and physical therapist 4 months after the onset of symptoms. Electroneuromyogram results indicated fibrillation potentials in the right abductor pollicis brevis. The remainder of the needle examination was "silent at rest with normal motor unit potentials on volition." Motor conduction latency was prolonged at the left median wrist/abductor pollicis brevis on the right. Sensory nerve action potentials revealed no response at the right median wrist/second digit.

Case Study Questions

1. Fibrillation potentials in the right abductor pollicis as a singular finding may be the result of which of the following?
   a. Median neuropathy
   b. Median neuropathy at the elbow
   c. Median neuropathy in the forearm
   d. All of the above

2. The positive median nerve Tinel sign at the wrist and Phalen sign point to pathology near which landmark?
   a. Wrist
   b. Forearm
   c. Elbow
   d. Shoulder

3. Which of the following is true of fasciculations?
   a. Often visible to the eye
   b. May be a sign of motor neuron disease
   c. May be benign
   d. All of the above

4. Which of the following shows the three items in order of severity?
   a. Neurapraxia, neurotmesis, axonotmesis
   b. Neurotmesis, axonotmesis, neurapraxia
   c. Axonotmesis, neurapraxia, neurotmesis
   d. Axonotmesis, neurotmesis, neurapraxia

5. Which of the following is an example of a diagnosis that produces bizarre high-frequency ("dive bomber") discharges?
   a. Myotonia
   b. Amyotrophic lateral sclerosis
   c. Polio
   d. C5 radiculopathy

References

1. Seddon HJ. A classification of nerve injuries. *Br Med J.* 1942; 2:237.
2. Seddon HJ. Three types of nerve injury. *Brain.* 1943;86:237.
3. Dyck PJ. Quantitative sensory testing: a consensus report from the Peripheral Neuropathy Association. *Neurology.* 1993; 43:1050–1052.
4. Neilson VK. Sensory and motor nerve conduction in the median nerve in normal subjects. *Acta Med Scand.* 1973;194: 435–443.
5. Fisher MA. AAEM Minimonograph #13: H reflexes and F waves: physiology and indications. *Muscle Nerve.* 1992;15: 1223–1233.
6. Weber GA. Nerve conduction studies and their clinical applications. *Clin Podiatr Med Surg.* 1990;7(1):151–178.

7. Oh SJ, Eslami T, Nishihira T, et al. Electrophysiological and clinical correlation in myasthenia gravis. Trans Am Neurol Assoc. 1982;12:348–354.

8. Pavesi G, Cattaneo L, Tinchelli S, Mancia D. Masseteric repetitive nerve stimulation in the diagnosis of myasthenia gravis. *Clin Neurophysiol.* 2001;112:1064–1069

9. Buchthal F, Rosenfalck P. Electrophysiological aspect of myopathy with particular reference to progressive muscular dystrophy. In: Bourne GH, Golarz MN, eds. *Muscular Dystrophy in Man and Animals.* New York: Hafner; 1963: 193–262.

10. Josefsson JO, Thesleff S. Electromyographic findings in experimental botulinum intoxication. *Acta Physiol Scand.* 1961;51:63.

11. Dabby R, Sadeh M, Herman O, et al. Clinical electrophysiological and pathologic findings in 10 patients with myotonic dystrophy 2. *Isr Med Assoc J.* 2011;13(12): 745–747.

12. Wettstein A. The origin of fasciculations in motoneuron disease. *Ann Neurol.* 1979;3:295–300.

13. Lagueny A. Single fiber electromyography. *Rev Med Liege.* 2004;59(Suppl 1):141–149.

Chapter 13

Laboratory Investigation of Suspected Peripheral Neuropathy

Stephen J. Carp, PT, PhD, GCS

"The investigation of nature is an infinite pasture ground where all may graze, and where the more bite, the longer the grass grows, the sweeter is its flavor and the more it flourishes."

—Aldous Huxley (1894–1963)

Objectives

On completion of this chapter, the student/practitioner will be able to:

- To gain appreciation of the hypothesis-oriented algorithm for clinicians as a method of improving efficiency and timeliness of the evaluation process for patients with suspected peripheral neuropathy.
- To be able to differentiate screening versus diagnostic laboratory testing.
- To use clinical laboratory testing results as an important adjuvant to the diagnostic process.
- To begin to correlate laboratory data with the physical examination to add to, remove, or confirm the differential diagnoses.

Key Terms

- Laboratory values
- Hypothesis-Oriented Algorithm for Clinicians (HOAC)
- Laboratory testing
- Screening
- Electrodiagnostic testing

Introduction

For most presentations of suspected peripheral neuropathy, the logical starting point for the diagnostician is the patient interview and review of prior laboratory, electrodiagnostic, and radiographic data. Visual and audible clues provided by the patient during the taking of the medical/surgical history and history of the present illness and hard data from the prior diagnostic workup allow the clinician to begin to develop a differential diagnosis list. The **Hypothesis-Oriented Algorithm for Clinicians (HOAC)** and the later iteration, HOAC II[1] provide a logical diagnostic framework

for the clinician. Initial "clinical scripts" provide clues enabling the clinician to begin to develop a list of differential diagnoses. The clinician can then eliminate from, add to, or confirm the list of differential diagnoses through the application and analysis of additional evaluative data obtained from performing the physical examination, ordering additional radiological and **laboratory testing,** or asking qualifying questions to the patient about the history presented. The HOAC framework allows for a systematic and orderly search for the differential diagnoses rather than the "shotgun" method of ordering batteries of tests and measures and performing unnecessary physical examination tests and

Diagnostic Algorithm for Suspected Peripheral Neuropathy

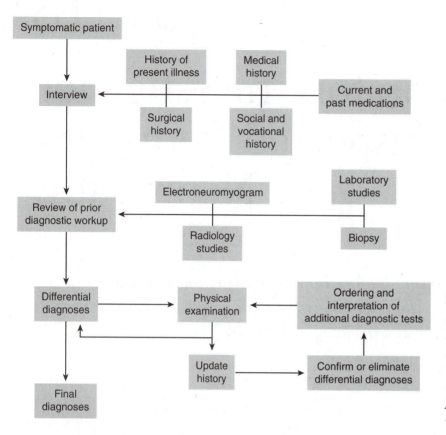

Figure 13-1 Example of a diagnostic algorithm for the evaluation of suspected peripheral neuropathy. The algorithm was developed by the author and reflects the Hypothesis-Oriented Algorithm developed by Rothstein et al. *(From Rothstein JM, Echternach JL, Riddle DL. The hypothesis-oriented algorithm for clinicians II (HOAC II): a guide for patient management. Phys Ther. 2003;83(5):455–470.)*

measures. As research continues to improve the sensitivity and specificity of diagnostic utilities, the use of frameworks such as the HOAC will improve the cost-effectiveness and timeliness of diagnostic work (Fig. 13-1).

Adjuvant to the physical examination, the clinician relies on additional tests and measures to provide data to help narrow, add to, or confirm the differential list of neuropathic diagnoses. These include the electroneuromyogram, radiographic studies, autonomic testing, biopsy, and laboratory testing.

Electroneuromyogram studies are a very important part of the diagnostic workup. Abnormal electrodiagnostic studies provide unequivocal information to the diagnostician that there is a neuropathic diagnosis (normal studies cannot prove or disprove a neurological diagnosis—small myelinated and unmyelinated fibers cannot be assessed by typical **electrodiagnostic testing**). Electrodiagnostic studies also assist the clinician in determining the neurological extent of the abnormal process, including uni-, hemi-, para-, or quadri-limb involvement; systemic or local; mononeuropathy, multiple mononeuropathies, or systemic neuropathy; and involvement of roots, cords, or peripheral nerve branches. Lastly, the electroneuromyogram provides the clinician with the neurological extent of the

injury—neurapraxia, axonotmesis, or neurotmesis—and the type of nerve involved—sensory, autonomic, or motor or a combination.

Radiographic studies have an important but limited role in the workup of suspected peripheral neuropathies. Magnetic resonance imaging (MRI) has assumed the dominant role in radiological diagnostics of spinal stenosis and brachial and lumbosacral plexopathies. Flat plate radiographs, computed tomography (CT), and MRI are useful in identifying offending structures in entrapment neuropathies. Central lesions associated with chronic inflammatory demyelinating polyradiculoneuropathy may be seen with MRI. Imaging studies help identify primary tumors related to paraneoplastic syndrome and other cancer-induced neuropathies. However, many diagnoses that result in motor, sensory, and autonomic neuropathies are best evaluated with tools other than radiography.

Autonomic function testing is useful in specific circumstances, especially in neuropathies in which autonomic failure is the predominant manifestation. Autonomic testing assists the clinician in determining sympathetic and parasympathetic nervous system involvement, the location as either local or systemic and preganglionic or postganglionic, and the severity of the manifestation. Examples of autonomic function testing are the quantitative sudomotor axon reflex test and the simple "tilt test."

Nerve biopsy, an invasive procedure with often persistent (2 to 3 weeks or longer) symptoms after biopsy, is used to assist with the confirmation of a host of neuropathic disorders, including vasculitides, sarcoidosis, heredity neuropathy, Farber disease, and leprosy.

Because of the spectrum of available laboratory testing, tests should be ordered on the basis of **screening,** confirmation, or eliminating a differential diagnosis. Except for basic screening tools, there is no clinical laboratory order set that fits all patients with suspected peripheral neuropathy. In this chapter, we review the basic battery of screening laboratory tools and discuss disease-specific tests to assist with narrowing the differential diagnosis list. We review basic screening and neurological laboratory testing and discuss the diagnostic, functional, and interventional implications of the test results.

Laboratory Screening Tests

Advances in understanding of the pathogenesis and progress of disease have led to a spectral systems' view of illness rather than an isolated system etiology, such as a disease being of purely neurological, integument, or orthopedic origin. For this reason, after the interview and review of previously ordered diagnostic data, master diagnosticians and interventionists advocate one-time screening of all organ systems as a starting point of the diagnostic inquiry. Screening tests, whether part of the physical examination, imaging database, or laboratory workup, are useful adjuncts in evaluating the patient's overall state of health, medical conditions, and potential contraindications to therapy by adding to, eliminating, or confirming differential diagnoses.

As a caveat, there are limitations to laboratory testing. As with all diagnostic tests, each laboratory screening test has a percentage of false-positive and false-negative results. Over-the-counter, prescription, and illegal medications may affect **laboratory values.** Some tests must be ordered for a specific time of day and either fasting or nonfasting. Reference ranges and processing of samples may vary by laboratory. Many laboratory tests have no predictive value. For instance,

coronary risk screen laboratory assessments all may be "negative" one day, and the individual may have a myocardial infarction the next day. The positive predictive value of a test is directly related to the prevalence of the disease in the community. The more prevalent the disease, the more valid the measure; the less prevalent the disease, the less valid the measure. A diagnosis can rarely, if ever, be made based on laboratory testing alone. The reliability, and to a lesser extent the validity, of the diagnostic process depends on the clinical decision-making skills, the use of evidence-based inquiry, and the clinical expertise of the diagnostician.

Complete Blood Count

Screening tests may be ordered individually or ordered in group format such as the complete blood count (CBC) or metabolic panel. These tests typically are not diagnostic; rather, they are ordered to provide a cursory glimpse of the health of all corporal systems. Because possible etiologies for peripheral nerve injury include dysfunction related to all corporal systems, it is intuitive to perform, at a minimum, a screen of each corporal system.

The CBC is an evaluation of components typically found in venous blood. It is not a measure of the function of these components. For instance, an individual may have a normal red blood cell count but may have a disease resulting in abnormal oxygen transport. The components of the CBC include white blood cell (WBC) count, red blood cell (RBC) count, hemoglobin (Hgb), hematocrit (Hct), and platelets (Table 13-1).

WBC count volume screens the immune system and assists in identifying the presence of inflammatory processes. An increase in WBC count greater than 11×10^3 is called leukocytosis. Leukocytosis occurs in the presence of infection—primarily bacterial. Leukocytosis is also seen with leukemia, severe trauma, inflammatory disease, significant tissue necrosis, and pregnancy. WBC counts less than 5×10^3 are known as leukopenia and are associated with chemotherapy, radiation, bone marrow failure, chronic infection, and HIV. WBC count differential estimates the percentage of different types of WBCs (leukocytes) being produced. Distinctive patterns of WBCs are produced

Table 13-1 Complete Blood Count Normal Values					
	WBC Count (cells/mL)	RBC Count (mL/μL)	Hematocrit (%)	Hemoglobin (g/dL)	Platelet Count (cells/μL)
Men	4,000–10,000	4.7–5.5	43–49	14.4–16.6	15,000–410,000
Women	4,000–10,000	4.1–4.9	38–44	12.2–14.7	15,000–410,000

WBC, White blood cell; RBC, red blood cell.
Pagana K, Pagana T. *Mosby's Rapid Reference to Diagnostic and Laboratory Tests.* St. Louis: Mosby; 2000

by different disease states. The differential count is expressed as a percentage of the total number of WBCs. The absolute number of each type of WBC is obtained by multiplying the percentage of one type by the total WBC count.[2]

RBC count measures the quantity of RBCs in a given volume of blood. RBCs carry the functional unit of oxygenation, Hgb. Anemia is the most common cause of a low RBC count. The etiologies of anemia are many and include acute or chronic blood loss, destruction of RBCs, decreased production of RBCs, and molecular defects in the shape of RBCs such as seen with sickle cell anemia. An elevated RBC count is known as polycythemia.[2]

Hct measures the percent, by volume, of packed RBCs in a centrifuged volume of blood. Hct percentages often correlate with Hgb values. Hgb is a measure in grams of Hgb found in 1 dL of whole blood and is often represented in grams. Hgb and Hct are used to assess hydration, anemia, and polycythemia. Low Hct and Hgb levels are typically indicative of anemia, chronic inflammatory illness, or hemodilution. Elevated levels may be indicative of chronic hypoxemia as seen with chronic obstructive pulmonary disease and pulmonary fibrosis, polycythemia vera, and residing at high altitudes.[2]

Platelets circulate in the blood and assist with the clotting cascade. Platelets form "plugs" in the walls of ruptured blood vessels to stem the tide of leakage. Normal platelet values are 150,000 to 400,000 per microliter of blood. Thrombocytosis occurs when the platelet count is elevated greater than 1 million per microliter of blood. Causes of thrombocytosis include neoplasm, inflammation, infection, and polycythemia vera. Thrombocytosis increases the risk of clot formation. Thrombocytopenia occurs when there are less than 150,000 platelets per microliter of blood.[2] Causes of thrombocytopenia include neoplasm, viral infection, nutritional deficiency, drug interaction, radiation, chemotherapy, aplastic anemia, HIV, and idiopathic thrombocytopenia.[2,3] Thrombocytopenia may lead to internal or external hemorrhage of blood vessels, ecchymoses, purpura, and petechiae.[4]

Abnormal results of the CBC in conjunction with symptoms of peripheral neuropathy may assist with the diagnostic path. For instance, abnormalities in the WBC count may lead the diagnostician to look for a space-occupying abscess that may result in compression of a peripheral nerve or a neoplasm with resultant paraneoplastic syndrome. Elevated platelets may lead to nerve infarction; diminished platelets may lead to internal hemorrhage resulting in space-occupying hematoma. Thrombocytopenia may also be indicative of nutritional deficiencies that may result in systemic neuropathy. A chronically low Hgb and Hct may be indicative of "anemia of chronic illness," such as rheumatoid arthritis, cancer, systemic lupus erythematosus,

Table 13-2	Basic Metabolic Panel Normal Values
Test	**Normal Value**
Sodium	136.0–145.0 mEq/L
Potassium	3.5–5.0 mEq/L
Carbon dioxide	23.0–33.0 mEq/L
Blood urea nitrogen	10.0–20.0 mg/dL
Creatinine	0.6–1.2 mg/dL
Glucose	70.0–110.0 mg/dL
Chloride	98.0–106.0 mEq/L

and diabetes—all with implications of neuropathic symptoms.

Basic Metabolic Panel

The constituents of the basic metabolic panel (BMP) are defined by *Current Procedure Terminology* (CPT) codes.[5] The BMP replaces the antiquated panels such as the SMA-6, SMA-12, chemistry panel, chemistry screen, and SMAC-12. The BMP is a group of eight tests and consists of serum concentrations of sodium, potassium, chloride, calcium, blood urea nitrogen (BUN), creatinine, glucose, and carbon dioxide. Venous blood samples obtained after a 10- to 12-hour fast are used for assessment (Table 13-2).[2]

Sodium (Na$^+$) is an electrolyte metal that is important in the development and propagation of action potentials in nerve, in muscle contraction, in controlling osmotic gradients, and in many aspects of cellular function. Normal values range from 136.0–145.0 mEq/L.[3] Sodium blood levels are affected by diet, medications, activity, and disease processes.[3] Elevated sodium is referred to as hypernatremia; decreased sodium is referred to as hyponatremia. Abnormalities in sodium blood concentrations result in many potential impairments. Fluid concentrations within and external to cells are dependent on sodium concentration. Action potential dysfunction may result in cardiac arrhythmia, muscle weakness, loss of sensation, mental status changes, and potential intracranial hemorrhage with coma and possible death.[5] No specific exercise guidelines are available for individuals with hypernatremia or hyponatremia.

Potassium (K$^+$) is an electrolyte that is strongly associated with optimal neuromuscular function. Even minor changes in blood potassium concentrations may have a severe impact on health. Normal values range from 3.5 to 5.0 mEq/L. Hypokalemia, or decreased potassium concentrations, may produce ventricular arrhythmia including fibrillation, cardiac irritability, ST-T segment depression, dizziness, low blood pressure, and a decreased left ventricular ejection fraction. Hyperkalemia, or elevated potassium concentration, may produce nausea, vomiting, and electrocardiogram changes including arrhythmia.[5] Because of the small window of acceptable blood potassium concentrations, individuals with even minor elevated or decreased potassium levels should not exercise.

Carbon dioxide (CO_2) content is a measure of the concentration of CO_2 in blood. Knowledge of the concentration assists with evaluating pH and electrolyte status. CO_2 also is an indirect measurement of bicarbonate (HCO_3), which is regulated by the kidneys. Because CO_2 assists with regulation of pH, abnormalities may produce alkalosis or acidosis.[3]

Blood urea nitrogen (BUN) and creatinine are both regulated by the kidneys. Renal failure causes metabolite wastes to accumulate in the blood, which can be measured to assess renal function. BUN is formed in the liver and is the end product of dietary protein breakdown. It is filtered by the kidney and excreted in urine. BUN concentration is directly related to kidney function and the metabolic function of the liver. Smaller changes in BUN concentration may be a reflection of dietary protein intake.[3] In individuals with combined liver and kidney disease, the BUN concentration may be normal secondary to a combined cause of poor hepatic function creating less BUN and poor renal function resulting in poor excretion. Creatinine is the by-product of normal muscle metabolism and represents a gradient between production by muscle and clearance by the kidney. Because muscle mass is relatively constant, changes in creatinine concentrations are most likely related to kidney function. Similar to BUN, it is regulated by the kidney and is used as a marker for kidney function.[4]

Blood glucose (BG) or blood sugar (BS) is a measurement of the BS level. Evaluation of this concentration must always be based on the time of day the sample was taken and whether or not it was a fasting sample. Hypoglycemia, a decreased BG level, may be secondary to starvation, insulinoma, or insulin (or oral diabetes medication) overdose. Hyperglycemia, an elevated BG concentration, may be due to one of various diabetes diagnoses or acute stress.[6]

Chloride (Cl^-) is an electrolyte controlled by the kidneys. Because the concentration varies with fluid status, Cl^- levels are often used to determine levels of hydration. Cl^- also assists with acid-base metabolism.[5]

Abnormalities in the BMP may also affect the diagnostic process when searching for possible etiologies of neuropathy. Fluid overload may lead to compressive neuropathies. Hypokalemia or hyperkalemia may affect action potential associated with sensory, autonomic, and motor nerves resulting in dysfunction. Chronic kidney disease with associated elevated BUN and creatinine is strongly associated with peripheral neuropathy. Hyperglycemia associated with diabetes is the leading cause of motor and sensory neuropathy worldwide.

Laboratory Diagnostic Testing

Specialized laboratory tests, alone or in combination with other tests and measures, are ordered to rule in or rule out specific pathology or, if a diagnosis is already confirmed, may be used to assess severity of the disease or to measure progression or improvement of the disease.

Hemostasis

Hemostasis, also called clotting studies and bleeding time, is used to determine the body's ability to initiate the clotting cascade and how rapidly the cascade occurs and to diagnose specific primary clotting diagnoses such as hemophilia. Hemostatic studies may also be used to assess the effectiveness and dosage of anticoagulant therapy used as prophylaxis against clot in various diagnoses such as atrial fibrillation, valvular replacement, arterial thoracic outlet syndrome, and deep vein thrombosis.[7] Common hemostatic studies include the international normalized ratio (INR), prothrombin time (PT), and activated partial thromboplastin time (APTT).[2,4] The INR was developed as a method to express PT in a standard format, eliminating laboratory variability.[3] The INR is the ratio of the individual's result to the reference range, correcting for variability in the PT testing hardware reagents and materials. The PT evaluates thrombin production. The APTT assesses the production and use of clotting factors. Aberrant clotting times, whether extensive or diminished, disease based or intervention based, may result in neuropathy secondary to possible internal hematoma formation or nerve/cord ischemia owing to infarct.

Inflammation

The presence and severity of inflammation can be measured in a nonspecific method using erythrocyte sedimentation rate (ESR) and C-reactive protein (CRP). ESR is the rate that RBCs settle by gravity in a given volume of unclotted plasma in 1 hour. The test is based on the premise that inflammation and necrotic processes lead to an alteration in blood cell proteins, resulting in an aggregation within the RBCs making them denser than RBCs in individuals without inflammation or necrosis.[2] The faster the cells fall, the higher the ESR and the greater the inflammation. ESR may be used as a screening test for systemic inflammatory diseases such as rheumatoid arthritis, systemic lupus erythematosus, and infection.[8] It is often used as a screening tool to differentiate rheumatic diseases from complaints organic in nature.[5] ESR may also be used to assess the effectiveness of medications given to decrease inflammation.[7] CRP was originally believed to quantify inflammation specifically associated with coronary artery disease, but subsequent studies have shown that acute and chronic musculoskeletal conditions may also lead to an elevated CRP, reducing the sensitivity of the test for coronary artery disease.[5]

Although elevated serum CRP concentration has been shown to be associated with even mild neuropathy,[9,10] it is not very useful as a diagnostic tool because of the lack of specificity of the test. However, the ESR and CBC remain useful as a screening tool for rheumatological and infectious diseases that may result in neuropathy.[10]

Cardiac Enzymes

Enzymes are typical organic catalysts that facilitate chemical reactions within cells but are not destroyed in the process. Normally, these enzymes are found within cells, but damage to cells, especially to the cell walls, may cause leakage into the bloodstream. Some enzymes are present in all cells; some are present in specific organs. Identifying these unique enzymes in the bloodstream can often tell us which organ has been injured. Cardiac enzymes are monitored following episodic chest pain or suspected myocardial infarction. These enzymes change in a predictable waxing and waning pattern that allows diagnosticians not only to identify that a cardiac event has occurred (in correlation with the electrocardiogram, echocardiogram, and angiography) but also possibly to pinpoint the actual time the event occurred.[2] Enzyme creatine kinase (CK) is a sensitive marker for myocardial infarction but not very specific because this particular enzyme is also found in skeletal muscle and may be elevated after muscle injury or disease.[3] The CK-MB is a particular CK enzyme found primarily in the heart. The CK-MB and CK are measured in suspected cardiac injury, and if the CK-MB exceeds 5.0% of the CK, there is a strong likelihood that cardiac injury has occurred.[3] The volume of CK-MB in the bloodstream is correlated with the quantity of coronary damage.[2,11] Serum CK begins increasing 3 to 8 hours after a cardiac event, peaks in 10 to 30 hours, and returns to normal in 3 to 5 days. CK-MB begins increasing 4 to 8 hours after a cardiac event, peaks in 12 to 24 hours, and returns to normal in 2 to 3 days.[3] Lactic acid dehydrogenase (LDH) is an extracellular enzyme distributed to most internal organs. LDH begins increasing 1 to 2 days after a cardiac event, peaks in 3 to 5 days, and returns to normal in 8 to 14 days.[3]

A cardiac workup including enzymes, electrocardiogram, stress testing, and imaging studies is often useful in at-risk patients with face, neck, jaw, scapular, arm, and forearm symptoms that may be cardiac in origin but may also be due to gastrointestinal or cervical/thoracic radicular symptoms.

Liver Enzymes

Poor liver function places a patient at risk for multiorgan dysfunction syndrome because of a higher risk of organ exposure to bacteria and toxins normally filtered by the liver. Because the liver has many functions, there is not one test to assess liver function; a battery of tests must be used. Liver tests are typically divided into two types: tests diagnostic of liver disease and tests that measure a particular liver function. An example of a test used to diagnose the cause of liver damage is the test for gamma-glutamyltransferase (GGT). This test is a very sensitive indicator of hepatobiliary tract disease.[3] GGT is elevated after alcohol ingestion and in hepatitis, primary or metastatic liver malignancy, and cirrhosis.[3] An example of a liver test measuring liver function is alanine aminotransferase (ALT), which is a strong indicator of hepatocellular damage (Table 13-3).[8]

Because of the spectrum of hepatic and biliary functions, these organs are affected by many disease processes that may also result in neuropathic symptoms. For instance, chronic alcohol abuse eventually leads to liver disease and quite possibly motor and sensory neuropathy. Purposeful, accidental, or environmental exposure to toxins such as arsenic and mercury may initially manifest as abnormalities in liver function but may also result in neuropathic symptoms. HIV and AIDS may manifest as concomitant liver failure and peripheral neuropathy.

Immunological Tests

Immunological testing results have a broad range of potential implications. These tests are used in the diagnosis of immune disorders and allergic reactions, infectious disease, rheumatological diagnoses, and neoplastic diseases.[2,3] Immunoglobulins, antibodies that are produced in response to antigens, are divided into five classes (IgG, IgA, IgM, IgD, and IgE). In testing, each of the classes of globulins is divided via electrophoresis into different fractions.[3] The pattern of fractions is uniquely elevated in response to specific illnesses. Rheumatoid factor is seen in persons with and without rheumatoid arthritis, but most adults with rheumatoid arthritis do exhibit it.[3] Antinuclear antibodies are nonspecific antibodies that react with antigens in all organs. A positive response is not specific for a particular disease, but a negative response rules strongly against the diagnosis of a rheumatological disease. Antinuclear antibodies are used more as a conformational test rather than for diagnosis.[12]

Immunological testing has a large role in confirming diagnoses associated with signs and symptoms of peripheral neuropathy. Many rheumatological diseases including rheumatoid arthritis, systemic lupus erythematosus, and the spondyloarthropathies have a high association with neuropathic symptoms. Immunological testing is used to confirm the diagnosis of these diseases as well as infectious entities such as Guillain-Barré syndrome (GBS) and the Miller-Fischer variation of GBS. Paraneoplastic syndrome, paraneoplastic

Table 13-3 Laboratory Tests for Liver and Biliary Disease

Panel	Test	Normal Range	Comment
Bilirubin	Direct serum bilirubin	0.1–0.3 mg/dL	Increased with biliary obstruction
	Indirect serum bilirubin	0.2–0.8 mg/dL	Increased with bile duct dysfunction, primary liver disease, cirrhosis
	Total bilirubin	0.1–2.0 mg/dL	Increased in cirrhosis, hepatitis, anemia, transfusion reaction, hepatic malignancy
	Urine bilirubin	0.0 mg/dL	
Serum proteins	Albumin	3.5–5.5 g/dL	Decreased in malnutrition states, Crohn's disease, anorexia, bulimia, burns, liver disease
	Globulin	2.5–3.5 g/dL	Increased in hepatitis
	Total	6.0–8.0 g/dL	See albumin
	A:G	1.5:1–2.5:1	Ratio reverses chronic liver disease
	Transferrin	250–300 µg/dL	Decreases with liver disease; increases with iron deficiency
	Alpha-fetoprotein	6–20 ng/mL	Cancer-associated antigen
Serum enzymes	AST	8–20 U/L	Increased in liver damage and primary muscle disease (i.e., Duchenne)
	ALT	5–35 U/L	See AST
	LDH	45–90 U/L	See AST
	GGT	5–38 U/L	See AST
	ALP	30–85 U/L	Increased in primary liver cancer, rheumatoid arthritis, biliary obstruction
Ammonia	Blood ammonia	<75 µg/dL	Increased in liver dysfunction

A:G, Albumin-to-globulin ratio; AST, aspartate aminotransferase; ALT, alanine aminotransferase; LDH, lactate dehydrogenase; GGT, gamma-glutamyltransferase; ALP, alkaline phosphatase.

encephalomyelitis, and subacute sensory neuronopathy are associated with antineuronal nuclear antibody type I.[3] Immunological testing also has a significant role in the diagnosis of suspected vasculitic neuropathy. Herpes zoster infections may be detected by varicella-zoster virus–specific IgM antibody in blood; this antibody appears only during active episodes of chickenpox or herpes zoster and not while the virus is dormant.[13]

Urinalysis

Urine is best described as the end product of a host of metabolic processes in the body, and examination of the urine can provide a host of information about health and disease. Urine is an extremely complex substance, 95% liquid and 5% solids, with primary constituents of water, sodium chloride, and urea with smaller concentrations of protein, glucose, ketones, blood, and minute concentrations of more than 1000 chemicals (Table 13-4).[8] Urine should be pale yellow in color owing to the presence of urochrome, a chemical found in food and that is also a by-product of bile metabolism. Color other than pale yellow is often the result of food intake (carrots, rhubarb, beats, grape juice), medications (antiplatelet drugs, levodopa, laxitives), or disease (hepatic failure, disseminating intravascular coagulation).[14] Bleeding from the urinary tract may result in urine ranging in color from beet red to bright red depending on the source of bleeding.

Table 13-4 Urinalysis, Microscopic Examination of Sediment, and Chemical Content

Urinalysis	Examination of Sediment	Chemical Content
Color: Pale yellow to amber-yellow	Casts: Negative	Ketones: Negative
Turbidity: Clear to slightly hazy	Red blood cells: Negative or rare	Blood: Negative
Specific gravity: 1.015–1.025	Crystals: Negative	Bilirubin: Negative
pH: 4.5–8	White blood cells: Negative or rare Epithelial cells: Rare	Nitrate for bacteria: Negative Leukocyte esterase: Negative

Specific gravity is a measure of urine concentration. Diluted urine has a low specific gravity, and concentrated urine has a high specific gravity. Abnormal specific gravity with normal hydration status may indicate renal disease.[2] The presence of red blood cells is indicative of occult blood.[2] The presence of myoglobinuria is typically related to skeletal muscle injury.[3] Glucose may be found in the urine if the concentration of blood glucose exceeds the ability of the renal tubules to reabsorb it, resulting in "urine spillage."[3] Slight sugar concentrations found in the urine may not be pathological; stress and heavy, sugary meals may lead to spillage.[8] Ketonuria is due to the use of fats as the primary source of energy and is an early indication of possible diabetic coma.[5] Urine may also be screened for prescription, over-the-counter, and illegal drugs.[8]

Urinalysis is a useful adjunct in identifying diagnoses related to peripheral neuropathy. Urinalysis can be used to assist with the diagnoses of metabolic abnormalities, diabetes, renal disease, and clotting abnormalities.

Culture

Normal flora abounds on the skin, in the mouth, and in the gastrointestinal tract. In some pathological conditions, these bacteria "escape" and enter the bloodstream leading to the potential of life-threatening metastatic infection. Heart valves, bones, joints, and internal organs all may be seeded by septicemia. Blood culturing is the random sampling of blood and culturing it to determine if bacterial growth occurs. Because the chance of obtaining a bacterium from one sampling is small, blood cultures are often drawn three times, increasing the chance of encountering a pathogen. For blood culturing to be effective, samples must be drawn before the initiation of antibiotics.[8]

Rapid Plasma Reagin

Syphilis is a sexually transmitted disease caused by the organism *Treponema pallidum*. The rapid plasma reagin (RPR) looks for nonspecific antibodies in the blood of a patient that may indicate the presence of the bacteria. The RPR level is also a titer and can be used to track the progress of the disease over time and its response to antibiotic therapy. The test is most sensitive (90% to 100%) in infections present for at least 1 month and less sensitive in newly acquired infections or infections present for months.[15]

Syphilis, although not directly associated with peripheral neuropathy, is often on the differential diagnosis list because of the gummatous and late (tertiary) neurosyphilis complication. Gummatous syphilis, also known as late benign syphilis, begins an average of 15 years after untreated infection acquisition and is characterized by the formation of chromic gummas, soft tumor-like balls of inflammation that vary in size and location. They often affect skin, bone, and liver but may appear anywhere. Owing to the potential location adjacent to peripheral nerve, gummas may result in compressive or tensile neuropathies. Late neurosyphilis occurs 4 to 25 years after acute infection. Tabes dorsalis, a complication of late neurosyphilis, affects the posterior white column of the spinal cord resulting in decreased proprioception and kinesthetic and vibratory sense. Functionally, patients with tabes dorsalis have loss of gross and fine motor control, ataxia, frequent falls, and gait dysfunction. These symptoms mimic many systemic peripheral neuropathies.[15]

Table 13-5	Relationship of Hemoglobin A$_{1c}$ Percentage and Mean Blood Sugar	
Hemoglobin A$_{1c}$ (%)	**Mean Blood Sugar (mg/dL)**
6	135
7	170
8	205
9	240
10	275
11	310
12	345

Hemoglobin A$_{1c}$

Finger-stick BS provides only a "snapshot" of BG concentrations. Hgb A$_{1c}$ provides a 3-month view of mean BG concentrations. Glucose molecules "stick" to the proteins within RBCs, and because these cells live for an average of 3 months, laboratory assessment of the number of glucose molecules attached to the proteins in the RBC provides an excellent long-term view of glucose control. In most laboratories, the normal range is 4.0% to 5.9%. In patients with diabetes, acceptable Hgb A$_{1c}$, indicating good control, is less than 7.0%. The American Association of Clinical Endocrinologists recommends a goal of less than 6.5%. Poorly controlled is defined as greater than 8.0% (Table 13-5).[16] Numerous studies have documented data showing that poorly controlled diabetes is directly related to the early onset of peripheral neuropathy and the severity of the signs and symptoms.

CASE STUDY

DB is a 62-year-old man who was referred to a physical therapist with a diagnosis of falls. His medical history includes hypertension, type 2 diabetes mellitus, and hypercholesterolemia. Vital signs at the evaluation included a heart rate of 72, blood pressure 132/88, respiratory rate of 16, and oxygen saturation of 98% on room air. A fasting finger-stick blood sugar was 102 mg/dL. Physical examination revealed no focal, unilateral, or patterned motor weakness with strength 5/5 throughout. Tone was normal. No neurological deficits were noted except for decreased vibration and kinesthetic sense in both lower extremities from the knees to the toes and impaired balance tests: Romberg eyes closed 8 seconds and a Timed Up and Go balance assessment of less than expected for the age group. Observational gait examination revealed a mildly wide-based gait pattern with shortened stride bilaterally and decreased arm swing. DB did not use any assistive devices.

Case Study Questions

1. The therapist can rule out diabetes mellitus as a possible cause of DB's falls for which of the following reasons?
   a. There is no documented focal motor weakness.
   b. The finger-stick blood sugar value was in the normal range: 102 mg/dL.
   c. The blood pressure was mildly elevated.
   d. The therapist cannot, with the current information presented, rule out diabetes as a cause of the falls.

2. To assist with "ruling in" diabetes as a cause for the falls, which laboratory test would be most indicated?
   a. Hemoglobin A_{1c}
   b. Urinalysis
   c. Repeat finger-stick blood sugar
   d. Complete blood count

3. To rule out anemia as a cause for the falls, which laboratory test would be most indicated?
   a. Hemoglobin A_{1c}
   b. Urinalysis
   c. Repeat finger-stick blood sugar
   d. Complete blood count

4. To rule out a urinary tract infection as a cause for the falls, which laboratory test would be most indicated?
   a. Hemoglobin A_{1c}
   b. Urinalysis
   c. Repeat finger-stick blood sugar
   d. Complete blood count

5. The hemoglobin A_{1c} test looks "back" at the blood sugar concentration for a period of how long?
   a. 1 hour
   b. 1 day
   c. 1 month
   d. 3 months

References

1. Rothstein JM, Echternach JL, Riddle DL. The hypothesis-oriented algorithm for clinicians II (HOAC II): a guide for patient management. *Phys Ther.* 2003;83(5):455–470.
2. Pagana K, Pagana T. *Mosby's Rapid Reference to Diagnostic and Laboratory Tests.* St. Louis: Mosby; 2000.
3. Fischbach F. *Nurses' Quick Reference to Common Laboratory and Diagnostic Tests.* 3rd ed. Philadelphia: Lippincott Williams & Wilkins; 2002.
4. Tsai H. Advances in the pathogenesis, diagnosis, and treatment of thrombotic thrombocytopenic purpura. *J Am Soc Nephrol.* 2003;14:1072–1081.
5. Goodman CC, Boissonnault WG, Fuller KS. *Pathology: Implications for the Physical Therapist.* 2nd ed. Philadelphia: Saunders; 2003.
6. Rother KI. Diabetes treatment—bridging the divide. *N Engl J Med* 2007;356(15):1499–1501.
7. Poller L, Keown M, Chauhan N, et al. European Concerted Action on Anticoagulation. Correction of displayed international normalized ratio on two point-of-care test whole-blood prothrombin time monitors (CoaguChek Mini and TAS PT-NC) by independent international sensitivity index calibration. *Br J Haematol.* 2003;122(6):944–949.
8. Goodman C, Snyder T. *Differential Diagnosis in Physical Therapy.* Philadelphia: Saunders; 1990.
9. Lloyd-Jones DM, Liu K, Tian L, Greenland P. Narrative review: assessment of C-reactive protein in risk prediction for cardiovascular disease. *Ann Intern Med.* 2006;145(1):35–42.
10. Carp SJ, Barbe MF, Barr AE. Serum biomarkers as signals for risk and severity of work-related musculoskeletal injury. *Biomark Med.* 2008;2:67–79.
11. Wallimann T, Wyss M, Brdiczka D, Nicolay K, Eppenberger HM. Intracellular compartmentation, structure and function of creatine kinase isoenzymes in tissues with high and fluctuating energy emends: the 'phosphocreatine circuit' for cellular energy homeostasis. *Biochem J.* 1992;281(1):21–40.
12. Kavanaugh A, Tomar R, Reveille J, Solomon DH, Homburger HA. Guidelines for clinical use of the antinuclear antibody test and tests for specific autoantibodies to nuclear antigens. *Arch Pathol Lab Med.* 2000;124:71–81.
13. Johnson RW, Dworkin RH (2003). Treatment of herpes zoster and postherpetic neuralgia. *BMJ* 2003;326(7392):748–750.
14. Nicolle LE. Uncomplicated urinary tract infection in adults including uncomplicated pyelonephritis. *Urol Clin North Am.* 2008;35(1):1–12.
15. Kent ME, Romanelli F. Reexamining syphilis: an update on epidemiology, clinical manifestations, and management. *Ann Pharmacother.* 2003;42(2):226–236.
16. American Diabetes Association. Standards of medical care in diabetes—2007. *Diabetes Care.* 2007;30(Suppl 1):S4–S41.

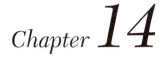

Chapter 14

The Examination: Evaluation of the Patient With Suspected Peripheral Neuropathy

Stephen J. Carp, PT, PhD, GCS

"Seize the moment of excited curiosity on any subject to solve your doubts; for if you let it pass, the desire may never return and you may remain forever in ignorance."

—William Wirt (1772–1834)

Objectives

On completion of this chapter, the student/practitioner will be able to:

- Develop an evidenced-based evaluative algorithm for assessment of suspected peripheral neuropathy.
- Develop sufficient knowledge of the cognitive components of the peripheral neuropathy evaluation to enable the practicing therapist to develop valid and reliable psychomotor components of the evaluation.
- Identify important signs and symptoms that may relate to peripheral neuropathy.

Key Terms

- Assessment
- Evaluation
- Peripheral neuropathy

Introduction

The physical examiner encountering a patient with suspected **peripheral neuropathy** has four primary challenges. The first challenge is to obtain a thorough, comprehensive, and valid oral history of the chief complaint, history of the present illness, past medical history, past surgical history, current and past medications, family history, and review of systems. The second challenge is to perform, as directed by the oral history, a comprehensive physical and functional examination. The third challenge is to review and incorporate key diagnostic findings such as blood indices, radiological data, and electroneuromyogram results into the clinical decision-making algorithm. The fourth challenge is to complete the clinical decision-making algorithm by identifying functional problems and developing time-based functional goals and a goal-oriented intervention.

The Chief Complaint

Following the development of the patient-therapeutic relationship, a good probing question for the part of the interview inquiring about the chief complaint is "So, what brought you here to see me today?" Such an open-ended question encourages the patient to talk. Typically, a patient with neuropathy relates an onset of one or a combination of the following: motor weakness, falls, tonal changes, dyscoordination, sensory loss, ataxia, or autonomic complaints. The practitioner should listen closely to the order in which the patient expresses his or her complaints. Typically, the complaints are presented in the order of the ones that have the most functional impact to ones that have the least functional impact.

History of the Present Illness

Following the patient's brief explanation of what brought him or her to the clinic for **evaluation,** the practitioner should begin to search for the history of the present illness. Patients often describe their symptoms with simple but descriptive adjectives and phrases, such as "burning," "tingling," "clumsiness," "loss of balance," "dizziness," "ache," and "knifelike pain." Practitioners should always focus on the time frame of the onset of symptoms. Arbitrary but very useful boundaries have been established to determine if a symptom is acute, subacute, or chronic. Categorizing symptoms as acute (present for days to 4 weeks), subacute (present for 4 weeks to 2 months), or chronic (present for greater than 2 months) is often helpful in establishing differential diagnoses. For instance, neuropathy related to Guillain-Barré syndrome[1-3] often develops in less than 4 weeks. Diabetic neuropathy may take years to develop fully and manifests as a chronic condition. Paraneoplastic neuropathies may evolve as subacute or chronic neuropathies.[4-6]

There may be confusion related to the perception of the onset of the neuropathy. Often a patient presents to a practitioner because of an exacerbation or worsening of symptoms rather than the onset of symptoms. Inherited and some viral neuropathies often begin in childhood, but the patient presents only when there is a functional loss.[7,8] Pointed questions often assist with the diagnostic process, such as the following: "Did you play sports as a child?"; "Did you walk differently from the other children when you were a child?"; "Could you run as fast as the other children?"; "Did you often have ankle sprains as a child?"

Location of onset is important. Most neuropathies have a neural length relationship; the symptoms tend to initiate farthest from the body core—that is, the hands and feet. Sensory symptoms in the trunk, buttocks, thighs, shoulders, and arms or proximal motor symptoms such as difficulty rising from a chair, climbing steps, or reaching overhead as presenting symptoms may suggest an inflammatory demyelinating polyneuropathy.[9]

Past Medical and Surgical Histories

Review of the past medical and surgical histories of a patient with neuropathy should focus on four key areas. First, the examiner should ask the patient to relate all current and past medical issues, including dates of diagnosis. From this list, the examiner identifies any diagnoses that may directly or secondarily result in a complication of peripheral neuropathy. The date of diagnosis of the disease does not always equate with the onset of the disease, but the date of diagnosis provides the examiner with a reference especially when searching for time-related neuropathies. Examples include diabetes mellitus, cancer, and peripheral vascular disease; less obvious examples are malabsorption syndromes and inflammatory bowel disease such as Crohn's disease and irritable bowel syndrome, which may lead to vitamin deficiencies and resultant peripheral neuropathy.

Second, the examiner should ask the patient to list all surgeries and dates of surgeries. The examiner is searching for surgeries that may directly or indirectly relate to peripheral neuropathies, such as carpal tunnel syndrome, back fusion or laminectomy, brachial plexus neurolysis, and vascular bypass. Gastric bypass surgeries have been linked with essential vitamin deficiencies leading to peripheral neuropathy.

Third, the examiner should ask the patient for a list of current and recently prescribed and over-the-counter medications or herbals including dosages. Because this list often requires a bit of work by the patient, the office scheduler can ask the patient to prepare this list before the office visit and examination. Many medications have a dose-related complication of peripheral neuropathy. The examiner also can ask the patient about recreational drug usage during the discussion of medications. Nitrous oxide and cocaine have been linked to peripheral neuropathy.[10-18]

Finally, after obtaining the medical, surgical, and medication histories, the examiner should "triangulate" these data to see if any data point was inadvertently excluded. For instance, if the patient is taking an antiplatelet medication and there is nothing in the medical or surgical history that explains this medication, further questioning is indicated (Table 14-1).[19-38]

Social and Occupational Histories

The examiner takes a social history to identify potential barriers to a successful intervention and to identify hobbies, occupations, habits, and behaviors that may have induced the peripheral neuropathy. Table 14-2 outlines hobbies and occupations that may involve sustained exposure to neurotoxic chemical compounds that may result in signs and symptoms of peripheral neuropathy.[39-54] For example, neurotoxic hexacarbons are found in the paint and solvents used by automobile painters. Similar hexacarbons are found in furniture stains and paint removers used by furniture makers and refinishers. Welders may exhibit high levels of central and peripheral neurotoxic lead. Habits and behaviors

Table 14-1 Medications That May Result in Peripheral Neuropathy

Procainamide	Almitrine	Gold salts
Phenytoin	Isoniazid	Suramin
Cisplatin	Chloroquine	Misonidazole
Pyridoxine excess	Nitrous oxide	Amiodarone
Colchicine	Vinca alkaloids	Thalidomide
Dapsone	Paclitaxel	Metronidazole
Didanosine	Nitrofurantoin	Perhexiline
Disulfiram	Zalcitabine	Stavudine
Doxorubicin	Tacrolimus	Sildenafil
Ethambutol		

Data compiled from Ziconotide: new drug. Limited analgesic efficacy, too many adverse effects. *Prescrire Int.* 2008;17(97):179–182; Biondi DM. Is migraine a neuropathic pain syndrome? *Curr Pain Headache Rep.* 2006;10(3):167–178; Brouwers EE, Huitema AD, Boogerd W, Beijnen JH, Schellens JH. Persistent neuropathy after treatment with cisplatin and oxaliplatin. *Acta Oncol.* 2009;48(6):832–841; Castro M. Peripheral sensory neuropathy—fighting cold with cold. *Lancet Oncol.* 2008;9(5):415–416; Dees EC, O'Neil BH, Lindley CM, et al. A phase I and pharmacologic study of the combination of bortezomib and pegylated liposomal doxorubicin in patients with refractory solid tumors. *Cancer Chemother Pharmacol.* 2008;63(1):99–107; Doherty SD, Hsu S. A case series of 48 patients treated with thalidomide. *J Drugs Dermatol.* 2008;7(8):769–773; Eksioglu E, Oztekin F, Unlu E, Cakci A, Keyik B, Karadavut IK. Sacroiliitis and polyneuropathy during isotretinoin treatment. *Clin Exp Dermatol.* 2008;33(2):122–124; Gdynia HJ, Muller T, Sperfeld AD, et al. Severe sensorimotor neuropathy after intake of highest dosages of vitamin B6. *Neuromuscul Disord.* 2008;18(2):156–158; Hoque R, Chesson AL Jr. Pharmacologically induced/exacerbated restless legs syndrome, periodic limb movements of sleep, and REM behavior disorder/REM sleep without atonia: literature review, qualitative scoring, and comparative analysis. *J Clin Sleep Med.* 2010;6(1):79–83; Kautio AL, Haanpaa M, Leminen A, Kalso E, Kautiainen H, Saarto T. Amitriptyline in the prevention of chemotherapy-induced neuropathic symptoms. *Anticancer Res.* 2009;29(7):2601–2606; Koh C, Kwong KL, Wong SN. Mercury poisoning: a rare but treatable cause of failure to thrive and developmental regression in an infant. *Hong Kong Med J.* 2009;15(1):61–64; Kumarasamy N, Venkatesh KK, Cecelia AJ, et al. Spectrum of adverse events after generic HAART in southern Indian HIV-infected patients. *AIDS Patient Care STDS.* 2008;22(4):337–344; Moore A, Pinkerton R. Vincristine: can its therapeutic index be enhanced? *Pediatr Blood Cancer.* 2009;53(7):1180–1187; Nakamura Y, Tajima K, Kawagoe I, Kanai M, Mitsuhata H. Efficacy of traditional herbal medicine, Yokukansan on patients with neuropathic pain. *Masui.* 2009;58(10):1248–1255; O'Connor TL, Kossoff E. Delayed seizure associated with paclitaxel-Cremophor el in a patient with early-stage breast cancer. *Pharmacotherapy.* 2009;29(8):993–996; Pierce DA, Holt SR, Reeves-Daniel A. A probable case of gabapentin-related reversible hearing loss in a patient with acute renal failure. *Clin Ther.* 2008;30(9):1681–1684; Qi X, Chu Z, Mahller YY, Stringer KF, Witte DP, Cripe TP. Cancer-selective targeting and cytotoxicity by liposomal-coupled lysosomal saposin C protein. *Clin Cancer Res.* 2009;15(18):5840–5851; Selvarajah D, Gandhi R, Emery CJ, Tesfaye S. Randomized placebo-controlled double-blind clinical trial of cannabis-based medicinal product (Sativex) in painful diabetic neuropathy: depression is a major confounding factor. *Diabetes Care.* 2010;33(1):128–130; Singh S, Mukherjee KK, Gill KD, Flora SJ. Lead-induced peripheral neuropathy following ayurvedic medication. *Indian J Med Sci.* 2009;63(9):408–410; and Toyooka K, Fujimura H. Iatrogenic neuropathies. *Curr Opin Neurol.* 2009;22(5):475–479.

Table 14-2 Hobbies and Occupations That May Predispose to Peripheral Neuropathy

Occupation/Hobby	Neuropathic Toxin
Oral surgeons, dentists, dental hygienists	Nitrous oxide
Cabinet makers, house painters, industrial/auto painters	Hexacarbons
Agricultural workers (farmers, harvesters, researchers)	Organophosphates
Dry cleaners, rubber workers, tire manufacturers	Trichloroethylene
Manufacturers of batteries, plastics	Lead
Welders, firearms instructors, demolition crews	Lead
Painters, roofers, plumbers, refinishers	Lead
Glassmakers, glassblowers	Lead
Copper smelters, tree sprayers, taxidermists, jewelers	Arsenic
Plastic industry workers	Acrylamide
Rayon industry workers	Carbon disulfide
Data entry clerks, typists, low-force/high-repetition activities	Compressive, inflammatory

Data compiled from Occupational Medicine Physician's Guide to Neuropathy in the Workplace Part 3: Case Presentation. *J Occup Environ Med.* 2009;51(7):861–862; Gimranova GG, Bakiirov AB, Karimova LK. Complex evaluation of work conditions and health state of oil industry workers [in Russian]. *Med Tr Prom Ekol.* 2009;(8):1–5; Goffeng LO, Heier MS, Kjuus H, Sjoholm H, Sorensen KA, Skaug V. Nerve conduction, visual evoked responses and electroretinography in tunnel workers previously exposed to acrylamide and N-methylolacrylamide containing grouting agents. *Neurotoxicol Teratol.* 2008;30(3):186–194; Huang CC. Polyneuropathy induced by n-hexane intoxication in Taiwan. *Acta Neurol Taiwan.* 2008;17(1):3–10; Krajnak K, Waugh S, Johnson C, Miller R, Kiedrowski M. Vibration disrupts vascular function in a model of metabolic syndrome. *Ind Health.* 2009;47(5):533–542; Kutlu G, Gomceli YB, Sonmez T, Inan LE. Peripheral neuropathy and visual evoked potential changes in workers exposed to n-hexane. *J Clin Neurosci.* 2009;16(10):1296–1299; Lagueny A. Drug induced neuropathies. *Rev Prat.* 2008;58(17):1910–1916; Lansdown AB. Critical observations on the neurotoxicity of silver. *Crit Rev Toxicol.* 2007;37(3):237–250; Ling SK, Cheng SC, Yen CH. Stonefish envenomation with acute carpal tunnel syndrome. *Hong Kong Med J.* 2009;15(6):471–473; Majersik JJ, Caravati EM, Steffens JD. Severe neurotoxicity associated with exposure to the solvent 1-bromopropane (n-propyl bromide). *Clin Toxicol (Phila).* 2007;45(3):270–276; Matsuoka M. Neurotoxicity of organic solvents—recent findings. *Brain Nerve.* 2007;59(6):591–596; Ohnari K, Uozumi T, Tsuji S. Occupation and carpal tunnel syndrome. *Brain Nerve.* 2007;59(11):1247–1252; Pelclova D, Urban P, Ridzon P, et al. Two-year follow-up of two patients after severe thallium intoxication. *Hum Exp Toxicol.* 2009;28(5):263–272; Puriene A, Janulyte V, Musteikyte M, Bendinskaite R. General health of dentists. Literature review. *Stomatologija.* 2007;9(1):10–20; Sauni R, Paakkonen R, Virtema P, et al. Vibration-induced white finger syndrome and carpal tunnel syndrome among Finnish metal workers. *Int Arch Occup Environ Health.* 2009;82(4):445–453; and Sethi PK, Khandelwal D. Cadmium exposure: health hazards of silver cottage industry in developing countries. *J Med Toxicol.* 2006;2(1):14–15.

may lead to risk of peripheral neuropathy. Smoking often leads to neoplasms of the face, neck, jaw, and lung possibly resulting in paraneoplastic peripheral neuropathy. Excessive alcohol ingestion is linked to nutritional and vitamin deficiencies, which are linked to peripheral neuropathy. Cocaine use may lead to vasculitic neuropathy secondary to hypertension (Table 14-3).[39–54]

Table 14-3 Habits and Behaviors That May Predispose to Peripheral Neuropathy

Habit/Behavior	Neuropathic Toxin
Paint eating	Lead
Tobacco ingestion (cigarette, cigar, pipe, snuff, chew)	Carcinogen
Excess alcohol	Vitamin deficiency
Sexual preference	HIV
Medications and vitamin B_6	Toxic
Intravenous drug use	HIV
Cocaine use	Hypertension
Nitrous oxide use	Cobalamin deficiency
Vegan diet	Cobalamin deficiency
Excessive keyboarding and video games	Compressive and inflammatory

Data compiled from Occupational Medicine Physician's Guide to Neuropathy in the Workplace Part 3: Case Presentation. *J Occup Environ Med.* 2009;51(7):861–862; Gimranova GG, Bakiirov AB, Karimova LK. Complex evaluation of work conditions and health state of oil industry workers [in Russian]. *Med Tr Prom Ekol.* 2009;(8): 1–5; Goffeng LO, Heier MS, Kjuus H, Sjoholm H, Sorensen KA, Skaug V. Nerve conduction, visual evoked responses and electroretinography in tunnel workers previously exposed to acrylamide and N-methylolacrylamide containing grouting agents. *Neurotoxicol Teratol.* 2008;30(3):186–194; Huang CC. Polyneuropathy induced by n-hexane intoxication in Taiwan. *Acta Neurol Taiwan.* 2008;17(1):3–10; Krajnak K, Waugh S, Johnson C, Miller R, Kiedrowski M. Vibration disrupts vascular function in a model of metabolic syndrome. *Ind Health.* 2009;47(5):533–542; Kutlu G, Gomceli YB, Sonmez T, Inan LE. Peripheral neuropathy and visual evoked potential changes in workers exposed to n-hexane. *J Clin Neurosci.* 2009;16(10):1296–1299; Lagueny A. Drug induced neuropathies. *Rev Prat.* 2008;58(17):1910–1916; Lansdown AB. Critical observations on the neurotoxicity of silver. *Crit Rev Toxicol.* 2007;37(3):237–250; Ling SK, Cheng SC, Yen CH. Stonefish envenomation with acute carpal tunnel syndrome. *Hong Kong Med J.* 2009;15(6):471–473; Majersik JJ, Caravati EM, Steffens JD. Severe neurotoxicity associated with exposure to the solvent 1-bromopropane (n-propyl bromide). *Clin Toxicol (Phila).* 2007;45(3):270–276; Matsuoka M. Neurotoxicity of organic solvents—recent findings. *Brain Nerve.* 2007;59(6):591–596; Ohnari K, Uozumi T, Tsuji S. Occupation and carpal tunnel syndrome. *Brain Nerve.* 2007;59(11):1247–1252; Pelclova D, Urban P, Ridzon P, et al. Two-year follow-up of two patients after severe thallium intoxication. *Hum Exp Toxicol.* 2009;28(5):263–272; Puriene A, Janulyte V, Musteikyte M, Bendinskaite R. General health of dentists. Literature review. *Stomatologija.* 2007;9(1):10–20; Sauni R, Paakkonen R, Virtema P, et al. Vibration-induced white finger syndrome and carpal tunnel syndrome among Finnish metal workers. *Int Arch Occup Environ Health.* 2009;82(4):445–453; and Sethi PK, Khandelwal D. Cadmium exposure: health hazards of silver cottage industry in developing countries. *J Med Toxicol.* 2006;2(1):14–15.

Review of Systems

The review of systems is typically performed as a question-and-answer session directed by the examiner. Unless asked, the patient may not connect minor symptoms from distant or seemingly unrelated sites to the neuropathic complaint. In addition, some patients may be unwilling to offer information about potentially embarrassing symptoms related to reproductive, genitourinary, or gastrointestinal systems unless asked. Table 14-4 lists examples of probing system health inquiries. Affirmative answers should be explored further to obtain additional data. The review of systems is important as an adjunct tool to evaluate the possible etiology of the peripheral neuropathy (Table 14-5).[55–67]

Physical Examination

Information garnered from the chief complaint, history of the present illness, past medical and surgical histories, medications, social and occupational histories, and

Table 14-4 Examples of Health Systems Probing Questions

System	Question
Cardiac	Do you have chest pain? Do you have difficulty walking up steps? Do you become short of breath when you lie down?
Cancer	Have you ever been diagnosed or treated for cancer? Do you have any unusual lumps or moles?
Endocrine	Are you often unexpectedly tired? Do you have excessive thirst? Do you feel more tired than usual?
Gastrointestinal	How is your appetite? Do you ever notice bloody stools? Does your belly hurt? Do you have regular bowel movements?
Genitourinary	Do you urinate excessively? Are you incontinent? Are there any sexual concerns?
Integument	Do you have any skin wounds that are not healing? Do you have any rashes?
Musculoskeletal	Do you have joint or muscle pain? Do you feel stiff? Do you feel weak? Have you fallen recently?
Pulmonary	Do you have breathing issues? Do you get short of breath with minimal activity? Do you wheeze when you breathe?
Sensory	Have you noticed any recent visual or hearing changes? Do you have any numb areas on your body?

Table 14-5	Neuropathies Associated With System Impairment
System	Neuropathy (or Possible Neuropathic-like Symptoms)
Cardiac	Mitral valve prolapse, arrhythmia, coronary artery disease
Endocrine	Diabetic, hypothyroid
Gastrointestinal	Amyloid, chronic inflammatory demyelinating polyneuropathy
Genitourinary	Amyloid
Integument	Diabetic
Musculoskeletal	Compressive, tensile, connective tissue disease, traumatic
Neurological	Compressive, tensile, neoplastic, repetitive strain
Pulmonary	Sarcoid, paraneoplastic
Sensory	Inherited neuropathies, amyloid, chemotoxic, Refsum disease, Fabry disease

Data from Aboussouan LS, Lewis RA, Shy ME. Disorders of pulmonary function, sleep, and the upper airway in Charcot-Marie-Tooth disease. *Lung.* 2007;185(1):1–7; Coste TC, Gerbi A, Vague P, Maixent JM, Pieroni G, Raccah D. Peripheral diabetic neuropathy and polyunsaturated fatty acid supplementations: natural sources or biotechnological needs? *Cell Mol Biol (Noisy-le-grand).* 2004;50(7):845–853; Di Nardo G, Blandizzi C, Volta U, et al. Review article: molecular, pathological and therapeutic features of human enteric neuropathies. *Aliment Pharmacol Ther.* 2008;28(1):25–42; Freeman R. Autonomic peripheral neuropathy. *Neurol Clin.* 2007;25(1):277–301; Lacigova S, Bartunek L, Cechurova D, et al. Influence of cardiovascular autonomic neuropathy on atherogenesis and heart function in patients with type 1 diabetes. *Diabetes Res Clin Pract.* 2009;83(1):26–31; Manzella D, Paolisso G. Cardiac autonomic activity and Type II diabetes mellitus. *Clin Sci (Lond).* 2005;108(2):93–99; Maule S, Papotti G, Naso D, Magnino C, Testa E, Veglio F. Orthostatic hypotension: evaluation *Cardiovasc Hematol Disord Drug Targets.* 2007;7(1):63–70; Mehta A, Ricci R, Widmer U, et al. Fabry disease defined: baseline clinical manifestations of 366 patients in the Fabry Outcome Survey. *Eur J Clin Invest.* 2004;34(3):236–242; Oka N, Sugiyama H, Kawasaki T, Mizutani K, Matsui M. Falls in peripheral neuropathy [in Japanese]. *Rinsho Shinkeigaku.* 2005;45(3):207–210; Sacco IC, Bacarin TA, Canettieri MG, Hennig EM. Plantar pressures during shod gait in diabetic neuropathic patients with and without a history of plantar ulceration. *J Am Podiatr Med Assoc.* 2009;99(4):285–294; Said G. Familial amyloid polyneuropathy: mechanisms leading to nerve degeneration. *Amyloid.* 2003;10(Suppl 1):7–12; Vial C, Bouhour F. Vasculitis multiple mononeuropathies [in French]. *Rev Prat.* 2008;58(17):1896–1899; and Yeung H, Krentz HB, Gill MJ, Power C. Neuropsychiatric disorders in HIV infection: impact of diagnosis on economic costs of care. *AIDS.* 2006;20(16):2005–2009.

review of systems influences the examiner's algorithm of the planned physical examination for peripheral nerve injury. The physical examination can help confirm a suspected diagnosis garnered from the interview, or the physical examination may prompt additional interview questions.

Vital Signs

Standard vital signs should be taken with all new patients, not only patients with suspected peripheral neuropathy. Heart rate, respiration rate, blood pressure, and oxygen saturation provide a momentary perspective into the patient's general health and act as a screening tool for potential issues not yet discovered by the primary care physician. A finger-stick blood sugar test should also be added to the list of vital signs. Although limited in scope, reliability, and validity in diagnosing an impairment, the finger-stick blood sugar can act as a screening tool for potential hyperglycemic impairments as well as provide feedback to patients who have a diagnosis of diabetes regarding their blood control. Lastly, visual analog scales (or happy/sad face or Oucher scales for children) have proved reliable in assessing pain.[68–70] The visual analog scale can be expanded to include anterior and posterior corporal figures on which the patient can mark the location and type of pain symptoms.

Postural Examination and Corporal Presentation

Peripheral neuropathy, with possible impact on the efferent and afferent systems, may stress the joints and muscles and induce sufficient pain to alter posture. In addition, postural changes resulting from habit, trauma, degeneration, or illness may secondarily affect the peripheral nervous system leading to sensory, motor, and autonomic signs and symptoms. Maintenance of correct posture requires motor and somatosensory systems that are strong, flexible, and easily adaptable to environmental change.

Postural **assessment** begins informally with first patient contact and expands as an integral and definitive part of the physical examination. To assess posture accurately, the patient should be adequately undressed and should not wear shoes or socks. Adaptive equipment such as orthoses and assistive equipment such as walkers, canes, or crutches should be noted. Standing and sitting posture should be assessed in the normal or relaxed state, which is often difficult for the patient to assume when being watched. A plumb line or plastic postural assessment screen often aids the postural examination (Figs. 14-1 and 14-2).

Postural assessment begins with a visual screening of symmetry. In the anteroposterior view, is the head straight on the shoulders? Is the jaw in midline? Is the neck line, as defined by the upper trapezius line, symmetrical on both sides? Are both acromion processes elevated equally? Are the waist angles equal, and are the arms hung equidistant from the hips? Are the carrying angles of the elbows equal? Is the internal/external rotation of the shoulders equal as represented by palm position? Is the spine straight with normal cervical, thoracic, and lumbosacral curves? Is there a scoliosis? Are the anterior superior iliac spines equal in elevation? Are the patellae of the knees pointing straight ahead? Are the knees straight? Is there genu valgus or varus? Are the arches present in both feet,

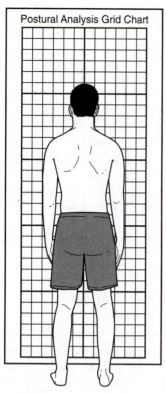

Figure 14-1 Postural assessment using a postural screen: posterior view. Postural screen validity is enhanced thorugh the use of static postural graphical screens or through the use of two-dimensional videography.

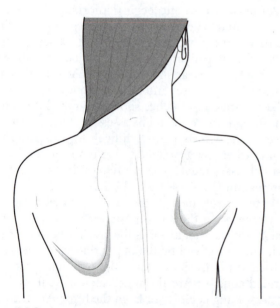

Figure 14-2 Asymmetrical position of scapulae as seen with intrinsic scapular muscle weakness. Visual screening is a necessary component of the physical examination. Overt postural abnormalities may result in only small changes in articular range of motion and muscle strength.

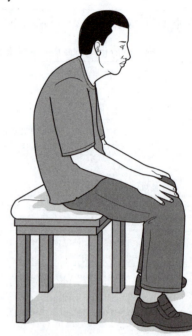

Figure 14-3 Habitual slouched chair posture may result in axial and articular dysfunction, which often progresses to nerve impingement syndromes. Long-standing postural abnormalities in sitting, standing, or supine/prone may result in chronic soft tissue changes leading to nerve injury related to aberrant compressive or tensile forces.

and do they appear equal? Are all muscle groups symmetrical in size and location? In the mediolateral view, note the position of the head. Is it forward on the trunk as measured through an imaginary line passing from the earlobe to the anterior portion of the acromion process? Are the scapulae protracted? Is the sternal angle depressed or exaggerated? Are the thoracic kyphosis and lumbar lordosis normal, exaggerated, or depressed? Do the knees exhibit recurvatum?

Posture in the sitting position should also be assessed anteroposteriorly and mediolaterally. Structural anatomy impairments noted in standing should also be noted in sitting. In addition, poor sitting posture as directed by habit or impairment, such as a flattened lumbar lordosis, exaggerated thoracic curve, flattened cervical lordosis, forward head, and protracted scapulae, may lead to axial and articular dysfunction resulting in nerve impingement (Figs. 14-3 and 14-4).

Integument Examination

Examination of the integument typically follows the postural assessment. The entire body should be scanned as well as the oral mucosa. Skin ulcerations—chronic, acute, or healing—may be associated with diabetic neuropathy or vasculopathy.[71] These ulcerations are typically neural and vascular–length dependent and are often found on the legs, ankles, feet, and hands. However, poorly healing traumatic injures may be

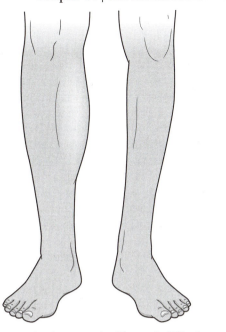

Figure 14-4 Muscle wasting of calf muscle. Wasting noted in the gastrocsoleus complex.

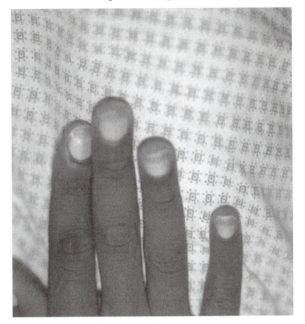

Figure 14-5 Mees lines are typical of arsenic or thallium intoxication. *From Goldsmith, Adult and Pediatric Dermatology, F.A. Davis, Philadelphia, 1997, page 535.*

found anywhere on the body, especially over areas that are often injured during daily life such as the shins, elbows, and hips. Cellulitis is associated with diabetic vasculopathy[71] and can be found anywhere on the body. The cellulitis may be primary—directly related to trauma—or secondary—that is, "seeded" from a distant skin opening or infected site. Purpura and livedo reticularis are often associated with vasculitides.[72,73] Alopecia may be a sign of hypothyroidism, systemic lupus erythematosis, or thallium intoxication.[74–76] Mees lines are associated with arsenic or thallium intoxication.[77–82] Clubbing of the fingertips is associated with inflammatory lung disease, lung cancer, liver disease, and inflammatory bowel disease.[83–86] White nails may be associated with POEMS (polyneuropathy, organomegaly, endocrinopathy, monoclonal gammopathy, and skin changes) (Figs. 14-5).[87–90]

Integument examination continues with pulse assessment. Upper extremity pulses—radial and brachial—and lower extremity pulses—femoral, popliteal, dorsalis pedis, and posterior—should be assessed and graded. Diminished pulse may indicate vascular impingement as seen with arterial thoracic outlet syndrome or peripheral vascular disease.

Peripheral edema has many etiologies, but a few may have an impact on the diagnosis of peripheral neuropathy. Venous thoracic outlet syndrome results in acute or chronic subclavian vein obstruction by a neighboring structure and may result in brachial plexus compression. Lower extremity edema may be caused by a lower abdominal space-occupying lesion that may also affect the lumbosacral plexus. Edema in a pregnant woman may be related to positional dependency or

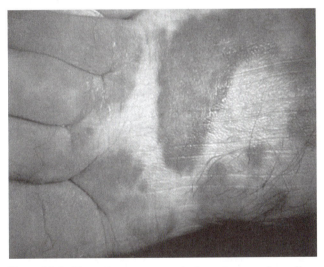

Figure 14-6 Kaposi's sarcoma, oral ulcerations, and needle tracks are integument signs of potential HIV infection. *From Goldsmith, Adult and Pediatric Dermatology, F.A. Davis, Philadelphia, 1997, page 414.*

may be secondary to eclampsia or preeclampsia. The edema may be of sufficient magnitude to have a structural impact on a neighboring peripheral nerve.[91,92]

Edematous articular joints may indicate infection, joint effusion, trauma, or neuropathic joints. Painful axial joints may indicate discitis, disc herniation, spinal stenosis, or compression fracture; all of these etiologies are capable of resulting in radicular peripheral nerve symptoms.

The presence of needle tracks on the arms or legs, oral ulcerations, and Kaposi's sarcoma may indicate HIV infection/AIDS (Fig. 14-6).

Salivary gland swelling may indicate Sjögren syndrome.[93,94] Lymphadenopathy may indicate an acute or subacute viral or bacterial infection.

Musculoskeletal Examination

The musculoskeletal system consists of bones, joints, fascias, ligaments, tendons, and entheses. Documenting muscle strength, articular range of motion (ROM), axial ROM, and two-joint muscle lengths is intrinsic to all examinations. Valid measurements of the musculoskeletal system provide an initial baseline data source to serve three purposes: to help with diagnosis and prognosis, to determine improvement or deterioration of function in follow-up assessments, and to assess the efficacy of intervention.

Manual muscle testing (MMT) has been validated, primarily with larger muscles, in many clinical studies.[95–98] To facilitate interrater reliability, the examiner should use a standard method of examination and standardized semantics of grading. Standardization must include patient position, locus of resistance, and locus of stabilization. Examiners should develop a pattern of MMT that includes at least one muscle from each central and peripheral myotome. A form-based assessment is recommended to prompt the examiner as to which muscle to assess. When the MMT is complete, the examiner may look at the data to determine if the pattern of weakness is unilateral, upper extremity versus lower extremity, central myotome dependent, peripheral myotome dependent, or asymmetrical. Intrinsic hand muscles and gross grasp are best assessed via pinch and grasp dynamometers (Fig. 14-7).

Axial and articular active range of motion (AROM) and passive range of motion (PROM) are best assessed via cardinal plane measurements with a goniometer. AROM should be performed first and followed with PROM measurements if the AROM deviates from what is expected. With limitations in PROM, the examiner should note the end-feel of the blockage. End-feel may be bony, as with normal full extension of the elbow joint; capsular, as with attempts at hyperextension of the metacarpophalangeal joints; springy, as with blockage by a piece of fractured articular cartilage or loose body; spongy, as with limitations via joint effusion; empty, as limited by the patient's unwillingness to allow the joint to be moved further because of pain or fear; spasm secondary to muscle contraction or tone; and neural, as exemplified by the sensation felt by the patient of a neural tethering. In addition to limited movement patterns found with cardinal plane goniometry, the examiner should look for evidence of joint hypomobility and hypermobility by examining the structure of the joint capsule and associated collateral and extra-articular and interarticular ligaments. Joint hypermobility secondary to traumatic lesions, such as lesions often seen in the medial collateral ligament of overhead baseball pitchers, may also result in compression or tensile neuropathies of local peripheral nerves (the ulnar nerve in the case of baseball pitchers). Limitations in articular or axial ROM may result from peripheral neuropathy secondary to articular manifestations of neural tethering, space-occupying lesions, inflammation, or poorly healed or aligned fracture.

Two-joint muscles, muscles whose proximal and distal attachments cross two joints, should also be examined for length. The biceps brachii and the triceps brachii in the upper extremity and the rectus femoris, hamstring group, and gastrocnemius in the lower extremity may exhibit passive insufficiency with attempts to stretch the muscle across two joints. The passive insufficiency may be sufficient to restrict functional articular motion and result in tensile stresses to peripheral nerves at the terminus of range of motion.

Neurological Examination

The comprehensive neurological examination provides the examiner with direct evidence of motor, sensory, and autonomic involvement secondary to nerve injury. The examiner uses the data provided by the neurological examination to determine if the symptoms are upper motor neuron, lower motor neuron, or mixed; to define the extent of the impairment; to collect final data before the functional examination; and to aid in diagnosis and prognosis. As with muscle strength testing, an algorithm-based and evidence-driven examination greatly adds to the reliability of the neurological examination.

Sensory System Examination

The sensory system examination is the most difficult portion of the neurological examination not only because of the inherent reliability and validity issues but also because it is driven by the patient's perception, understanding, and cooperation. In addition, the

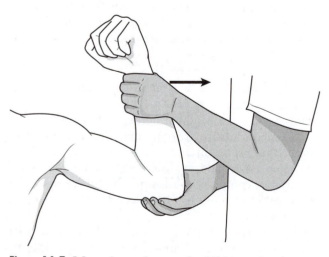

Figure 14-7 Manual muscle test of a 5/5 biceps brachii.

presence of a peripheral or central neuropathy may lead to a confused perception and localization of sensory symptoms on the part of the patient. Regardless of these barriers, a meticulously performed sensory system examination may provide enormous benefits with determination of diagnosis, prognosis, and extent of the illness.

At a minimum, the sensory system examination should include an assessment of the following modalities: light touch, sharp, vibration, and proprioception. Additional modalities that may be assessed include temperature and deep pressure. Light touch may be assessed with a wisp of cotton; sharp, with a safety pin; vibration, with a tuning fork; hot and cold, with test tubes filled with hot and cold water, respectively; and deep pressure, with a finger.

The examination should be performed with the patient first in the supine position and then in the prone position. Tested areas must be exposed. Confounding sensory data such as draping sheets, air blowing from fans, and ambient music should be controlled. The examiner needs to provide the patient with adequate instruction about the testing method before beginning the examination. A corporal representation form often helps the examiner document the results of the testing.

Large-fiber sensory testing is often the most difficult to perform. The use of a tuning fork for vibratory sense is straightforward. A representative "education" of the patient as to what sensation is elicited by the tuning fork—typically performed on the chin, mandible, or acromion—is followed by the testing. A symmetrical touching of bony prominences is performed beginning in the feet and working proximally, constantly querying the patient as to whether the intensity is equal symmetrically and if the intensity is equal to the "normative" intensity at the location. The testing pattern typically begins at the fifth metatarsal head on the right, fifth metatarsal head on the left, first metatarsophalangeal joint on the right, first metatarsophalangeal joint on the left, navicular on the right, and so on. Following the testing over two bony prominences, the tuning fork needs to be re-excited. Proprioception, the sense of the position of parts of the body relative to other neighboring parts of the body, is a more difficult modality to assess reliably than the tactile sensory modalities. Examiners use a variety of testing methods—all with relevancy but all with confounding and uncontrolled variables and with less than hoped for reliability. Some examiners passively position one extremity and ask the patient, with eyes closed, to mimic the position with the contralateral extremity. This method requires the patient to have greater than 3/5 motor strength and normal tone in all muscles in the contralateral extremity. The Romberg and Sharpened Romberg for the trunk and lower extremities and the pronator drift for the trunk and upper extremities

are nonspecific screening tests that, if positive, may indicate impairment in the sensorimotor, visual, or vestibular systems.[98–105]

Postural tone, if abnormal, may be indicative of upper motor neuron, lower motor neuron, basal ganglia, extrapyramidal, or medication-induced impairments. Spasticity, characterized by hyperactive deep tendon reflexes, obligatory posturing, a patterned response to hypertonicity, associated reactions, and a clasp-knife response to quick stretch by the examiner, is associated with upper motor neuron lesions—lesions occurring above the level of the anterior horn cell. Hypotonus, as related to nerve injury, is characterized by diminished or absent deep tendon reflexes, "floppy" extremities, and an empty response to quick stretch by the examiner and is associated with lower motor neuron lesions—lesions below and at the level of the anterior horn cell. Rigidity—characterized by increased tone in a nonpatterned distribution in the limbs, trunk, and face; a cogwheeling response to quick stretch by the examiner; bradykinesia; and festination—is associated with basal ganglia and extrapyramidal impairments. Rigidity may also be traumatic or medication-induced.

With movement of the extremities and the axial skeleton, the nervous system slides and glides relative to surrounding structures and is subject to stretch. A healthy nervous system can tolerate this loading, whereas low levels of stretch in nerves with epineural or perineural scarring secondary to chronic inflammation or nerves compressed by local structures are sufficient to generate ectopic impulses from an inflamed nerve. The ectopic impulses typically travel distally in the radicular distribution.[106,107] This increased mechanosensitivity is the key characteristic that is evaluated in many clinical provocation tests, such as Spurling's test for cervical radiculopathy, Tinel's sign, and the straight leg–raising test for lumbar radiculopathy.

The straight leg–raising test[108–110] and the femoral nerve test[109] in the lower extremity and the various upper limb neural tension tests[111–116] were designed to evaluate the mechanosensitivity of the sciatic nerve, femoral nerve, brachial plexus, median nerve, radial nerve, and ulnar nerve. A neurodynamic test is considered positive if symptoms can be reproduced and if symptoms can be altered by structural differentiation.[111,112] Structural differentiation uses static and active movement at a site remote to the entrapment area to load further or unload the nervous system.[112–115] An example is the addition of contralateral cervical lateral bend away from horizontal adduction of the arm; this tests the median nerve. The reliability of upper and lower limb neurodynamic testing has been explored widely. Most of these studies investigated whether symptom reproduction occurred at a consistent point through ROM. The overall view is that ROM measurement at the point of symptom reproduction is reliable (Table 14-6).

Table 14-6 Large-Fiber Neuropathies Resulting in Loss of Proprioceptive and Kinesthetic Function

Chemotoxic disorders	Pyrinuron Metronidazole Cisplatin Vitamin B_6 Nitrous oxide	Immune-mediated disorders	Paraneoplastic neuropathy Sensory neuropathy associated with sicca syndrome Idiopathic sensory neuropathy Diabetic neuropathy Guillain-Barré syndrome Miller-Fisher variant of Guillain-Barré syndrome Chronic inflammatory demyelinating polyneuropathy Multiple sclerosis
Infectious disorders	Tabes dorsalis Diphtheritic polyneuropathy HIV neuropathy		

Data compiled from Azhary H, Farooq MU, Bhanushali M, Majid A, Kassab MY. Peripheral neuropathy: differential diagnosis and management. *Am Fam Physician.* 2010;81(7):887–892; Schroder A, Linker RA, Gold R. Plasmapheresis for neurological disorders. *Expert Rev Neurother.* 2009; 9(9):1331–1339; Zhang Q, Gu Z, Jiang J, et al. Orthostatic hypotension as a presenting symptom of the Guillain-Barre syndrome. *Clin Auton Res.* 2010;20(3):209–210; Compston A. Primary sensory neuropathy with muscular changes associated with carcinoma. Editorial. *Brain.* 2009; 132(Pt 8):1995–1996; Isoda A, Sakurai A, Ogawa Y, et al. Chronic inflammatory demyelinating polyneuropathy accompanied by chronic myelomonocytic leukemia: possible pathogenesis of autoimmunity in myelodysplastic syndrome. *Int J Hematol.* 2009;90(2):239–242; Amlie-Lefond C, Jubelt B. Neurologic manifestations of varicella zoster virus infections. *Curr Neurol Neurosci Rep.* 2009;9(6):430–434; Lunn MP, Willison HJ. Diagnosis and treatment of inflammatory neuropathies. *J Neurol Neurosurg Psychiatry.* 2009;80(3):249–258; Isoda A, Sakurai A, Ogawa Y, et al. Chronic inflammatory demyelinating polyneuropathy accompanied by chronic myelomonocytic leukemia: possible pathogenesis of autoimmunity in myelodysplastic syndrome. *Int J Hematol.* 2009;90(2):239–242; Neiman J, Haapaniemi HM, Hillbom M. Neurological complications of drug abuse: pathophysiological mechanisms. *Eur J Neurol.* 2000;7(6):595–606; O'Connor G, McMahon G. Complications of heroin abuse. *Eur J Emerg Med.* 2008;15(2):104–106; O'Sullivan JM, McMahon G. Descending polyneuropathy in an intravenous drug user. *Eur J Emerg Med.* 2005;12(5):248–250; Ziconotide: new drug. Limited analgesic efficacy, too many adverse effects. *Prescrire Int.* 2008;17(97):179–182; Biondi DM. Is migraine a neuropathic pain syndrome? *Curr Pain Headache Rep.* 2006;10(3):167–178; Brouwers EE, Huitema AD, Boogerd W, Beijnen JH, Schellens JH. Persistent neuropathy after treatment with cisplatin and oxaliplatin. *Acta Oncol.* 2009;48(6):832–841; Castro M. Peripheral sensory neuropathy—fighting cold with cold. *Lancet Oncol.* 2008;9(5):415–416; Dees EC, O'Neil BH, Lindley CM, et al. A phase I and pharmacologic study of the combination of bortezomib and pegylated liposomal doxorubicin in patients with refractory solid tumors. *Cancer Chemother Pharmacol.* 2008;63(1):99–107; Doherty SD, Hsu S. A case series of 48 patients treated with thalidomide. *J Drugs Dermatol.* 2008; 7(8):769–773; Huang CC. Polyneuropathy induced by n-hexane intoxication in Taiwan. *Acta Neurol Taiwan.* 2008;17(1):3–10; Coste TC, Gerbi A, Vague P, Maixent JM, Pieroni G, Raccah D. Peripheral diabetic neuropathy and polyunsaturated fatty acid supplementations: natural sources or biotechnological needs? *Cell Mol Biol (Noisy-le-grand).* 2004;50(7):845–853; Di Nardo G, Blandizzi C, Volta U, et al. Molecular, pathological and therapeutic features of human enteric neuropathies. *Aliment Pharmacol Ther.* 2008;28(1):25–42; Freeman R. Autonomic peripheral neuropathy. *Neurol Clin.* 2007;25(1):277–301; Lacigova S, Bartunek L, Cechurova D, et al. Influence of cardiovascular autonomic neuropathy on atherogenesis and heart function in patients with type 1 diabetes. *Diabetes Res Clin Pract.* 2009;83(1):26–31; Manzella D, Paolisso G. Cardiac autonomic activity and Type II diabetes mellitus. *Clin Sci (Lond).* 2005;108(2):93–99; Cheer K, Shearman C, Jude EB. Managing complications of the diabetic foot. *BMJ.* 2009;339:b4905; Brown PJ, Zirwas MJ, English JC 3rd. The purple digit: an algorithmic approach to diagnosis. *Am J Clin Dermatol.* 2010;11(2):103–116; Kluger N, Frances C. Cutaneous vasculitis and their differential diagnoses. *Clin Exp Rheumatol.* 2009;27(1 Suppl 52): S124–138; and Cohen PR. Primary alopecia neoplastica versus secondary alopecia neoplastica: a new classification for neoplasm-associated scalp hair loss. *J Cutan Pathol.* 2009;36(8):917–918.

Because the sensory symptoms of various disease processes vary in their location, reliable sensory mapping is extremely useful in assisting with the diagnosis. Cobalamin deficiency often manifests as sensory disturbances in the upper extremity.[117] Guillain-Barré syndrome[1,2] and chronic inflammatory demyelinating polyneuropathy[118,119] also often begin in the hands. Unilateral upper extremity involvement may be due to an isolated mononeuropathy, such as ulnar neuropathy at the elbow, or a more complicated brachial plexus neuropathy.

Examiners should not omit the trunk when performing a sensory examination. Length-dependent neuropathies such as seen with diabetes often result in sensory symptoms not only in the typical stocking-glove distribution but also along the anterior truncal wall 2 to 4 cm bilateral of midline.[120] The distal intercostals and abdominal sensory nerves may also be affected by length-dependent neuropathies.[119,120]

Radicular diseases such as thoracic intervertebral stenosis, thoracic compression fractures, and thoracic disc herniations may result in sensory symptoms along the trunk wall.[119]

Assessment of the autonomic nervous system is difficult to perform in the office, in the clinic, or at the bedside. A hallmark sign of autonomic dysfunction is orthostatic hypotension.[121] Orthostatic hypotension is defined as a systolic blood pressure 20 mm Hg or greater or a diastolic blood pressure 10 mm Hg or greater with standing after maintaining supine position at least 5 miniutes.[121,122] In patients with emerging autonomic dysfunction, cardiovagal function may be sufficiently intact to provide a chronotropic response to heart rate to maintain cardiac output. With long-standing autonomic disease, this response fails to materialize, and diminished consciousness and potential for fall result.[121–123] Tests involving greater risk to the patient or tests requiring additional equipment,

Box 14-1

Neuropathies Associated With Autonomic Dysfunction or Disease

Drug-induced neuropathies: paclitaxel, amiodarone, cisplatin, vincristine

Alcohol neuropathy

Miller-Fisher variation of Guillain-Barré syndrome

Guillain-Barré syndrome

Paraneoplastic autonomic neuropathy

Familial amyloid polyneuropathies

Porphyria

Chemotoxic neuropathies: thallium, arsenic, mercury, organic solvents, hexacarbons

Diabetic polyneuropathy

Data compiled from Azhary H, Farooq MU, Bhanushali M, Majid A, Kassab MY. Peripheral neuropathy: differential diagnosis and management. *Am Fam Physician.* 2010;81(7):887–892; Schroder A, Linker RA, Gold R. Plasmapheresis for neurological disorders. *Expert Rev Neurother.* 2009;9(9):1331–1339; Compston A. Primary sensory neuropathy with muscular changes associated with carcinoma. Editorial. *Brain.* 2009;132(Pt 8):1995–1996; Layzer R, Wolf J. Myeloma-associated polyneuropathy responding to lenalidomide. *Neurology.* 2009;73(10):812–813; Lunn MP, Willison HJ. Diagnosis and treatment of inflammatory neuropathies. *J Neurol Neurosurg Psychiatry.* 2009;80(3):249–258; Tatum WO, Bui DD, Grant EG, Murtagh R. Pseudo-Guillain-Barre syndrome due to "whippet"-induced myeloneuropathy. *J Neuroimaging.* 2010;20(4):400–401; Dees EC, O'Neil BH, Lindley CM, et al. A phase I and pharmacologic study of the combination of bortezomib and pegylated liposomal doxorubicin in patients with refractory solid tumors. *Cancer Chemother Pharmacol.* 2008;63(1):99–107; Doherty SD, Hsu S. A case series of 48 patients treated with thalidomide. *J Drugs Dermatol.* 2008;7(8):769–773; Eksioglu E, Oztekin F, Unlu E, Cakci A, Keyik B, Karadavut IK. Sacroiliitis and polyneuropathy during isotretinoin treatment. *Clin Exp Dermatol.* 2008;33(2):122–124; Cheer K, Shearman C, Jude EB. Managing complications of the diabetic foot. *BMJ.* 2009;339:b4905; Brown PJ, Zirwas MJ, English JC 3rd. The purple digit: an algorithmic approach to diagnosis. *Am J Clin Dermatol.* 2010;11(2):103–116; Kluger N, Frances C. Cutaneous vasculitis and their differential diagnoses. *Clin Exp Rheumatol.* 2009;27(1 Suppl 52):S124–138; and Cohen PR. Primary alopecia neoplastica versus secondary alopecia neoplastica: a new classification for neoplasm-associated scalp hair loss. *J Cutan Pathol.* 2009;36(8):917–918.

such as postganglionic sudomotor tests, tilt tests, and Valsalva, are better performed in an autonomic reflex laboratory (Box 14-1).

Deep Tendon Stretch Examination

The deep tendon stretch reflex (DTR) is an excellent test to assist the examiner in determining upper motor neuron versus lower motor neuron origin of neuropathic symptoms. The examiner should score each tendon tap and compare for symmetry, asymmetry, or unilateral responses. Hyperreflexic responses to tendon tap, especially responses accompanied by a positive Babinski sign and clonus, are often indicative of an upper motor neuron lesion. Hyperreflexic response with the absence of a positive Babinski sign or clonus is rare but may be indicative of amyotrophic lateral

sclerosis.[124] Hyporeflexic responses are often associated with lower motor neuron dysfunction. Hyporeflexia may be mononeuropathic or multineuropathic. As a caveat, early DTR responses to acute upper motor neuron injury such as hemorrhagic or thrombotic stroke, traumatic brain injury, and spinal cord injury may often manifest as hyporeflexic but typically evolve to hyperreflexia.[124–126]

Babinski and Clonus Testing

The Babinski and clonus tests are used, often in conjunction with the DTR examination, to assist the examiner in determining if the symptoms are upper motor neuron or lower motor neuron. Sensitivity for the Babinski test has been reported to range from 35% to 96%, and sensitivity for the clonus test has been reported to range from 56% to 100%.[127–129]

Tinel's Sign

Tinel's sign, named for the French physician Jules Tinel (1879–1952), is often tested in conjunction with neurodynamic testing.[130,131] Tapping of an inflamed, irritated, entrapped, or reinnervating peripheral nerve may lead to radicular symptoms in the sensory distribution of the nerve tested. Tinel's sign has a fairly high sensitivity (70% to 90%) for diagnosis of carpal tunnel syndrome and ulnar neuropathy at the level of the elbow.[130–132]

Cranial Nerve Examination

Cranial nerve examination is an integral part of the examination of a patient with suspected peripheral nerve injury (Table 14-7). Anosmia, or loss of smell, is associated with the common diagnoses of diabetic and hypothyroid-induced peripheral neuropathy[1] and with the less common diagnoses of cobalamin deficiency[117] and Refsum disease.[133] Optic neuritis is often the presenting sign in chronic inflammatory demyelinating polyradiculopathy.[5,9] A large pupil that constricts poorly to light and near vision resulting in a tonic response with poor redilation are signs of tonic pupil, which is seen in conjunction with widespread or limited neuropathies such as associated with Guillain-Barré syndrome,[3,14] Sjögren syndrome,[93,94] cancer,[134] and chronic inflammatory demyelinating polyneuropathy.[5,9] Facial weakness, with or without pain, is usually associated with connective tissue diseases such as Sjögren syndrome[93] and mixed connective tissue disorder.[135–137] True facial weakness is often associated with a focal seventh nerve injury, acquired inflammatory demyelinating disease, sarcoidosis, and amyotrophic lateral sclerosis (Box 14-2).[138–144]

Balance Assessment

Postural stability in the dynamic and static state requires a complex interaction between the somatosensory system, the vestibular system, and the visual system within a framework of appropriate musculoskeletal indices and cognition. The goal of the balance

Table 14-7 Cranial Nerve Testing

Nerve	Testing
Olfactory	• Test each nostril separately by placing stimuli under one nostril and occluding the other nostril. Stimuli should be nonirritating, such as cinnamon, toothpaste, or clove.
Optic	• Visual acuity is tested in each eye separately via the Snellen eye chart and the near card. • Visual fields are assessed by asking the patient to cover one eye while the examiner tests the other. The examiner wiggles a finger in each of the four quadrants, and the patient is asked to state whether he or she sees the finger in the periphery. • Pupillary light reflex is tested as the patient stares into the distance as the examiner shines the penlight obliquely into each pupil. Pupillary constriction should be noted via the consensual and direct responses.
Oculomotor, trochlear, abducens	• Inspect for ptosis, eye position, and nystagmus. Pupil size should be measured with shape and asymmetry noted. The examiner tests ocular movements by standing 1 m in front of the patient and asking the patient to follow the target with eyes only. The target is moved in an "H" shape, and the patient is asked to report diplopia. Nystagmus should be noted. • The accommodation reflex is testing by moving the target toward the patient's nose. As the eyes converge, the pupils should constrict.
Trigeminal	• Light touch is tested in the three divisions of the trigeminal nerve on each side of the face using a cotton wisp. For pain and temperature, a pin (pain) and test tubes of hot and cold water (temperature) are used. • The corneal reflex is tested with a wisp of cotton. • Muscles of mastication (temporalis, masseter) should be inspected for atrophy and symmetry. Palpate the temporalis and masseter as the patient clenches the jaw. The pterygoids can be tested by asking the patient to open the mouth against resistance and move the jaw side outside against resistance. The jaw reflex can be tested by placing a finger over the patient's chin and tapping the finger with a reflex hammer.
Facial	• Inspect for facial asymmetry, involuntary movements, and fasciculation. The patient shuts eyes tightly; compare each side. • The patient grins; compare nasolabial grooves. • The patient frowns, shows teeth, puffs out cheeks.
Vestibulocochlear	• With one of the patient's ears covered, whisper numbers in the other ear and ask the patient to repeat the numbers. Conduct the Rinne test and Weber test. • Weber test: Lateralization. Place 512/1,024 Hz (256 if deaf) vibrating fork on top of patient's head/forehead. "Where do you hear sound coming from?" Normal reply is midline. • Rinne test: Air vs. bone conduction. Place 512/1,024 Hz (256 if deaf) vibrating fork on mastoid behind ear. Ask the patient to state when he or she stops hearing it. When the patient stops hearing it, move the vibrating fork to the patient's ear so that he or she can hear it. Normal: air conduction (ear) better than bone conduction (mastoid).
Glossopharyngeal	• Perform the gag response test to both sides of the soft palate. Assess palatal articulation "KA" and guttural articulation "GO."
Accessory	• From behind, examine the upper trapezius for symmetry. • Perform manual muscle test of the upper trapezius and sternocleidomastoid bilaterally.
Hypoglossal	• Inspect the tongue for atrophy, fasciculations, or asymmetry with protrusion.

assessment is to identify individuals who, through their impairments, are at risk for falling and require further assessment and ultimately intervention. Peripheral neuropathy may affect many of the matrices of balance: the somatosensory system, the vestibular system, the visual system, and the musculoskeletal system. A balance screen should have simple and easily understood measurement tools that reliably and validly identify fall risk for a given population. Many reliable and well-validated population-specific tools are available.[145–148]

Cognitive Examination

The most validated of the short forms of cognitive assessment is the Mini-Mental State Examination (MMSE).[149–152] The MMSE provides the examiner with data related to the cognitive ability of the patient. If the MMSE score is lower than expected, the patient should be referred for additional cognitive and psychomotor assessment. The Beck Depression Inventory is another validated test to determine the presence of depression in the patient.[153–156] The 36-Item Short

Box 14-2

Potential Etiologies of True or Apparent Facial Weakness Associated With Peripheral Neuropathy

Acoustic neuroma

Amyotrophic lateral sclerosis

Bell palsy (facial nerve palsy)

Botulism toxin injection

Chronic inflammatory demyelinating polyradiculopathy

Erb palsy

Gelsolin amyloidosis

HIV

Liposuction

Lyme disease

Mastoiditis/mastoidectomy

Myasthenia gravis

Parotid gland excision

Pseudobulbar palsy

Sarcoidosis

Tangier disease

Facial trauma

Data compiled from Bagger-Sjoback D, Remahl S, Ericsson M. Long-term outcome of facial palsy in neuroborreliosis. *Otol Neurotol.* 2005;26(4):790–795; Chernoff WG, Parnes LS. Tuberculous mastoiditis. *J Otolaryngol.* 1992;21(4):290–292; Ellis SL, Carter BL, Leehey MA, Conry CM. Bell's palsy in an older patient with uncontrolled hypertension due to medication nonadherence. *Ann Pharmacother.* 1999;33(12):1269–1273; Gonzalez-Garcia R, Rodriguez-Campo FJ, Escorial-Hernandez V, et al. Complications of temporomandibular joint arthroscopy: a retrospective analytic study of 670 arthroscopic procedures. *J Oral Maxillofac Surg.* 2006;64(11):1587–1591; Rainsbury JW, Whiteside OJ, Bottrill ID. Traumatic facial nerve neuroma following mastoid surgery: a case report and literature review. *J Laryngol Otol.* 2007;121(6):601–605; Smith IM, Mountain RE, Murray JA. An out-patient review of facial palsy in the community. *Clin Otolaryngol Allied Sci.* 1994;19(3):198–200; and Witt RL. Facial nerve function after partial superficial parotidectomy: an 11-year review (1987–1997). *Otolaryngol Head Neck Surg.* 1999;121(3):210–213.

The functional examination is typically scaffolded—beginning with basic movement patterns that are prerequisites for more complicated patterns and activities. Scoring is typically nominal either dependent or independent or with further delineation such as maximal assist, moderate assist, minimal assist, contact guard, or independent. The examiner should also note if adaptive equipment such as bracing, prosthetics, hearing aids, and orthoses are used by the patient during the testing. The examiner should also note assistive equipment used by the patient at home or work, such as walkers, crutches, elevated toilet seats, shower chairs, and stair glides. The typical functional examination starting point is bed mobility. Can the patient move to the right, left, up, and down in bed? Transfers are assessed next. Can the patient transfer from bed to chair to standing and back to bed? Can the patient transfer onto a toilet or into a bathtub? The examiner can use visual gait analysis or, if available, quantified measurements of gait performed in a structured gait analysis laboratory to determine impairments in any one or more of the basic subsets of gait. Functionally, is the patient able to dress and undress, perform basic hygiene skills, and don and doff requisite adaptive equipment independently? Fine motor coordination should be assessed. Validated measures such as the Disabilities of the Arm, Shoulder and Hand (DASH), Developmental Test of Visual-Motor Integration, and Goodenough Draw-a-Person Test are helpful in measuring fine motor coordination.[161–167] Standardized functional capacity evaluations provide validated information about a patient's ability to return safely to his or her job.

Validated, generalized functional outcome measures and standardized assessment tools such as the Functional Independence Measure, SF-36, DASH, and the Rancho are useful for documentation of performance and for assessing improvement or regression of symptoms and assessing the efficacy of intervention.

Form Health Survey (SF-36) is another validated tool that measures quality of life indices.[157–160]

Functional Examination

Peripheral neuropathy may result in functional impairments. Focal or patterned motor weakness may lead to an inability to perform fine and gross motor movement patterns satisfactorily resulting in loss of an ability to accomplish activities of daily living. Secondary impairments resulting from weakness, loss of endurance, articular and axial joint dysfunction, and disuse atrophy may exacerbate the functional loss. Loss of somatosensory afferent feedback may lead to loss of static and dynamic standing balance, dyscoordination of the extremities, and neuropathic joints. Loss of protective sensation may lead to integument injury.

CASE STUDY

JJ is a 40-year-old construction worker who specializes in old paint removal, wood preparation, priming, and painting. He has been performing this type of work for the past 20 years. His hobbies include running, reading, and playing sports with his children. Recently, he has experienced general numbness in his hands and feet, occasional loss of balance, and a perception of mild confusion and forgetfulness. His laboratory work, including hemoglobin, hematocrit, platelets, white blood cells, chemistries, blood sugar, and urine analysis, all came back "normal." Magnetic resonance imaging of his brain, ECG, and chest x-ray were also "normal." JJ's primary physician referred him to physical therapy for balance assessment and treatment. He reports no medications but has used nitrous oxide in the past as a recreational drug.

Case Study Questions

1. After taking the history as detailed in the case study, would the therapist consider a vestibulopathy as a possible etiology of the balance disorder?
   a. No, because the patient also complains of numb hands and feet
   b. Yes, because the patient could have two unrelated diagnoses
   c. No, because patients with vestibulopathies never have cognitive impairment
   d. Yes, because patients with vestibulopathies often have cognitive impairment

2. Which of the following in JJ's history is a possible risk factor for neuropathy?
   a. Paint removal
   b. Running
   c. Television watching
   d. Playing with his children

3. Risk factors of lead intoxification include which of the following?
   a. Loss of balance, sensory disturbances of the hands and feet, cognitive impairments
   b. Blindness, ulcerative colitis, muscle weakness
   c. Cognitive loss, tremor, skin ulcers
   d. Muscle tenderness, hair loss, cognitive impairments

4. If the therapist thinks that lead intoxification belongs on the differential list, the therapist should ask the physician to order which of the following tests?
   a. Repeat brain magnetic resonance imaging
   b. Cardiac enzymes
   c. Serum lead levels
   d. Blood urea nitrogen

5. Based on the history alone, additional differential diagnoses may include which of the following?
   a. An undiagnosed neoplasm
   b. Multiple sclerosis
   c. Nitrous oxide exposure secondary to recreational use
   d. All of the above

References

1. Azhary H, Farooq MU, Bhanushali M, Majid A, Kassab MY. Peripheral neuropathy: differential diagnosis and management. *Am Fam Physician.* 2010;81(7):887–892.
2. Schroder A, Linker RA, Gold R. Plasmapheresis for neurological disorders. *Expert Rev Neurother.* 2009;9(9):1331–1339.
3. Zhang Q, Gu Z, Jiang J, et al. Orthostatic hypotension as a presenting symptom of the Guillain-Barre syndrome. *Clin Auton Res.* 2010;20(3):209–210.
4. Compston A. Primary sensory neuropathy with muscular changes associated with carcinoma. Editorial. *Brain.* 2009;132(Pt 8):1995–1996.
5. Isoda A, Sakurai A, Ogawa Y, et al. Chronic inflammatory demyelinating polyneuropathy accompanied by chronic myelomonocytic leukemia: possible pathogenesis of autoimmunity in myelodysplastic syndrome. *Int J Hematol.* 2009;90(2):239–242.
6. Layzer R, Wolf J. Myeloma-associated polyneuropathy responding to lenalidomide. *Neurology.* 2009;73(10):812–813.
7. Amlie-Lefond C, Jubelt B. Neurologic manifestations of varicella zoster virus infections. *Curr Neurol Neurosci Rep.* 2009;9(6):430–434.
8. Lunn MP, Willison HJ. Diagnosis and treatment of inflammatory neuropathies. *J Neurol Neurosurg Psychiatry.* 2009;80(3):249–258.
9. Isoda A, Sakurai A, Ogawa Y, et al. Chronic inflammatory demyelinating polyneuropathy accompanied by chronic myelomonocytic leukemia: possible pathogenesis of autoimmunity in myelodysplastic syndrome. *Int J Hematol.* 2009;90(2):239–242.
10. Jameson M, Roberts S, Anderson NE, Thompson P. Nitrous oxide-induced vitamin B(12) deficiency. *J Clin Neurosci.* 1999;6(2):164–166.
11. Linstedt U, Jaeger H, Petry A. The neuropathy of the autonomic nervous system. An additional anesthetic risk in diabetes mellitus [in German]. *Anaesthesist.* 1993;42(8):521–527.
12. Ogundipe O, Pearson MW, Slater NG, Adepegba T, Westerdale N. Sickle cell disease and nitrous oxide-induced neuropathy. *Clin Lab Haematol.* 1999;21(6):409–412.
13. Richardson PG. Peripheral neuropathy following nitrous oxide abuse. *Emerg Med Australas.* 2010;22(1).88–90.
14. Tatum WO, Bui DD, Grant EG, Murtagh R. Pseudo-Guillain-Barre syndrome due to "whippet"-induced myeloneuropathy. *J Neuroimaging.* 2010;20(4):400–401.
15. Gay D, Singh A. Cocaine-induced reflex sympathetic dystrophy. *Clin Nucl Med.* 2000;25(11):863–865.
16. Neiman J, Haapaniemi HM, Hillbom M. Neurological complications of drug abuse: pathophysiological mechanisms. *Eur J Neurol.* 2000;7(6):595–606.
17. O'Connor G, McMahon G. Complications of heroin abuse. *Eur J Emerg Med.* 2008;15(2):104–106.
18. O'Sullivan JM, McMahon G. Descending polyneuropathy in an intravenous drug user. *Eur J Emerg Med.* 2005;12(5):248–250.
19. Ziconotide: new drug. Limited analgesic efficacy, too many adverse effects. *Prescrire Int.* 2008;17(97):179–182.
20. Biondi DM. Is migraine a neuropathic pain syndrome? *Curr Pain Headache Rep.* 2006;10(3):167–178.
21. Brouwers EE, Huitema AD, Boogerd W, Beijnen JH, Schellens JH. Persistent neuropathy after treatment with cisplatin and oxaliplatin. *Acta Oncol.* 2009;48(6):832–841.
22. Castro M. Peripheral sensory neuropathy—fighting cold with cold. *Lancet Oncol.* 2008;9(5):415–416.
23. Dees EC, O'Neil BH, Lindley CM, et al. A phase I and pharmacologic study of the combination of bortezomib and pegylated liposomal doxorubicin in patients with refractory solid tumors. *Cancer Chemother Pharmacol.* 2008;63(1):99–107.
24. Doherty SD, Hsu S. A case series of 48 patients treated with thalidomide. *J Drugs Dermatol.* 2008;7(8):769–773.
25. Eksioglu E, Oztekin F, Unlu E, Cakci A, Keyik B, Karadavut IK. Sacroiliitis and polyneuropathy during isotretinoin treatment. *Clin Exp Dermatol.* 2008;33(2):122–124.

26. Gdynia HJ, Muller T, Sperfeld AD, et al. Severe sensorimotor neuropathy after intake of highest dosages of vitamin B6. *Neuromuscul Disord*. 2008;18(2):156–158.

27. Hoque R, Chesson AL Jr. Pharmacologically induced/ exacerbated restless legs syndrome, periodic limb movements of sleep, and REM behavior disorder/REM sleep without atonia: literature review, qualitative scoring, and comparative analysis. *J Clin Sleep Med*. 2010;6(1):79–83.

28. Kautio AL, Haanpaa M, Leminen A, Kalso E, Kautiainen H, Saarto T. Amitriptyline in the prevention of chemotherapy-induced neuropathic symptoms. *Anticancer Res*. 2009;29(7):2601–2606.

29. Koh C, Kwong KL, Wong SN. Mercury poisoning: a rare but treatable cause of failure to thrive and developmental regression in an infant. *Hong Kong Med J*. 2009;15(1):61–64.

30. Kumarasamy N, Venkatesh KK, Cecelia AJ, et al. Spectrum of adverse events after generic HAART in southern Indian HIV-infected patients. *AIDS Patient Care STDS*. 2008; 22(4):337–344.

31. Moore A, Pinkerton R. Vincristine: can its therapeutic index be enhanced? *Pediatr Blood Cancer*. 2009;53(7):1180–1187.

32. Nakamura Y, Tajima K, Kawagoe I, Kanai M, Mitsuhata H. Efficacy of traditional herbal medicine, Yokukansan on patients with neuropathic pain. *Masui*. 2009;58(10): 1248–1255.

33. O'Connor TL, Kossoff E. Delayed seizure associated with paclitaxel-Cremophor EL in a patient with early-stage breast cancer. *Pharmacotherapy*. 2009;29(8):993–996.

34. Pierce DA, Holt SR, Reeves-Daniel A. A probable case of gabapentin-related reversible hearing loss in a patient with acute renal failure. *Clin Ther*. 2008;30(9):1681–1684.

35. Qi X, Chu Z, Mahller YY, Stringer KF, Witte DP, Cripe TP. Cancer-selective targeting and cytotoxicity by liposomal-coupled lysosomal saposin C protein. *Clin Cancer Res*. 2009;15(18):5840–5851.

36. Selvarajah D, Gandhi R, Emery CJ, Tesfaye S. Randomized placebo-controlled double-blind clinical trial of cannabis-based medicinal product (Sativex) in painful diabetic neuropathy: depression is a major confounding factor. *Diabetes Care*. 2010;33(1):128–130.

37. Singh S, Mukherjee KK, Gill KD, Flora SJ. Lead-induced peripheral neuropathy following ayurvedic medication. *Indian J Med Sci*. 2009;63(9):408–410.

38. Toyooka K, Fujimura H. Iatrogenic neuropathies. *Curr Opin Neurol*. 2009;22(5):475–479.

39. Occupational Medicine Physician's Guide to Neuropathy in the Workplace Part 3: Case Presentation. *J Occup Environ Med*. 2009;51(7):861–862.

40. Gimranova GG, Bakiirov AB, Karimova LK. Complex evaluation of work conditions and health state of oil industry workers [in Russian]. *Med Tr Prom Ekol*. 2009;(8):1–5.

41. Goffeng LO, Heier MS, Kjuus H, Sjoholm H, Sorensen KA, Skaug V. Nerve conduction, visual evoked responses and electroretinography in tunnel workers previously exposed to acrylamide and N-methylolacrylamide containing grouting agents. *Neurotoxicol Teratol*. 2008;30(3): 186–194.

42. Huang CC. Polyneuropathy induced by n-hexane intoxication in Taiwan. *Acta Neurol Taiwan*. 2008;17(1): 3–10.

43. Krajnak K, Waugh S, Johnson C, Miller R, Kiedrowski M. Vibration disrupts vascular function in a model of metabolic syndrome. *Ind Health*. 2009;47(5):533–542.

44. Kutlu G, Gomceli YB, Sonmez T, Inan LE. Peripheral neuropathy and visual evoked potential changes in workers exposed to n-hexane. *J Clin Neurosci*. 2009;16(10): 1296–1299.

45. Lagueny A. Drug induced neuropathies. *Rev Prat*. 2008; 58(17):1910–1916.

46. Lansdown AB. Critical observations on the neurotoxicity of silver. *Crit Rev Toxicol*. 2007;37(3):237–250.

47. Ling SK, Cheng SC, Yen CH. Stonefish envenomation with acute carpal tunnel syndrome. *Hong Kong Med J*. 2009;15(6): 471–473.

48. Majersik JJ, Caravati EM, Steffens JD. Severe neurotoxicity associated with exposure to the solvent 1-bromopropane (n-propyl bromide). *Clin Toxicol (Phila)*. 2007;45(3):270–276.

49. Matsuoka M. Neurotoxicity of organic solvents—recent findings. *Brain Nerve*. 2007;59(6):591–596.

50. Ohnari K, Uozumi T, Tsuji S. Occupation and carpal tunnel syndrome. *Brain Nerve*. 2007;59(11):1247–1252.

51. Pelclova D, Urban P, Ridzon P, et al. Two-year follow-up of two patients after severe thallium intoxication. *Hum Exp Toxicol*. 2009;28(5):263–272.

52. Puriene A, Janulyte V, Musteikyte M, Bendinskaite R. General health of dentists. Literature review. *Stomatologija*. 2007;9(1):10–20.

53. Sauni R, Paakkonen R, Virtema P, et al. Vibration-induced white finger syndrome and carpal tunnel syndrome among Finnish metal workers. *Int Arch Occup Environ Health*. 2009; 82(4):445–453.

54. Sethi PK, Khandelwal D. Cadmium exposure: health hazards of silver cottage industry in developing countries. *J Med Toxicol*. 2006;2(1):14–15.

55. Aboussouan LS, Lewis RA, Shy ME. Disorders of pulmonary function, sleep, and the upper airway in Charcot-Marie-Tooth disease. *Lung*. 2007;185(1):1–7.

56. Coste TC, Gerbi A, Vague P, Maixent JM, Pieroni G, Raccah D. Peripheral diabetic neuropathy and polyunsaturated fatty acid supplementations: natural sources or biotechnological needs? *Cell Mol Biol (Noisy-le-grand)*. 2004;50(7):845–853.

57. Di Nardo G, Blandizzi C, Volta U, et al. Molecular, pathological and therapeutic features of human enteric neuropathies. *Aliment Pharmacol Ther*. 2008;28(1):25–42.

58. Freeman R. Autonomic peripheral neuropathy. *Neurol Clin*. 2007;25(1):277–301.

59. Lacigova S, Bartunek L, Cechurova D, et al. Influence of cardiovascular autonomic neuropathy on atherogenesis and heart function in patients with type 1 diabetes. *Diabetes Res Clin Pract*. 2009;83(1):26–31.

60. Manzella D, Paolisso G. Cardiac autonomic activity and Type II diabetes mellitus. *Clin Sci (Lond)*. 2005;108(2): 93–99.

61. Maule S, Papotti G, Naso D, Magnino C, Testa E, Veglio F. Orthostatic hypotension: evaluation *Cardiovasc Hematol Disord Drug Targets*. 2007;7(1):63–70.

62. Mehta A, Ricci R, Widmer U, et al. Fabry disease defined: baseline clinical manifestations of 366 patients in the Fabry Outcome Survey. *Eur J Clin Invest*. 2004;34(3):236–242.

63. Oka N, Sugiyama H, Kawasaki T, Mizutani K, Matsui M. Falls in peripheral neuropathy [in Japanese]. *Rinsho Shinkeigaku*. 2005;45(3):207–210.

64. Sacco IC, Bacarin TA, Canettieri MG, Hennig EM. Plantar pressures during shod gait in diabetic neuropathic patients with and without a history of plantar ulceration. *J Am Podiatr Med Assoc*. 2009;99(4):285–294.

65. Said G. Familial amyloid polyneuropathy: mechanisms leading to nerve degeneration. *Amyloid*. 2003;10(Suppl 1): 7–12.

66. Vial C, Bouhour F. Vasculitis multiple mononeuropathies [in French]. *Rev Prat*. 2008;58(17):1896–1899.

67. Yeung H, Krentz HB, Gill MJ, Power C. Neuropsychiatric disorders in HIV infection: impact of diagnosis on economic costs of care. *AIDS*. 2006;20(16):2005–2009.

68. Feise RJ, Menke JM. Functional Rating Index: literature review. *Med Sci Monit*. 2010;16(2):RA25–36.

69. Longo UG, Loppini M, Denaro L, Maffulli N, Denaro V. Rating scales for low back pain. *Br Med Bull*. 2010;94: 81–144.

70. McWilliams LA, Saldanha KM, Dick BD, Watt MC. Development and psychometric evaluation of a new measure of pain-related support preferences: the Pain Response Preference Questionnaire. *Pain Res Manag*. 2009;14(6): 461–469.

71. Cheer K, Shearman C, Jude EB. Managing complications of the diabetic foot. *BMJ*. 2009;339:b4905.

72. Brown PJ, Zirwas MJ, English JC 3rd. The purple digit: an algorithmic approach to diagnosis. *Am J Clin Dermatol*. 2010;11(2):103–116.

73. Kluger N, Frances C. Cutaneous vasculitis and their differential diagnoses. *Clin Exp Rheumatol*. 2009; 27(1 Suppl 52):S124–138.

74. Cohen PR. Primary alopecia neoplastica versus secondary alopecia neoplastica: a new classification for neoplasm-associated scalp hair loss. *J Cutan Pathol*. 2009;36(8): 917–918.

75. Mounsey AL, Reed SW. Diagnosing and treating hair loss. *Am Fam Physician*. 2009;80(4):356–362.

76. Trueb RM. Systematic approach to hair loss in women. *J Dtsch Dermatol Ges*. 2010; 8(4):284–297, 284–298.

77. Ceyhan AM, Yildirim M, Bircan HA, Karayigit DZ. Transverse leukonychia (Mees' lines) associated with docetaxel. *J Dermatol*. 2010;37(2):188–189.

78. Chauhan S, D'Cruz S, Singh R, Sachdev A. Mees' lines. *Lancet*. 2008;372(9647):1410.

79. Huang TC, Chao TY. Mees lines and Beau lines after chemotherapy. *Can Med Assoc J*. 2010;182(3):E149.

80. Lu CI, Huang CC, Chang YC, et al. Short-term thallium intoxication: dermatological findings correlated with thallium concentration. *Arch Dermatol*. 2007;143(1):93–98.

81. Seavolt MB, Sarro RA, Levin K, Camisa C. Mees' lines in a patient following acute arsenic intoxication. *Int J Dermatol*. 2002;41(7):399–401.

82. Zhao G, Ding M, Zhang B, et al. Clinical manifestations and management of acute thallium poisoning. *Eur Neurol*. 2008;60(6):292–297.

83. Marrie TJ, Brown N. Clubbing of the digits. *Am J Med*. 2007;120(11):940–941.

84. Nguyen K, Aronowitz P. Drumstick digits: a case of clubbing of the fingers and toes. *J Hosp Med*. 2010; 5(3):196.

85. Spicknall KE, Zirwas MJ, English JC 3rd. Clubbing: an update on diagnosis, differential diagnosis, pathophysiology, and clinical relevance. *J Am Acad Dermatol*. 2005;52(6): 1020–1028.

86. Wu JY, Shih JY. Leg pains, clubbing of digits and lung mass: what is your call? *Can Med Assoc J*. 2008;178(4): 395–396.

87. Gandhi V, Nagral A, Philip S, Malkani RH, Pimputkar R. Reversal of nail changes after liver transplantation in a child. *Indian J Gastroenterol*. 2009;28(4):154–156.

88. Huang CC, Sun PL. Superficial white onychomycosis caused by *Trichophyton verrucosum*. *Int J Dermatol*. 2008; 47(11):1162–1164.

89. Ruwan KP, Parakramawansha C, Wijeweera I, Ratnatunga N, Sumanasekara WG. A case of POEMS syndrome with mixed hyaline vascular and plasma cell type Castleman's disease. *Ceylon Med J*. 2009;54(2):68–69.

90. Savage SA, Navarini AA, Trueb RM. Dyskeratosis congenita; psoriasis. *Ther Umsch*. 2010;67(4):153–165.

91. Mondelli M, Rossi S, Monti E, et al. Long term follow-up of carpal tunnel syndrome during pregnancy: a cohort study

92. Smith MW, Marcus PS, Wurtz LD. Orthopedic issues in pregnancy. *Obstet Gynecol Surv*. 2008;63(2):103–111.

93. Giuca MR, Bonfigli D, Bartoli F, Pasini M. Sjogren's syndrome: correlation between histopathologic result and clinical and serologic parameters. *Minerva Stomatol*. 2010; 59(4):149–157.

94. Kang JH, Lin HC. Comorbidities in patients with primary Sjogren's Syndrome: a registry-based case-control study. *J Rheumatol*. 2010; 37(6):1188–1194.

95. Cuthbert SC, Goodheart GJ Jr. On the reliability and validity of manual muscle testing: a literature review. *Chiropr Osteopat*. 2007;15:4.

96. Li RC, Jasiewicz JM, Middleton J, et al. The development, validity, and reliability of a manual muscle testing device with integrated limb position sensors. *Arch Phys Med Rehabil*. 2006;87(3):411–417.

97. Perry J, Weiss WB, Burnfield JM, Gronley JK. The supine hip extensor manual muscle test: a reliability and validity study. *Arch Phys Med Rehabil*. 2004;85(8):1345–1350.

98. Savic G, Bergstrom EM, Frankel HL, Jamous MA, Jones PW. Inter-rater reliability of motor and sensory examinations performed according to American Spinal Injury Association standards. *Spinal Cord*. 2007;45(6): 444–451.

99. Anderson NE, Mason DF, Fink JN, Bergin PS, Charleston AJ, Gamble GD. Detection of focal cerebral hemisphere lesions using the neurological examination. *J Neurol Neurosurg Psychiatry*. 2005;76(4):545–549.

100. Pullen RL Jr. Neurologic assessment for pronator drift. *Nursing*. 2004;34(3):22.

101. Henriksson NG, Johansson G, Olsson LG, Ostlund H. Electric analysis of the Romberg test. *Acta Otolaryngol*. 1966; Suppl 224:272+.

102. Jansen EC, Larsen RE, Olesen MB. Quantitative Romberg test. Measurement and computer calculation of postural stability. *Ugeskr Laeger*. 1978;140(44):2715–2717.

103. Njiokiktjien C, de Rijke W. The recording of Romberg' test and its application in neurology. *Agressologie*. 1972; 13(Suppl C):1–7.

104. Reicke N. The Romberg head-shake test within the scope of equilibrium diagnosis [in German]. *HNO*. 1992;40(6): 195–201.

105. Rogers JH. Romberg and his test. *J Laryngol Otol*. 1980; 94(12):1401–1404.

106. Masear VR, Colgin S. The treatment of epineural scarring with allograft vein wrapping. *Hand Clin*. 1996;12(4): 773–779.

107. Palazzi S, Palazzi JL. Neurolysis in compressive neuropathies. *Int Surg*. 1980;65(6):509–514.

108. Davis DS, Quinn RO, Whiteman CT, Williams JD, Young CR. Concurrent validity of four clinical tests used to measure hamstring flexibility. *J Strength Cond Res*. 2008; 22(2):583–588.

109. Mens JM, Pool-Goudzwaard A, Beekmans RE, Tijhuis MT. Relation between subjective and objective scores on the active straight leg raising test. *Spine (Phila Pa 1976)*. 2010; 35(3):336–339.

110. Rebain R, Baxter GD, McDonough S. A systematic review of the passive straight leg raising test as a diagnostic aid for low back pain (1989 to 2000). *Spine (Phila Pa 1976)*. 2002; 27(17):E388–395.

111. Kreitz BG, Cote P, Yong-Hing K. Crossed femoral stretching test. A case report. *Spine (Phila Pa 1976)*. 1996; 21(13):1584–1586.

112. Davis DS, Anderson IB, Carson MG, Elkins CL, Stuckey LB. Upper limb neural tension and seated slump tests: the

false positive rate among healthy young adults without cervical or lumbar symptoms. *J Man Manip Ther.* 2008;16(3): 136–141.

113. Heebner ML, Roddey TS. The effects of neural mobilization in addition to standard care in persons with carpal tunnel syndrome from a community hospital. *J Hand Ther.* 2008; 21(3):229–240; quiz 241.

114. Nawrot P, Nowakowski A, Kubaszewski L. The usefulness of the provocative tests in nerve monitoring after operative treatment of upper limb neuropathy. *Chir Narzadow Ruchu Ortop Pol.* 2007;72(2):105–115.

115. Rubinstein SM, van Tulder M. A best-evidence review of diagnostic procedures for neck and low-back pain. *Best Pract Res Clin Rheumatol.* 2008;22(3):471–482.

116. Sanders RJ, Hammond SL, Rao NM. Diagnosis of thoracic outlet syndrome. *J Vasc Surg.* 2007;46(3):601–604.

117. Schiff M, Ogier de Baulny H, Bard G, et al. Should transcobalamin deficiency be treated aggressively? *J Inherit Metab Dis.* 2010; 33(3):223–229.

118. Hantson P, Kevers L, Fabien N, Van Den Bergh P. Acute-onset chronic inflammatory demyelinating polyneuropathy with cranial nerve involvement, dysautonomia, respiratory failure, and autoantibodies. *Muscle Nerve.* 2010;41(3): 423–426.

119. Jacobs BC, Willison HJ. Peripheral neuropathies: biomarkers for axonal damage in immune-mediated neuropathy. *Nat Rev Neurol.* 2009;5(11):584–585.

120. Goldberg A, Russell JW, Alexander NB. Standing balance and trunk position sense in impaired glucose tolerance (IGT)-related peripheral neuropathy. *J Neurol Sci.* 2008; 270(1–2):165–171.

121. Pop-Busui R. Cardiac autonomic neuropathy in diabetes: a clinical perspective. *Diabetes Care.* 2010;33(2):434–441.

122. Spallone V, Morganti R, Fedele T, D'Amato C, Maiello MR. Reappraisal of the diagnostic role of orthostatic hypotension in diabetes. *Clin Auton Res.* 2009;19(1): 58–64.

123. Villavicencio-Chavez C, Miralles Basseda R, Gonzalez Marin P, Cervera AM. Orthostatic and postprandial hypotension in elderly patients with chronic diseases and disability: prevalence and related factors. *Rev Esp Geriatr Gerontol.* 2009;44(1):12–18.

124. Pop-Busui R. Cardiac autonomic neuropathy in diabetes: a clinical perspective. *Diabetes Care.* 2010;33(2):434–441.

125. Spallone V, Morganti R, Fedele T, D'Amato C, Maiello MR. Reappraisal of the diagnostic role of orthostatic hypotension in diabetes. *Clin Auton Res.* 2009;19(1): 58–64.

126. Villavicencio-Chavez C, Miralles Basseda R, Gonzalez Marin P, Cervera AM. Orthostatic and postprandial hypotension in elderly patients with chronic diseases and disability: prevalence and related factors. *Rev Esp Geriatr Gerontol.* 2009;44(1):12–18

127. Berger JR, Fannin M. The "bedsheet" Babinski. *South Med J.* 2002;95(10):1178–1179.

128. Ditunno JF, Bell R. The Babinski sign: 100 years on. *BMJ.* 1996;313(7064):1029–1030.

129. Ghosh D, Pradhan S. "Extensor toe sign" by various methods in spastic children with cerebral palsy. *J Child Neurol.* 1998;13(5):216–220.

130. Bruske J, Bednarski M, Grzelec H, Zyluk A. The usefulness of the Phalen test and the Hoffmann-Tinel sign in the diagnosis of carpal tunnel syndrome. *Acta Orthop Belg.* 2002; 68(2):141–145.

131. Howard M, Lee C, Dellon AL. Documentation of brachial plexus compression (in the thoracic inlet) utilizing provocative neurosensory and muscular testing. *J Reconstr Microsurg.* 2003;19(5):303–312.

132. Lifchez SD, Means KR Jr, Dunn RE, Williams EH. Intra- and inter-examiner variability in performing Tinel's test. *J Hand Surg Am.* 2010;35(2):212–216.

133. Levin KH. Variants and mimics of Guillain Barre Syndrome. *Neurologist.* 2004;10(2):61–74.

134. Sodhi M, Stoller JK. Small cell carcinoma with paraneoplastic polyneuropathy and tumor embolization: a case report and literature review. *Respiration.* 2010;79(1): 77–80.

135. Cortes S, Chambers S, Jeronimo A, Isenberg D. Diabetes mellitus complicating systemic lupus erythematosus—analysis of the UCL lupus cohort and review of the literature. *Lupus.* 2008;17(11):977–980.

136. Mellgren SI, Goransson LG, Omdal R. Primary Sjogren's syndrome associated neuropathy. *Can J Neurol Sci.* 2007; 34(3):280–287.

137. Tzioufas AG, Voulgarelis M. Update on Sjogren's syndrome autoimmune epithelitis: from classification to increased neoplasias. *Best Pract Res Clin Rheumatol.* 2007;21(6): 989–1010.

138. Bagger-Sjoback D, Remahl S, Ericsson M. Long-term outcome of facial palsy in neuroborreliosis. *Otol Neurotol.* 2005;26(4):790–795.

139. Chernoff WG, Parnes LS. Tuberculous mastoiditis. *J Otolaryngol.* 1992;21(4):290–292.

140. Ellis SL, Carter BL, Leehey MA, Conry CM. Bell's palsy in an older patient with uncontrolled hypertension due to medication nonadherence. *Ann Pharmacother.* 1999;33(12): 1269–1273.

141. Gonzalez-Garcia R, Rodriguez-Campo FJ, Escorial-Hernandez V, et al. Complications of temporomandibular joint arthroscopy: a retrospective analytic study of 670 arthroscopic procedures. *J Oral Maxillofac Surg.* 2006;64(11): 1587–1591.

142. Rainsbury JW, Whiteside OJ, Bottrill ID. Traumatic facial nerve neuroma following mastoid surgery: a case report and literature review. *J Laryngol Otol.* 2007;121(6):601–605.

143. Smith IM, Mountain RE, Murray JA. An out-patient review of facial palsy in the community. *Clin Otolaryngol Allied Sci.* 1994;19(3):198–200.

144. Witt RL. Facial nerve function after partial superficial parotidectomy: an 11-year review (1987–1997). *Otolaryngol Head Neck Surg.* 1999;121(3):210–213.

145. Boswell-Ruys CL, Sturnieks DL, Harvey LA, Sherrington C, Middleton JW, Lord SR. Validity and reliability of assessment tools for measuring unsupported sitting in people with a spinal cord injury. *Arch Phys Med Rehabil.* 2009;90(9):1571–1577.

146. Clark RA, Bryant AL, Pua Y, McCrory P, Bennell K, Hunt M. Validity and reliability of the Nintendo Wii Balance Board for assessment of standing balance. *Gait Posture.* 2010;31(3):307–310.

147. Delbaere K, Close JC, Mikolaizak AS, Sachdev PS, Brodaty H, Lord SR. The Falls Efficacy Scale International (FES-I). A comprehensive longitudinal validation study. *Age Ageing.* 2010;39(2):210–216.

148. MacIntyre NJ, Stavness CL, Adachi JD. The Safe Functional Motion test is reliable for assessment of functional movements in individuals at risk for osteoporotic fracture. *Clin Rheumatol.* 2010;29(2):143–150.

149. Bassuk SS, Murphy JM. Characteristics of the Modified Mini-Mental State Exam among elderly persons. *J Clin Epidemiol.* 2003;56(7):622–628.

150. Fabrigoule C, Lechevallier N, Crasborn L, Dartigues JF, Orgogozo JM. Inter-rater reliability of scales and tests used to measure mild cognitive impairment by general practitioners and psychologists. *Curr Med Res Opin.* 2003; 19(7):603–608.

151. Koch HJ, Gurtler K, Fischer-Barnicol D, Szecsey A, Ibach B. Determination of reliability of psychometric tests in psychiatry using canonical correlation. *Psychiatr Prax.* 2003; 30(Suppl 2):157–160.

152. Marinus J, Visser M, Verwey NA, et al. Assessment of cognition in Parkinson's disease. *Neurology.* 2003;61(9): 1222–1228.

153. Burkhart BR, Rogers K, McDonald WD, McGrath R, Arnoscht O. The measurement of depression: enhancing the predictive validity of the Beck Depression Inventory. *J Clin Psychol.* 1984;40(6):1368–1372.

154. Byerly FC, Carlson WA. Comparison among inpatients, outpatients, and normals on three self-report depression inventories. *J Clin Psychol.* 1982;38(4):797–804.

155. Lightfoot SL, Oliver JM. The Beck Inventory: psychometric properties in university students. *J Pers Assess.* 1985;49(4): 434–436.

156. Meites K, Lovallo W, Pishkin V. A comparison of four scales for anxiety, depression, and neuroticism. *J Clin Psychol.* 1980;36(2):427–432.

157. Brazier JE, Walters SJ, Nicholl JP, Kohler B. Using the SF-36 and Euroqol on an elderly population. *Qual Life Res.* 1996;5(2):195–204.

158. Jacobson AM, de Groot M, Samson JA. The evaluation of two measures of quality of life in patients with type I and type II diabetes. *Diabetes Care.* 1994;17(4):267–274.

159. Jenkinson C, Wright L, Coulter A. Criterion validity and reliability of the SF-36 in a population sample. *Qual Life Res.* 1994;3(1):7–12.

160. Bloch MH, Sukhodolsky DG, Leckman JF, Schultz RT. Fine-motor skill deficits in childhood predict adulthood tic severity and global psychosocial functioning in Tourette's syndrome. *J Child Psychol Psychiatry.* 2006;47(6):551–559.

161. Desrosiers J, Hebert R, Bravo G, Dutil E. Upper extremity performance test for the elderly (TEMPA): normative data and correlates with sensorimotor parameters. Test d'Evaluation des Membres Superieurs de Personnes Agees. *Arch Phys Med Rehabil.* 1995;76(12):1125–1129.

162. Gagnon C, Mathieu J, Desrosiers J. Standardized finger-nose test validity for coordination assessment in an ataxic disorder. *Can J Neurol Sci.* 2004;31(4):484–489.

163. Neuhauser G. The value of motor tests in neuro-developmental diagnosis. *Fortschr Med.* 1975;93(25): 1159–1166.

164. Peters LH, Maathuis KG, Kouw E, Hamming M, Hadders-Algra M. Test-retest, inter-assessor and intra-assessor reliability of the modified Touwen examination. *Eur J Paediatr Neurol.* 2008;12(4):328–333.

165. Poeta LS, Rosa-Neto F. Motor assessment in school-aged children with indicators of the attention deficit/hyperactivity disorder. *Rev Neurol.* 2007;44(3):146–149.

166. Pothmann R, Kurbjuhn A. Assessment of fine motor skills in young children and school children. *Fortschr Med.* 1989; 107(28):592–595.

167. Spano M, Mercuri E, Rando T, et al. Motor and perceptual-motor competence in children with Down syndrome: variation in performance with age. *Eur J Paediatr Neurol.* 1999;3(1):7–13.

Chapter **15**

Overview of Rehabilitation Intervention for Peripheral Nerve Injury

Stephen J. Carp, PT, PhD, GCS

"Leave all the afternoon for exercise and recreation, which are as necessary as reading. I will rather say more necessary because health is worth more than learning."

—Thomas Jefferson (1743–1826)

Objectives

On completion of this chapter, the student/practitioner will be able to:

- Explain the concept of International Classification of Functioning, Disability and Health within the context of treating a patient with peripheral neuropathy and the commonality of terms when discussing this diagnosis with other health care practitioners.
- Discuss the use of the Hypothesis-Oriented Algorithm for Clinicians as a model for evaluating patients with peripheral neuropathy.
- Identify three paradigm shifts within health care that affect the provision of rehabilitation services to patients with peripheral neuropathy.
- Describe the focus of therapeutic intervention by rehabilitation services professionals for patients with peripheral neuropathy.

Key Terms

- Disability and Health
- Hypothesis-Oriented Algorithm for Clinicians
- International Classification of Functioning
- Intervention

Introduction

Medicine is undergoing an accelerated change in theory, practice, documentation, and reimbursement. Rehabilitation services are not immune to these paradigm shifts. The key to being a successful provider of health care services is effective management of this change. In the past few years, rehabilitation services moved from older disability models such as Nagy to the World Health Organization's International Classification of Function, **Disability and Health**. Documentation for many of us has moved from pen and paper to keyboard. The medical record, once a collection of thousands of paper medical charts, is becoming a secured (hopefully!) connection to the Internet. Diagnosis, previously the isolated domain of physicians, is now being performed by therapists. Therapists working in the inpatient and outpatient arenas are struggling with decreased lengths of stay and lower facility reimbursement.

Physical and occupational therapy **intervention** for diagnoses related to peripheral neuropathy is provided within the aforementioned constraints and process shifts. Great clinical strides have occurred in recent years with the publication of many excellent peer-reviewed, evidenced-based studies related to the many possible impairments associated with peripheral neuropathy. One example is the "sickness behavior" observed in many clients with neuropathy. Sickness behavior is a downstream effect of the elevation of serum proinflammatory mediators resulting in anorexia, sleep disturbances, anemia, and depression. Lifelong learning is mandatory for all practicing therapists.[1]

This chapter begins with a discussion of the **International Classification of Functioning,** Disability and Health (ICF); continues with a short discussion of the use of the **Hypothesis-Oriented Algorithm for Clinicians** (HOAC), which is a succinct and rational method of evaluating patients with neuropathy; and ends with a brief overview of the various therapeutic interventions used to treat patients with peripheral neuropathy. Later chapters expound on each of these interventions.

International Classification of Functioning, Disability and Health

Functional limitations and disability are universal experiences that affect people of all ages, races, cultures, economic levels, and locations. Most persons will experience functional limitation or disability secondary to an acute or chronic physical or mental illness, trauma, or disease at some point in life. Restoring function and limiting disability is an important adjunct to the complex medical and surgical care offered throughout the continuum of health care services.

Physical and occupational therapy are health care professions involved in ameliorating functional loss and disability across the health care continuum. Therapists assist in identifying persons with functional limitation or disability, collect pertinent data, take histories, evaluate, assess function, identify problems, develop functional goals, and develop and implement a treatment plan (see the next section on "Hypothesis-Oriented Algorithm for Clinicians"). Services are performed in collaboration with other health care professionals such as physicians, nurses, social workers, psychologists, pharmacists, and respiratory therapists; with community agencies such as religious organizations, support groups, foundations, and agencies; and with the patient's family members and social support structure. Therapists are often the primary provider of services for many musculoskeletal and neurological conditions. For others, such as developmental disabilities or internal structural issues, therapists are members of the care team.

With the collaborative nature of health care, common language, terminology, and classifications must be used as descriptors of patient problems. In many areas of the United States and the world, the International Classification of Diseases (ICD) is still used.[2] This classification system and its many iterations does not meet the need of physical therapists who, by the nature of the rehabilitation spectrum, require a more functional-based system than the diagnosis-based ICD. Even with the shift away from the ICD system, reimbursement often remains tied to the ICD system, and payment, based on a diagnosis, omits the broad spectrum of severity of functional involvement that can occur with a particular diagnosis.

With the development and implementation of the International Classification of Functioning, Disability and Health (ICF),[3] therapists can now rely on a universal classification system that is equally responsive to all health care personnel in all health care locations along the continuum. The ICF contains lists of categories organized in two different parts: Functional and Disability and Contextual Factors. The Functional and Disability category is further subdivided into Body Function and Structures and Activities and Participation. The Contextual Factors category is also subdivided into Environmental Factors and Personal Factors. Within the hierarchical grading system of the ICF classification, the ICF categories are designated by the letters "B" for body function, "S" for body structure, "D" for domains representing the component activity and participation, and "E" for environmental factors. The grading system is followed by a numeric code stating the chapter (1 digit), followed by the second number (1 digit) and the third and fourth levels (1 digit each) (Table 15-1). The ICF can be employed as a common

Table 15-1	Classification Rubric for Structure and Function of the International Classification of Functioning, Disability and Health	
Parts	Part 1: Functioning and Disability	Part 2: Contextual Factors
Components	Body Functions and Structures Activities and Participation	Environmental Factors Personal Factors
Domains and Categories	Items levels 1st 2nd 3rd 4th	Items levels 1st 2nd 3rd 4th

framework across the curriculum and used by all health care personnel to provide a detailed diagnostic and functional description of the patient's illness in a standard terminology format. Such a set description can provide a definition of widely accepted lists of ICF categories for therapist interventions.

Hypothesis-Oriented Algorithm for Clinicians

In 1986, Rothstein and Echternach[4] published a clinical decision and documentation guide called the Hypothesis-Oriented Algorithm for Clinicians (HOAC), which offered rehabilitation clinicians a pragmatic, evidenced-based approach to patient assessment, intervention, and management (since updated as the Hypothesis-Oriented Algorithm for Clinicians II[5]). Since the publication of these seminal works, radical changes have continued to occur in the U.S. health care system. For example, there is now widespread discussion of the importance of physical therapists developing diagnoses.[6] In addition, therapists are often required by insurers to refer and use practice guides and guidelines developed through peer-reviewed evidence.[7] We argue that what is needed is a patient management system that involves the patient in decision making and can be used to provide payers with better justifications for interventions, including occasions when therapists may disagree with practice guidelines. Compatibility with the patient management model in the *Guide to Physical Therapist Practice*, including the formulation of diagnoses, is also desirable.[8] The use of the HOAC provides the necessary scaffolding to allow the practicing therapist to accomplish many of these measures. This tool is especially useful in patients with suspected peripheral neuropathy.

Clinical scripts are pieces of evidence from the subjective portion of the evaluation or from the review of the concurrent available data, including laboratory values, radiographic reports, consultations, and neuro-diagnostic testing, that prompt the clinician to add to or remove items from the differential diagnosis list and ultimately assist with confirmation of the differential diagnosis list. Clinical scripts may be classified as patient-identified problems (PIPs) or non–patient-identified problems (NPIPs). A PIP may be concurrent. An example of a current PIP is "my left knee buckles ascending steps" or "my right little finger and ring finger are numb." PIPs may also be anticipated, such as "if my numbness gets any worse I may not be able to type" or "so far I have not fallen down, but I can see this happening soon if I do not get help."

NPIPs are problems that are identified by the therapist and often the patient is unaware of the potential association of the finding with pathology. For example, a patient may attend rehabilitation services for therapy related to a fractured ankle, but the therapist identifies weakness in the contralateral ankle. Another example would be a review of laboratory data reveals an aberrant hemoglobin A_{1c} test.

Testing criteria are identified by the therapist to confirm, add to, or remove items from the differential diagnosis list. Through the use of testing criteria based on best evidence such as sensitivity and specificity, the practitioner can narrow the differential diagnosis list and eventually arrive at the correct diagnosis. Testing criteria are used to examine the correctness of the hypothesis related to problems that currently exist. For NPIPs and PIPs that are anticipated, the therapist establishes predictive criteria, which, if met, indicate that problems most likely will be avoided because the risk factors were reduced or eliminated. To justify any predictive criterion, the therapist must use appropriate clinical decision making: best evidence or clinical expertise.

Following the use of testing criteria to narrow the differential diagnosis list to the true diagnosis, the therapist can develop a problem list identified by the testing criteria including the functional examination, the patient's concerns, and any risk factors identified throughout the evaluation process. The problem list provides the therapist and the patient with talking points to assist with determining a mutually agreed-on list of short-term and long-term goals and approximate time frames for accomplishment. Goals must be objective, functional, and measurable. Behavioral, problem-solving, and outcome goals should be included in the goal list. Each identified problem must have a related short-term or long-term goal. An intervention is then developed for each goal. Lastly, an ongoing schedule of reassessments should be established to provide feedback about the effectiveness of the intervention in meeting the pre-established treatment goals.

Overview of Intervention

Coordination, Communication, and Documentation

According to the *Guide to Physical Therapist Practice*, an "intervention" is defined as "the purposeful and skilled interaction of a therapist and the patient/client and, when appropriate, with other individuals involved in the patient's clinical care, using various physical therapy procedures and techniques to produce changes in the condition consistent with the diagnosis and prognosis."[8] An intervention consists of five components: coordination, communication, documentation, patient-related instruction, and direct interventions.

Coordination, communication, and documentation among health care professionals and the patient allow for a well-defined, goal-oriented, coordinated intervention from many professionals across the health care continuum. Persons with peripheral neuropathic illness often not only have impairments related to function but also have economic, social, administrative, financial, medical, and relationship issues. Along with therapist consultation, patients may also be involved in regular consultation with their primary physician, physician specialist, nurse, case manager, counselor, social worker, and others. Communication must be unimpeded and timely to allow proper coordination of all services.

Historically, health care was provided in a context of a "disease-centered model," in which most decisions about a patient's care were made unilaterally by the health care professional.[9] The disease model focused on the particular illness rather than the patient as a whole. Treatment goals were set by the health care practitioner rather than in collaboration with the patient. This model was predicated on the patient complying with 100% adherence to the teaching and recommendations of the health care professional. Lack of program adherence was seen as a fault of the patient rather than as a process issue, a lack of communication on the part of the health care professional, or contradictory learning and teaching styles of the patient and health care professional. Over the past decade, outcome data suggested flaws with the authoritarian delivery of teaching, and recommendations for a patient-therapist collaborative model have been advanced.[10]

Discussions of a collaborative treatment model have been evolving since the early 1980s in response to validated outcome studies and social, cultural, and political changes.[11] Patient-therapist collaboration is the cornerstone to patient-centered care. The characteristics of a collaborative relationship include an open and trusting relationship, power sharing, and a willingness to negotiate. Patient-centered care has been associated with increased patient and therapist satisfaction, improved outcome measure scores, and adherence.[12,13] Rothstein and Echternach[4] list the development of the patient-therapist collaborative relationship as a prerequisite to the diagnostic process.

Patient education is an important part of the intervention and must be performed in a collaborative mode. Through the development of the patient-therapist relationship, the therapist must determine the preferred learning style of the patient and reflect this in the method of delivery of the teaching materials. Is the patient a visual learner? Does the patient prefer a cognitive or spiritual approach? Is the patient a minimalist learner, or does the patient require ancillary information?

A common confounding variable impacting teaching is the overestimation the reading and comprehension ability of patients. Recommendations for the presentation of health-related information range from fifth grade to eighth grade reading levels.[14] The use of validated tools such as the Fog index can assist the therapist in determining the reading level of teaching handouts.[15] Educational materials may be presented to the patient in the following ways: orally, handwritten or typed, preprocessed handouts and brochures, custom-made presentations, Web addresses and links, and textbooks. Copies of all teaching materials should be placed in the medical record. Many physical therapists now use telemedicine processes such as live video chats to follow up with patients. Notes should be taken during these sessions and placed in the medical record. In most areas of the United States, financial pressures on the patient, created by higher copays, higher deductibles, and lack of insurance for outpatient rehabilitation services, have added to the importance of teaching and the home program. Many patients cannot afford to attend outpatient therapy three or four times per week. Often the norm of treatment is one visit per week with a comprehensive home program and exercise/performance log with frequent telephone or e-mail communication between the therapist and the patient. The importance of a well-written home program is obvious.

The book *Cognition and Curriculum* by Eisner[16] containing research on cognition has become a significant reference point in debates about teaching and curriculum making in the United States. Perhaps best described as a "cognitive pluralist," Eisner argues that cognition is frequently approached as a phenomenon that deals with knowing rather than feeling. For Eisner, knowledge cannot be just a verbal construct (and constrained by the structures of language). This approach counters the practice of many health care professionals who teach patients only in the verbal domain. Rather, knowledge is an intensely variable and personal "event," something acquired via a combination of one's senses—visual, auditory, tactile, olfactory, gustatory—assembled according to a personal schema and then made public—typically expressed by the same sensory modalities used in the initial acquisition.

Table 15-2 Eisner's Five Philosophical Orientations That Guide Lesson Design

Philosophical Orientation	Definition	Example
Cognitive process	Teaches the patient how to find the data, how to read the data, and how to translate the data to one's personal need. Little emphasis on providing clinical information to the patient. Teaches the patient how to acquire evidence-based data and incorporate it into his or her lifestyle.	A therapist is asked by a patient's family member for information on trigeminal neuralgia. The therapist gives the family member the name of a support group, a website address, and two journal articles. The therapist asks the family member to call the therapist if he has questions.
Academic rationalism	A classic approach to learning. Teaches the "history" of the subject. Little practical application but provides a conceptual framework for understanding the topic.	A patient has a rotator cuff issue. The therapist discusses at length the history of physical therapy intervention for tendonitis: heat, massage, electrical stimulation, interferential therapy, manual therapy. Uses evidence-based language.
Technological	Focuses on practical and technical behaviors to facilitate the patient becoming impairment-free. Home programs, behavioral modification techniques, precautions.	The therapist demonstrates, provides, and allows the patient to demonstrate a home program of exercises for his chronic shoulder pain that includes frequency and duration.
Social adaptation and social reconstruction	Patient teaching with a goal of societal improvement. How may I impact this patient's health in a way that benefits society?	The therapist demonstrates the impact of maintaining a "healthy" hemoglobin A_{1c} to minimize complications related to diabetes and to decrease future health care dollars spent.
Personal relevance	Focuses on what is personally important to the patient. "One of my patients had a similar problem. At home he ..." Used for temporal confidence building, easing anxiety.	"One of my patients had a similar type of surgery ... he is now doing extremely well."

Adapted from Eisner EW. *Cognition and Curriculum: A Basis for Deciding What to Teach.* New York: Longman; 1982.

For health care professionals, the key to developing knowledge within the patient is to create a varied and stimulating environment in which patients become immersed in the subject matter. Therapists also need to encourage patients to try make meaning—to read (or conceptualize) the situation. Patients do this by constructing images derived from the material the senses provide and refining the senses as a primary means for expanding consciousness—translating the data into usable components. Patients require access to the experience of different forms of representation or symbol systems, such as verbal, reading, video, reference sources, and personal experience. Trying to make sense of these, being encouraged to draw on them and play with them, nurtures the imagination and allows patients to be more creative in their responses to the situations in which they find themselves. Patients should also be encouraged to become lifelong learners of their chronic diseases, to search out reputable sources of information and discuss the cogent findings with their health care practitioner.

Eisner's five philosophical orientations that guide lesson design are an extremely important part of the preactive teaching process. Cognitive, academic rationalism, technological, social adaptation and reconstruction, and personal relevance are philosophical orientations that may be employed by the therapist to teach the patient. Based on knowledge gained during the development of the patient-therapist collaborative relationship, the therapist can best define how to present the teaching information to the patient (Table 15-2).

With some peripheral neuropathies, such as those caused by prolonged hyperglycemia or exposure to environmental or medication toxins, the primary therapeutic intervention is to control risk factors. After assessing the patient's learning style, the therapist should use aspects of the Eisner philosophical orientation to guide teaching of home instructions and risk factor modification An example of diabetic neuropathy risk factor modification taught through the cognitive domain may be the therapist providing the patient with a website that provides a discussion of the relationship between an elevated hemoglobin A_{1c} and the progression of neuropathy. The academic rationalism approach may be used to discuss with the patient the history of treatment of diabetes from ancient times to today. The technological approach may be providing information related to insensate foot precautions, daily foot examinations, and a recommendation for monofilament examination every 6 months. The social adaptation and social reconstruction approach may be to discuss the lifetime cost of treating a patient with good diabetes control versus the cost of treating a patient with poor control. Lastly, the therapist may use a personal relevance approach to risk factor modification providing exemplars of good diabetes control in patients.

In many instances, interdisciplinary communication is accomplished through the use of the medical record. President George W. Bush established a goal to have a universal electronic medical record (EMR) by 2014.[17] In 2009, President Obama launched an initiative, the Health Information Technology for Economic and Clinical Health Act, to move the United States from a paper to paperless system of medical documentation (the EMR) beginning with the Department of Veterans Affairs health care system and then expanding to all of the health care continuum.[18]. The bill included a $17.2 billion incentive to assist with funding widespread adoption and "meaningful use" of "certified" EMR technology. The legislation ties the payments specifically to the achievement of advances in health care processes and outcomes. The American Physical Therapy Association cited its support of the electronic health record in physical therapy through a position statement adopted by the House of Delegates in 2008.[19] Proliferation and promotion of the EMR offers many opportunities to enhance clinical efficiency, patient safety, case management, interprofessional dialogue, interfacility dialogue, research, and outcomes assessment. To date, the initiative is progressing slowly because of implementation cost and the difficulty of multiple systems "talking" to each other in a common language. At the present time, in many instances, obtaining a checking account balance from a bank in the United States while on vacation in Europe is much easier than obtaining a medical record from the primary care practitioner if one is hospitalized 10 miles from home.

Direct Intervention: Behavioral Concerns

Patients with peripheral neuropathic diagnoses present with an unusually wide spectrum of behavioral concerns, clinical impairments, functional deficits, pain, and risk factors. In the development of a goal-based treatment plan, each of these areas of potential deficits may become a confounding variable with regard to attainment of treatment goals. This textbook contains chapters addressing each of these areas.

To address behavioral concerns best, the therapist must be aware of the difference between diagnosis and illness. The diagnosis is the cellular component of a pathology resulting in impairment. An intertrochanteric hip fracture diagnosis is defined as a trauma or pathology impacting the area of the femur between the greater and lesser trochanters resulting in loss of bone continuity. The hip fracture illness includes the resultant bed mobility, gait, and transfer dysfunctions; the loss of income because of inability to work; pain; the

transportation burden; and the need for adaptive and assistive equipment. Illness incorporates the functional, social, and behavioral implications of the diagnosis for the patient and the patient's family. Rehabilitation interventions must be directed not only at the diagnosis but also the illness. Each impairment associated with the illness must be designated as a problem and have a corresponding goal and intervention.

A wealth of information exists regarding issues of patients experiencing emotional illness related to neuropathic diagnoses.[20-23] Emotional response to injury or illness is a personal reaction to the illness and varies greatly from individual to individual and from one diagnosis to another.[20] Emotional response may be secondary to pain, impact on the patient's social structure, loss of work, loss of independence, disability, and having a "diagnosis."[21] The frequency of an emotional response to a neuropathic illness or injury that affects the patient's functioning has been estimated to be 50%.[22] The severity of the response to injury or illness may range from minimal to overwhelming. The emotional response to an illness must be identified, noted, and addressed by the treating therapist. Emotional responses, valid or aberrant, have the potential to be a confounding variable in the journey to meet clinical goals.

Most of the research to date uses a cohort of subjects with diabetic peripheral neuropathic pain.[20-22] The primary challenge to patients with neuropathic pain is the management of the condition precipitating the pain, such as blood sugar control in persons with diabetes and inflammation in persons with a rheumatological diagnosis. However, disorders associated with emotional pain, especially depression and anxiety, also greatly complicate the clinician's efforts to attain optimal outcomes for patients with neuropathy. Jain et al.[19] reviewed the high rate of comorbidity between diabetic peripheral neuropathic pain and depression and anxiety with a focus on why this pattern of comorbidity exists and which management tools the clinician can use to assist with goal accomplishment. There are many physiological similarities between neuropathic pain and depression and anxiety, and these are reviewed in Chapter 19. Numerous therapist-assessed and self-reporting tools are available to assist the therapist in identifying an emotional component to the neuropathic diagnosis and the severity of the component. Therapist awareness of these issues assists with program adherence and intervention. Examples include tools associated with neuropathy severity (Toronto Clinical Neuropathy Score), pain quantity and quality (Visual Analogue Scale), pain score (Brief Pain Inventory), quality of life and health status measures (EuroQol Instrument 5 Domains), sleep quantity and quality (Medical Outcomes Sleep Study Scale), anxiety and depression associated with hospital stay (Hospital Anxiety and Depression Scale), and general health and quality of life (Short Form 36 Health Survey and the Health Assessment Questionnaire).[23]

Depression and anxiety are also common comorbidities in patients with peripheral neuropathies secondary to chemotherapy drugs. Medications with side effects of peripheral neuropathy include taxanes, platinum-based drugs, vinca alkaloids, and thalidomide. Chemotherapy-induced peripheral neuropathy may last for months or years after treatment and can affect functional performance and quality of life. Tofthagen[22] investigated the effects of chemotherapy-induced peripheral neuropathy and neuropathic pain on the lives of patients with cancer. Semistructured, private interviews with participants were conducted, and transcripts were reviewed for symptoms and effects. Participants often had difficulty describing neuropathic symptoms but reported simultaneous pain or discomfort and loss of sensation in the upper and lower extremities. Injuries secondary to numbness, muscle weakness, and loss of balance were reported. Neuropathic symptoms interfered with many aspects of daily life, and participants voiced feelings of frustration, depression, and loss of life purpose as a result of inability to perform and participate in enjoyable activities. The results of this study emphasize the importance of ongoing assessment and communication with patients about their experiences with peripheral neuropathies.

Direct Intervention: Clinical Concerns

Direct interventions are selected based on the findings of the evaluation and examination of the patient, diagnosis, prognosis, problem list, patient-therapist collaborative goals, anticipated outcomes, time frames, and anticipated length of service. Direct interventions are performed with or on the patient. Direct intervention and teaching represent the largest segments of patient care provided by rehabilitative therapists (Box 15-1). An intervention is most effective when addressing functional needs that are mutually agreed on by the patient and therapist. The most successful intervention schemas are schemas that combine evidence-based and clinical expertise–based knowledge and experience. The following interventional principles should be incorporated into any comprehensive rehabilitation program.

Principle 1: Control Inflammation and the Downstream Components: Pain, Scarring, Edema, Angiogenesis

High repetition–low force and low repetition–high force injuries to soft tissue result in an immediate migration of macrophages and monocytes to the site of injury. These cells express proinflammatory cytokines that activate the inflammatory cascade. Pain, edema (secondary to increased vascular permeability), angiogenesis, scarring, and other "healing" activities develop at the injured site. Eventually, anti-inflammatory cytokines are expressed that "turn off"

Box 15-1

Intervention Principles

Control inflammation and the downstream components: pain, scarring, edema, angiogenesis
Increase flexibility
Strengthen weakened muscles
Correct posture
Improve movement quality
Analyze and integrate entire kinetic chain
Incorporate neuromuscular rehabilitation
Improve functional outcome
Maintain or improve overall health and fitness
Provide patient education: home program, risk factor modification, knowledge of diagnosis and pathology
Incorporate patient self-management
Ensure a safe return to function to a maximum level of independent function

---

the inflammatory cascade.[23] If pathological activity and irritation continue at the injured site and the inflammatory cascade is left unchecked, chronic pain and disability may result. The rehabilitation therapist has many modalities available that control the downstream effects of the proinflammatory cytokines. These are easily remembered with the mnemonic PRICEMEM: protection, rest, ice, compression, elevation, manual therapy, early motion, and medications.

Protection: Protection is the removal of the offending stimulus. If the offending stimulus is repetitive strain from keyboard typing, this is removed. If the offending stimulus is throwing a baseball, this is removed.

Rest: Rest is the absence of an offending stimulus and not the absence of movement. Prolonged immobilization may have a deleterious impact on bone, ligament, nerve, and muscle. Rest is the prescription of selective motions that will not exacerbate the impairment but allow for normal, or as close to normal as possible, functioning. Rest may be defined as bracing an injured area; wrapping to control edema; non–weight-bearing to protect an injured bone; avoidance of lifting to prevent back pain exacerbation; and avoidance of particular motions, such as overhead shoulder elevation, in persons with venous thoracic outlet syndrome.

Ice: Cold thermal therapies are an important adjunct to controlling the acute inflammatory process and inflammation developed during the therapeutic rehabilitation process.

Compression: Compression, via wrapping, massage, positioning, or a pneumatic device, helps prevent and alleviate edema associated with increased capillary permeability.

Elevation: Used with ice and compression, elevation assists with decreasing edema associated with inflammation. For elevation to be most effective, consider the heart as the fulcrum for the flow of accumulated fluid. For elevation to be most successful as a modality to decrease edema, the edematous part should be elevated above the heart.

Manual therapy: Manual therapy has many positive impacts on inflammation. Stimulation of the large-fiber afferents assists with pain control. The mechanical effect of joint movement assists with regaining joint motion. Prescribed forces and force vectors assist with remodeling of connective tissue. Nerve glides and slides are an important modality in assisting with preventing intraneural and extraneural scarring commonly seen with inflamed peripheral nerves.

Early motion: Early motion is helpful with reducing the muscle atrophy associated with rest, assists with maintaining joint function, and assists with preventing ligamentous "creeping."

Medications: Although not within the realm of physical therapy practices in most locations, the judicious use of steroid and nonsteroidal medications assists with controlling and limiting the inflammatory cascade.

Principle 2: Increase Flexibility

With the scarring that is a consequence of the inflammatory cascade, loss of flexibility—articular, single muscle, two joint muscle, and nerve—is an expected complication of injury. Posture and strength are dependent on proper joint mechanics and range of motion. With a primary peripheral nerve injury, nerve glides and slides within the symptom-free range are of tantamount importance in the rehabilitation plan. Care must be taken when performing articular or muscle stretching to avoid tension to injured neural tissue.

Principle 3: Correct Posture

With injury, the adaptive shortening and lengthening of tissues coupled with protective and painful positioning leads to learning of abnormal, and, if untreated, obligatory, posturing. The restoration of proper posture in standing, sitting, and lying down assists with alleviating abnormal torque and joint positioning on the axial and appendicular systems. "Retraining" correct posture can often be aided by popular therapeutic techniques such as Alexander technique, yoga, Feldenkris, Pilates, and Tai Chi Chuan.

Principle 4: Improve Movement Quality

Byl[24] and Coq et al.[25] showed that peripheral injury may result in alteration of the central maintenance components of motor control leading to a loss of coordination and function. As part of a coordinated plan of intervention, movement quality cannot be ignored. Classic principles of motor acquisition, training, and learning should be employed when there is identified loss of motor control.

Principle 5: Analyze and Integrate the Entire Kinetic Chain

The movement at one joint often depends on the quality of motion and the afferent feedback of the large myelinated afferent sensory fibers from the distal and proximal joints. A comprehensive rehabilitation plan encompassing all links along the kinetic chain improves outcomes. Emerging research indicates improper sequencing and activation of motor responses along the kinetic chain to perturbation may be disease-specific.[26]

Principle 6: Incorporate Neuromuscular Rehabilitation

Neuromuscular rehabilitation is the method of training the enhancement of subconscious motor responses to normal and aberrant perturbations by simultaneously stimulating afferent signals and central mechanisms responsible for dynamic and static motor control. The goal of this therapy is to improve the ability of the central nervous system to sequence, control the amplitude of firing, and use proper agonist/antagonist control of the muscle response to balance loss and postural changes.

Principle 7: Improve Optimal Function

Short-term and long-term rehabilitation goals must be functional, objective, and measurable. To meet this end, clinical interventions must be functionally directed. This emphasis on function is an enhancement of past goals and plans that were written solely to improve metrics such as manual muscle test grade or a degree measurement of articular range of motion. All interventions should include a therapeutic functional progression along with an exercise progression.

Principle 8: Maintain or Improve Overall Fitness and Health

Whenever possible, the treating therapist should address, along with the functional limitation, the downstream impact of risk factors such as inactivity, improper nutrition, tobacco usage, obesity, and an increased fall risk. As a result of the paradigm shift from the Nagy model to the ICF, standards changes from The Joint Commission, and amendments to state practice acts, the scope of rehabilitation therapy services has expanded to include addressing risk factors and practices that may affect health.

Principle 9: Provide Patient Education: Home Program, Risk Factor Modification, Knowledge of Diagnosis, Pathology

Patient-therapist collaboration is the cornerstone of the therapeutic relationship. The therapist and patient work together through the diagnostic journey, the development of mutually agreed-on goals, the spectrum of the treatment plan, and the schedule for reassessment. As part of the intervention, the therapist and patient constantly discuss the path from impairment to health and from disability to functional independence. The therapist helps mold the patient into an educated consumer of health care, and the patient assists with educating the therapist about the patient's perceptions of illness and disability. The patient is taught to self-manage his or her condition and how to prevent reoccurrences. The home program, an extension of the clinical relationship, consists of the exercise prescription, treatment goals and time frames, risk factor modification, and precautions. A trusting therapeutic relationship promotes program adherence.

Principle 10: Incorporate Patient Self-Management

Many of the patients therapists treat have chronic or relapsing conditions. As part of the therapeutic intervention, illness self-management skills are taught to the patient. Self-management skills include disease-specific knowledge of medication, prevention, acute response to exacerbation, healthy lifestyle choices, and intervention.

Principle 11: Ensure a Safe Return to a Maximum Level of Independent Function

A focus of patient teaching is safety. The Joint Commission has taken the lead via the National Patient Safety Goals encouraging the development of safety as a goal for every patient in the United States. From hand washing to fall prevention to documentation standards mandating the identification of at-risk suicidal patients, the National Patient Safety Goals encourage therapists to promote a risk-free assessment and intervention environment.

Principle 12: Coordination of Care

This is a general principle for all persons providing health care. All care, regardless of the provider, must be communicated to the health care stakeholders of the patient. These stakeholders vary by patient and episode of care. In most cases, the primary care physician, as the gatekeeper of the patient's care, should be informed of all therapeutic interventions. In other instances, therapists may need to communicate cogent findings to nurses, specialists, social workers, case managers, insurance companies, and other rehabilitation professionals—all within the scope of patient privacy legislation.

evidence of early chronic kidney disease, elevated cholesterol and triglycerides, a hemoglobin A$_{1c}$ of 8.6, and a blood sugar of 230 mg/dL.

JJ also has a chronic wound on his right heel. A recent ankle-brachial index of the involved ankle was 0.72 indicating a significant level of vascular disease.

Case Study Questions

1. After reading the patient history, the very first thing Kristin should do with this patient is which of the following?
   a. Take his vital signs
   b. Review his medications and dosages
   c. Speak with his primary care physician
   d. Develop a trusting patient-therapist collaborative relationship

2. Which of the following should be considered an illness and not a diagnosis?
   a. Insulin-dependent diabetes mellitus
   b. Peripheral vascular disease
   c. Chronic arterial vascular wound
   d. Inability to work secondary to gait instability

3. In developing a written home program and written educational material for JJ, Kristin should develop these at which grade level?
   a. Undergraduate college
   b. 12th grade
   c. Eighth grade
   d. Second grade

4. The use of specific tests and measures to add to, remove from, and confirm items on the differential diagnosis list is called which of the following?
   a. Hypothesis-oriented algorithm for clinicians
   b. International Classification of Functioning, Disability and Health
   c. Nagy model
   d. Patient-centered model of health care

5. The first principle in the treatment of peripheral nerve injuries is which of the following?
   a. Control pain
   b. Control inflammation
   c. Maintain function
   d. Bracing for rest

CASE STUDY

Kristin is a physical therapist in a hospital-based outpatient practice. Her first patient of the day is JJ, a 40-year-old man with a chief complaint of gait dysfunction secondary to large-fiber afferent sensory neuropathy related to his 15-year history of insulin-dependent diabetes. JJ admits to lack of compliance with his diabetic regimen and medications. Kristin reviewed his most recent laboratory tests and noted

References

1. Carp SJ, Barbe MF, Barr AE. Serum biomarkers as signals for risk and severity of work-related musculoskeletal injury. *Biomark Med.* 2008;2:67–79.
2. International Statistical Classification of Diseases and Related Health Problems: ICD-1. Geneva, Switzerland: World Health Organization; 1992.
3. International Classification of Functioning, Disability and Health: ICF. Geneva, Switzerland: World Health Organization; 1999.

4. Rothstein JM, Echternach JL. Hypothesis-oriented algorithm for clinicians: a method for evaluation and treatment planning. *Phys Ther.* 1986;66:1388–1394.

5. Rothstein JM, Echternach JL. Hypothesis-oriented algorithm for clinicians II (HOAC II): a guide for patient management. *Phys Ther.* 2003;83(5):455–470.

6. Delitto A, Snyder-Mackler L. The diagnostic process: examples in orthopedic physical therapy. *Phys Ther.* 1995;75:203–211.

7. Feder G, Eccles M, Grol R, et al. Clinical guidelines: using clinical guidelines. *BMJ.* 1999;318:728–730.

8. American Physical Therapy Association. Guide to Physical Therapist Practice. Second edition. American Physical Therapy Association. *Phys Ther.* 2001;81(1):9–746.

9. Stanton MW. Expanding patient-centered care to empower patient and assist providers. Publication No. 02-0024. http://archive.ahrq.gov/research/findings/factsheets/patient-centered/ria-issue5/ria-issue5.html. Accessed August 14, 2011.

10. Steiner JF, Earnest MA. The language of medication taking. *Ann Intern Med.* 2000;132:926–930.

11. Hook M. Partnering with patients—a concept ready for action. *J Adv Nurs.* 2006;56:133–143.

12. Wolf DM, Lehman L, Quinlin R, Zullo T, Hoffman L. Effect of patient-centered care on paitent satisfaction and quality of care. *J Nurs Care Qual.* 2008;23:316–321.

13. Fuentes JN, Mislowack A, Bennett J, Paul L, Gilbert TC, Fontan G. The physician-patient working alliance. *Patient Educ Couns.* 2007;66:29–36.

14. Weiss SM, Smith-Siomone SY. Consumer and health literacy: The need to better design tobacco-cessation product packaging, labels, and inserts. *Am J Prev Med* 2010;38(3 Suppl):S403–413.

15. Bogert J. In defense of the Fog index. *Bulletin of the Association for Business Communication.* 1985;48(2):9–11.

16. Eisner EW. *Cognition and Curriculum: A Basis for Deciding What to Teach.* New York: Longman; 1982.

17. Bush GW. 2004 State of the Union Address. January 20, 2004. http://www.c-span.org/Transcripts/SOTU-2004.aspx. Accessed August 14, 2011.

18. American Physical Therapy Association. Support of electronic health record in physical therapy. HOD P06-08-13-11. http://www.APTA.org. Accessed August 14, 2011.

19. Jain R, Jain S, Raison CL, Maletic V. Painful diabetic neuropathy is more than pain alone: examining the role of anxiety and depression as mediators and complicators. *Curr Diab Rep.* 2011;4:275–284.

20. Paliakov I, Toth C. The impact of pain in patients with polyneuropathy. *Eur J Pain.* 2011;15(10):1015–1022.

21. Stankovic Z, Jasovic-Gasic M, Zamaklar M. Psycho-social and clinical variables associated with depression in patients with type 2 diabetes. *Psychiatr Danub.* 2011;23(1):34–44.

22. Tofthagen C. Patient perceptions associated with chemotherapy-induced peripheral neuropathy. *Clin J Oncol Nurs.* 2010;14(3):E22–28.

23. Barbe MF, Barr AE. Inflammation and pathophysiology of work-related musculoskeletal disorders. *Brain Behav Immun.* 2006;20:423–429.

24. Byl NN. Focal hand dystonia: a historical perspective from a clinical scholar. *J Hand Ther.* 2009;22(2):105–108.

25. Coq JO, Barr AE, Strata F, et al. Peripheral and central changes combine to induce motor behavioral deficits in a moderate repetition task. *Exp Neurol.* 2009;220(2):234–245.

26. Horak FB, Imitrova D, Nutt JG. Directional specific postural instability in subjects with Parkinson's disease. *Exp Neurol.* 2005;193:504–521.

Chapter 16

Manual Therapy Techniques for Peripheral Nerve Injuries

SCOTT BURNS, PT, DPT, OCS, FAAOMPT, AND BILL EGAN, PT, DPT, OCS, FAAOMPT

"Healing is a matter of time, but it is sometimes also a matter of opportunity."
—HIPPOCRATES (460 B.C.–370 B.C.)

Objectives

On completion of this chapter, the student/practitioner will be able to:

- Verbalize the concepts of manual therapy.
- Understand the basic techniques of neural mobilization.
- Describe key manual therapy techniques.

Key Words

- Manual therapy
- Neurodynamic tests
- Passive movement

Introduction

Manual therapy encompasses treatment interventions involving the application of skilled **passive movement** techniques. Several types of clinicians are trained in and apply manual therapy, including chiropractors, osteopaths, and physical therapists. There is moderate evidence that manual therapy, when included as part of a multimodal rehabilitation program, is effective in the management of many common musculoskeletal disorders.[1] In the past, manual therapy had mostly focused on interventions targeting joint articulations or soft tissue. Over the past 25 years, manual therapy techniques and systems have emerged that purport to assess and mobilize neural tissue directly.[2] Research in the form of high-quality clinical trials and observational studies investigating the effectiveness of manual therapy for peripheral nerve injuries has also emerged. As a result, clinicians frequently use manual therapy in the management of peripheral nerve injuries. This chapter begins with an overview of concepts related to manual therapy assessment and management directed toward neural tissue and peripheral nerve injuries. For each region, we focus on key manual therapy techniques, especially techniques supported by evidence from the peer-reviewed literature, for common peripheral nerve injuries. Several excellent texts written by experts and pioneers in the field of manual therapy related to neural tissue are available.[2-5] The reader is directed to these texts for further information and more detailed coverage of this topic.

Manual therapy for peripheral nerve injuries begins with the assessment and clinical examination of the patient. For patients with peripheral nerve injuries, the clinician should first perform standard orthopedic and neurological testing to assist with making the diagnosis. Specific to manual therapy, clinicians can examine the joint articulations and soft tissue structures surrounding the injured nerve, also known as the neural tissue interface or neural container. Manual therapy interventions can be directed to impairments of these interfacing tissues as one method of treatment for peripheral nerve injuries. Manual therapists can also attempt to palpate the nerve in question directly, when possible.[6,7] Nerves are not normally sensitive to mechanical pressure, and increased sensitivity can alert the clinician to an underlying disorder.

To help with the examination and diagnosis of peripheral nerve injuries, clinicians can use tests and positions that selectively apply tension to particular peripheral nerves based on anatomical and biomechanical principles. These tests have been referred to as neural tension tests and more recently as **neurodynamic tests.**[2] The term "neurodynamic" has been used to reflect that these tests are not simply an assessment of the length or flexibility of the nerve, but rather assess the sliding and gliding of the nerve within its interfacing tissues. The most commonly known and used neurodynamic test is the straight leg raise. The straight leg raise increases the tension applied to the lower lumbar nerve roots and sciatic nerve and is used in the assessment of lumbar radiculopathy. If the clinician finds a limitation of movement with the neural tension test compared with the uninvolved side or the test directly reproduces the patient's symptoms, the test is considered positive.[8] A positive neural tension test, in isolation, does not indicate a peripheral nerve injury. It is also well recognized that in certain pain disorders, such as whiplash-associated disorders, there is a frequent occurrence of central pain sensitization.[9] Central pain sensitization can lead to false-positive test results, including neural tension tests.[10]

Aside from mobilizing the interfacing tissues, the manual therapist can also attempt to mobilize the nerve directly with either passive or active interventions. The neurodynamic test position frequently is used to initiate the intervention. Techniques for directly mobilizing nerves can be performed as a static or prolonged hold or in an oscillatory fashion known as neural flossing or gliding. The latter techniques are recommended at first, especially in the management of acute nerve injuries, because there is less potential for further damage to the nerve or irritation of the patient's condition compared with static stretching of an injured nerve. When a nerve is elongated, there is a decrease in the nerve's vascular supply because of the "wringing-out" effect occurring during elongation of the nerve and nerve bed.[3] Neural mobilization techniques can be further classified based on the intent of the technique. Techniques that place tension or stretch on both the distal and the proximal end are known as "tensioners."[11] Techniques that place tension on one end of the nerve while simultaneously releasing or slackening the other end of the nerve are known as "sliders." In vitro and in vivo studies have shown that sliders cause a greater excursion of the nerve throughout its interfacing tissues.[11] Conversely, tensioners place a greater strain on the nerve. It is recommended that neural mobilization techniques begin with sliders given the less strain and greater excursion of the nerve. Combined manual therapy techniques can also be performed in which the interfacing tissue is mobilized while the nerve is placed in stretch or while the neural tissue is actively or passively mobilized. Specific examples of the various types of manual therapy techniques for peripheral nerve injuries are described throughout this chapter.

The mechanisms of how manual therapy techniques produce beneficial effects such as a reduction in pain and improvement in function are poorly understood. The mechanical effect of manual therapy has been the predominant theory for many years, including the notion that displaced joint articulations can be realigned or put back in place. Similarly, it was thought that neural mobilization techniques had their beneficial effects from stretching shortened neural tissue, releasing scarring and adhesions around injured nerve, or improving the gliding of the nerve within its interfacing tissues. Current research concerning the mechanisms of manual therapy now supports alternative theories.[12] Pain modulation through either peripherally or centrally mediated nervous system effects is now thought to be the predominant mechanism by which manual therapy acts. Nonspecific effects, such as the patient's expectations, the patient-provider relationship, and the placebo effect, cannot be ignored because they have been shown to be powerful modulators of the clinical outcome.[13] Manual therapy interventions are rarely used in isolation. Most research has shown that manual therapy is most effective when combined with a multimodal program involving active and patient-centered interventions such as education, advice, and exercise.[14]

Common Disorders

Cervical Radiculopathy

Cervical radiculopathy is defined as a lesion or disease of the cervical nerve root and is most often attributed to cervical disc herniation or spondylosis.[15] The prevalence of cervical radiculopathy has been estimated at 3.3 per 1,000 cases with the peak incidence in the fourth or fifth decade of life.[16] Men are typically more affected with cervical radiculopathy than women.[17] Cervical radiculopathy commonly manifests with upper extremity pain or paresthesias, neck pain, headaches, or scapulothoracic region pain.[18]

The diagnosis of cervical radiculopathy is traditionally made with magnetic resonance imaging (MRI)[19,20] or electromyography.[21,22] The shortcomings of the diagnostic utility of imaging in spinal conditions when used in isolation has been well documented, and clinicians should also use an accurate clinical examination to diagnose cervical radiculopathy.[15] Wainner et al.[23] identified a test item cluster of four variables for the diagnosis of cervical radiculopathy. The four variables include the Spurling test, neck distraction test, upper limb neurodynamic test with median nerve bias, and ipsilateral cervical rotation of 60° or less. The presence of all four of these variables yields a positive likelihood ratio of 30.3, which shifts the post-test probability of cervical radiculopathy being present on electromyography to 90%. In the study by Wainner et al.,[23] the supine upper limb neurodynamic test with median nerve bias was best at ruling out the presence of cervical radiculopathy with a sensitivity of 97%. Additional findings on the physical examination that are associated with cervical radiculopathy include diminished deep tendon reflexes, sensory deficits, and motor weakness.[24]

Manual therapy interventions in the management of cervical radiculopathy frequently include manipulation of the cervical and thoracic spine regions (Fig. 16-1).[25–28] Manipulation of the thoracic spine region is recommended as the initial intervention to avoid potential exacerbation of the radiculopathy from techniques targeting the cervical spine (Fig. 16-2).

There is moderate evidence for the effectiveness of thoracic spine manipulation in the treatment of neck pain including radiculopathy.[18,25,27,28] In a case series, Cleland et al.[29] reported 91% of patients experienced

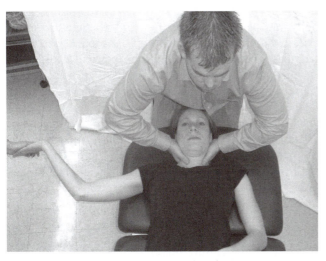

Figure 16-1 Cervical lateral glide manual mobilization.

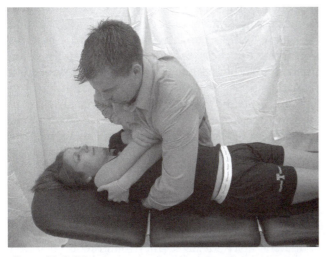

Figure 16-2 Thoracic spine thrust manipulation in supine.

clinically meaningful improvements in pain and function at 6-month follow-up. The patients were treated using a multimodal approach including cervical lateral glides in upper limb neurodynamic test position, thoracic spine manipulation, intermittent mechanical traction, and deep neck flexor strengthening. In another case series, 83% of patients had significant reduction in disability scores following a multimodal treatment approach including intermittent cervical traction, thoracic spine manipulation, and deep neck flexor strengthening.[30]

Intermittent cervical traction has been advocated in the treatment of patients with cervical radiculopathy.[26,31] Raney et al.[26] identified predictive variables of patients who will respond favorably to cervical traction and exercise. In this trial, 68 patients received six sessions of intermittent cervical traction and strengthening exercises (two times per week for 3 weeks). Of the subjects, 44% reported a perceived recovery of "a great deal better" or "a very great deal better." Five predictive variables were identified, including peripheralization of lower cervical (C4–7) with mobility testing, positive shoulder abduction test, age 55 years or older, positive upper limb neurodynamic test with median nerve bias, and positive neck distraction test. A positive upper limb neurodynamic test with median nerve bias and a positive neck distraction test are included in the test-item cluster for detecting the presence of cervical radiculopathy.[23] The age of the patient and peripheralization of symptoms with mobility testing of C4–7 correlate to other signs and symptoms that may be related to cervical radiculopathy.[16]

Young et al.[32] investigated the outcomes of a manual therapy and exercise approach with or without intermittent cervical traction. The study comprised 81 patients randomly assigned into one of two groups. Group 1 included manual therapy, exercise, and intermittent cervical traction, whereas group 2 included manual therapy, exercise, and sham cervical traction. The manual therapy techniques used in this study were either thrust or nonthrust techniques directed to the upper and middle thoracic spine. In addition to the thoracic techniques, at least one nonthrust mobilization was directed at the cervical spine. The cervical spine nonthrust techniques included retraction, rotations, and lateral glides in the upper limb neurodynamic position or posterior-to-anterior mobilizations. In this trial, the therapist was able to choose the manual therapy techniques based on patient response and centralization or reduction of symptoms. The exercises included in this trial featured deep neck flexion, scapular stabilization, and cervical retraction or extension. At least one of the exercises was used during the treatment session. The subjects in group 1 also received mechanical intermittent cervical traction for 15 minutes with the on/off cycle set at 50/10. The traction force started at 20 pounds or 10% of the patient's body weight, whichever was less. The force was progressively increased by 2 to 5 pounds each visit. Both groups experienced clinically meaningful improvements in pain and function at immediate-term and short-term follow-up, but there were no differences between groups.

There is a moderate amount of evidence to support the use of manual therapy techniques directed to the cervical or thoracic spine in patients with cervical radiculopathy.[18,25,27,28,30] Several studies demonstrate the effectiveness of intermittent cervical traction[26,30,31]; however, when intermittent cervical traction was combined with manual therapy and exercise, there were no significant differences.[18]

Thoracic Outlet Syndrome

Thoracic outlet syndrome (TOS) describes a constellation of upper extremity symptoms that occur when the neurovascular structures that pass through the thoracic outlet become compressed.[33] Three main types of TOS have been identified: neurogenic, venous, and arterial.[33,34] In this chapter, we focus on neurogenic TOS because it involves the peripheral nervous system. Neurogenic TOS accounts for nearly 95% of all cases[33] and occurs when the nerve roots of the brachial plexus become entrapped as they course through the triangle formed by the first rib and the anterior and middle scalene muscles. There are two variations of neurogenic TOS: "true" and "disputed" or symptomatic.[34,35] True neurogenic TOS is rare and typically manifests with clinical findings isolated within the C8–T1 dermatome.[34] Disputed or symptomatic neurogenic TOS accounts for nearly 90% of TOS-related surgeries in the United States.[36] Disputed neurogenic TOS may be associated with a traumatic onset or the presence of a cervical rib.

Clinical signs of neurogenic TOS include pain or weakness in the neck, shoulder, or upper extremity[34]; altered scapular or glenohumeral position and strength; presence of a cervical rib; and possibly traumatic onset.[34,35] Terao et al.[37] reported that in patients with TOS the inclination of the clavicle on the involved side is 3° lower compared with the uninvolved side. Another useful clinical examination tool is the cervical rotation lateral flexion (CRLF) test to assess for an elevated first rib, which may apply pressure on the neurovascular bundle.[38] The CRLF test begins with the patient in the seated position. The examiner passively rotates the head away from the affected side and then flexes the neck toward the sternum. The test is considered positive if there is a noticeable decrease in range of motion (ROM) combined with a hard end-feel. A positive CRLF test may warrant manual therapy techniques directed at the first rib in patients with TOS.[39]

TOS may have several different clinical manifestations. Given that there are several different variations without clear diagnostic criteria, the literature is difficult to interpret. Caution is required when generalizing treatments to all patients with TOS. There is relatively little consensus on the appropriate management of patients with TOS.[33,35,40] General management strategies include postural education, relaxation exercises, manual therapy, and active exercise programs.[39,41]

There is little evidence for the use of manual therapy techniques in the management of TOS.[39,41] Hooper et al.[39,42] provide an excellent review of pathology, examination, and management of patients with TOS. These authors recommend the use of first rib mobilization techniques, glenohumeral mobilization, manual scalene stretch, and neural mobilization.[39] Additionally, the patient is instructed in self-mobilization techniques of the involved first rib. Smith[40] advocated for use of manual therapy techniques directed at the shoulder girdle and sternoclavicular joint, manual stretching of the scalene and pectoral muscles, scapular mobilization, and mobilization of the ipsilateral first and second ribs in the management of patients with TOS. Smith[40] described a treatment protocol including manual therapy techniques in conjunction with postural and body mechanics re-education and therapeutic exercises. Manual therapy techniques aimed at restoring scapula-humeral rhythm and proper scapular kinematics have also been recommended.[35] In a case series, Buonocore et al.[43] reported that a program using massage and manual cervical traction techniques resulted in the abolishment of all resting symptoms in 13 patients with TOS. Revel and Amor[44] reported 76% of patients had excellent to good outcomes with a multimodal approach including massage techniques directed at the cervicothoracic region and passive mobilizations of the upper quarter.

Lateral Epicondylalgia

Although more commonly known as lateral epicondylitis and tennis elbow, lateral epicondylalgia is a more appropriate term because there are no inflammatory cells associated with the condition.[45,46] Occasionally, lateral elbow pain results from or is partially attributed to entrapment neuropathies of the radial nerve around the elbow such as radial tunnel syndrome. Clinicians can assess for these entrapment neuropathies using standard neurological testing and nerve conduction velocity and electromyography studies. Clinicians can also use a neurodynamic test for the radial nerve to assist with the diagnosis of radial tunnel syndrome or involvement of the radial nerve in patients with lateral elbow pain. The diagnostic accuracy of this test for radial nerve entrapment has not been studied. The test is considered positive if there is restricted ROM compared with the uninvolved side or if the test reproduces the patient's chief complaint. Yaxley and Jull[47] assessed the radial nerve tension test in 20 patients with unilateral lateral epicondylalgia. They found reduced ROM with the test in the involved arm compared with the uninvolved arm in all patients. Additionally, 55% of the patients' symptoms were reproduced with the test. The authors postulated that irritation of the radial nerve could be a source or contributing factor to the symptoms of lateral epicondylalgia.

If the radial neurodynamic test is positive, clinicians can consider mobilization of the radial nerve as either an active or a passive treatment intervention. Clinicians can also use manual therapy techniques directed toward the cervical spine, thoracic spine, elbow, and wrist to address impairments of the tissues interfacing with the radial nerve. There is no high-quality research supporting the effectiveness of neural mobilization techniques in the management of lateral epicondylalgia or radial nerve entrapment. In a case report, Ekstrom and Holden[48] described a patient with a 4-month history of lateral elbow pain. The patient had a positive radial nerve tension test, and the authors attributed her symptoms to mild entrapment of the radial nerve. A multimodal program including radial nerve mobilization was successful in relieving the patient's symptoms.

Cubital Tunnel Syndrome

Cubital tunnel syndrome is the second most common upper extremity nerve compression syndrome after carpal tunnel syndrome (CTS),[49] with an annual incidence estimated at 0.8%.[50] Originally described in 1954 by Feindel and Stratford,[51] cubital tunnel syndrome typically manifests with medial elbow pain, sensory complaints within the ulnar nerve distribution of the hand, and possibly weakness. In severe cases, wasting of the intrinsic musculature of the hand may be present.[49] Initially, symptoms tend to be intermittent in nature, but as severity increases they may become constant.

A thorough history and assessment of risk factors is key in the clinical diagnostic process of cubital tunnel syndrome. Several risk factors have been identified for individuals who develop cubital tunnel syndrome. Cubital tunnel syndrome has been estimated to affect up to 64% of individuals whose primary occupation involves computer or repetitive related tasks as well as musicians.[52] Descatha et al.[50] followed 600 subjects for 3 years to determine predictive variables for individuals most likely to develop cubital tunnel syndrome. "Holding a tool in position" (odds ratio, 4.1; confidence interval, 1.4 to 12.0) and obesity (odds ratio, 4.3; confidence interval, 1.2 to 16.2) were the only predictive factors identified. The presence of medial epicondylitis, CTS, radial tunnel syndrome, or cervicobrachial neuralgia also increased the chances of developing cubital tunnel syndrome. Electrodiagnostic testing is a common method of diagnosing cubital tunnel syndrome. Four commonly used provocative tests performed during physical examination include Tinel's sign, elbow flexion, direct pressure to the area, and elbow flexion plus direct pressure.[53] Elbow flexion coupled with direct manual pressure over the ulnar nerve at the cubital tunnel has a sensitivity of 91% making it the best screening test.

Common nonsurgical interventions for cubital tunnel syndrome include bracing, activity modification, night splinting, and patient education.[49] Surgery is recommended only for severe or recalcitrant cases. Svernlöv et al.[54] performed a high-quality randomized trial for the conservative treatment of cubital tunnel syndrome. They randomly assigned 70 patients with mild to moderate cubital tunnel syndrome, based on clinical findings, into three groups. The three groups were night splinting, active neural gliding exercises, and a control group. All three groups received advice and education about the condition and ways to modify activities to avoid placing strain on the ulnar nerve. At 6-month follow-up, 90% of the patients were improved with no differences between groups on any outcome measures. This study speaks to the self-limiting nature of this condition; most patients with mild to moderate symptoms can experience improvement with simple advice. Manual therapy is an option in the management of cubital tunnel syndrome, although there is limited evidence at this time. In a case series of seven patients with mild to moderate cubital tunnel syndrome, Oskay et al.[55] reported significant reductions in pain, provocative testing, and disability in a treatment program that included neural mobilizations and traditional physical interventions. These results were maintained over a 12-month follow-up. In a case report, Coppieters et al.[56] described an impairment-based approach including manual therapy and neural mobilizations. In this case, a 17-year-old student had a traumatic onset of cubital tunnel syndrome. She presented with medial elbow pain, symptoms in the ulnar nerve distribution, negative electrodiagnostic testing, and cervicothoracic segmental dysfunctions. The patient was treated for 6 sessions consisting of neural gliding, cervicothoracic thrust, and nonthrust manipulation, with an additional home exercise program. The home exercise program consisted of neural gliding and strengthening exercises. The patient reported no pain or disability at 6-week and 10-month follow-up evaluations.

Carpal Tunnel Syndrome

CTS is the most common peripheral neuropathy in the upper extremity with an estimated prevalence of 3.8%.[57] The diagnosis of CTS is typically made with electrodiagnostic testing; however, clinical diagnosis is possible. Wainner et al.[58] developed a clinical prediction rule to assist in the clinical identification of CTS. They identified five predictor variables, including shaking of the hands for relief, wrist ratio index greater than 0.67, Symptom Severity Scale score greater than 1.9, age older than 45 years, and diminished sensation over the thumb (median nerve distribution). The presence of all five variables yielded a positive likelihood ratio of 18.3, which shifts the post-test probability to 90% for the diagnosis of CTS. In this study, electrophysiological testing was used as the reference standard. The wrist ratio index is the measurement of the anteroposterior wrist width divided by the mediolateral wrist width. This value has been purported to estimate the size of the carpal canal with larger ratios (greater than 0.70) predisposing individuals to CTS.[59] Additional impairments have been associated with patients with CTS including forward head posture and decreased cervical ROM.[60]

Treatment of CTS may range from conservative care to surgical management. Numerous interventions have shown short-term efficacy in the conservative management of CTS.[61] There is strong to moderate evidence for oral steroids, steroid injections, ultrasound, electromagnetic field therapy, night splints, and ergonomic modifications.[62] Emerging evidence has demonstrated the possible efficacy of manual therapy in the treatment of patients with CTS.[63–67] Manual therapy techniques used in CTS include neural mobilizations, carpal bone mobilization, and soft tissue mobilization.

Neural mobilization is a form of manual therapy in which forces are directed at nervous tissue.[68] Coppetiers and Butler[11] outline two separate neural mobilization techniques termed "sliders" or "tensioners." "Sliders" refers to gliding the nerve through its sheath by selectively placing the joints in certain positions. "Tensioners" refers to keeping one end of the nerve fixed and then placing the joints in position to produce tension within the nerve. The two separate techniques apply different amounts of strain or excursion through the nerve. A "tensioning" technique produces roughly 50% of the excursion and nearly seven times the amount of strain on the nerve compared with a "sliding" technique.[11] In systematic reviews regarding the efficacy of neural mobilization, the results are often inconclusive regarding clinical outcomes[69]; however, typically only tensioning techniques were included, and most often these techniques were part of an exercise program. In a clinical trial, 40 female subjects were randomly assigned to receive manual neurodynamic tensioning mobilizations or a sham treatment.[68] At 3 weeks, the temporal summation of the ulnar nerve was reduced, indicating a possible neurophysiological effect of tensioning neurodynamic mobilizations. The outcomes of the two groups in this study did not differ in terms of pain or disability. In this study, neural mobilization using "tensioning" techniques produced an effect on the nervous system as detected by quantitative sensory testing; however, there was no change in clinical outcomes compared with sham. It is unclear what effect sliding techniques have on clinical outcomes or neurophysiological parameters. The equivocal evidence regarding the use of neural mobilizations in this population may be due partly to the heterogeneity of the application of the techniques.[69]

Other manual therapy techniques, such as carpal bone mobilizations or soft tissue techniques, are purportedly effective in patients with CTS. Tal-Akabi and Rushton[64] compared the results of neural mobilization, carpal bone mobilization, and no treatment in patients with CTS. In this study, both neural mobilization and carpal bone mobilization produced better outcomes compared with no treatment. There was no significant difference between the two intervention groups. Surgical interventions ultimately were performed in 85% of the patients in the control group compared with 28% and 14% of patients in the neural and carpal bone mobilization groups, respectively. Moraska et al.[66] compared general massage to the upper quadrant versus targeted massage therapy to the potential median nerve entrapment sites of the upper extremity. Targeted massage resulted in a 17.3% increase in grip strength compared with 4.8% for general massage. Some providers advocated for the use of instrumented soft tissue mobilization techniques. Burke et al.[63] investigated instrumented soft tissue mobilization compared with traditional soft tissue mobilization implemented by the clinician's hands. The authors concluded that there was no difference in outcomes with the two techniques.

Given that patients with CTS exhibit greater forward head posture and decreased cervical spine ROM, it seems plausible that a treatment approach targeting the cervical and thoracic spine may be useful. A study reported that 48.6% of female patients with CTS reported a successful outcome immediately following a manual therapy treatment program including targeted soft tissue mobilization techniques, lateral cervical glides, and manual sliding neural mobilization techniques.[70] In this study, success was defined at a perceived recovery rating of +5 or greater on the Global Rating of Change scale, which represents a "quite a bit better" rating or greater by the patient. Another case study reported a complete recovery of pain and disability using thrust manipulation techniques that targeted the cervical spine and elbow over a 4-week period. The role of manual therapy in the management of CTS appears promising; however, more high-quality trials are required to determine the effectiveness of manual therapy techniques in this population.

Lumbar Radiculopathy

Lumbar radiculopathy is a common peripheral nerve injury in the lower quarter region.[71] In patients younger than age 50, lumbar radiculopathy usually arises secondary to lumbar herniated discs. In patients older than 50, radiculopathy is more commonly associated with degenerative lateral canal stenosis. Some clinicians distinguish between lumbar radiculitis involving leg or nerve root pain only versus radiculopathy that involves leg pain with neurological signs. The clinical diagnosis of lumbar radiculopathy is associated with lancinating leg pain; loss of sensation, reflexes, and motor function; and positive nerve root tension signs.[72] With radiculopathy, the patient's pain distribution does not always follow the classic dermatomal distribution.[73] The straight leg–raise test is the most commonly used clinical test in the assessment of lumbar radiculopathy. However, this test is more applicable to rule out a radiculopathy because it is a sensitive test but not very specific. Although the methodological quality of studies investigating this test is poor, the well or crossed straight leg–raise test is purported to have greater specificity to help rule in radiculopathy. Similarly, the neurological tests of sensation, reflexes, and motor function help to rule in a radiculopathy but do not serve as adequate screening tests for radiculopathy because of their low sensitivity. The most commonly affected nerve roots in lumbar radiculopathy are the L4–S1 nerve roots. Upper lumbar radiculopathies are rare—their recognition should alert the clinician to the possibility of a space-occupying lesion, such as metastatic cancer.

Physical therapy management of lumbar radiculopathies frequently consists of traction, manual therapy, and exercise. As with other regions, interventions can be directed toward treating the neural interface, directly mobilizing neural tissue, or a combination of both. Evidence for conservative or manual therapy management of lumbar radiculopathy is scarce. A systematic review of literature addressing conservative management of a lumbar radiculopathy resulting from lumbar herniated disc revealed moderate to weak evidence in favor of traction, manipulation, and stabilization exercises.[74] Highlights of some of the higher quality research in support of manual therapy for lumbar radiculopathy follow.

Mechanical diagnosis and therapy (MDT), also known as the McKenzie method, is widely used throughout the world in the management of spinal conditions.[75] With this method, clinicians ask patients to perform movements of the spine including static, single, and repeated movements in various planes of motion while assessing the patient's signs and symptoms (Fig. 16-3).

The key sign associated with MDT is the centralization phenomenon. Centralization is defined as a retreat of the patient's symptoms in a distal-to-proximal fashion that occurs during testing and remains afterward.[76] An example is in a patient with an S1 radiculopathy who performs repeated lumbar extension in standing. If the pain was reported in the calf region at baseline and retreated proximally to the buttock region during the exercise and stayed in the buttock region after the completion of the testing, the patient's symptoms would be classified as centralized. With this intervention, the patient is prescribed exercises with the addition of manual therapy procedures as needed

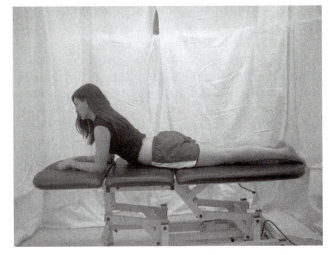

Figure 16-3 Prone lumbar extension exercise.

in the direction that achieved centralization. Patients are also educated about how to avoid positions during their daily activities that cause their radicular symptoms to worsen or move toward the periphery. The importance of the centralization sign is that patients who achieve centralization have a more favorable prognosis in terms of recovery of function, decreased pain, and return to work status compared with patients who do not achieve centralization.[76] MDT and directional exercise have been studied for patients with low back pain, and the results have been favorable compared with control groups. Despite these findings, MDT and directional exercise have not been specifically studied in patients with lumbar radiculopathy.[77] Nevertheless, it is recommended that repeated directional motion testing be completed in patients presenting with lumbar radiculopathy before considering other interventions. If the patient's symptoms centralize, exercises and manual therapy procedures into the direction that produced centralization should be used because of the favorable prognosis.[77] Not all patients with lumbar radiculopathy achieve centralization with directional exercises, and the exact percentage of patients who can be classified as achieving centralization varies widely across studies.

Fritz et al.[78] performed a prospective randomized controlled trial investigating the use of an extension-oriented exercise treatment compared with the same treatment with the addition of mechanical lumbar traction. The study enrolled 64 patients 19 to 60 years old with clinical signs of lumbar radiculopathy. Both groups received the extension-oriented treatment consisting of instruction in repeated lumbar extension exercises in standing and prone and lumbar posterior-to-anterior nonthrust manipulation. Patients were instructed as needed to shift their pelvis laterally during the exercises to promote extension. Therapists could also apply overpressure while the patient performed prone extension to promote extension ROM. Patients were instructed to perform the extension exercises every 4 to 5 hours at home in addition to receiving supervised treatment in the clinic. Patients were also told to maintain a neutral lumbar lordosis throughout their daily activities and to avoid lumbar flexion. This treatment was provided a maximum of nine times over a 1-week period. The traction group received mechanical lumbar traction in a prone position. Traction was performed on a three-dimensional adjustable traction table with a traction force 40% to 60% of the patients' body weight for 12 minutes. Clinicians adjusted the force and the direction of the traction to achieve centralization of the patients' symptoms. Patients in the traction group received 12 treatments over a 6-week period including traction four times per week during the first 2 weeks. At the 2-week and 6-week follow-up evaluations, both groups achieved clinically and statistically significant improvement in pain and function with no difference between groups. Further subgroup analysis found that patients who had a positive crossed straight leg–raise test or had symptom peripheralization with lumbar extension had substantially better outcomes if they received traction. Patients who achieved centralization with extension achieved clinically and statistically better outcomes regardless of group assignment. A larger prospective study is under way to investigate this question further, but the results suggest that a subgroup of patients with lumbar radiculopathy benefit from traction.[79]

McMorland et al.[80] compared spinal thrust manipulation with microdiskectomy in a group of patients with lumbar radiculopathy secondary to lumbar disc herniation. Patients were included if they had symptoms for at least 3 months' duration and had failed conservative treatment, positive neurological findings, and MRI findings consistent with lumbar disc herniation. There were 20 patients randomly assigned to the spinal manipulation group consisting of a lumbar thrust manipulation in side-lying, education, and participation in a core stabilization program and 20 patients randomly assigned to receive a microdiskectomy. At 6 weeks after surgery, the patients were provided with a similar education and exercise program as the manipulation group. At 12-week follow-up evaluation, both groups had achieved clinically and statistically significant improvement in pain and function with no difference between the groups. Of the 20 patients in the manipulation group, 8 eventually crossed over to surgery. Although this was considered a pilot study, the results are interesting in that some patients who had failed other forms of nonsurgical care were able to benefit from spinal manipulation. It has been proposed that radiculopathy, including positive neurological findings, is a contraindication to manipulation or that these patients do not benefit from manipulation (see Fig. 16-4).[81] This study showed that some patients

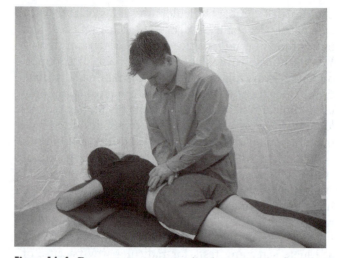

Figure 16-4 Posterior-to-anterior lumbar manual mobilization.

could potentially benefit with a low risk of harm. The authors of the study were careful to position the patients so as not to cause peripheralization of the patient's symptoms during the manipulation. We support this idea and attempt manipulation in patients with lumbar radiculopathy only if the position and techniques can be accomplished without peripheralizing the patient's symptoms.

Patients older than 50 years of age who have lumbar radiculopathy are more likely to have degenerative lateral canal stenosis compared with lumbar disc herniation. There are few high-quality trials investigating conservative treatment for patients with lumbar spinal stenosis. Rates of surgery, including spinal fusion, for lumbar spinal stenosis have been steadily increasing over the past decade.[82] Given the frequent comorbidities in older adults with spinal stenosis, complications arising from surgery have been increasing as well. Effective nonsurgical management options for patients with spinal stenosis are crucial. In a high-quality randomized controlled trial, Whitman et al.[83] compared an exercise-based physical therapy program with a multimodal physical therapy program. These investigators randomly assigned 58 patients with lumbar spinal stenosis to receive supervised flexion-oriented exercises plus a level walking program or manual therapy, exercises, and an unloaded treadmill walking program. Manual therapy was individually tailored and targeted the impairments found during the examination (Fig. 16-5).

Techniques included lumbar thrust and nonthrust manipulation and procedures aimed at improving hip mobility. Exercise was designed to promote lumbar spine flexion, lumbar core stabilization, and hip muscle flexibility. Groups received in-clinic treatment two times per week for 6 weeks and were prescribed a home exercise program. Both groups achieved clinically and

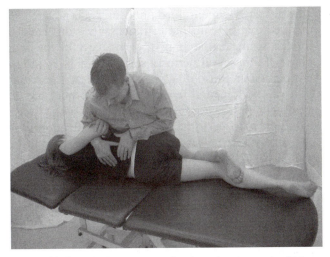

Figure 16-5 Side-lying rotary lumbar thrust manipulation.

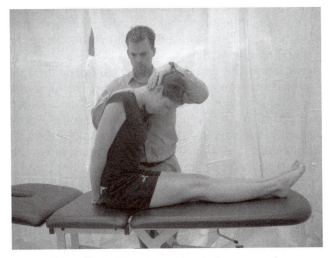

Figure 16-6 Clinician-assisted slump stretch.

statistically meaningful improvement in pain and function at 6-week and 1-year follow-up evaluations, with the multimodal physical therapy group achieving significantly better outcomes. It is difficult to separate the effects of the manual therapy from the other interventions in this study. In our opinion, key manual therapy techniques for patients with lumbar radiculopathy resulting from lumbar stenosis include lumbar manipulation (thrust or nonthrust) and hip stretching/mobilization. It is important during these procedures to ensure that the patient's symptoms do not peripheralize during the technique.

Few studies have investigated the effects of direct neural mobilization in patients with lumbar radiculopathy. Cleland et al.[84] performed a pilot randomized controlled trial comparing slump stretching with stabilization exercises for 30 patients with low back and leg pain (Fig. 16-6).

Patients who met the inclusion criteria for the study had low back pain with symptoms distal to the buttocks and a positive slump test. Patients were excluded if they had positive neurological findings or a positive straight leg raise of less than 45°. Also, patients could not show signs of peripheralization or centralization during repeated directional lumbar ROM testing. Patients in both groups received standardized lumbar stabilization exercises and posterior-to-anterior nonthrust manipulation directed to the lumbar spine two times per week for 3 weeks. Patients in the slump stretching group also received passive stretching in the slump position for five bouts of 30 seconds in addition to performing this exercise at home for two bouts of 30 seconds per day. Both groups achieved improvement in pain and function at the completion of the study, but the slump stretching group achieved clinically and statistically greater improvements. The slump stretch group showed a greater degree of centralization of leg symptoms at the end of the treatment. The patients in this study did not have acute radiculopathy, and their symptoms did not change with repeated motion testing. The patients in this study represent a subgroup of patients with chronic leg pain that likely started as an acute radiculopathy. Proponents of neural mobilization have recommended that exercises or passive treatments do not begin with procedures that place tension on the nerve at both the proximal and the distal ends,[85] particularly in the acute phase where performing "tensioners" could have an adverse effect because of the decrease in blood circulation while in the fully stretched position. It is recommended that patients initially perform gentle neural "flossing" exercises in an oscillatory fashion.

Piriformis Syndrome

Piriformis syndrome is a controversial diagnosis because of the commonality of signs and symptoms between piriformis syndrome and other conditions, particularly lumbar radiculopathy. There is currently no accepted standard for the clinical diagnosis of piriformis syndrome, and it remains a diagnosis of exclusion. Piriformis syndrome is thought to arise from anatomical anomalies where the sciatic nerve pierces the piriformis muscle or from indirect compression of the sciatic nerve in the region of the piriformis caused by trauma or repetitive strain.[86] Clinicians should examine the lumbar, sacroiliac, and hip joint regions before ruling in piriformis syndrome as a potential diagnosis. Repeated lumbar movement testing as mentioned earlier should be conducted in attempts to find directions that either centralize or peripheralize the patient's pain. If the patient's symptoms can be centralized with repeated lumbar movement, the diagnosis of piriformis syndrome is unlikely. Tests that purportedly rule in piriformis syndrome as a diagnosis include the flexion, adduction, internal rotation (FAIR) test, straight leg raise, and direct palpation of the piriformis muscle belly.[87] For the FAIR test, the patient is in side-lying and the clinician passively flexes, adducts, and internally rotates with patient's top leg. The test is positive if it reproduces symptoms in the piriformis region. A systematic review of the literature reported that the following signs were most common among studies investigating the diagnosis of piriformis syndrome: buttock pain, external tenderness over the greater sciatic notch, aggravation of the pain through sitting, and augmentation of the pain with maneuvers that increase piriformis muscle tension.[86] Nonrandomized, observational studies reported some benefit from the injection of the piriformis muscle with botulinum toxin to reduce muscle spasms and relieve pressure on the sciatic nerve.[88] High-quality trials of physical and manual therapy interventions are lacking. General strategies include stretching and direct mobilization of the piriformis muscle. In addition to treating the muscle, sciatic neural mobilization using neural flossing or exercises could be attempted. A case report in the literature indicates that a possible cause of piriformis syndrome is motor control dysfunction of the lower extremity whereby the hip and femur on the affected side excessively adducts and internally rotates during functional activities.[89] In theory, this movement dysfunction places strain on the piriformis muscle which is an external rotator of the hip. In the case report, correction of this dysfunction with movement re-education and strengthening exercises for the hip external rotators and gluteal muscles was beneficial for the patient.

Hamstring Strains

Although hamstring injuries predominantly involve muscle strain from sudden high-velocity eccentric contraction of the hamstrings during athletic activities, there have been reports in the literature of sciatic nerve involvement.[90] During the injury, the sciatic nerve could become overstretched resulting in a tension neuropathy. Additionally, the acute inflammatory response in the region of the injured muscle tissue could lead to bleeding and scarring around the sciatic nerve. It has also been proposed that lumbar spine dysfunction, either as a predisposing factor or as a result of the injury, is associated with hamstring injury, and the lumbar dysfunction could result in concomitant sciatica.[91] It has been recommended that all patients with hamstring injuries receive an evaluation of the lumbar spine, pelvis, and hip joints to assess for impairments that could be contributing to the signs and symptoms of hamstring injury.[92] In the evaluation of patients with hamstring injury, the slump test has been recommended to evaluate the patient for sciatic neural irritation.[90] In an experimental study, Kornberg and Lew[93] reported that Australian football players who had sustained a grade I hamstring injury and also had a positive slump test were able to return to play more quickly if they received slump stretching in addition to traditional management compared with a group of players

who did not. As mentioned previously, it is now recommended that patients perform neural flossing exercises for the sciatic nerve at first, particularly in the acute phase of injury, and perform static neural stretching as a progression and only as needed to clear the patient fully of sciatic neural tension signs. Another potential treatment option for hamstring-related sciatic neural irritation is to perform soft tissue mobilization while the patient actively stretches the hamstring and flosses the nerve.

Meralgia Paresthetica

Entrapment of the lateral femoral cutaneous nerve in the inguinal region, also known as meralgia paresthetica, involves paresthesias, numbness, and burning in the peripheral nerve's field.[94] Common causes include obesity, diabetes, direct trauma, pregnancy, radiation, and direct pressure on the nerve from restrictive clothing and utility belts. Clinical diagnosis involves testing sensation in the nerve's field, palpating the nerve in the lateral inguinal region, and neural tension testing. For neural tension testing, the patient is in prone, and the knee is passively flexed; this places tension on the upper lumbar nerve roots and femoral nerve. The hip can be adducted to apply further tension to the lateral femoral cutaneous nerve.[3] Typical treatment involves patient education to alter any direct compression on the nerve from restrictive clothing or belts, injections, and surgery as a last resort.[94] Manual therapy treatment could be directed toward the soft tissue in the anterior thigh and inguinal region. Assessment and manual therapy management of upper lumbar dysfunction could also be potentially beneficial because the lateral femoral cutaneous nerve receives its supply from the upper lumbar spine. Direct mobilization of the nerve involves knee flexion in an oscillatory fashion either actively by the patient or passively by the clinician. Active neural flossing while performing soft tissue mobilization of the anterior thigh or inguinal region is another potentially useful option.

Neuropathies of the Foot and Ankle Region

Aside from diabetic peripheral neuropathy, peripheral nerve injuries of the foot and ankle region are uncommon. There is no evidence from high-quality randomized trials in the literature concerning manual therapy for peripheral nerve injuries in the foot and ankle region. The major peripheral nerves of the lower leg, including the posterior tibial, peroneal, and sural nerves, can be evaluated for neuropathy using history and physical examination. Part of the physical examination could involve neural tension testing, making use of the anatomical course of the nerve around the foot and ankle region.[95-98] For example, to tension the tibial nerve selectively, the ankle can be placed in dorsiflexion and eversion during the straight leg–raise test. To apply tension to the peroneal nerve, the ankle can be placed in plantar flexion and inversion. Manual therapy management of peripheral nerve injuries about the foot and ankle can involve mobilization of the surrounding structures, direct mobilization of the nerve, or a combination of the two. Based on the examination findings, tissues that interface with the injured nerve could be targeted with manual therapy interventions. For example, in patients with plantar heel pain associated with posterior tibial neuropathy, also known as tarsal tunnel syndrome, the subtalar joint can be passively manipulated. For direct neural mobilization, the posterior tibial nerve can be mobilized using passive ankle dorsiflexion with eversion. For a combination manual therapy technique, the subtalar joint can be manipulated while the tibial nerve is on stretch. In another example, the manual therapist can address the superficial peroneal nerve, which can be injured during an inversion ankle sprain.[99] For this injury, the proximal and distal tibiofibular joint can be passively manipulated. The superficial peroneal nerve can be directly mobilized with passive ankle plantar flexion with inversion. The distal tibiofibular joint can be mobilized with the superficial peroneal nerve on stretch.

CASE STUDY

BR, a 52-year-old man who works as a computer programmer for a large software company, presents to outpatient therapy with a chief complaint of a 3-month history of numbness in his right (dominant hand), which worsens with computer activity and sleep. An electroneuromyography examination revealed slowing of the median nerve through the carpal tunnel and mild denervation potentials in the thenar compartment musculature. His symptoms were assessed with the Symptom Severity Score with a result of 2.2. His medical history is otherwise benign. BR does not take any prescriptive medications.

Case Study Questions

1. The clinical prediction rule developed by Wainner et al.[58] identified five predictor variables to assess the possibility of a CTS diagnosis. Which of the following items is not part of the prediction rule?
   a. Weakness of the ipsilateral digiti minimi muscle
   b. Shaking of the hand for relief
   c. A Symptom Severity Scale score of greater than 1.9 and age older than 45 years
   d. Wrist ratio index greater than 0.67

2. Which of the following tests is the "gold standard" test for diagnosing CTS?
   a. Disability of the Arm, Shoulder and Hand (DASH) assessment
   b. Electroneuromyography
   c. Phalen's test
   d. Symptom Severity Scale score of greater than 1.9 and age older than 45 years

3. Manual therapy techniques used in the treatment of carpal tunnel syndrome include all of the following except which one?
   a. Carpal bone mobilization
   b. Lumbar thrust maneuver
   c. Neural mobilization
   d. Soft tissue mobilization

4. Given that patients with CTS syndrome exhibit greater forward head posture and decreased cervical spine ROM, which of the following therapeutic techniques may be useful?
   a. Cervical ROM
   b. Postural retraining
   c. Thoracic manipulation
   d. All of the above

5. "Sliders" and "tensioners" are two types of which of the following?
   a. Manipulative thrusts of the thoracic spine
   b. Manipulative thrust of the cervical spine
   c. Neurodynamic treatment techniques
   d. Mobilization techniques for the carpal bones

References

1. Bronfort G, Haas M, Evans R, Leininger B, Triano J. Effectiveness of manual therapies: the UK evidence report. *Chiropr Osteopat*. 2010;18:3.
2. Butler DS. *The Sensitive Nervous System*. 1st ed. Adelaide, South Australia: Noigroup Publications; 2000.
3. Shacklock M. *Clinical Neurodynamics: A New System of Neuromusculoskeletal Treatment*. Oxford, UK: Butterworth-Heinemann; 2005.
4. Maitland G, Hengeveld E, Banks K, English K. *Maitland's Vertebral Manipulation*. 7th ed. Oxford, UK: Butterworth-Heinemann; 2005.
5. Butler D. *Mobilisation of the Nervous System*. 1st ed. Edinburgh: Churchill Livingstone; 1991.
6. Schmid AB, Brunner F, Luomajoki H, et al. Reliability of clinical tests to evaluate nerve function and mechanosensitivity of the upper limb peripheral nervous system. *BMC Musculoskelet Disord*. 2009;10:11.
7. Walsh J, Hall T. Reliability, validity and diagnostic accuracy of palpation of the sciatic, tibial and common peroneal nerves in the examination of low back related leg pain. *Man Ther*. 2009;14(6):623–629.
8. Wainner RS, Fritz JM, Irrgang JJ, et al. Reliability and diagnostic accuracy of the clinical examination and patient self-report measures for cervical radiculopathy. *Spine*. 2003; 28(1):52–62.
9. Nijs J, Van Houdenhove B, Oostendorp RAB. Recognition of central sensitization in patients with musculoskeletal pain: application of pain neurophysiology in manual therapy practice. *Man Ther*. 2010;15(2):135–141.
10. Scott D, Jull G, Sterling M. Widespread sensory hypersensitivity is a feature of chronic whiplash-associated disorder but not chronic idiopathic neck pain. *Clin J Pain*. 2005;21(2):175–181.
11. Coppieters MW, Butler DS. Do "sliders" slide and "tensioners" tension? An analysis of neurodynamic techniques and considerations regarding their application. *Man Ther*. 2008;13(3):213–221.
12. Bialosky JE, Bishop MD, Price DD, Robinson ME, George SZ. The mechanisms of manual therapy in the treatment of

musculoskeletal pain: a comprehensive model. *Man Ther.* 2009;14(5):531–538.

13. Bialosky JE, Bishop MD, Cleland JA. Individual expectation: an overlooked, but pertinent, factor in the treatment of individuals experiencing musculoskeletal pain. *Phys Ther.* 2010;90(9):1345–1355.

14. Gross AR, Hoving JL, Haines TA, et al. Manipulation and mobilisation for mechanical neck disorders. *Cochrane Database Syst Rev.* 2004;(1):CD004249.

15. Wainner RS, Gill H. Diagnosis and nonoperative management of cervical radiculopathy. *J Orthop Sports Phys Ther.* 2000;30(12):728–744.

16. Radhakrishnan K, Litchy WJ, O'Fallon WM, Kurland LT. Epidemiology of cervical radiculopathy. A population-based study from Rochester, Minnesota, 1976 through 1990. *Brain.* 1994;117(Pt 2):325–335.

17. Eubanks JD. Cervical radiculopathy: nonoperative management of neck pain and radicular symptoms. *Am Fam Physician.* 2010;81(1):33–40.

18. Young IA, Michener LA, Cleland JA, Aguilera AJ, Snyder AR. Manual therapy, exercise, and traction for patients with cervical radiculopathy: a randomized clinical trial. *Phys Ther.* 2009;89(7):632–642.

19. Larsson EM, Holtås S, Cronqvist S, Brandt L. Comparison of myelography, CT myelography and magnetic resonance imaging in cervical spondylosis and disk herniation. Pre- and postoperative findings. *Acta Radiol.* 1989;30(3):233–239.

20. Song K, Choi B, Kim G, Kim J. Clinical usefulness of CT-myelogram comparing with the MRI in degenerative cervical spinal disorders: is CTM still useful for primary diagnostic tool? *J Spinal Disord Tech.* 2009;22(5):353–357.

21. Eisen A. The utility of proximal nerve conduction in radiculopathies: the cons. *Electroencephalogr Clin Neurophysiol.* 1991;78(3):171–172; discussion 167.

22. Cho SC, Ferrante MA, Levin KH, Harmon RL, So YT. Utility of electrodiagnostic testing in evaluating patients with lumbosacral radiculopathy: an evidence-based review. *Muscle Nerve.* 2010;42(2):276–282.

23. Wainner RS, Fritz JM, Irrgang JJ, et al. Reliability and diagnostic accuracy of the clinical examination and patient self-report measures for cervical radiculopathy. *Spine.* 2003;28(1):52–62.

24. Childs JD, Cleland JA, Elliott JM, et al. Neck pain: clinical practice guidelines linked to the International Classification of Functioning, Disability, and Health from the Orthopedic Section of the American Physical Therapy Association. *J Orthop Sports Phys Ther.* 2008;38(9):A1–A34.

25. Cleland JA, Childs JD, Fritz JM, Whitman JM, Eberhart SL. Development of a clinical prediction rule for guiding treatment of a subgroup of patients with neck pain: use of thoracic spine manipulation, exercise, and patient education. *Phys Ther.* 2007;87(1):9–23.

26. Raney NH, Petersen EJ, Smith TA, et al. Development of a clinical prediction rule to identify patients with neck pain likely to benefit from cervical traction and exercise. *Eur Spine J.* 2009;18(3):382–391.

27. Cleland JA, Mintken PE, Carpenter K, et al. Examination of a clinical prediction rule to identify patients with neck pain likely to benefit from thoracic spine thrust manipulation and a general cervical range of motion exercise: multi-center randomized clinical trial. *Phys Ther.* 2010;90(9):1239–1250.

28. Cleland JA, Fritz JM, Whitman JM, Heath R. Predictors of short-term outcome in people with a clinical diagnosis of cervical radiculopathy. *Phys Ther.* 2007;87(12):1619–1632.

29. Cleland JA, Whitman JM, Fritz JM, Palmer JA. Manual physical therapy, cervical traction, and strengthening exercises in patients with cervical radiculopathy: a case series. *J Orthop Sports Phys Ther.* 2005;35(12):802–811.

30. Waldrop MA. Diagnosis and treatment of cervical radiculopathy using a clinical prediction rule and a multimodal intervention approach: a case series. *J Orthop Sports Phys Ther.* 2006;36(3):152–159.

31. Moeti P, Marchetti G. Clinical outcome from mechanical intermittent cervical traction for the treatment of cervical radiculopathy: a case series. *J Orthop Sports Phys Ther.* 2001;31(4):207–213.

32. Young IA, Michener LA, Cleland JA, Aguilera AJ, Snyder AR. Manual therapy, exercise, and traction for patients with cervical radiculopathy: a randomized clinical trial. *Phys Ther.* 2009;89(7):632–642.

33. Brooke BS, Freischlag JA. Contemporary management of thoracic outlet syndrome. *Curr Opin Cardiol.* 2010;25(6):535–540.

34. Povlsen B, Belzberg A, Hansson T, Dorsi M. Treatment for thoracic outlet syndrome. *Cochrane Database Syst Rev.* 2010;(1):CD007218.

35. Watson LA, Pizzari T, Balster S. Thoracic outlet syndrome part 2: conservative management of thoracic outlet. *Man Ther.* 2010;15(4):305–314.

36. Wilbourn AJ. The thoracic outlet syndrome is overdiagnosed. *Arch Neurol.* 1990;47(3):328–330.

37. Terao T, Ide K, Taniguchi M, et al. The management of patients with thoracic outlet syndrome (TOS) and an assistant diagnosis to discriminate between TOS and cervical spondylosis [in Japanese]. *No Shinkei Geka.* 2008;36(7):615–623.

38. Lindgren KA, Leino E, Manninen H. Cervical rotation lateral flexion test in brachialgia. *Arch Phys Med Rehabil.* 1992;73(8):735–737.

39. Hooper T, Denton J, McGalliard M, Brismee J, Sizer P. Thoracic outlet syndrome: a controversial clinical condition. Part 2: non-surgical and surgical management. *J Man Manip Ther.* 2010;18(3):132–138.

40. Smith KF. The thoracic outlet syndrome: a protocol of treatment. *J Orthop Sports Phys Ther.* 1979;1(2):89–99.

41. Vanti C, Natalini L, Romeo A, Tosarelli D, Pillastrini P. Conservative treatment of thoracic outlet syndrome. A review of the literature. *Eura Medicophys.* 2007;43(1):55–70.

42. Hooper T, Denton J, McGalliard M, Brismee J, Sizer P. Thoracic outlet syndrome: a controversial clinical condition. Part 1: anatomy, and clinical examination/diagnosis. *J Man Manip Ther.* 2010;18(2):75–83.

43. Buonocore M, Manstretta C, Mazzucchi G, Casale R. The clinical evaluation of conservative treatment in patients with the thoracic outlet syndrome [in Italian]. *G Ital Med Lav Ergon.* 1998;20(4):249–254.

44. Revel M, Amor B. Rehabilitation of cervico-thoraco-brachial outlet syndromes [in French]. *Phlebologie.* 1983;36(2):157–165.

45. Vicenzino B, Cleland JA, Bisset L. Joint manipulation in the management of lateral epicondylalgia: a clinical commentary. *J Man Manip Ther.* 2007;15(1):50–56.

46. Waugh EJ. Lateral epicondylalgia or epicondylitis: what's in a name? *J Orthop Sports Phys Ther.* 2005;35(4):200–202.

47. Yaxley GA, Jull GA. Adverse tension in the neural system. A preliminary study of tennis elbow. *Aust J Physiother.* 1993;39(1):15–22.

48. Ekstrom RA, Holden K. Examination of and intervention for a patient with chronic lateral elbow pain with signs of nerve entrapment. *Phys Ther.* 2002;82(11):1077–1086.

49. Szabo RM, Kwak C. Natural history and conservative management of cubital tunnel syndrome. *Hand Clin.* 2007;23(3):311–318.

50. Descatha A, Leclerc A, Chastang J, Roquelaure Y. Incidence of ulnar nerve entrapment at the elbow in repetitive work. *Scand J Work Environ Health.* 2004;30(3):234–240.

51. Feindel W, Stratford J. The role of the cubital tunnel in tardy ulnar palsy. *Can J Surg*. 1958;1(4):287–300.

52. Pascarelli EF, Hsu YP. Understanding work-related upper extremity disorders: clinical findings in 485 computer users, musicians, and others. *J Occup Rehabil*. 2001;11(1):1–21.

53. Novak CB, Lee GW, Mackinnon SE, Lay L. Provocative testing for cubital tunnel syndrome. *J Hand Surg Am*. 1994; 19(5):817–820.

54. Svernlöv B, Larsson M, Rehn K, Adolfsson L. Conservative treatment of the cubital tunnel syndrome. *J Hand Surg Eur Vol*. 2009;34(2):201–207.

55. Oskay D, Meriç A, Kirdi N, et al. Neurodynamic mobilization in the conservative treatment of cubital tunnel syndrome: long-term follow-up of 7 cases. *J Manipulative Physiol Ther*. 2010;33(2):156–163.

56. Coppieters MW, Bartholomeeusen KE, Stappaerts KH. Incorporating nerve-gliding techniques in the conservative treatment of cubital tunnel syndrome. *J Manipulative Physiol Ther*. 2004;27(9):560–568.

57. Atroshi I, Gummesson C, Johnsson R, et al. Prevalence of carpal tunnel syndrome in a general population. *JAMA*. 1999; 282(2):153–158.

58. Wainner RS, Fritz JM, Irrgang JJ, et al. Development of a clinical prediction rule for the diagnosis of carpal tunnel syndrome. *Arch Phys Med Rehabil*. 2005;86(4):609–618.

59. Johnson EW, Gatens T, Poindexter D, Bowers D. Wrist dimensions: correlation with median sensory latencies. *Arch Phys Med Rehabil*. 1983;64(11):556–557.

60. De-la-Llave-Rincón AI, Fernández-de-las-Peñas C, Palacios-Ceña D, Cleland JA. Increased forward head posture and restricted cervical range of motion in patients with carpal tunnel syndrome. *J Orthop Sports Phys Ther*. 2009;39(9): 658–664.

61. Hirata H. Carpal tunnel syndrome and cubital tunnel syndrome [in Japanese]. *Rinsho Shinkeigaku*. 2007;47(11): 761–765.

62. Huisstede BM, Hoogvliet P, Randsdorp MS, et al. Carpal tunnel syndrome. Part I: effectiveness of nonsurgical treatments—a systematic review. *Arch Phys Med Rehabil*. 2010;91(7):981–1004.

63. Burke J, Buchberger DJ, Carey-Loghmani MT, et al. A pilot study comparing two manual therapy interventions for carpal tunnel syndrome. *J Manipulative Physiol Ther*. 2007;30(1): 50–61.

64. Tal-Akabi A, Rushton A. An investigation to compare the effectiveness of carpal bone mobilisation and neurodynamic mobilisation as methods of treatment for carpal tunnel syndrome. *Man Ther*. 2000;5(4):214–222.

65. Valente R, Gibson H. Chiropractic manipulation in carpal tunnel syndrome. *J Manipulative Physiol Ther*. 1994;17(4): 246–249.

66. Moraska A, Chandler C, Edmiston-Schaetzel A, et al. Comparison of a targeted and general massage protocol on strength, function, and symptoms associated with carpal tunnel syndrome: a randomized pilot study. *J Altern Complement Med*. 2008;14(3):259–267.

67. Baysal O, Altay Z, Ozcan C, et al. Comparison of three conservative treatment protocols in carpal tunnel syndrome. *Int J Clin Pract*. 2006;60(7):820–828.

68. Bialosky JE, Bishop MD, Price DD, et al. A randomized sham-controlled trial of a neurodynamic technique in the treatment of carpal tunnel syndrome. *J Orthop Sports Phys Ther*. 2009;39(10):709–723.

69. Medina McKeon JM, Yancosek KE. Neural gliding techniques for the treatment of carpal tunnel syndrome: a systematic review. *J Sport Rehabil*. 2008;17(3):324–341.

70. Fernández-de-Las-Peñas C, Cleland JA, Ortega-Santiago R, et al. Central sensitization does not identify patients with

carpal tunnel syndrome who are likely to achieve short-term success with physical therapy. *Exp Brain Res*. 2010;207(1–2): 85–94.

71. Van Boxem K, Cheng J, Patijn J, et al. 11. Lumbosacral radicular pain. *Pain Pract*. 2010;10(4):339–358.

72. van der Windt DA, Simons E, Riphagen II, et al. Physical examination for lumbar radiculopathy due to disc herniation in patients with low-back pain. *Cochrane Database Syst Rev*. 2010;(2):CD007431.

73. Murphy DR, Hurwitz EL, Gerrard JK, Clary R. Pain patterns and descriptions in patients with radicular pain: does the pain necessarily follow a specific dermatome? *Chiropr Osteopat*. 2009;17:9.

74. Hahne AJ, Ford JJ, McMeeken JM. Conservative management of lumbar disc herniation with associated radiculopathy: a systematic review. *Spine*. 2010;35(11): E488–504.

75. May S, Donelson R. Evidence-informed management of chronic low back pain with the McKenzie method. *Spine J*. 2008;8(1):134–141.

76. Werneke M, Hart DL. Centralization phenomenon as a prognostic factor for chronic low back pain and disability. *Spine*. 2001;26(7):758–764; discussion 765.

77. Long A, Donelson R, Fung T. Does it matter which exercise? A randomized control trial of exercise for low back pain. *Spine*. 2004;29(23):2593–2602.

78. Fritz JM, Lindsay W, Matheson JW, et al. Is there a subgroup of patients with low back pain likely to benefit from mechanical traction? Results of a randomized clinical trial and subgrouping analysis. *Spine*. 2007;32(26):E793–800.

79. Fritz JM, Thackeray A, Childs JD, Brennan GP. A randomized clinical trial of the effectiveness of mechanical traction for sub-groups of patients with low back pain: study methods and rationale. *BMC Musculoskelet Disord*. 2010;11:81.

80. McMorland G, Suter E, Casha S, du Plessis SJ, Hurlbert RJ. Manipulation or microdiskectomy for sciatica? A prospective randomized clinical study. *J Manipulative Physiol Ther*. 2010; 33(8):576–584.

81. Chou R, Qaseem A, Snow V, et al. Diagnosis and treatment of low back pain: a joint clinical practice guideline from the American College of Physicians and the American Pain Society. *Ann Intern Med*. 2007;147(7):478–491.

82. Deyo RA, Mirza SK, Martin BI, et al. Trends, major medical complications, and charges associated with surgery for lumbar spinal stenosis in older adults. *JAMA*. 2010;303(13): 1259–1265.

83. Whitman JM, Flynn TW, Childs JD, et al. A comparison between two physical therapy treatment programs for patients with lumbar spinal stenosis: a randomized clinical trial. *Spine*. 2006;31(22):2541–2549.

84. Cleland JA, Childs JD, Palmer JA, Eberhart S. Slump stretching in the management of non-radicular low back pain: a pilot clinical trial. *Man Ther*. 2006;11(4):279–286.

85. Nee RJ, Butler D. Management of peripheral neuropathic pain: integrating neurobiology, neurodynamics, and clinical evidence. *Phys Ther Sport*. 2006;7(1):36–49.

86. Hopayian K, Song F, Riera R, Sambandan S. The clinical features of the piriformis syndrome: a systematic review. *Eur Spine J*. 2010;19(12):2095–2109.

87. Fishman LM, Dombi GW, Michaelsen C, et al. Piriformis syndrome: diagnosis, treatment, and outcome—a 10-year study. *Arch Phys Med Rehabil*. 2002;83(3):295–301.

88. Fishman LM, Konnoth C, Rozner B. Botulinum neurotoxin type B and physical therapy in the treatment of piriformis syndrome: a dose-finding study. *Am J Phys Med Rehabil*. 2004; 83(1):42–50; quiz 51–53.

89. Tonley JC, Yun SM, Kochevar RJ, et al. Treatment of an individual with piriformis syndrome focusing on hip muscle

strengthening and movement reeducation: a case report. *J Orthop Sports Phys Ther.* 2010;40(2):103–111.

90. Turl SE, George KP. Adverse neural tension: a factor in repetitive hamstring strain? *J Orthop Sports Phys Ther.* 1998; 27(1):16–21.

91. Hoskins W, Pollard H. The management of hamstring injury—part 1: issues in diagnosis. *Man Ther.* 2005;10(2): 96–107.

92. Hoskins W, Pollard H. Hamstring injury management—part 2: treatment. *Man Ther.* 2005;10(3):180–190.

93. Kornberg C, Lew P. The effect of stretching neural structures on grade one hamstring injuries. *J Orthop Sports Phys Ther.* 1989;10(12):481–487.

94. Harney D, Patijn J. Meralgia paresthetica: diagnosis and management strategies. *Pain Med.* 2007;8(8):669–677.

95. Alshami AM, Souvlis T, Coppieters MW. A review of plantar heel pain of neural origin: differential diagnosis and management. *Man Ther.* 2008;13(2):103–111.

96. Alshami AM, Babri AS, Souvlis T, Coppieters MW. Biomechanical evaluation of two clinical tests for plantar heel pain: the dorsiflexion-eversion test for tarsal tunnel syndrome and the windlass test for plantar fasciitis. *Foot Ankle Int.* 2007;28(4):499–505.

97. Coppieters MW, Alshami AM, Babri AS, et al. Strain and excursion of the sciatic, tibial, and plantar nerves during a modified straight leg raising test. *J Orthop Res.* 2006;24(9): 1883–1889.

98. Alshami AM, Babri AS, Souvlis T, Coppieters MW. Strain in the tibial and plantar nerves with foot and ankle movements and the influence of adjacent joint positions. *J Appl Biomech.* 2008;24(4):368–376.

99. Nitz AJ, Dobner JJ, Kersey D. Nerve injury and grades II and III ankle sprains. *Am J Sports Med.* 1985;13(3):177–182.

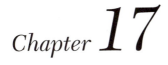

The Role of Physical Agents in Peripheral Nerve Injury

JAMES W. BELLEW, PT, EdD, AND EDWARD MAHONEY, PT, DPT, CWS

"When health is absent Wisdom cannot reveal itself, Art cannot become manifest, Strength cannot be exerted, Wealth is useless and Reason is powerless."

—HEROPHILOS (300 B.C.)

Objectives

On completion of this chapter, the student/practitioner will be able to:

- Discuss the role of physical agents in patient intervention.
- List the physical agents available to the practicing therapist and note their therapeutic indications.
- Describe the various forms of therapeutic electrical stimulation.
- Develop evidence-based knowledge of the indications, contraindications, and applications of physical agents.

Key Terms

- Electrical stimulation
- Modality
- Pain modulation
- Physical agents

Introduction

The inherent potential of the peripheral nervous system to undergo autogenic repair after injury or insult is a compelling impetus both to individuals experiencing damage or loss of function and to the practitioners addressing the associated symptoms and impairments. Although it is known that injured peripheral axons have the ability to regenerate, restoration of functional ability remains less than optimal. Nevertheless, pursuit of effective and meaningful recovery remains paramount.

Physical agents, or therapeutic modalities, represent a spectrum of adjunctive therapies used to complement or supplement other interventions, such as exercise, joint or tissue mobilization, strengthening, or stretching. Collectively, physical agents and the interventions they supplement comprise the more comprehensive intervention plan. Advances in understanding of the biophysical effects of physical agents have spurred their continued use in rehabilitation.[1-6] Although injured peripheral nerves have demonstrated the ability to regenerate, physical agents impart specific and selective responses to mediate tissue healing that have led practitioners to select physical agents for peripheral nerve injury (PNI) intervention.[7]

Physical Agents

Role of Physical Agents

Physical agents are complementary, or adjunctive, interventions used with other treatment strategies to increase the probability that a desired therapeutic effect will be realized. For example, the use of **electrical stimulation** (ES) at a wound bed may be used to attract cells, such as fibroblasts, or influence the orientation of endothelial cells to promote and potentiate wound healing.[1,8,9] Physical agents are not intended to supplant more skilled and selective interventions provided by practitioners. Rather, physical agents represent a viable supplementary class of tools for influencing healing of injured tissue.

What Are Physical Agents?

Physical agents are means of delivering and using for therapeutic purpose one or more of several types of physical energies. Therapeutic benefits are derived from the transfer of these energies to patients to stimulate tissue responses that may not be realized through other interventions. Physical agents traditionally include thermal modalities (e.g., heat and cold), electromagnetic modalities (e.g., ES and diathermy), light modalities (e.g., laser or infrared), and mechanical modalities (e.g., traction, compression, and ultrasound [US]). Table 17-1 summarizes the classes and types of physical agents with representative examples of clinical uses.

Physical Agents for Peripheral Nerve Injury

Compared with central nerve injury, PNI has received much less attention from neuroscientists. This is likely

Table 17-1   Classes of Physical Agents and Clinical Uses

Class of Agent	Type	Examples
Electromagnetic	Electricity	High-volt pulsed current; direct current; microcurrent; TENS
	Electromagnetic waves	Short-wave or pulsed diathermy; PEMF; ultraviolet radiation
	Light	Laser; infrared
Thermal	Thermotherapy (i.e., heat)	Hot pack; Fluidotherapy; continuous-wave US or diathermy
	Cryotherapy (i.e., cold)	Cold or ice pack
Mechanical	Sound	Continuous or pulsed US
	Traction	Manual or mechanical traction
	Compression	Intermittent pneumatic compression; compression wraps
	Hydrotherapy (i.e., water)	Whirlpool

PEMF, pulsed electromagnetic field; TENS, transcutaneous electrical nerve stimulation; US, ultrasound.

due to the pervasive view that healing can occur in peripheral nerves secondary to Schwann cell activity, whereas oligodendrocytes of the central nervous system (CNS) do not demonstrate such repair.[10,11] Interventions aimed at accelerating regeneration and improving reinnervation are of great interest. Herein lies the impetus for the use of physical agents for PNI—acceleration of healing. To date, a substantial amount of evidence in animal models suggests efficacy for the use of physical agents. Such evidence in humans remains elusive, but this has not discouraged interest and use of physical agents for PNI.

Electrical Stimulation

ES following PNI has long been considered to promote nerve regeneration, decrease pain associated with injury, and maintain denervated skeletal muscle. The literature is replete with optimistic evidence of nerve regeneration after ES of injured peripheral nerves. However, most of this evidence comes from animal models. Such evidence has not been produced in humans.

Regeneration of Nerve

In the 1980s, using rat and rabbit models, low-frequency alternating current (AC) after crush injury was reported to accelerate the return of reflex foot withdrawal and contractile force in reinnervated muscles.[12–14] These findings served as the impetus for investigations assessing the effects of ES on nerve regeneration and reinnervation, and much of this information has come from Gordon et al.[7,12,15–18] Gordon's group found that after continuous low-frequency (20 pps) stimulation of the proximal nerve stump for 2 weeks, all motor neurons that regenerated their axons into the distal stump eventually regenerated into the appropriate endoneurial tubes. A comparison between stimulated and nonstimulated nerve regeneration showed that low-frequency stimulation promoted axon regeneration of all motor neurons over a 25-mm distance within 3 weeks in contrast to 8 to 10 weeks in the nonstimulated nerves.[15] The same 1-hour stimulation of the proximal nerve stump accelerated sensory nerve regeneration, while directing the axons into the correct sensory nerve pathways.[19]

To find a more clinically feasible intervention for nerve regeneration, Gordon's group progressively shortened the stimulation to 1 hour, applied immediately after surgical repair of the nerve transection. The degree of regeneration was not diminished. Similarly robust findings after 1 hour of stimulation either before or after nerve suture have been reported more recently.[12,20]

From earlier evidence of accelerated regeneration after ES, investigation of human patients with compressive nerve injury from carpal tunnel syndrome (CTS) and loss of greater than 50% of functional motor units of the median eminence was undertaken.[7,17]

Direct ES of the median nerve proximal to and immediately after surgical release for 1 hour at 20 pps was effective in promoting reinnervation of muscles within 9 months. This result is in stark contrast to the nonsignificant return of functional motor units in control patients who did not receive stimulation.

Collectively, the aforementioned findings demonstrate accelerated axon regeneration in rats and accelerated muscle reinnervation in humans.[7,12,15,17,18,21] The findings that were the result of 1 hour of stimulation applied directly to the proximal nerve and immediately after surgical repair indicate a relatively narrow window of time. If the noted acceleration can be effective in accelerating axon regeneration sufficiently to extend the window of opportunity for regeneration, ES may become a viable intervention to aid and augment recovery of function after PNI.[18] Reports from human subjects are sparse at this stage of research, which leaves the future use of ES for nerve regeneration questionable but hopeful.

Bottom line for nerve regeneration after ES: ES has been associated with several findings indicative of nerve regeneration. However, these findings occurred largely under experimental conditions with rodents where nerve injury is easily induced, reproducible, and well controlled. There remains a large divide between the evidence for regeneration in animals and the functional recovery in humans. Although the volumes of laboratory data touting regeneration of nerve and effects of ES are encouraging, these findings have yet to be realized in clinical situations with humans and remain essentially intangible for clinical use.

Modulation of Pain

Neuropathic pain secondary to injury or pathology to peripheral nerves pose a considerable challenge. Transcutaneous electrical nerve stimulation (TENS) has been used in the management of pain associated with peripheral neuropathy with widely varying results. Prior studies of TENS on neuropathic pain are largely from populations with diabetic peripheral neuropathy, with TENS reported to reduce pain in 50% to 75% of patients.[22–24]

Three systematic and meta-analytic reviews published in 2010 and prior studies describing TENS with neuropathic pain in humans are available.[25–30] In a review of relevant randomized controlled trials of TENS for painful diabetic neuropathy, Jin et al.[26] determined only 3 of 130 studies met appropriate inclusion criteria.[28–30] Likewise, Pieber et al.[27] identified only 15 relevant studies using ES for painful diabetic neuropathy from 3,801 hits during a data search for "diabetic neuropathy." Dubinsky and Miyasaki[25] determined only 3 of 263 articles met their criteria. Collectively, these reviews concluded that TENS yielded positive benefits for pain relief lasting up to 12 weeks with no adverse effects. Complete relief of pain

was observed in 16% to 36% of patients receiving TENS. TENS appeared to be helpful in patients who failed to show benefit from amitriptyline, a conventional first-line pharmacological intervention.[28,29] More surprising was the observation that the combination of TENS and amitriptyline resulted in greater pain relief than TENS alone.[28]

Treatment conditions across reviewed studies were similar because they extended from the same research group.[28,29,31] A biphasic, exponentially decaying waveform using a 4-msec pulse duration and an amplitude 35 mA or less and 23 to 35 volts was administered 30 minutes per day for 4 weeks.[1] Patients self-selected a frequency between 2 and 70 pps. Nearly 85% of the patients receiving TENS reported substantial reduction of pain, and 36% reported complete resolution.[28] Changes in pain before treatment compared with after treatment were not noted in the sham-treatment group. However, when the sham group later received TENS, a significant reduction in pain was observed in 70% of the subjects (Fig. 17-1).[29] Prior human studies of TENS for painful diabetic neuropathy reported benefit lasting up to 12 weeks; however, the long-term effect of TENS is unknown. Forst et al.[30] performed a double-blind randomized study examining 12 weeks of TENS versus placebo for mild to moderate painful diabetic neuropathy. Of the TENS group, 70% reported improvement versus only 29% in the placebo group, with benefit noted in the TENS group for up to 12 weeks. A retrospective analysis by Julka et al.[31] on the

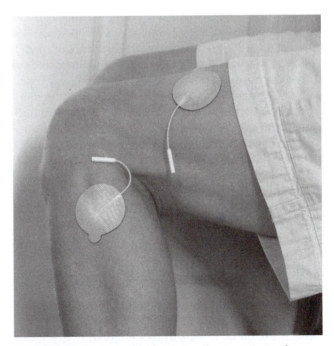

Figure 17-1 Electrode configuration for treatment of neuropathic pain using TENS electrodes placed proximal to the patella over the vastus lateralis and medialis oblique, over the neck of the fibula, and over the proximal gastrocnemius distal to the popliteal fossa.[28,29]

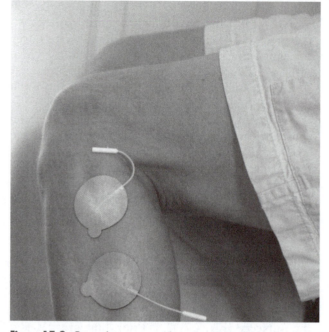

Figure 17-2 Stimulation over the common peroneal nerve for treatment of painful diabetic peripheral neuropathy.[30]

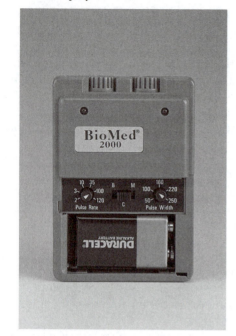

Figure 17-3 A basic TENS unit with controls for pulse frequency, duration, and amplitude may be used to treat painful diabetic neuropathy. (*From Michlovitz S, Bellew J, Nolan T. Modalities for Therapeutic Intervention. 5th ed. Philadelphia: FA Davis; 2011.*)

long-term benefit of TENS used questionnaire data regarding pain. Over an average use of 1.7 years, 76% of the patients using TENS reported a 44% ± 4% subjective reduction of pain with use of TENS (Fig. 17-2).

Information regarding stimulation parameters may be gathered from rat models. Somers and Clemente[32] reported that high-frequency (100 pps) stimulation or a combination of high-frequency (100 pps) and low-frequency (20 pps) stimulation to the contralateral limb of rats with unilaterally induced neuropathic pain prevents the onset of mechanical allodynia. This appears to occur via distinctly different alterations in dorsal horn neurotransmitter content, which suggests that the mechanism of action of high-frequency stimulation or a combination of high-frequency and low-frequency stimulation may be unique.[32] The TENS stimulator used by Somers and Clemente was a readily available conventional model, allowing for easy replication of the stimulus parameters with most types of basic TENS stimulators (Fig. 17-3).

A combination of high-frequency and low-frequency TENS has also been shown to decrease pain associated with type II complex regional pain syndrome—a chronic condition that can develop after PNI.[33] TENS has shown varying results in rats, with some rats demonstrating an increase in pain threshold.[34] TENS administered contralateral to the nerve injury yielded the most benefit. Specifically, high-frequency TENS (100 pps) reduced the onset of mechanical allodynia, whereas low-frequency TENS (20 pps) reduced the onset of thermal allodynia.[33] Clinical administration of TENS for neuropathic pain may yield greater

therapeutic benefits by delivering both high-frequency and low-frequency stimulation. Although many TENS units maintain a constant frequency, interferential currents employing a reciprocal or integral sweep from low frequency to high frequency may be used to deliver both high-frequency and low-frequency TENS. More recent data support this variation for modulation of pain.[35,36]

Frequency Rhythmic Electrical Modulation System

To date, frequency rhythmic electrical modulation system (FREMS) has shown promising results for the treatment of painful peripheral neuropathy, but it is still considered a novel intervention **modality.** FREMS is high-voltage, biphasic current delivered with a variable (i.e., rhythmic) pulse frequency, pulse duration, and amplitude. Results from a double-blind, randomized, placebo-controlled, crossover study supported the use of FREMS for peripheral neuropathy.[37] After treatment, day and night pain scores, vibratory perception threshold, monofilament testing, and motor nerve conduction velocity (NCV) improved compared with baseline and remained significantly improved at 4 months. Conversely, none of these parameters improved significantly in the placebo group. Conti et al.[38] used the same study design to assess the effects of FREMS on cutaneous blood flow. Transcutaneous oxygen tension did not change in the initial 3 weeks of treatment but at 4 months was significantly higher than baseline. Conti et al. suggested that improvement in peripheral neuropathy was the result of increased local blood flow; however, more research is needed to test this hypothesis.

Bottom line on ES for pain associated with peripheral neuropathy: Three extensive reviews of TENS on painful diabetic neuropathy deemed only a modicum of studies from hundreds to be worthy of review, evidencing the lack of quality data from which to draw clinical conclusions.[25–27] Current data generally support the inclusion of TENS in the comprehensive management of painful neuropathy. More specifically, a combination of high-frequency and low-frequency stimulation may be most effective. Largely enhanced by the lack of adverse effects with TENS, a recommendation to support use of TENS can be loosely made based on the limited number of prior studies.

Preservation of Denervated Muscle

Use of ES for increasing strength, volitional recruitment, re-education, and function in normally innervated but weak skeletal muscle is well known and supported. Use in denervated muscle or muscle awaiting reinnervation secondary to PNI is less certain, with few studies offering contradictory results.[39–41] As such, ES for denervated muscle after PNI continues to be scrutinized and remains highly controversial.[42] It is unclear whether nerve growth is suppressed or impaired with ES, and this is a dividing point for individuals on either side of this issue.

The differentiation between muscle denervated by injury to the peripheral nerve versus denervation secondary to injury of the CNS, as seen in stroke or spinal cord injury, must be distinguished. Direct injury to the peripheral nerve results in a lower motor neuron lesion, whereas injury to the CNS leaves an intact lower motor neuron below the level of CNS injury. This differentiation is critical. With an intact lower motor neuron, and assuming appropriate stimulus parameters, ES elicits muscular contraction by depolarizing the peripheral nerve as the neurolemma maintains a lower threshold for excitation than the muscle membrane (sarcolemma). With an injury to the lower motor neuron, ES may evoke a muscular contraction by direct stimulation and depolarization of the higher threshold sarcolemma. The stimulus parameters required for the latter differ vastly from the former. Specifically, the pulse duration required to evoke a muscular contraction in muscle denervated by lower motor neuron injury often exceeds 1 msec, a duration not offered on many clinical stimulators. Consequently, many clinicians are unable to offer effective ES to patients with PNI. Additionally, the intensity of the current required to depolarize the sarcolemma versus the neurolemma is significantly greater and is often painful. These two factors underlie much of the unsatisfactory results from stimulation of denervated muscle after PNI.

After denervation, human skeletal muscle, similar to an injured nerve, exhibits strategies to promote recovery and reinnervation.[43] ES is thought to facilitate these strategies; however, direct stimulation of denervated skeletal muscle has shown conflicting results. A study published in 2010 by Gigo-Benato et al.[39] examined direct transcutaneously administered cathodal stimulation to denervated anterior tibialis muscles of rats. ES accentuated muscle atrophy and impaired neuromuscular functional recovery in rats compared with nonstimulated controls. Impaired healing after ES was also reported by Baptista et al.,[44] who compared high-frequency TENS (100 pps, pulse duration 80 μsec) and low-frequency TENS (4 pps, pulse duration 240 μsec) in mice after sciatic crush injury. ES resulted in signs of impaired regeneration, including axonal edema, thinner myelinated fibers, and irregular cytoarchitecture with more pronounced impairment in the high-frequency group. These findings are particularly noteworthy because the TENS was delivered using surface electrodes and parameters consistent with those commonly employed in humans when administering high-frequency (i.e., conventional) or low-frequency (i.e., acupuncture) TENS.[45]

The literature is not without contradiction. Dow et al.[46] initially reported ES reduced changes in muscle function related to denervation. However, after prolonged denervation, the same protocol failed to produce optimistic findings suggesting that ES may not attenuate factors hindering regeneration following a delayed reinnervation.[47] That the intrinsic rate of endogenous reinnervation of injured nerve is slow underlies the significance of this evidence. Although ES may render some therapeutic benefit in the initial period after injury, application following prolonged denervation may not yield such results.

Bottom line for ES to preserve denervated muscle: A 2007 review of ES in patients with neurological conditions concluded that evidence neither supports nor refutes the use of ES for increasing strength after PNI.[48] Studies with low methodological quality and large variations in the response of humans to ES make a more conclusive understanding infeasible. Given the continued clinical interest in the use of ES for denervated muscle, this conclusion is concerning. There is renewed interest in using ES during gait or other activities to provide function; however, these applications often involve upper motor neuron injury and cannot be extrapolated to lower motor neuron injury stemming from PNI.[49–51] Clinicians are left to make decisions from limited and poorly designed studies or are left to draw conclusions from other populations.[48]

Ultrasound

Use of therapeutic US for PNI has been studied for two distinct effects: (1) reduction of pain and improved function and (2) facilitation of nerve regeneration.[52]

Therapeutic US is classified as thermal or nonthermal. The physiological effects realized from thermal or continuous US generally reflect the thermal effects observed with other thermal agents with two exceptions: (1) The depth of effect is greater with US than other thermal agents except short wave diathermy, and (2) the effect is more pronounced in tissues with higher collagen content because these tissues retain more sound energy.[52,53] Because peripheral nerves possess high levels of collagen and subcellular organelles throughout the axon, an interest in the use of US for nerve healing has encouraged further study.[54-56] Nonthermal or pulsed US imparts the effects of cavitation, microstreaming, and acoustic streaming, which are believed to facilitate endogenous mechanisms of tissue healing. Understanding of these mechanisms in PNI is unclear.

Studies in animal models using continuous US after PNI have shed light on the potential for healing.[57,58] Mourad et al.[57] treated rats with complete axonotmetic denervation 3 days after a crush injury with continuous US ranging from 0.25 to 5.0 W/cm^2. Compared with control rats, the US-treated group demonstrated a significantly greater rate of recovery in function with the most improvement seen in the rats receiving 1-minute applications of 0.25 W/cm^2 US at 1.0 MHz or 2.25 MHz. Similar findings were reported by Hong et al.[58] who examined recovery of measures of electrophysiological function (compound motor action potential [CMAP], NCV, and distal motor latency [DML]) following continuous thermal US at 0.5 W/cm^2 and 1.0 W/cm^2 in rats with compression neuropathy. The recovery rate of DML did not improve, but CMAP and NCV showed significantly faster recovery rates compared with untreated controls. However, these improvements occurred only in the nerves receiving US at 0.5 W/cm^2. With 1.0 W/cm^2, the recovery rate of the CMAP was slower than in the untreated leg, and no significant changes were noted in recovery rate for NCV and DML. These findings of efficacy for continuous low-intensity US (i.e., less than 1.0 W/cm^2) were supported by Lowdon et al.[59] comparing 0.5 W/cm^2 and 1.0 W/cm^2. Collectively, these studies indicate that US less than 1.0 W/cm^2 can facilitate recovery, whereas US greater than 1.0 W/cm^2 can retard recovery.

Use of low-intensity pulsed US (LIPUS; less than 1.0 W/cm^2) has consistently shown accelerated regeneration of peripheral nerve in rats despite the lack of understanding of the precise mechanisms.[60-63] US was studied in rats after complete nerve transection and surgical placement of a grafted nerve conduit to guide axonal sprouting and regeneration. Using 400 mW/cm^2 applied 2 minutes per day for 8 weeks beginning 24 hours after injury, Park et al.[62] demonstrated a nearly 50% greater rate of nerve regeneration, greater axon diameter, and thicker myelin in rats treated with US.

The effect of LIPUS on isolated Schwann cells from proximal nerve stumps of rats has also been studied because Schwann cells appear to aid in myelinating axons and directional guidance of neurons—events critical to regeneration.[64] Following daily 5-minute applications of LIPUS at 100 mW/cm^2 for 14 days, Zhang et al.[63] reported that treated Schwann cells increased cell proliferation and expression of neurotrophic growth factors (neurotrophin-3 and brain-derived neurotrophic factor) versus control cells. Additional support for the regenerative effects of LIPUS is available.[60,61,65] Raso et al.[65] reported a significantly greater rate of functional recovery and nerve fiber density after crush injury of the sciatic nerve in rats versus untreated injured controls. US was delivered daily for 2 minutes at 400 mW/cm^2 for 10 days beginning the day after injury. After 5 minutes of LIPUS at 300 mW/cm^2 and 1 MHz administered 12 times over 2 weeks, Chang et al.[61] reported a significantly greater number and area of regenerated axons.

Clinical use of US for PNI in humans has been primarily for CTS. However, only a few randomized controlled studies exist. Improvements in median NCV and pain were reported by Ebenbichler et al.[66] after pulsed US at 1.0 W/cm^2 applied 15 minutes daily for 2 weeks versus sham US in mild to moderate CTS. Piravej and Boonhong[67] reported the benefit of continuous low-intensity (0.5 W/cm^2) US on CTS after 10-minute treatments administered 5 days per week for 4 weeks. Both the US group and the control group, who received diclofenac and sham US, showed significant improvements in sensory nerve action potentials, in addition to a significant difference noted in the US group. In contrast, Oztas et al.[68] compared US (1.5 W/cm^2 or 0.8 W/cm^2) with sham US and reported no significant change in clinical or neurophysiological measures. US therapy (pulsed 1.0 W/cm^2) for CTS was also compared with low-level laser therapy (LLLT) with both groups showing benefit, but greater improvement was noted in the US group.[69]

From collective examination of studies regarding use of US for CTS, two factors appear to affect efficacy of US: the duration and severity of symptoms and the power of the US.[52,66,68,70] In mild to moderate symptoms of lesser duration, treatment benefits appear to be derived from US. As the severity and duration of CTS increase, the benefits of US decrease or are absent. For intensity, data suggest low-intensity, less than 1.0 W/cm^2. Studies of both continuous and pulsed US using power less than 1.0 W/cm^2 have demonstrated improvement in nerve function after injury. Use of continuous US with less than 1.0 W/cm^2 power is unlikely to result in a true thermal effect on the treated tissues. Changes in tissue, cell, and membrane activity secondary to the mechanical effects of US likely underlie the observed effects.

Bottom line for US and PNI: Considerable evidence exists suggesting accelerated regeneration and recovery of function after administration of continuous and pulsed US in rat models. The degree to which these findings can be translated to recovery of PNI in humans is speculative. We are not aware of any quality evidence for the regeneration of peripheral nerve in humans after treatment with US. For compressive neuropathy secondary to CTS, low-intensity US (less than 1.0 W/cm²) may attenuate symptoms, but evidence for improved neurophysiological performance remains equivocal. Limited evidence suggests improved measures in neurophysiological function that may reflect change in cell and membrane function, alteration of intercellular communication, or increase in local circulation.

Laser

LLLT is widely used and accepted in several European countries as an adjunctive intervention for tissue healing. Acceptance and use of LLLT in the United States have been less robust since its initial approval for use in CTS in 2002. However, much discussion continues with regard to the use of LLLT for tissue healing, based on the purported ability of LLLT to augment or enhance the body's natural processes of healing. Conclusive evidence to support widespread use of LLLT in patients with PNI remains elusive. Much of the lack of evidence may be complicated by the limited populations for which laser has been approved; poor quality of study design; variable treatment techniques; variable assessment and outcome measures; and variations in equipment used, including wavelength and energy density or power.

Clinical interest in the use of laser for PNI stems from observed responses in the metabolic activity of tissues and cells, such as fibroblasts, endothelial cells, osteoclasts, and neurons, exposed to laser energy in primarily animal models and in a few human studies. Acute LLLT has shown decreased production of bradykinin, reduced levels of prostaglandin E_2, increased secretion of endogenous opioids, increased production of serotonin and nitric oxide, and increased axonal sprouting and nerve cell regeneration.[71–80]

Laser energy, or photoenergy, emits packets of light energy, called photons, that are absorbed by receptor chromophores within the mitochondria and cell membrane of tissues irradiated with laser energy.[81,82] Absorption of photoenergy increases cellular metabolism and increases the oxidative production of adenosine triphosphate (ATP)—a process known as photobiomodulation. In the presence of injury, ATP is used to synthesize DNA, RNA, proteins, and enzymes; facilitate cellular mitosis; and increase synthesis of growth factors to repair compromised tissue.

As with ES for PNI, most evidence regarding LLLT has been derived from animal models. Based on rat studies, LLLT for repair of incomplete PNI is proposed to (1) increase the rate of axonal growth and myelination, (2) prevent or limit degeneration in the corresponding motor neurons of the spinal cord, (3) offer immediate protective effects to increase functional activity of the injured nerve, (4) maintain functional activity of injured nerve over time, and (5) minimize scar formation.[5]

Data from animal studies suggest that LLLT significantly improves recovery of PNI.[83–86] More specifically, low-power lasers (632.8 nm and 780 nm wavelength) attenuate retrograde degeneration of neurons in the corresponding segments of the spinal cord.[85] Shamir et al.[84] examined the effect of 780 nm helium-neon (HeNe) laser after complete rat sciatic nerve transection with anastomosis. LLLT demonstrated increased regenerative processes and accelerated axon growth, findings supported by more recent study.[87,88] Consistent findings have also been reported after end-to-end anastomosis followed by laser irradiation. In this use, the laser-treated groups had faster recovery of motor function and remyelination.[89] However, not all studies support the use of LLLT after PNI. Reis et al.[90] examined the effects of gallium-aluminum-arsenide (GaAlAs) laser (660 Nm) on rats after neurotmesis and epineural anastomosis and reported no significant changes in functional outcomes.

Compelled by optimistic findings in animal models, Rochkind et al.[87] performed a randomized, double-blind, placebo-controlled study in 2007 and reported the effects of low-power 780-nm laser in humans with incomplete peripheral nerve and brachial plexus injuries for greater than 6 months. Patients with traumatic nerve injury were treated 5 hours per day for 21 days and later compared with controls. Outcome measures were taken after 21 days, 3 months, and 6 months. Motor function, recruitment of motor units, and sensory function improved significantly, with no changes in controls. These findings as well as findings by Rochkind et al. while examining LLLT for incomplete PNI suggest that at least partial recovery of nerve function results from acceleration of nerve conductivity, followed by increased myelination in existing nerve fibers and partial regeneration of new axons and new synaptic connections.[83,85,87,88,91]

LLLT for compressive nerve injury secondary to CTS remains the most studied, albeit still limited, application of LLLT for PNI. To date, results remain equivocal, with no preponderance of evidence available to support or refute its use.[70,92–95] Evcik et al.[94] performed a prospective, randomized, placebo-controlled trial to investigate the efficacy of laser therapy in the treatment of CTS and reported significant improvements in sensory nerve velocity and sensory and motor distal latencies in the laser-treated group versus controls. No difference was observed in pain and pinch grip between the laser-treated group and the control group. In contrast, Irvine et al.[92] compared LLLT with sham laser in 15 patients with CTS and reported no significant effect on parameters of electrophysiological function. Similarly, clinical and electrophysiological parameters in patients with rheumatoid arthritis and CTS showed no significant improvement after LLLT applied 5 days per week for 2 weeks.[95] Improvements in neurophysiological parameters were reported by Naeser et al.,[93] who compared LLLT with TENS with sham laser with TENS. Significant improvements in mean sensory latency and pain were noted, with no difference in mean motor latency. However, extensive criticism of the data analyses of Naeser et al. leave considerable doubt as to the credibility of their observations.[96,97]

In response to PNI, muscle tissue demonstrates an accelerated degradation of myoprotein, atrophy, and decreased contractile mechanics. Through mechanisms of photobiostimulation, LLLT is thought to attenuate degeneration of muscle until axonal regeneration results in reinnervation.[5] Increased synthesis of creatine kinase, an enzyme involved in the supply of energy to skeletal muscle, and preservation of acetylcholine receptors observed after administration of LLLT in denervated rat muscle suggest a protective effect of laser.[98,99] The synthesis of high-energy phosphates via increased mitochondrial rephosphorylation of ATP is thought to preserve muscle integrity in the initial period after denervation injury by limiting the natural degenerative processes that occur in muscle. Data from rat models suggest that LLLT initiated as early as possible after injury may temporarily prevent denervation-induced biochemical changes as well as the potential restoration of muscle function.[5,98,99] There appear to be no deleterious consequences with muscle stemming from laser irradiation after PNI. Although these findings suggest a protective effect of laser, the research has yet to be substantiated in humans. Consequently, authors researching LLLT for PNI have suggested that more recent evidence from rat models should be a strong impetus for broader clinical trials in humans.[99–101]

Given the growing clinical interest in LLLT and continuing LLLT research, greater understanding of the effect of laser energy for PNI is imminent. Continuing research and technological advancements make LLLT a burgeoning area of physical agents. Technological advancements have made possible the concurrent administration of therapeutic ES with LLLT. Underlying this advancement are the observed findings and potential for healing for ES and laser when delivered as monotherapies. Newly approved by the U.S. Food and Drug Administration (FDA) for increasing local blood flow and **pain modulation,** combined therapy with ES and laser delivers electrical and light energy (Fig. 17-4).[102]

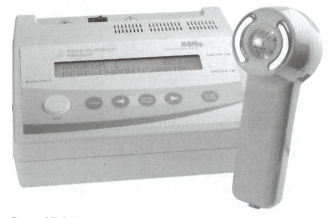

Figure 17-4 The simultaneous delivery of laser and electrical energy to evoke the biophysical responses of each modality (*MR4; Multi Radiance Medical, Solon, Ohio*).

Bottom line for laser and PNI: LLLT appears to be a viable intervention for PNI. A comprehensive 2005 review reported that all but two experimental studies showed LLLT to enhance recovery from severely injured peripheral nerve.[100] Likewise, a 2004 meta-analysis reported laser therapy to have an overall mean treatment effect size of 1.81 for tissue repair and 1.11 for pain control (an effect size of 0.8 or more indicates a large effect size) and that LLLT is a highly effective agent for tissue repair and pain.[78] Although findings for the use of laser therapy for PNI at first glance appear promising, these results are largely from animal models and limited randomized controlled trials. Such promising findings in humans are sparse. Postulated benefits for humans are predicated on speculative use from observed responses in animal and isolated cell studies. Because of the lack of substantial evidence in humans, the specific use of LLLT for PNI in humans can be neither fully endorsed nor completely refuted. Laser therapy may one day prove to be an effective intervention, but until then, endorsement is made via hopeful optimism.

Pulsed Electromagnetic Field

Pulsed electromagnetic field (PEMF) energy produced by diathermy devices passes through bodily tissues with minimal reflection at tissue interfaces or at bone, whereby minimal traces of energy accumulate at these interfaces as it occurs with US.[103] Gradually, absorption of energy by deeper tissues causes increased cellular activity.[103] Biological effects of PEMF include increased microvascular perfusion, changes in voltage-dependent ion-ligand binding, and alteration of cell membrane function and cellular activity.[104–109] PEMF therapy for 40 to 45 minutes and set to 600 pps has been shown to increase local blood flow significantly in healthy subjects without pathology and in patients with diabetic ulceration.[110,111] Increased cell mitosis and growth, expression of growth factors in fibroblasts and nerve cells, activity of macrophages, and phosphorylation and protein synthesis have been observed after PEMF therapy.[112-114] Despite lack of understanding of the mechanisms underlying these effects, PEMF therapy for PNI has continued.

Initial studies of PEMF therapy for regeneration of PNI in cats and rats showed promising results, but such results in humans were not examined until more recently. Use of PEMF in patients with refractory CTS and patients with diabetic neuropathy was studied in two separate randomized, double-blinded, placebo-controlled trials by Weintraub et al.[3,4] No effect of PEMF was noted in measures of neuropathic pain in patients with diabetic neuropathy. However, nearly one third of the subjects demonstrated an increase in epithelial nerve fiber density after 3 months—an effect not observed in the sham group. This finding suggested regenerative capabilities of PEMF and has provided the impetus for continued interest in PEMF. Subjects with refractory CTS receiving PEMF reported significant short-term and long-term pain relief, while also demonstrating a modest 10% improvement in distal nerve conduction latencies. In both studies, the authors concluded that although neurophysiological measures showed only modest change, little doubt exits that PEMF yields neurobiological effects that hold great promise. Use of PEMF therapy in patients with chronic diabetic polyneuropathy was examined by Musaev et al. in 2003.[115] Significant improvement in conduction of peripheral nerves and reflex excitability of functionally diverse motor neurons in the spinal cord and increased amplitudes of muscle potentials and the number of functioning motor neurons were observed after 10 applications of PEMF therapy.

At the time of this writing, we are unaware of any studies examining PEMF therapy in humans after transected PNI or more extensive studies in compressive nerve pathology. Although initial results from patients with diabetic neuropathy and compressive pathology following CTS appear encouraging, much more evidence is needed to support the widespread use of PEMF therapy for PNI in humans.

Bottom line for PEMF and PNI: Evidence for PEMF therapy for PNI is limited and appears largely related to as yet unclear cellular and hemodynamic events (i.e., increased perfusion). The limited evidence in humans stems from compressive neuropathy and mild ischemic neuropathy, conditions where increased local perfusion may underlie observed benefits. Changes in cell activity and increased local blood flow do not appear to be unique to PEMF. At this time, there is insufficient evidence to support use of PEMF as a therapeutic intervention for PNI in humans.

Monochromatic Infrared Energy

The most widely used physical agent for the treatment of peripheral neuropathy at the present time is infrared light. Monochromatic infrared energy (MIRE) is delivered at a single wavelength (890 nm long, at a rate of 292 times per second) from a pad containing 60 superluminous GaAlAs diodes by a therapeutic device manufactured by Anodyne Therapy, LLC (Tampa, Florida).[116] Since it was approved by the FDA for the reduction of pain and increasing circulation, numerous investigations have been performed on the effectiveness of MIRE.

The primary outcome measure of studies assessing MIRE has generally been restoration of protective sensation, and some cases have included wound recurrence, quality of life, number of falls, and fear of falling as outcome measures. Although earlier studies examined the effects of MIRE on wound healing, the first published study specifically aimed at determining the effectiveness of MIRE on the reversal of peripheral neuropathy was published by Kochman in 2002.[117] Following six treatments of MIRE, 48 of 49 patients had improved sensation, with all demonstrating improvement in 12 weeks. Similar results were reported by Prendergast et al.[118] Following 10 treatments in 2 weeks, 96% of all subjects had a reduced severity grade of sensory impairment after the treatments with MIRE.

A primary limitation of the previous studies is the lack of a control group without which improvements secondary to placebo cannot be ruled out. Without a control group treated with a sham device, it is difficult to determine how much of the improvement in sensation could be attributed to a placebo effect. Leonard et al.[119] addressed this issue by performing a double-blind, randomized, placebo-controlled study in patients with type 1 or type 2 diabetes who were insensate to the 5.07 Semmes Weinstein monofilament (SWM).[119] Subjects were treated with MIRE on one limb and a sham device on the other for 2 weeks, followed by active treatments to both limbs over the next 2 weeks. Although sham treatment did not improve sensitivity as measured by the number of insensate sites, 2 weeks of sham treatment did result in significantly reduced Michigan Neuropathy Screening Instrument scores, indicating an improvement of peripheral neuropathy. In subjects considered to have more severe conditions (i.e., insensate to 6.65 SWM), there was no significant improvement in sensation, pain, or neuropathic symptoms, but balance did improve moderately.

Two potential issues with the study by Leonard et al. were the short treatment duration and use of only two sizes of monofilaments. It may be argued that if treatment were for a longer duration or if smaller increments of monofilament were used, the potential effects of MIRE would have been more apparent. Arnall et al.[120] addressed these issues studying patients with diabetes treated for 8 weeks with a combination of infrared and visible red light. Six monofilaments, rather than two, were used, which improved the ability to detect small changes in sensation. A sham device was not used; however, the contralateral limb received no treatment and served as a control. Subjects initially sensitive to the 5.07 SWM showed no significant improvements in sensation in either the treatment or the control limb. In patients insensate to the 5.07 SWM at baseline, improvement was noted; however, only changes in the treatment group were significant. Arnall et al. likewise examined the effects of infrared light on the perception of vibratory sensation and found no significant changes in the subject's ability to perceive vibration after infrared light therapy.

Numerous retrospective studies are frequently cited in support of MIRE for the reversal of peripheral neuropathy. Using questionnaire data from patients with diabetic peripheral neuropathy that had improved with MIRE, Powell et al.[121] concluded that MIRE reduced the incidence of diabetic foot ulcerations when comparing the incidence of ulceration in their own study with the incidence reported in a previous study. Extrapolation to the general population of patients with diabetic neuropathy is impossible because patients who did not benefit from MIRE were excluded. Additionally, only 57% of eligible participants responded to the survey, so no conclusion can be made regarding whether the remaining participants fared as well or did not respond because they were less satisfied with the results. DeLellis et al.[122] reviewed records of 1,047 patients with peripheral neuropathy. Based on physician documentation, 99% were insensate to the 5.07 SWM in two or more places on both feet before the initiation of MIRE. After MIRE, 56% of patients regained protective sensation, and the number of insensate sites was significantly lessened. Similarly to additional studies of MIRE, there was no control group, which must be considered when interpreting the results. A comparable retrospective chart review of 2,239 patients who had received MIRE for peripheral neuropathy revealed a 67% reduction in pain and a 66% reduction in the number of insensate sites.[123] Although the results are impressive, the possibility of a placebo effect must be considered because this study was nonblinded and nonrandomized, and lacked a control group.

The functional benefits of MIRE, specifically the rate of falls in elderly patients with peripheral neuropathy, have been examined.[124] A health questionnaire of 252 patients reporting symptomatic reversal of peripheral diabetic neuropathy was used. Based on survey results, a reduction in fear of falling and number of falls and an increase in quality-of-life rating were apparent 1 month and 1 year after neuropathy improved. No objective measures of balance were assessed. Additionally, fear of falling has been implicated as a risk factor for falls, and the finding that participants were less fearful alludes to the functional relevance of this study.

Despite promising results from other studies, several placebo-controlled trials have not found such efficacy for MIRE. A double-blind, placebo-controlled trial assessing the effect of MIRE on sensation in 39 patients with peripheral neuropathy showed no significant difference between the active and placebo groups at 4 weeks because both groups demonstrated statistically significant improvements in the mean number of sites sensitive to the 5.07 SWM.[125] Similar findings were also noted at 8 weeks. Results of this placebo-controlled study suggest that MIRE offers no greater benefit than placebo treatment for peripheral neuropathy.

A placebo-controlled double-blinded study by Franzen-Korzendorfer et al.[126] also failed to demonstrate efficacy for MIRE. In this study, patients had each leg randomly assigned to the sham or active treatment group. At the conclusion of the study, there were no significant differences in pain or sensation levels between the active and sham groups. Additionally, pain scores did not change for either group. Sensation did significantly improve from baseline for both the control and sham groups, again suggesting a placebo effect. Perhaps the largest placebo-controlled study examining the effectiveness of MIRE was a double-blinded, sham-controlled study by Lavery et al.[127] involving 60 patients. In contrast to other studies that assigned one limb to the active group and the other to the control group, this study had two distinct groups statistically similar at baseline. Six different outcome measures were assessed. No significant differences were noted between groups after 3 months of treatment.

Bottom line for MIRE for peripheral neuropathy: Use of MIRE for the restoration of impaired sensation in patients with peripheral neuropathy remains contentious. Despite early, largely industry-funded, primarily noncontrolled studies that demonstrated positive effects of MIRE, more recent placebo-controlled studies have failed to yield such positive results. Because a placebo effect seems to be a strong possibility, further investigations of MIRE for the treatment of neuropathy should be large, independent studies with a sham control group.

CASE STUDY

While playing football, SC received a violent blow from a helmet to his right arm just distal to the acromion. He felt his arm immediately "weaken" and was pulled from the game. Initial assessment identified a "rotator cuff strain," and SC was prohibited from practice or playing until the arm healed. After 3 weeks of rest, the arm was not improving, and he saw a physical therapist. The therapist, after evaluation, thought the injury was neurological and referred SC to a neurologist for an electroneuromyography assessment. The needle examination revealed an axonotmetic lesion of the right axillary nerve with significant weakness of the right deltoid muscle. SC was referred back to the physical therapist for intervention.

Case Study Questions

1. SC, after researching "nerve injury" on the Internet, requested of the physical therapist that ES be performed to his shoulder. "From what I read online, electrical stimulation is the best tool to speed nerve regeneration," explained SC to his therapist. The therapist's best response would be:
   a. "Unfortunately, evidence the effectiveness of electrical stimulation in human studies is poor. There are more effective interventions we should try."
   b. "I am not convinced, but let's try it."
   c. "Most evidence is from rodent studies and is easily translated into human results."
   d. "Electrical stimulation worked for a friend of mine; let's try it."

2. Three systematic and meta-analytic reviews published in 2010 describing TENS with neuropathic pain are available. Which of the following statements is not true?
   a. TENS and amitriptyline are more effective than TENS alone.
   b. TENS promotes positive pain relief for up to 12 weeks with no adverse effects.
   c. Complete pain relief was found in 16% to 36% of patients who used TENS.
   d. Pain relief with TENS treatment lasted up to 10 years.

3. Which of the following statements regarding the use of ES to preserve denervated muscle is true?
   a. ES, performed twice per day, is an effective modality to maintain functional sarcomeres.
   b. A 2007 review of ES neither supports nor refutes the use of ES for the preservation of functional sarcomeres in denervated muscle.
   c. ES has no impact on preserving functional sarcomeres in denervated muscle.
   d. ES slows, but does not prevent, muscle atrophy in denervated muscle.

4. Which of the following statements best describes the use of US in the promotion of nerve regeneration?
   a. US is an effective modality to promote nerve regeneration in axonotmetic lesions.
   b. US is an effective modality to promote nerve healing in neurapraxic lesions.
   c. Although there is considerable evidence of the effectiveness of US in promoting nerve regeneration in a rat model, there is no quality evidence of the effectiveness in humans.
   d. For compressive neuropathy secondary to CTS, low-intensity US is a highly effective modality in aiding regeneration and improvement in functional performance.

5. Which of the following statements regarding findings of current research with LLLT and regeneration is true?
   a. LLLT has no effect on regeneration.
   b. Based on rat models and cellular models, LLLT is a promising agent as an intervention for nerve injury.
   c. Risk of complications makes LLLT an unsafe therapy.
   d. LLLT is a highly effective modality and always should be considered as a first-line modality for nerve injury.

References

1. Nuccitelli R. A role for endogenous electrical fields in wound healing. *Curr Top Dev Biol.* 2003;58:1–27.
2. Raja K, Garcia M, Isseroff R. Wound re-epithelialization: modulating keratinocyte migration in wound healing. *Front Biosci.* 2007;12:2849–2868.
3. Weintraub M, Cole S. A randomized controlled trial of the effects of a combination of static and dynamic magnetic fields on carpal tunnel syndrome. *Pain Med.* 2008;9(5):493–504.
4. Weintraub M, Herrmann D, Smith G, Backonja M, Cole S. Pulsed electromagnetic fields to reduce diabetic neuropathic pain and stimulate neuronal repair: a randomized controlled trial. *Arch Phys Med Rehabil.* 2009;90:1102–1109.
5. Rochkind S. Phototherapy in peripheral nerve injury for muscle preservation and nerve regeneration. *Photomed Laser Surg.* 2009;27(2):221–222.
6. Volkert W, Hassan A, Hassan M, et al. Effectiveness of monochromatic infrared photoenergy and physical therapy for peripheral neuropathy: changes in sensation, pain, and balance—a preliminary, multicenter study. *PhysOccup Ther Geriatr.* 2005;24(2):1–17.
7. Gordon T, Chan K, Sulaiman O, Udina E, Amirjani N, Brushart T. Accelerating axon growth to overcome limitations in functional recovery after peripheral nerve injury. *Neurosurgery.* 2009;65:A132–144.
8. McCaig C, Rajnicek A, Song B, Zhao M. Controlling cell behavior electrically: current views and future potential. *Physiol Rev.* 2005;85:943–978.
9. Erickson C, Nuccitelli R. Embyonic fibroblast motility and orientation can be influenced by physiological electrical fields. *J Cell Biol.* 1984;98:296–307.
10. Fenrich K, Gordon T. Axonal regeneration in the peripheral and central nervous systems—current issues and advances. *Can J Neurol Sci.* 2004;31:142–156.
11. Sulaiman O, Gordon T. Effects of short and long term Schwann cell denervation on peripheral nerve regeneration, myelination, and size. *Glia.* 2000;32:234–246.
12. Gordon T, Udina E, Verge M, de Chaves E. Brief electrical stimulation accelerates axon regeneration in the peripheral nervous system and promotes sensory axon regeneration in the central nervous system. *Motor Control.* 2009;13:412–441.
13. Nix W, Hopf H. Electrical stimulation of regenerating nerve and its effect on motor recovery. *Brain Res.* 1983;272:21–25.
14. Pockett S, Gavin R. Acceleration of peripheral nerve regeneration after crush injury in rat. *Neurosci Lett.* 1985;59:221–224.
15. Al-Majeed A, Neumann C, Brushart T, Gordon T. Brief electrical stimulation promotes the speed and accuracy of motor axonal regeneration. *J Neurosci Methods.* 2000;20:2602–2608.
16. Gordon A, Weistein M. Sodium salicylate iontophoresis in the treatment of plantar warts: case report. *Phys Ther.* 1969;49:869–870.

17. Gordon T, Brushart T, Amirjani N, Chan K. The potential of electrical stimulation to promote functional recovery after peripheral nerve injury: comparisons between rats and humans. *Acta Neurochir Suppl.* 2007;100:3–11.

18. Gordon T, Brushart T, Chan K. Augmenting nerve regeneration with electrical stimulation. *Neurol Res.* 2008;30: 1012–1022.

19. Brushart T, Jari R, Verge V, Rohde C, Gordon T. Electrical stimulation restores the specificity of sensory axon regeneration. *Exp Neurol.* 2005;194:221–229.

20. Franz C, Rustishauser U, Rafuse V. Intrinsic neuronal properties control selective targeting of regenerating motoneurons. *Brain.* 2008;131:1492–1505.

21. Havton L. A lumbosacral ventral root avulsion injury and repair model for studies of neuropathic pain in rats. *Methods Mol Bio.* 2012;851:185–193.

22. Cauthen J, Renner E. Transcutaneous and peripheral nerve stimulation for chronic pain states. *Surg Neurol.* 1975;4: 102–104.

23. Johansson F, Almay B, Von Knorring L, Terenius I. Predictors for the outcome of treatment with high-frequency transcutaneous electrical nerve stimulation in patients with chronic pain. *Pain.* 1980;9:55–61.

24. Meyler W, de Jongste M, Rolf C. Clinical evaluation of pain treatment with electrostimulation: a study on TENS in patients with different pain syndromes. *Clin J Pain.* 1994;10: 22–27.

25. Dubinsky R, Miyasaki J. Assessment: efficacy of transcutaneous electric nerve stimulation in the treatment of of pain in neurological disorders (an evidence-based review): report of the Therapeutics and Technology Assessment Subcommittee of the American Academy of Neurology. *Neurology.* 2010;74:173–176.

26. Jin D, Xu Y, Geng D, Yan T. Effect of transcutaneous electrical nerve stimulation on symptomatic diabetic neuropathy: a meta-analysis of randomized controlled trials. *Diabetes Res Clin Pract.* 2010;89:10–15.

27. Pieber K, Herceg M, Paternostro-Sluga T. Electrotherapy for the treatment of painful diabetic peripheral neuropathy: a review. *J Rehabil Med.* 2010;42:289–295.

28. Kumar D, Alvaro M, Julka I, Marshall H. Diabetic peripheral neuropathy: effectiveness of electrotherapy and amitriptyline for symptomatic relief. *Diabetes Care.* 1998;21:1322–1325.

29. Kumar D, Marshall H. Diabetic peripheral neuropathy: amelioration of pain with transcutaneous electrostimulation. *Diabetes Care.* 1997;20:1702–1705.

30. Forst T, Nguyen S, Forst S, Disselhoff B, Pohlmann T, Pfutzner A. Impact of low frequency transcutaneous electrical nerve stimulation on symptomatic diabetic neuropathy using the new Salutaris device. *Diabetes Nutr Metab.* 2004;17:163–168.

31. Julka I, Alvaro M, Kumar D. Beneficial effects of electrical stimulation on neuropathic symptoms in diabetes patients. *J Foot Ankle Surg.* 1988;37:191–194.

32. Somers D, Clemente F. Contra-lateral high or a combination of high- and low-frequency transcutaneous electrical nerve stimulation reduces mechanical allodynia and alters dorsal horn neurotransmitter content in neuropathic rats. *J Pain.* 2009;10(2):221–229.

33. Somers D, Clemente F. Transcutaneous electrical nerve stimulation for the management of neuropathic pain: the effects of frequency and electrode position on prevention of allodynia in a rat model of complex regional pain syndrom type II. *Phys Ther.* 2006;86(5):698–709.

34. Somers D, Clemente F. High-frequency transcutaneous electrical nerve stimulation alters thermal but not mechanical allodynia following chronic constriction injury

35. of the rat sciatic nerve. *Arch Phys Med Rehabil.* 1998;79: 1370–1376.

35. Bellew J. *Foundations of Electrotherapy.* 5th ed. Philadelphia: FA Davis; 2011.

36. Fuentes J, Olivo S, Magee D, Gross D. Effectiveness of interferential current therapy in the management of musculoskeletal pain: a systematic review and meta-analysis. *Phys Ther.* 2010;90(9):1219–1238.

37. Bosi E. Effectiveness of frequency-modulated electromagnetic neural stimulation in the treatment of painful diabetic neuropathy. *Diabetologia.* 2005;48:817–823.

38. Conti M. Frequency-modulated electromagnetic neural stimulation enhances cutaneous microvascular flow in patients with diabetic neuropathy. *J Diabetes Complications.* 2009;23:46–48.

39. Gigo-Benato D, Russo T, Geuna S, Domingues N, Salvini T, Parizotto A. Electrical stimulation impairs early functional recovery and accentuates skeletal muscle atrophy after sciatic nerve crush injury in rats. *Muscle Nerve.* 2010; 41:685–693.

40. McGinnis M, Murphy D. The lack of an effect of applied DC electric fields on peripheral nerve regeneration in the guinea pig. *Neuroscience.* 1992;51:231–244.

41. Marqueste T, Decherchi P, Dousset E, Berthelin F, Jammes Y. Effect of muscle electrostimulation on afferent activities from tibialis anterior muscle after nerve repair by self-anastamosis. *Neuroscience.* 2002;113:257–271.

42. Eberstein A, Eberstein S. Electrical stimulation of denervated muscle: is it worthwhile? *Med Sci Sports Exerc.* 1996;28(12):1463–1469.

43. Gosztonyi G, Naschold U, Grozdanovic Z, Stoltenburg-Didinger G, Gossrau R. Expression of Leu-19 (CD56-N-CAM) and nitric oxide synthase (NOS) I in denervated and reinnervated human skeletal muscle. *Microsc Res Techn.* 2001; 55:187–197.

44. Baptista A, Gomes J, Oliveira J, Santos S, Vannier-Santos M, Martinez A. High- and low-frequency transcutaneous electrical stimulation delay sciatic nerve regeneration after crush injury in the mouse. *J Peripher Nerv Syst.* 2008;13:71–80.

45. Bellew J. *Clinical Electrical Stimulaiton: Application and Techniques.* 5th ed. Philadelphia: FA Davis; 2011.

46. Dow D, Cederna P, Hassett C, Kostrominova T, Faulkner J, Dennis R. Number of contractions to maintain mass and force of a denervated rat muscle. *Muscle Nerve.* 2004;30(1): 77–86.

47. Dow D, Cederna P, Hassett C, Dennis R, Faulknet J. Electrical stimulation prior to delayed reinnervation does not enhance recovery in muscle of rats. *Restor Neurol Neurosci.* 2007;25:601–610.

48. Glinsky J, Harvey L, Van Es P. Efficacy of electrical stimulation to increase muscle strength in people with neurological conditions: a systematic review. *Physiother Res Int.* 2007;12(3):175–194.

49. Kern H, Hofer C, Modlin M, et al. Denervated muscles in humans: limitations and problems of currently used functional electrical stimulation training protocols. *Artif Organs.* 2002;26(3):216–218.

50. Mandl T, Meyerspeer M, Reichel M, et al. Functional electrical stimulation of long-term denervated, degenerated human skeletal muscle: estimating activation using T2-parameter magnetic resonance imaging methods. *Artif Organs.* 2008;32(8):604–608.

51. Modlin M, Forstner C, Hofer C, et al. Electrical stimulation of denervated muscles: first results of a clinical study. *Artif Organs.* 2005;29(3):203–206.

52. Michlovitz S. Is there a role for ultrasound and electrical stimulation following injury to tendon and nerve? *J Hand Ther.* 2005;18:292–296.

53. Michlovitz S, Bellew J, Nolan T. *Modalities for Therapeutic Intervention*. 5th ed. Philadelphia: FA Davis; 2011.
54. Bunge M, Williams A, Wood P, et al. Comparison of nerve cell and nerve cell plus Schwann cell cultures, with particular emphasis on basal lamina and collagen formation. *J Cell Biol*. 1980;84:184–202.
55. Lundborg G, Rydevik B. Effects of stretching the tibial nerve of the rabbit: a preliminary study of the intraneural circulation and barrier function of the perineurium. *J Bone Joint Surg (Br)*. 1973;55:390–401.
56. Rydevik B, Lundborg G, Nordborg C. Intraneural tissue reactions induced by internal neurolysis. *Scand J Plast Reconstr Surg*. 1976;10:3–8.
57. Mourad P, Lazar D, Curra F, et al. Ultrasound accelerates functional recovery after peripheral nerve damage. *Neurosurgery*. 2001;48(5):1136–1141.
58. Hong C, Liu H, Yu J. Ultrasound thermotherapy effect on the recovery of nerve conduction in experimental compression neuropathy. *Arch Phys Med Rehabil*. 1988;69:410–414.
59. Lowdon I, Seaber A, Urbaniak J. An improved method of recording rat tracks for measurements of the sciatic functional index of De Medinaceli. *J Neurosci Methods*. 1988;24:279–281.
60. Crisci A, Ferreira A. Low-intensity pulsed ultrasound accelerates the regeneration of the sciatic nerve after neurotomy in rats. *Ultrasound Med Biol*. 2002;28(10):1335–1341.
61. Chang C, Hsu S, Lin F, Chang H, Chang C. Low intensity ultrasound accelerated nerve regeneration using cell seeded poly (D,L-lactic acid-co-glycolic acid) conduits: an in-vivo and in-vitro study. *J Biomed Mater Res B Appl Biomater*. 2005;75:99–107.
62. Park S, Oh S, Seo T, Namgung U, Kim J, Lee J. Ultrasound-stimulated peripheral nerve regeneration within asymmetrically porous PLGA/Pluronic F127 nerve guide conduit. *J Biomed Mater Res*. 2010;94(2):359–366.
63. Zhang H, Lin X, Wan H, Li J, Li J. Effect of low-intensity pulsed ultrasound on the expression of neurotrophin-3 and brain-derived neurotrophic factor in cultured Schwann cells. *Microsurgery*. 2009;29(6):479–485.
64. Bhatheja K, Field J. Schwann cells: origins and role in axonal maintenance and regeneration. *Int J Biochem Cell Biol*. 2006;38:1995–1999.
65. Raso V, Barbieri C, Mazzer N, Fasan V. Can therapeutic ultrasound influence the regeneration of peripheral nerves? *J Neurosci Methods*. 2005;142:185–192.
66. Ebenbichler G, Resch K, Funovics M, Nicolakis P, Wiesinger G, Fialka V. Ultrasound treatment for treating carpal tunnel syndrome: randomized "sham" controlled trial. *BMJ*. 1998;316:7315.
67. Piravej K, Boonhong J. Effect of ultrasound thermotherapy in mild to moderate carpal tunnel syndrome. *J Med Assoc Thai*. 2004;87(Suppl 2):S100–106.
68. Oztas O, Turan B, Bora I, Karakaya M. Ultrasound therapy effects in carpal tunnel syndrome. *Arch Phys Med Rehabil*. 1998;79:1540–1544.
69. Bakhtiary A, Rashidy-Pour A. Ultrasound and laser therapy in the treatment of carpal tunnel syndrome. *Aust J Physiother*. 2004;50:147–151.
70. Piazzini D, Aprile I, Ferrara P, et al. A systematic review of conservative treatment of carpal tunnel syndrome. *Clin Rehabil*. 2007;21:299–314.
71. Pinheiro A, Gerbi ME. Photoengineering of bone repair processes. *Photomed Laser Surg*. 2006;24:169–178.
72. Passerella S, Casamassima E, Molinari S, et al. Increase of proton electrochemical potential and ATP synthesis in rat liver mitochondria irradiated in vitro by helium-neon laser. *FEBS Lett*. 1984;175:95–99.
73. Loevschal H, Arenholt-Bindslev D. Effect of low level diode laser irradiation of human oral mucosa fibroblasts in vitro. *Lasers Surg Med*. 1994;14:347–354.
74. Karu T. Molecular mechanisms of the therapeutic effects of low intensity laser radiation. *Lasers Life Sci*. 1989;2:53–74.
75. Mognato M, Squizzato F, Facchin F, Zaghetto L, Corti L. Cell growth modulation of human cells irradiated in vitro with low-level laser therapy. *Photomed Laser Surg*. 2004;22:523–526.
76. Moor P, Ridgway T, Higbee R, Howard E, Lucroy M. Effect of wavelength on low-intensity laser irradiation-stimulated cell proliferation in vitro. *Lasers Surg Med*. 2005;36:8–12.
77. Ferreira D, Zângaro R, Villaverde A, et al. Analgesic effect of He-Ne (632.8 nm) low-level laser therapy on acute inflammatory pain. *Photomed Laser Surg*. 2005;23(2):177–181.
78. Enwemeka C, Parker J, Dowdy D, Harkness E, Sanford L, Woodruff L. The efficacy of low-power lasers in tissue repair and pain control: a meta-analysis study. *Photomed Laser Surg*. 2004;22(4):323–329.
79. Byrnes K, Waynant R, Ilev I, et al. Light promotes regeneration and functional recovery and alters the immune response after spinal cord injury. *Lasers Surg Med*. 2005;36(3):171–185.
80. Yu W, Naim J, McGowan M, et al. Photomodulation of oxidative metabolism and electron chain enzymes in the rat liver mitochondria. *Photochem Photobiol*. 1997;66:866–871.
81. Abergel R, Meeker C, Lam T, Dwye R, Lesavoy M, Uitto J. Control of connective tissue metabolism by lasers: recent developments and future prospects. *J Am Acad Dermatol*. 1984;11:1142–1150.
82. Karu T. Molecular mechanisms of the therapeutic effects of low intensity laser radiation. *Lasers Life Sci*. 1989;2:53–74.
83. Rochkind S, Nissan M, Barr-Nea L, Razon N, Schwartz M, Bartal A. Response of peripheral nerve to He-Ne laser: experimental studies. *Lasers Surg Med*. 1987;7:441–443.
84. Shamir M, Rochkind S, Sandbank J, Alon M. Double-blind randomized study evaluating regeneration of the rat transected sciatic nerve after suturing and postoperative lower power laser treatment. *J Reconstr Microsurg*. 2001;17:133–138.
85. Rochkind S, Rousso M, Nissan M, Villarreal M, Barr-Nea L, Reese DG. Systemic effects of low-power laser irradiation on the peripheral and central nervous system, cutaneous wounds, and burns. *Laser Surg Med*. 1989;9(2):174–178.
86. Anders J, Borke R, Woolery S, Van de Merwe W. Low power laser irradiation alters the rate of regeneration of the rat facial nerve. *Lasers Surg Med*. 1993;13:72–82.
87. Rochkind S, Droroy V, Alon M, Nissan M, Ouaknine GE. The treatment of incomplete peripheral nerve injuries using a new modality-laser phototherapy (780nm). *Photomed Laser Surg*. 2007;25:436–442.
88. Rochkind S, Leider-Trejo L, Nissan M, Shamir M, Kharenko O, Alon M. Efficacy of 780nm laser phototherapy on peripheral nerve regeneration after neurotube reconstruction procedure (double-blind randomized study). *Photomed Laser Surg*. 2007;25:137–143.
89. Gigo-Benato D, Geuna S, deCastro Rodrigues A, et al. Low power laser biostimulation enhances nerve repair after end-to-side neurorrhaphy. A double blind randomized study in the rat median nerve model. *Laser Med Sci*. 2004;19:57–65.
90. Reis F, Belchior A, Nicolau R, Fonseca T, Carvalho P. Effect of gallium-aluminum-arsenide laser therapy (660Nm) on recovery of the sciatic nerve in rats following neurotmesis

lesion and epineural anastomosis: functional analysis. *Braz J Phys Ther.* 2008;12:215–221.

91. Rochkind S. Stimulation effects of laser energy on the regeneration of traumatically injured peripheral nerves. *Morphogen Regen.* 1978;83:25–27.

92. Irvine J, Chong S, Amirjani N, Chan M. Double blind randomized controlled trial of low level laser therapy in carpal tunnel syndrome. *Muscle Nerve.* 2004;30:182–187.

93. Naeser M, Hahn K, Lieberman B. Carpal tunnel syndrome pain treated with low level laser and microamperes transcutaneous electrical nerve stimulation: a controlled study. *Arch Phys Med Rehabil.* 2002;83:978–987.

94. Evcik D, Kavuncu V, Cakir T, Subasi V, Yaman M. Laser therapy in the treatment of carpal tunnel syndrome: a randomized controlled trial. *Photomed Laser Surg.* 2007;25: 34–39.

95. Ekim A, Armagan O, Tascioglu F, Oner C, Colak I. Effect of low level laser therapy in rheumatoid patients with carpal tunnel syndrome. *Swiss Med Wkly.* 2007;137: 347–352.

96. Bodofsky E. Treating carpal tunnel syndrome with lasers and TENS. *Arch Phys Med Rehabil.* 2002;83:1806–1807.

97. Bodofsky E. Follow-up on low level laser and microvolt transcutaneous electric stimulation. *Arch Phys Med Rehabil.* 2003;84:1402–1403.

98. Bolognani L, Volpi N. *Low Power Laser Enzymology: Reactivation of Myosin ATPase by GaAs and HeNe Lasers.* Bari, Italy: Trani; 1991.

99. Rochkind S, Geuna S, Shainberg A. Phototherapy in peripheral nerve injury: effects on muscle preservation and nerve regeneration. *Int Rev Neurobiol.* 2009;87:445–464.

100. Gigo-Benato D, Geuna S, Rochkind S. Phototherapy for enhancing peripheral nerve repair: a review of the literature. *Muscle Nerve.* 2005;31:694–701.

101. Rochkind S. Phototherapy in peripheral nerve regeneration: from basic science to clinical study. *Neurosurg Focus.* 2009; 26(2):E8, 1–6.

102. FDA Clearance: K071445. Trade Name Device: LaserTENS, Multi Radiance Medical.

103. Dellagatta E, Nolan T. *Electromagnetic Waves: Laser, Diathermy, and Pulsed Electromagnetic Fields.* 5th ed. Philadelphia: FA Davis; 2011.

104. Glassman L, McGrath M, Bassett C. Effect of external pulsing electromagnetic fields on the healing of soft tissues. *Ann Plast Surg.* 1986;16:287–295.

105. Ryaby J. Clinical effects of electromagnetic and electric fields on fracture healing. *Clin Orthop.* 1984;355(Suppl): 205–215.

106. Weintraub M. Magnetotherapy: historical background with a stimulating future. *Clin Rev Phys Rehabil.* 2004;16: 96–108.

107. Cameron M. *Physical Agents in Rehabilitation.* 2nd ed. St. Louis: Saunders; 2003.

108. Chiabrera A, Grattarola M, Viviani R. Interaction between electromagnetic fields and cells: microelectrophoretic effect of ligands and surface receptors. *Bioelectromagnetics.* 1984;5: 173–178.

109. McLeod B, Liboff A. Dynamic characteristics of low membrane ions in multified configurations of low frequency electromagnetic radiation. *Bioelectromagnetics.* 1986;7: 177–189.

110. Mayrovitz H, Larsen P. A preliminary study to evaluate the effect of pulsed radio frequency field treatment on lower extremity peri-ulcer skin microcirculaiton of diabetic patients. *Wounds.* 1995;7(3):90–93.

111. Mayrovitz H, Larsen P. Effects of pulsed electromagnetic fileds on skin microvascular blood perfusion. *Wounds.* 1992;4(5):197–202.

112. Markov MS, Muechsam DJ, Pilla AA. *Modulation of Cell-Free Myosin Phosphorylation With Pulsed Radio Frequency Electromagnetic Fields.* Singapore: World Scientific; 1995.

113. Boonstra J, Skper S, Varons S. Regulation of Na+-K+ pump activity by nerve growth factor in chick embryo dorsal root ganglia cells. *J Cell Physiol.* 1982;113:452–455.

114. Rozengurt E, Mendoza S. Monovalent ion fluxes and the control of cell proliferation in cultured fibroblasts. *Ann N Y Acad Sci.* 1980;339:175–190.

115. Musaev A, Guseinva S, Imamverdieva S. The use of pulsed electromagnetic fields with complex modulation in the treatment of patients with diabetic polyneuropathy. *Neurosci Behav Physiol.* 2003;33(8):745–752.

116. Burke T. 5 Questions—and answers—about MIRE treatment. *Adv Skin Wound Care.* 2003;16:369–371.

117. Kochman A. Symptomatic reversal of peripheral neuropathy in patients with diabetes. *J Am Podiatr Med Assoc.* 2002;92: 125–130.

118. Prendergast JJ, Miranda G, Sanchez M. Improvement of sensory impairment in patients with peripheral neuropathy. *Endocr Pract.* 2004;10:24–30.

119. Leonard DR, Farooqi MH, Myers S. Restoration of sensation, reduced pain, and improved balance in subjects with diabetic peripheral neuropathy: a double-blind, randomized, placebo-controlled study with monochromatic near-infrared treatment. *Diabetes Care.* 2004;27:168–172.

120. Arnall DA, Nelson AG, López L, et al. The restorative effects of pulsed light therapy on significant loss of peripheral protective sensation in patients with long-term type 1 and type 2 diabetes mellitus. *Acta Diabetol.* 2006;43: 26–33.

121. Powell MW, Carnegie DE, Burke TJ. Reversal of diabetic peripheral neuropathy and new wound incidence: the role of MIRE. *Adv Skin Wound Care.* 2004;17:295–300.

122. DeLellis SL, Carnegie DH, Burke TJ. Improved sensitivity in patients with peripheral neuropathy: effects of monochromatic infrared photo energy. *J Am Podiatr Med Assoc.* 2005;95:143–147.

123. Harkless LB, DeLellis S, Carnegie DH, Burke TJ. Improved foot sensitivity and pain reduction in patients with peripheral neuropathy after treatment with monochromatic infrared photo energy—MIRE. *J Diabetes Complications.* 2006;20:81–87.

124. Powell MW, Carnegie DH, Burke TJ. Reversal of diabetic peripheral neuropathy with phototherapy (MIRE) decreases falls and the fear of falling and improves activities of daily living in seniors. *Age Ageing.* 2006;35(1):11–16.

125. Clifft JK, Kasser RJ, Newton TS, Bush AJ. The effect of monochromatic infrared energy on sensation in patients with diabetic peripheral neuropathy: a double-blind, placebo-controlled study. *Diabetes Care.* 2005;28:2896–2900.

126. Franzen-Korzendorfer H, Blackinton M, Rone-Adams S, McCulloch J. The effect of monochromatic infrared energy on transcutaneous oxygen measurements and protective sensation: results of a controlled, double-blind, randomized clinical study. *Ostomy Wound Manage.* 2008;54:16–31.

127. Lavery LA, Murdoch DP, Williams J, Lavery DC. Does Anodyne light therapy improve peripheral neuropathy in diabetes? A double-blind, sham-controlled, randomized trial to evaluate monchromatic infrared photoenergy. *Diabetes Care* 2008;31:316–321.

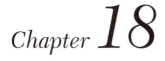

Chapter 18

Orthotic Intervention for Peripheral Neuropathy

Elizabeth Spencer Steffa, OTR/L, CHT

"Illness is the most heeded of all doctors. To goodness and wisdom we make only promises; to pain we obey."

—Marcel Proust (1871–1922)

Objectives

On completion of this chapter, the student/practitioner will be able to:

- List the indications for use of a splint in individuals with peripheral nerve injury.
- Describe the differences between static and dynamic splinting.
- Discuss common orthoses prescribed for individuals with median, ulnar, radial, and plexus injuries.
- Define the concept of three-point pressure.

Key Terms

- Contracture
- Dynamic splint
- Immobilization
- Safe position
- Serial casting
- Static splint
- Three-point pressure

Introduction

Using splinting to treat a peripheral nerve injury is important but often challenging. This chapter discusses the basic use of splinting forces as an intervention for brachial plexus, radial, median, and ulnar nerve injuries. Lower extremity nerve injuries are not addressed in this chapter; however, the basic splinting concepts may be translated to those nerve injuries as well.

All injuries to peripheral nerves result in possible motor loss and subsequent muscle imbalance creating the potential for further loss of function secondary to adaptive contractile and noncontractile tissue shortening and lengthening. The objectives of splinting include protection of injured tissues, enhancement of a healing environment, prevention or minimization of **contracture** formation, acting as a substitute for lost motor function, and facilitation and enhancement of functional daily activities. The prescription, fabrication, and fitting of a custom orthosis requires a strong understanding of the basic mechanical principles of splinting; knowledge of the mechanical properties of splinting materials; knowledge of deep and surface anatomy; knowledge of the impact of compressive, tensile, and shear forces on the integument; and a thorough understanding of the pathophysiology, diagnostics, and treatment of peripheral nerve injury. Therapists who use splinting should strive to practice with a "minimalistic" approach with emphasis on simplicity, cost accountability, flexibility, and sustainability in the attainment of splint effectiveness. This method of practice promotes patient satisfaction and compliance.[1] The ideal splint should be comfortable, lightweight, functional, easy to don and doff, and aesthetically "pleasing" to the patient while performing the function for which it was intended.

Splinting Mechanics and Terminology

The most frequently used splint for the appendicular skeleton is a **three-point pressure** splint. The proximal and distal forces occur in the same direction, and the middle force is in the opposite direction (Fig. 18-1). The wrist splint uses two points of pressure—one at the palm and the other along the proximal forearm—and an opposite directional point of force at the wrist (Fig. 18-2). The wrist splint is classified as a first-class lever.[2] Force is defined by type, such as push or pull; amount; application angle; and point of application.[3] The wrist splint has no moving parts and is commonly referred to as a **static splint.** This term and many other commonly used splinting terms are misleading. In 1992, the *American Society of Hand Therapists Splint*

Classification System was published in an effort to improve and standardize splinting nomenclature. The standard "wrist splint" is now classified as a "wrist extension **immobilization** splint, type 0."[1,4] The wrist extension immobilization splint, type 0, is fabricated at two thirds the length of the forearm and two thirds forearm circumference to distribute the force over a considerable surface area to minimize integument disruption and increase comfort as well as increase the splint strength. Because the distance of the lever arm (the distance between the opposite forces supplied by the splint) is an integral component of the force vector, the longer the lever arms, the greater resistance the splint can accommodate. The splint prevents wrist motion but does not limit finger flexion or extension. The splint allows full rotational motion and opposition of the thumb to the base of the little finger.

Splint design should prevent further injury and promote function whenever possible. Proper positioning of a weakened hand facilitates the maintenance of tissue length and permits a modicum of function. Speaking of the wrist extension immobilization splint, James described the **"safe position"** as follows: "The metacarpophalangeal joints are safe in flexion and most unsafe in extension; the PIP joints, conversely, are safe in extension and exceedingly unsafe if immobilized in flexion"[5] (Fig. 18-3).

The hand and wrist in the safe position splint shown in Figure 18-3 maintains wrist extension at 30°, which is the position of functional grip strength. The metacarpophalangeal (MCP) joints are in 90° flexion to maintain MCP ligament length and functional position. The proximal interphalangeal (PIP) joints are in extension to maintain extrinsic muscle length and prevent intrinsic muscle tightness. The thumb is placed in palmar abduction to maintain opposition potential to one or more digits in prehension. The MCP flexion, PIP extension immobilization splint is also called a type 1 splint.[4] The safe position splint is custom fitted to the flaccid hand and worn in the daytime and at night, but it is removed for skin care and hygiene or as permitted after a surgical repair. The splint is retained

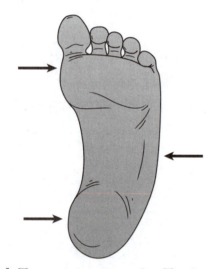

Figure 18-1 Three-point pressure splint. The three-point pressure system for the control of abnormal static positioning of a foot consists of two laterally directed forces—one at the area of the first metatarsal head and one at the medial border of the calcaneus—and one medially directed force just proximal to the base of the fifth metatarsal.

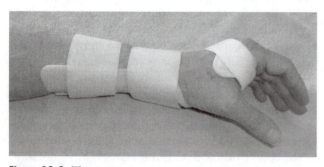

Figure 18-2 Three-point pressure wrist extension immobilization splint.

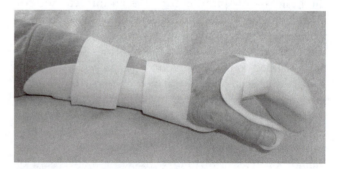

Figure 18-3 Safe position splint uses metacarpophalangeal flexion and interphalangeal extension immobilization in an intrinsic plus position.

as a nighttime splint as function begins to return or a functional daytime splint is used.

A **dynamic splint** is properly defined as a mobilization splint in flexion, extension, or rotation using some form of traction, such as rubber bands or springs. Rubber bands exhibit creep over time when subjected to a constant stress load. Creep results in a change in the force dynamics. Shorter thicker bands demonstrate less creep than longer thinner bands. Spring tension is not subject to creep and allows for the maintenance of the prescribed forces. Determination of proper length and tension is difficult to objectify and a hallmark of clinical expertise. An experienced therapist tends to use the proper length and tension, whereas an inexperienced therapist tends to fabricate dynamic splints with excessive forces applied to the soft tissues.[6] The rubber band tension is easy to change, does not easily snag on clothing, and is inexpensive. The springs are difficult to change, catch on clothing, and are more expensive. Collaboration, teamwork, and communication between the therapist and patient are important aspects of the determination of an appropriate tension prescribed in the dynamic splint. Increased tension may facilitate healing and function but may cause pain resulting in a negative impact on patient compliance.

Brachial Plexus Splinting

A preganglionic brachial plexus injury is an injury to the central nervous system occurring proximal to the neuron. A preganglionic injury has very poor capacity for recovery. A postganglionic brachial plexus injury involves the peripheral nervous system, and if the injury is neurapraxic or axonotmetic, the nerves are able to regenerate and are amenable to self-repair. Postganglionic neurotmetic lesions do not heal spontaneously and require surgical intervention for recovery (Figs. 18-4 and 18-5).[7] Preganglionic brachial plexus injury may be associated with head injury or incomplete spinal cord injury. Postganglionic plexus injuries typically result from forceful scapular depression, shoulder hyperhorizontal abduction, contralateral neck lateral flexion, or any combination of these motions.[8] Less common etiologies include injuries related to medication, infection, repetitive strain, or radiation. Plexus injuries secondary to a multiple trauma etiology may also include shoulder dislocation, fractures, or crush injuries. The splinting program must take into consideration individual cognitive or physical limitations. Knowledge of each individual nerve function and deficit is essential for splinting. Evaluation is ongoing because the injured or repaired nerves may regain function at different rates or may not recover at all. Recovery, especially with axonotmetic and neurotmetic lesions, is a prolonged process. Axonal regeneration may occur at a slow rate of 1 mm per month. Distal

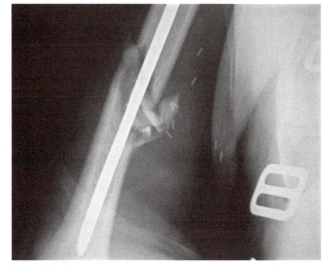

Figure 18-4 Plexus injury secondary to multiple trauma may also include shoulder dislocation, humeral fracture, or crush injury.

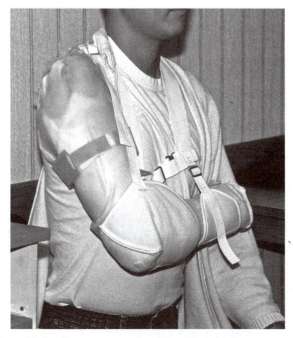

Figure 18-5 Plexus injury secondary to multiple trauma with shoulder dislocation, humeral fracture, or crush injury may require a hemisling support in addition to splinting.

muscles may require 24 months to reinnervate. In addition, atrophic changes may result in distal muscles awaiting reinnervation. Muscle scarring, arthropathy, chronic regional pain syndrome, and contracture all are common complications of proximal nerve lesions. Permanent loss of sarcomeres in the intrinsic hand muscles may occur if reinnervation does not occur within 6 months of injury.[9] Early splinting to position the injured plexus in the optimum posture for healing while allowing the spared muscles to function and maintenance of soft tissue length is essential for a favorable rehabilitation outcome.

Radial Nerve Splinting

The radial nerve innervates the triceps, extensor carpi radialis longus and brevis, brachioradialis, supinator, extrinsic finger extensors, and thumb extrinsic abductor muscles. Radial nerve injury commonly occurs with humeral fracture, elbow dislocation, and Monteggia fracture. Neuropathy may also result directly or indirectly from systemic disease.[10] For instance, tumor may directly compress the radial nerve or may indirectly injure the nerve via paraneoplastic syndrome, illness related to critical illness neuropathy or myopathy, or through the effects of chemotherapy medication or radiation. Proximal injury to the radial nerve may affect wrist, finger, and thumb extension and produce weakness of supination and thumb radial abduction.[9] The loss of wrist extension prevents tenodesis action and decreases finger use in power grip or grasp-release (Figs. 18-6 through 18-19).[11]

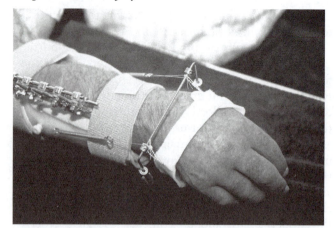

Figure 18-6 Radial nerve injury splinted with Phoenix wrist extension outrigger using spring tension following external fixator fracture stabilization. Proper outrigger alignment with the wrist joint is essential to prevent wrist joint compaction.

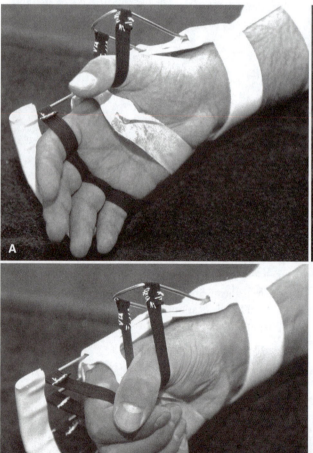

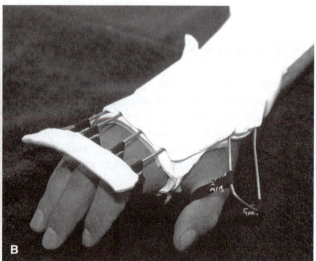

Figure 18-7 A–C, James Sellers, OTR, described the dorsal splint with elastic digit extension assist for radial nerve injury. The splint allows full finger flexion. The elastic extension assist requires hand sewing to replace.

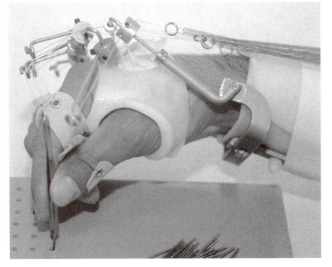

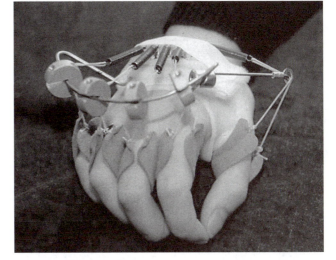

Figure 18-8 Following humeral fracture with radial nerve injury, a 34-year-old man was splinted for mobilization using combined Phoenix wrist and Rolyan adjustable outriggers to assist wrist and finger extension and allow full finger flexion. The wrist may go into flexion as needed for activities of daily living or fine motor tasks.

Figure 18-10 A hand-based finger and thumb extension splint was used as wrist motion returned to permit right dominant writing and keyboarding for a 21-year-old university student. She was able to complete all her classes despite her injury and extended recovery.

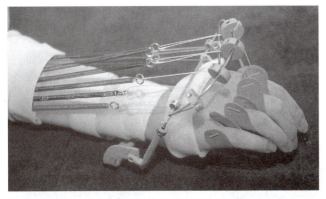

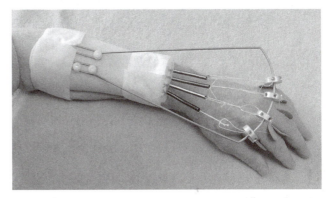

Figure 18-9 Radial nerve injury and humeral fracture following a motor vehicle accident was splinted with Phoenix wrist and digit extension mobilization.

Figure 18-11 The extended Phoenix outrigger is used with the lightest metacarpophalangeal extension assist force to decrease a tenodesis effect when performing activities of daily living (zipper pull, buttoning, or shoe tying) that require going in and out of wrist flexion.

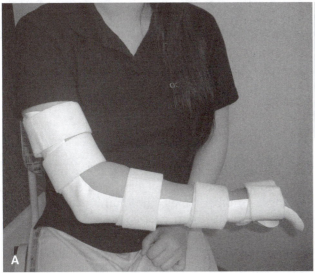

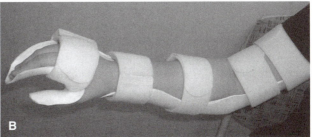

Figure 18-12 A and B, Elbow flexion/wrist/hand immobilization splint with finger intrinsic plus position and thumb supported in palmar abduction.

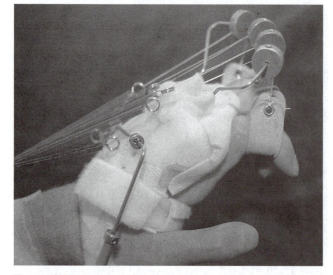

Figure 18-13 Proximal interphalangeal joint contractures treated with dynamic splinting.

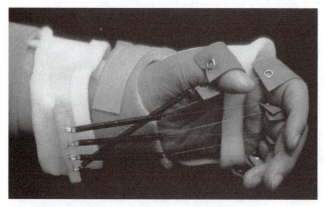

Figure 18-14 A 57-year-old man did not receive early splinting to maintain the hand and fingers in the safe position. He was referred to therapy for metacarpophalangeal flexion splinting after metacarpophalangeal capsulotomies but did not obtain functional return.

With radial nerve lesions, the wrist is splinted in 20° to 30° extension to assist functional grip strength. Based on the physical examination, the required splint may be a static immobilization splint or a dynamic mobilization splint. There are multiple opinions in the literature. Pearson[12] states that a static wrist immobilization splint without dynamic finger extension mobilization assist may be adequate for many patients with proximal radial nerve lesions with motor neuropathy. Fess and Philips[13] state that patients with nonfunctional radial nerve–innervated muscles should be treated with an external hand support. Dillingham et al.[14] recommend a hinged wrist orthosis with dynamic finger extension assists to compensate for muscular deficits resulting from the radial nerve injury.

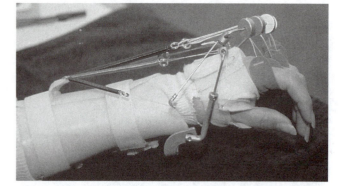

Figure 18-15 A 39-year-old woman sustained a traumatic shoulder dislocation with a lower brachial plexus injury. She was initially treated with upper arm immobilization to the chest wall to place the plexus in a "resting" position, which eliminated tensile forces. In addition, she was prescribed a safe splint and forearm hemisling. Because the median nerve sustained a neurapraxic injury and the radial nerve sustained axonal degeneration, conduction returned to the medial nerve before the radial nerve. She was fitted with a combined wrist and metacarpophalangeal extension mobilization splint with spring assist replacing the lost radial nerve function. Splinting allowed functional prehension and early use of the intrinsic hand muscles, which prevented muscle atrophy and joint contractures.

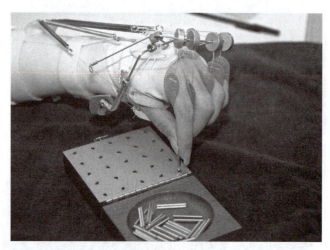

Figure 18-16 The splint also permitted wrist flexion, essential for many activities of daily living tasks, such as buttoning, manipulating objects at or below waist level, or using a zipper.

The "safe position" splint should be worn during the day and at night. The mobilization splint may use static lines for a tenodesis effect or elastic tension such as springs or rubber bands. The thumb may not need to be included in the outrigger because the thumb extensors and abductors are located on the dorsoulnar surface and are not on stretch when wrist extension is provided by the splint.[10] Mobilization splints are typically worn

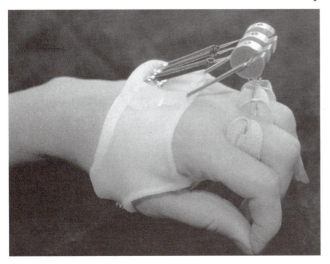

Figure 18-17 As radial nerve axonal regeneration occurred, the splint was converted into a hand-based metacarpophalangeal-mobilization splint for finger extension. Without the splint, a Wartenberg's sign could be elicited and, therefore, the quality of prehension in the index finger and thumb diminished.

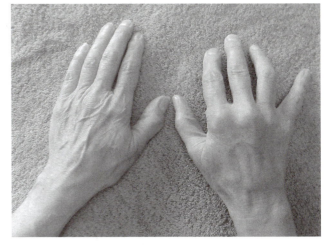

Figure 18-19 Wartenberg's sign—inability to adduct the extended little finger to the extended ring finger because of lack of intrinsic function.

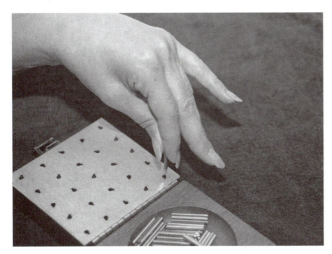

Figure 18-18 Diminished prehension associated with intrinsic weakness and a positive Wartenberg's sign.

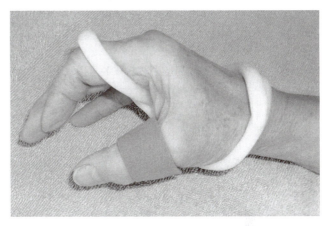

Figure 18-20 Metacarpophalangeal flexion and thumb sling in palmar abduction prevents contracture formation while permitting functional prehension.

during the daytime and changed to a static splint for nighttime wear.

Median Nerve Splinting

The median nerve innervates the extrinsic pronator muscles, radial wrist flexor, superficial digit flexors, index and long finger profundus flexors, and long thumb flexor through branches exiting early from the nerve (Figs. 18-20, 18-21, and 18-22). Thumb abduction and opposition are innervated from branches exiting distally. Palm and anterior digit tactile and kinesthetic/proprioception sensation are provided by

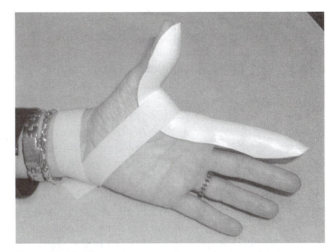

Figure 18-21 The web space splint is worn primarily at night to maintain thumb adductor length.

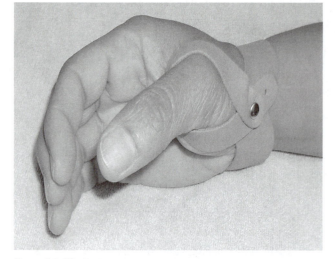

Figure 18-22 Soft leather thumb abduction splint allows tool use without palmar pressure.

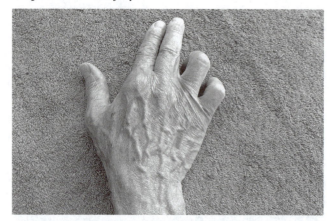

Figure 18-23 Ulnar claw deformity.

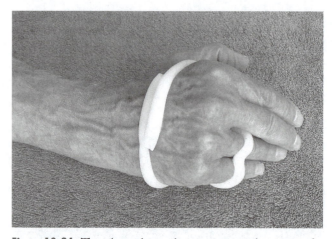

Figure 18-24 The ulnar claw splint maintains the ring and small finger metacarpophalangeal joints in flexion permitting active interphalangeal joint extension.

the median nerve except for the small finger and ulnar half of the ring finger.[15] Splinting for the high-level median nerve injury supports the radial fingers in MCP flexion and the thumb in palmar abduction opposition. High median nerve palsy typically limits flexion of the index finger distal interphalangeal (DIP) joint and the thumb interphalangeal joint decreasing functional tip prehension. Ring splints may be used to flex the distal joints of the index finger and thumb to prevent joint hyperextension and to improve tip prehension. The low-level median nerve injury splint is used to place the thumb in palmar abduction and to maintain opposition.[9] The unopposed adductor pollicis muscle may be positioned in a full thumb abduction web space splint to maintain the muscle length. The thumb may be held in palmar abduction with a soft daytime splint that permits functional grip on a handle or tool.

Median nerve compression at the wrist level—carpal tunnel syndrome (CTS)—is a neurological disorder and may result from trauma, distal radius fracture, hormone changes during pregnancy, endocrine disorders such as diabetes, or repetitive wrist motion. CTS is the most frequent compression neuropathy and occurs in 0.7% to 16% of the general population.[16] Evidence-based research has shown that night splinting alone reduces CTS symptom severity as measured by nerve conduction testing.[16] Evidence suggests splinting the wrist in neutral improves symptoms more than splinting the historical and often used 20° of wrist extension.[16] Surgical intervention provides better long-term outcomes than splinting alone.[17] Courts[18] found that using splinting in symptomatic individuals with CTS during pregnancy increased average grip strength by 5.4 pounds in each of the pinch strengths after just 1 week of splinting. When fabricating a static splint for clients with CTS, care should be taken to ensure

that holding straps are loosened at night to prevent possible compression secondary to the development of nighttime edema. Wider and softer straps may also decrease venous return compression.

Ulnar Nerve Splinting

The ulnar nerve innervates the flexi carpi ulnaris, the ring and little finger deep flexors and lumbricales, dorsal and palmar interossei, abductor and opponens digiti minimi, and adductor pollicis.[15] Loss of the intrinsic hand muscles produces an ulnar claw deformity with the MCP joints unable to flex and the PIP joints unable to extend, whereas the long flexors remain intact. The extrinsic extensors hyperextend the MCP joints, and the extrinsic flexors flex the PIP and DIP joints (Figs. 18-23 and 18-24). The volar capsular ligament structures may elongate and exacerbate the claw deformity. Clawing may not occur when the flexor digitorum is affected. Splinting the ring and little finger MCP joints in flexion permits active extension of the PIP joints and allows functional hand use for grasp and release. Anticlaw splinting is contraindicated if contractures are present and the MCP joints cannot be passively flexed or the interphalangeal joints cannot be passively extended. Early anticlaw splinting prevents contracture formation. An ulnar nerve injury proximal to the wrist may produce a weak interossei muscle creating Wartenberg's sign with the little finger in abduction.[15] A minimal "double ring" splint or soft "trapper" may be used to prevent overstretching with the little finger in abduction. Hyperflexion of the thumb when pinching produces Froment's sign secondary to a weak adductor pollicis muscle requiring flexor pollicis longus for power pinch.[19]

One of the most common etiologies of proximal ulnar lesions is cubital tunnel syndrome. Bozentka reported that cubital tunnel syndrome is the second most common peripheral compression neuropathy after CTS.[20] The etiology of cubital tunnel syndrome is varied and includes direct trauma, osseous fracture, and overuse. For cubital tunnel syndrome with ulnar nerve compression at the elbow, a soft daytime Neoprene splint and a nighttime anterior elbow splint at 20° flexion may be used.

Combined Peripheral Nerve Injures and Complications

Cases of delayed diagnosis or referral may require splinting to reduce contractures. Contractures of the interphalangeal joints are best treated using plaster of Paris **serial casting** to hold the joint at end range and to allow tissue cell growth. If the patient has sufficient cognitive and psychomotor skills, he or she may be instructed to change the casting every 2 or 3 days. However, replacement casts are applied by the splinting therapist in most instances (Fig. 18-25).

Forearm or hand trauma may result in more than one peripheral nerve injury. Combining splinting techniques for each of the injured nerves may be possible. Minimalistic splint design for the combined injury may allow preservation of functional hand use.

The clinical objectives of using splinting in patients with a diagnosis of peripheral nerve injury vary from protection, stabilization, lengthening shortened tissues, shortening lengthened tissues, rest, exercise, and preserving function. Splinting is an important primary and adjunct intervention for nerve injuries. Much of the process of splinting revolves around clinical decision making: Splint or no splint? Which type of splint? Dynamic or static? Material? Fastening mechanism? Wear schedule? An increasing number of evidenced-based publications address splinting. That being said, clinical expertise and experience remain important components in splinting intervention.

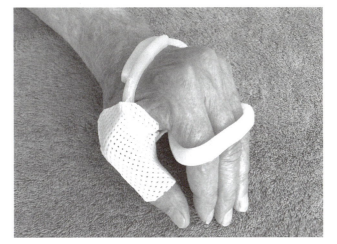

Figure 18-25 The combined ulnar and median nerve laceration injury was splinted with a hand-based splint for metacarpophalangeal flexion permitting active interphalangeal finger extension. The thumb spica is in palmar abduction. The splint is easily removed for hygiene.

CASE STUDY

Annie is a 50-year-old, previously healthy, right hand dominant woman who works as a certified public accountant. She sustained a traumatic cervical spine and brachial plexus injury to the right upper extremity as a result of a body surfing accident 1 year ago. Along with orthopedic and integument injuries, Annie sustained C7 through T1 spinal nerve traction injuries resulting in significant upper extremity weakness, sensory loss, and dysfunction. At 1 year after injury, the latissimus, pectoralis, triceps, and all distal muscle groups function at grade between 0/5 and 1/5. The three deltoid divisions, the rotator cuff, and the biceps function at grade 2+/5. Annie now presents with a flail wrist and hand. There is patchy loss of tactile sense throughout the entire upper extremity. Capillary refill is excellent. There is mild hand edema. She reports no improvement in muscle strength or sensation over the past 6 months. She underwent an unsuccessful brachial plexus surgical exploration 9 months ago.

Annie presents at the clinic with an over-the-counter sling and over-the-counter cloth glove on her right hand. She is experiencing right shoulder pain, which she attributes to the sling.

A custom, lightweight, thermoplastic, foam-lined orthosis was fabricated using a Step-Lock elbow joint. A prefabricated cock-up splint was fitted to the patient. An over-the-counter compressive sleeve extending from the fingertips to the wrist was provided to the patient. Lastly, a figure-of-eight harness was attached to the elbow orthosis to aid in suspension and ipsilateral limb comfort.

Case Study Questions

1. The purpose of the Step-Lock elbow joint is which of the following?
  a. Pain control
  b. Control of edema
  c. Skin protection
  d. Elbow positioning

2. The compressive glove will provide which function for the wrist and hand?
  a. Protection
  b. Decrease dependent edema
  c. Neither a nor b
  d. Both a and b

3. The therapist is addressing the shoulder pain by which of the following interventions?
  a. Compressive glove
  b. Figure-of-eight harness
  c. The locked elbow
  d. The wrist cock-up splint

4. Daily skin checks should be performed by the patient to assist with identifying which of the following?
  a. Edema
  b. Allergic reaction to the splinting materials
  c. Pressure ulcers
  d. All of the above

5. Additional educational teaching should be provided to the patient regarding which of the following?
  a. Insensate limb precautions
  b. Edema management
  c. Proper skin hygiene
  d. All of the above

References

1. Van Lede P. Minimalistic splint design: a rationale told in a personal style. *J Hand Ther.* 2002:192–201.
2. Janson JR. Mechanical principles. In: Fess EE, Gettle KS, Phillips CA, Jansen JR, eds. *Hand and Upper Extremity Splinting Principles and Methods.* 3rd ed. St Louis: Mosby; 2005:161–165.
3. Austin GP, Jacobs ML. Mechanical principles. In: Jacobs ML, Austin N, eds. *Splinting the Hand and Upper Extremity Principles and Process.* Philadelphia: Lippincott Williams & Wilkins; 2003:59–72.
4. American Society of Hand Therapists. *American Society of Hand Therapists Splinting Classification System.* Chicago: ASHT; 1992.
5. Fess EE. A history of splinting: to understand the present, view the past. *J Hand Ther.* 2002;15:97–132
6. Bell-Krotoski JA, Breger-Stanton DE. Biomechanics and evaluation of the hand. In: Macklin EJ, Callahan AD, Skirven TM, Schneider LH, Osterman AL, eds. *Rehabilitation of the Hand and Upper Extremity.* 5th ed. St Louis: Mosby; 2002:240–252.
7. Trumble TE. Brachial plexus injuries. In: *Principles of Hand Surgery and Therapy.* Philadelphia: Saunders; 2000:312–344.
8. Hentz DO. Traumatic brachial plexus injury. In: Green DP, Hotchkiss RN, Penderson WC, Wolfe SW, eds. *Green's Operative Hand Surgery.* Vol II. 5th ed. Philadelphia: Churchill Livingstone; 2005:1132–1199.
9. Robinson LR. Trauma rehabilitation. In: Robinson LR, Spencer Steffa EL, eds. *Diagnosis and Rehabilitation of Peripheral Nerve Injuries.* Philadelphia: Lippincott Williams & Wilkins; 2006:299–342
10. Colditz JC. Splinting for radial nerve palsy. *J Hand Ther.* 1987;1:18–19.
11. Hannah SD, Hudak PL. Splinting and radial nerve palsy: a single-subject experiment. *J Hand Ther.* 2001; 14:195–201.
12. Pearson SO. Splinting of the nerve injured hand. In: Skirven, T, Osterman A, Fedorczyk J, Amadio P (eds.): *Rehabilitation of the Hand,.* 5th ed. St. Louis: Mosby Elsevier; 2011: 567–601.
13. Fess EE, Philips CA: *Hand Splinting: Principles and Methods.* 2nd ed. St Louis: Mosby, 1978.
14. Dillingham TR, Olaje FH, Belandres PV, Thorn-Vogel MI. Orthosis for the complete median and radial nerve-injured war casualty. *J Hand Ther.* 1992; 5:212–217.
15. Kendall FP, McCreary EK, Provance PG. *Muscle Testing and Function.* 4th ed. Baltimore: Williams & Wilkins; 1993.
16. Gummesson AI, Johnsson R, McCabe SJ, Ornstein E. Severe carpal tunnel syndrome, potentially needing surgical treatment in a general population. *J Hand Surg Am.* 2003;28: 639–644.
17. Muller M, Tsui D, Schnuur R, Biddulph-Deisroth L, Hard J, MacDermid JC. Effectiveness of hand therapy interventions in primary management of carpal tunnel syndrome: a systematic review. *J Hand Ther.* 2004;17:210–225.
18. Courts RB. Splinting for symptoms of carpal tunnel syndrome during pregnancy. *J Hand Ther.* 1995;8:31–34.
19. Lund AT, Amadio PC. Treatment of cubital tunnel syndrome: perspectives for the therapist. *J Hand Ther.* 2006; 19:170–178.
20. Apfel E, Sigafoos GT. Comparison of range-of-motion constraints provided by splints used in the treatment of cubital tunnel syndrome—a pilot study. *J Hand Ther.* 2006;19: 384–391.

Chapter 19

Counseling and Behavior Modification Techniques for Functional Loss and Chronic Pain

AMY HEATH, PT, DPT, OCS

"Believe you can and you are halfway there."

—THEODORE ROOSEVELT (1858–1919)

Objectives

On completion of this chapter, the student/practitioner will be able to:

- Discuss the relationship between chronic pain and depression.
- Compare and contrast the various behavioral theories and their indication for use in a clinical setting.
- Discuss the term "positive psychology" as it relates to the treatment of chronic pain.
- Define the various methods of behavioral modification that may be applicable to the practicing therapist.

Key Terms

- Behavior therapy
- Depression
- Operant therapy
- Positive psychology

Introduction

Chronic pain and its concomitant functional loss requires a multimodal approach in management. Medical management seeks to resolve or decrease pain with medication, surgery, or a combination of both. Therapeutic management entails a variety of disciplines working together with the patient to help the patient better cope and function with chronic pain. "Counseling" and "behavior management" are umbrella terms used to describe strategies used by psychotherapy professionals working with patients with chronic pain.

It is well documented that pain is more than just a physiological response to a stimulus—pain is an experience. Included in this experience are psychological, emotional, sociological, financial, and environmental factors that influence an individual's perception of pain. This mulifaceted concept of pain is so well regarded that the Commission on Accreditation of Rehabilitation Facilities will accredit pain management facilities only if they have a mental health specialist on staff.[1] To complicate the matter further, individuals with chronic pain are often more likely to experience other psychological disturbances, such as depression.

Researchers have spent much money and time investigating the relationship (specifically the temporal relationship) between **depression** and chronic pain. To date, however, theorists have been able only to posit models relating the two. These models enlighten the psychology behind chronic pain and include the cognitive distortion model, in which individuals experiencing chronic pain have a "cognitive vulnerability" to depression, and the model of learned helplessness, in which individuals with chronic pain feel as though they cannot control their own outcomes (related to pain) and they develop an attitude of helplessness. The behavioral model, which embraces operant therapies as an intervention, presupposes that depression as a function of chronic pain occurs because of one or a combination of three reasons: (1) There are fewer positive reinforcers, (2) positive reinforcers that do exist no longer have an impact, or (3) the individual is incapable of gaining positive reinforcement. As a means to encompass components of each of these models, the chronic pain experience has evolved to capture the individual nature of each person's chronic pain experience.[2]

As is the case with any form of intervention, psychotherapeutic approaches to chronic pain and functional loss require a skilled professional. The counseling involved with this type of intervention strategy is derived from a positive regard for the client's personal experience, emphasizing empathy and respect.[3] A thorough assessment of the individual is required initially. This assessment can be used to guide treatment, diagnose any other psychological issues such as anxiety or depression, and build a rapport with the patient. Within the context of the assessment, it is critical for therapists to understand how the patient conceptualizes his or her pain. This information can be ascertained using standardized questionnaires and open-ended interview questions. Because of the complex nature of pain, questions may be directed toward personal values. A pertinent example is religiosity. Because some patients may see their pain as a punishment from a higher being, it is important to understand this information as a part of the individual's pain experience. If religiosity proves to be a component, it is imperative that the professional addressing these concerns is competent and knowledgable enough to address the issue properly. Standardized questionnaires can also assist in gathering patient information. The type of questionnaire chosen depends on the function, pain, and outcomes the therapist is targeting.

All of the information gathered from the initial assessment is essential to develop the patient's treatment plan and the psychological approach that will be used as an intervention. This chapter focuses on several types of psychotherapeutic interventions and the research that supports their use. Interventions that include behavioral modification strategies are addressed because these are likely to be used in conjunction with other therapies. Most of the research dealing with chronic pain does not specifically include chronic pain from a peripheral neuropathic etiology. However, neuropathic pain is similar to chronic pain from other origins in its individual chronic pain experiences—meaning that because of the multidimensional nature

of pain, it is a unique experience for each individual. Consequently, research about chronic pain may not be specific to peripheral neuropathy but is still valid, reliable, and informative.

Behavior Therapy

Psychological treatments are necessary when treating patients with chronic pain and the functional loss that may result. The question for clinicians providing these treatments is which intervention is more effective or appropriate? Answering this question is where differences in approaches become apparent. There is evidence to support the use of multiple approaches, but why choose one over the other? Determining the best course of treatment for a particular individual can best be determined by understanding the foundations of each approach. In this section, we review multiple psychological approaches, beginning with **operant therapy.** Operant therapy is an approach designed to address the gross motor and cognitive/subjective responses to clinical pain (Tables 19-1 and 19-2).[4]

In the late 1960s and early 1970s, Fordyce proposed a concept of clinical pain as more than just neurophysiological responses of the body. Based on Fordyce's earlier works, Sanders[4] defined pain as "an interacting cluster of individualized overt, covert, and neurophysiological responses capable of being produced by

Table 19-1	Multiple Response Conceptualization of Clinical Pain
Response Category	**Examples**
Neurophysiological ascending	Afferent A-delta and C nerve excitation
Neurophysiological supraspinal/cortical	Hypothalamic, limbic, somatosensory excitation
Neurophysiological descending	Efferent autonomic, pyramidal, extrapyramidal nerve excitation
Neurophysiological chemical	Chemical release of β-endorphin and enkephalin neuropeptides
Cognitive/subjective thoughts	Pain is horrible, unbearable, out of control
Cognitive/subjective feelings states	Perceptions of pain, fear/anxiety, anger, sadness/depression
Cognitive/subjective images	Visualizations of being crippled, having surgery, losing a job
Gross motor verbal	Moaning, crying/yelling, pain complaints
Gross motor nonverbal	Guarding, squeezing, limping, lying down, taking analgesics

Adapted from Sanders SH. Operant therapy with pain patients: evidence for its effectiveness. *Semin Pain Med.* 2003;1(2):90–98.

Table 19-2 Primary and Secondary Pain Responses and Antecedent and Consequent Stimuli by Acute and Chronic Pain States

Prevalent Antecedent Stimuli Initiating and Maintaining Responses	Pain Responses	Prevalent Consequent Stimuli Maintaining Responses
Acute state Tissue damage/irritation Environmental stressors Prior conditioned stimuli Pain response models	Neurophysiological Gross motor Cognitive/subjective	↓Subjective pain perception ↓Tissue damage/irritation ↓Environmental stressors ↑Social attention
Chronic state Environmental stressors Conditioned/distinctive stimuli Pain response models Tissue damage/irritation	Gross motor Cognitive/subjective Neurophysiological	↓Or avoid environmental stressors ↓Or avoid subjective pain perception ↓Or avoid drug withdrawal ↑Social attention ↑Economic gains ↓Or avoid tissue damage

Adapted from Sanders SH. Operant therapy with pain patients: evidence for its effectiveness. *Semin Pain Med.* 2003;1(2):90–98.

relevant tissue damage or irritation, and may also be produced and maintained by other antecedent or consequent stimulus conditions." Operant therapy addresses these antecedent or consequent stimulus conditions.

In the context of clinical pain, the stimulus conditions that are present before or after pain are behaviors that can be modified by the individual's environment or the effects of the behavior. Using operant therapy techniques, clinicians work to influence and manipulate both the environment and the consequences.[4] Clinicians manipulate the environment and consequences using rewards and punishments. Appropriate pain (well) behaviors are rewarded, and "inappropriate" pain behaviors are punished. Punishment is often a decrease in reinforcement from others, whereas well behaviors promote reinforcement.[5] This type of therapy is difficult when one considers the multiple environmental influences and the multitude of consequences that any one pain behavior may elucidate from any number of individuals. It is precisely because of this that operant therapies often include the individuals to whom the patient is most closely connected. Family therapies and psychodynamic approaches are often indicated for a comprehensive plan. The learned behaviors of the individual with pain can be unknowingly (or knowingly) reinforced by the individuals involved in the patient's care. The pain behaviors may result in more attention, more care, and distraction from other more negative consequences.[5]

With operant therapy, the individual and family and friends learn to identify the less desirable pain behaviors. The participants are taught to ignore the pain behaviors or to navigate another way to acknowledge the pain behavior while reinforcing well behavior.[6] Family therapy is especially beneficial when one considers the possible change in relationship dynamics that may result from functional loss or chronic pain.

Table 19-3 Impact of Chronic Pain on the Family: Two Dimensions

Person With Pain	Family Members
Pain that does not show	Inability to see or feel the pain
Fluctuating activity levels	Increased responsibility for maintaining the home and income
Isolation	Loss of personal support system
Lack of interest	Emotional outbursts of the person with pain
Doubt about the reality of the pain	Added daily stress
Loss of job, friends, and productivity	Loss of plans and hopes for the future

*Adapted from Cowan P, Kelly N, Pasero C, Covington E, Lidz C. Family manual. A manual for families of persons with pain. Rocklin, CA: American Chronic Pain Association; 1998.

According to Lewandowski et al.,[6] chronic pain can affect almost all areas of life and results in serious consequences for the family because often the individual with pain or functional loss depends emotionally and physically on others resulting in a change in family roles (Table 19-3).

One of the most difficult aspects of operant therapy is the patient's ability to comprehend the goal of treatment. For individuals with chronic pain, it is likely that the goal is not to "cure" the pain but to minimize it to "overcome disability and restore function, despite the continuation of some pain."[5] Despite the evidence in support of operant therapy, its use is still widely criticized.[6] Most criticism derives from the approach's inherent inability to be standardized. Its individualized approach makes its successes difficult to replicate. Additionally, it is argued that operant therapy alone is not as successful as when used in concert with another therapy, typically cognitive behavior therapy (CBT). In recent research, operant therapy (or behavior therapy) used in conjunction with CBT has proved to be the most successful in helping individuals with chronic pain.

Cognitive Behavior Therapy

Although the goals in behavior therapies are to decrease pain behaviors and promote well behaviors, the goal of CBT is to "moderate the demoralizing and potentially depressive experiences of the person in chronic pain and to encourage self-efficacy through psychological and physical behaviors that help enhance treatment outcomes."[7] CBT is not just one approach to chronic pain management—it is many different interventions with the goal of affecting an individual's pain experience through the alteration of the individual's pain-related thoughts and actions.[3] A few of these strategies include cognitive restructuring and reframing, developing skills to problem solve and cope, assertiveness training, reinterpretation of the pain experience, anxiety defusion, depression management, and other socioenvironmental interventions.[3,7] Similar to behavior therapy involving operant therapy principles, the rationale behind the use of CBT is that the individual's pain experience is not just neurophysiological but is the result of a combination of neurophysiological, gross motor, and cognitive/subjective factors.

Professionals using CBT as an intervention generally work with patients to educate them regarding factors that influence their perception of pain and helpful coping techniques. Therapists work to teach patients new ways of responding to pain and often encourage exercise and increased activity levels.[3] All of these strategies may be used with some patients, and only a few may be used with others. Similar to operant therapy, some people criticize the use of CBT because of the inability to structure one program to work with one, if not all, patients with chronic pain. However, despite this criticism, the outcomes-based research has proved this method of therapy to be effective.[7]

For patients with chronic pain, reinterpreting the pain experience can be extremely beneficial albeit challenging. For these people, distinguishing between pain, suffering, and pain behaviors gives them an opportunity to identify and name better the culprit of their negative experiences. According to Grant and Haverkamp,[3] "pain" is the sensation activated by stimulating nociceptors in the nervous system. "Suffering" is the affective response to the sensory experience, and "pain behaviors" are the actions elicited when people are suffering. Understanding how these concepts differ is the first step in being able to restructure one's own thoughts. In using language that differentiates between the neurophysiological, cognitive, and behavioral processes, the counselor can "challenge the reality of the patient's pain"[3] without defeating the patient. The goal of psychotherapeutic intervention is for the patient to gain a sense of control over the pain.[3] Cognitive restructuring, reframing, and reconceptualizing are strategies that can be very beneficial during episodes when pain levels increase. They can also be used in conjunction with other interventions, such as physical exercise, relaxation techniques, and other behavior modification and self-regulatory strategies for pain management.

Although it may seem counterintuitive, exercise is often suggested to patients experiencing chronic pain. As a result of chronic pain, individuals may decrease their activity as a means to avert the pain. However, exercise is actually a great way to prevent and overcome physical deconditioning, which serves to complicate further the neurophysiological aspect of the pain experience. It is important that exercise be closely monitored and supervised. Having the patient exercise as opposed to remaining sedentary can assist in demonstrating that the activity is not causing the patient harm but can help him or her feel better.[3]

Exercise is primarily viewed as a physical intervention; however, because of its "feel good" effects, it may also be viewed as an emotional intervention similar to anxiety defusion and depression management. Anxiety and depression are suspect in their relationship to chronic pain. It is sometimes difficult to determine which comes first—the emotional issues or the reported levels of increased pain. Either way it is essential that anxiety or depression or both are addressed in psychotherapeutic sessions for chronic pain. Addressing these emotional concerns can also aid in identifying common stressors, which can lead to more straightforward coping schemes.

Similar to concerns with operant strategies, significant consideration of the individual's socioenvironment is part of the CBT approach. Understanding the relationship dynamics between individuals with chronic pain and their loved ones can provide insight into the goals of the patient and what obstacles may stand in the way of the goals. Current research shows that chronic pain does not just affect the person with pain but also affects other loved ones by increasing dependency, shame, attention, or fear. All of these emotions should be managed with sensitivity; understanding how these emotions manifest themselves in the individual can be critical to achieving the goals of CBT.

Alternative Approaches

CBT and operant therapies are considered under the umbrella terms "counseling" and "behavior management" mentioned previously for psychotherapeutic approaches generally used by licensed professionals for patients with chronic pain. In addition to these two major approaches, there are alternative approaches that can be used, but they are used less frequently. These strategies are employed less frequently as a result of a lack of evidence to support their efficacy or a lack of understanding about how or why the strategy works. Although literature to support the success of these approaches is limited, this section discusses positive psychology, support groups and family therapies, and eye movement desensitization and reprocessing (EMDR).

Positive psychology is a relatively new area of growth in the psychological sciences. It is also an umbrella term incorporating many concepts ranging from an individual's personality traits, such as positive affect, optimism, hope, and gratitude, to an individual's spirituality and social support. Positive psychology is the scientific attempt at a greater understanding of how these concepts affect an individual's personal health—specifically, for our purposes, how the concepts of having a sense of coherence, self-efficacy, positive affect, optimisim, hope, gratitude, spirituality, and social support help an individual with chronic pain and the supporting rationale.[7,8]

The goal of positive psychology is to decrease negative depressive symptoms by increasing emotions to which individuals can respond in a positive sense.[9] Depressive symptoms frequently appear in concert with chronic pain sypmptoms.[2] Researchers theorize that positive psychology has a helpful effect as a result of biological, behavioral, or social processes.[8] From a neurobiological perspective, it is understood that positive psychology may affect the neuroendocrine and immune systems. Behaviorly and socially, positive psychology may affect how a person can prevent serious health issues and promote greater participation in his or her own rehabilitation processes.[8] Individuals with chronic pain who possess a positive psychological well-being may be better prepared to deal with their chronic pain.[7] Interventions that have been suggested for use but that are still in the infancy stage with regard to evidence ask individuals to identify their own stengths, their "blessings," and three doors that have opened as a result of their experience. Additionally, patients are encouraged to savor enjoyable activities in the hope that their positive psychological well-being will increase to manage and deal better with their chronic pain.[7]

In positive psychology, patients who perceive that they have a social or familial support system are often best able to manage their pain behaviors and continue to function with their impairment. As stated previously in this chapter, when an individual experiences chronic pain, the pain does not just affect the individual's life but also affects the lives of the people around him or her. There may be a change in the dynamic and function of relationships as a result of the individual's perception of pain and pain behaviors. The use of family therapy and support groups is advocated for as part of a comprehensive approach to chronic pain management. Family therapy generally includes partners, children, and caregivers. Within the therapy sessions, numerous psychotherapeutic approaches can be used, including CBT, operant therapy, and positive psychology. The parties are taught in the sessions the skills to identify pain behaviors and, based on the approach being used, to respond accordingly.[6,7] Support groups help individuals with chronic pain, and the people in their lives feel less alone in their chronic pain experience. Support groups can limit an individual's feeling of isolation, give the individual an arena to discuss any problems he or she may be having, and lead to increased motivation through social experience.[10] Both of these strategies can be a significant additive to a more well-rounded approach to chronic pain management.

The final alternative approach reviewed here is EMDR, an intervention that is designed to "bring the client into a more adaptive cognitive and emotional state."[11] The rationale supporting the use of EMDR is that chronic pain contains physical, cognitive, and emotional experiences. EMDR can work to address and reprocess these experiences to allow patients to cope better with the pain. Using EMDR requires a trained clinician to guide the individual. The steps for EMDR include focusing on the first pain event, pain sensations, or other pain-related distressing experiences. At this point, the clinician uses bilateral auditory, visual, or tactile sensory stimuli to decrease the intensity of the initial event, pain sensations, or other experiences. Next, the biliateral stimulation is used to strengthen positive responses, such as increased relaxation or decreased pain, as a means for the individual to reprocess the experiences himself or herself.[11]

These alternative approaches to chronic pain management in addition to the typical psychotherapeutic interventions may prove to help patients cope with their pain more readily as well as move forward in their ability to function within their societal role. None of these approaches have been proven to be better than the other, and, generally speaking, they are probably most successful when used together. There is no clear-cut approach to working with an individual with chronic pain—there are many factors to consider and many strategies with which to work.

Behavior Modification Strategies

In addition to psychotherapeutic approaches, multiple behavioral modification strategies exist that can be employed to assist individuals with chronic pain. These behavior modification strategies in particular are often used in conjunction with the counseling approaches discussed previously.

Relaxation training can encompass multiple strategies. It is also one of the most common techniques used to help individuals manage their pain.[3] According to Grant and Haverkamp,[3] "... relaxation techniques can include deep breathing, progressive muscle relaxation, relaxing imagery, cue-controlled relaxation, autogenic relaxation, or hypnosis." In addition to the sheer number of relaxation techniques that exist, the number of theories attempting to explain their use and success also contribute to their dominant presence within the treatment of chronic pain. Arena[12] reported that there are three primary theories explaining why relaxation strategies are effective. One theory states that with chronic pain comes an increase in stress on an individual's body. If the individual can learn how to control the stress by using relaxation strategies, the individual can help to decrease his or her own pain. The second theory states that increased muscle tension is a contributing factor to most pain, and if an individual can use relaxation techniques to decrease muscle tension, the individual should be able to decrease his or her pain. Finally, the third theory states that individuals with chronic pain have sympathetic nervous systems that are "stuck" in a flight-or-fight response. Given the appropriate relaxation strategy, the individual may be able to "unstick" himself or herself from this sympathetic nervous system response and decrease his or her pain.[12] In combination with other strategies, research has shown that relaxation techniques are helpful in controlling chronic pain experiences.

Whichever technique is used, one of the keys to success with this specific intervention is whether or not the patient can generalize the strategy to appropriate situations outside of the clinic or facility. A patient may be able to enact a relaxation strategy in the controlled environment of a health care professional's office. However, being able to identify stressors in day-to-day activities and apply the appropriate relaxation technique to decrease pain is a difficult task. The task of learning how to generalize can be overcome by practicing the technique in different situations.[12]

Another behavior modification strategy is biofeedback. Similar to other psychotherapeutic techniques, biofeedback can be used in conjunction with relaxation techniques. Biofeedback is used to draw the patient's attention, via auditory, visual, or tactile stimulation, to increased stress levels and muscle tension. By drawing the attention of the individual to these issues, the hope is that the individual can work to decrease the stress levels or muscle tension, generally by executing an additional technique such as one of the psychotherapeutic interventions or a relaxation intervention.[12] Despite the usefulness of biofeedback in drawing an individual's attention to areas of issue, there is some concern about its applicability because of its added expense and the fact that the individual must be trained to use it appropriately. Additionally, there is evidence to support the notion that general relaxation techniques, without the use of biofeedback, can be equally effective.[3,12]

The final behavior modification technique discussed in this section is activity planning and exercise. As mentioned previously, it may seem counterintuitive to individuals with chronic pain to increase their activity levels or exercise, but there is empirical evidence to support that doing so can have multiple positive effects.[3] The exercise and increased activity levels should be supervised by a health care clinician with the skill set to do so. Increasing activity levels and exercise can move the individual to a greater understanding of his or her body as well as the understanding that activity is *not* causing any increase in tissue damage despite what the pain experience may be. Additionally, increased activity and exercise can prevent further deconditioned states, which may serve to complicate the initial diagnosis of chronic pain.[3]

If increased activity or exercise is out of the question, then, at a minimum, individuals with chronic pain should be educated to plan their activities. An individual experiencing chronic pain often has times of the day that are worse than others, or there may be certain situations that may cause an increase in pain behaviors. Allowing individuals to understand and appreciate these nuances of their own pain experience can lead them to make better decisions about the timing of their activities. For instance, for a particular individual, if the pain experience is worse in the mornings than in the evening, it would be important for that individual to perform more rigorous activities in the morning when he or she is feeling better, leaving the less rigorous activities for the evening.

All of these behavior modification strategies may be employed with most, if not all, individuals with chronic pain. However, to facilitate the most success, the behavior modification strategies should not be used in isolation. Instead, incorporating the behavior modification strategies in with one (or more) of the psychotherapeutic interventions is likely to provide the most supportive environment to control pain and support a return to function for a patient with chronic pain.

Research

In 1999, Morley et al.[13] published a systematic review and meta-analysis of randomized controlled trials in which CBT and behavior therapy (operant therapy and relaxation training) were used as interventions for all forms of chronic pain, excluding headaches. In 2001, Van Tulder et al.[14] published an additional systematic review of trials in which behavioral treatments were employed for patients with chronic low back pain. As is the case with most systematic reviews and meta-analyses, there were many outcome measures used to capture what the original reasearchers intended to use as an objective measurement of pain, function, or well-being. Similarly, the interventions within the original research included a variety of techniques, often used in combination. Appreciating these caveats, it seems exceptional that the authors of the systematic reviews and meta-analyses were able to come to any conclusion at all. However, after grouping and organizing interventions and outcome measures, their conclusions were the same—psychological intervention, regardless of the approach, results in better outcomes for individuals compared with individuals who were placed on a waiting list and did not receive psychological intervention.[15]

Following the work of Morley et al.[13] and Van Tulder et al.,[14] McCracken and Turk[16] published a literature review, which indicated that combining behavior therapy and CBT also produces positive effects for all types of chronic pain, not just chronic low back pain. Hoffman et al.[15] published a meta-analysis of psychological interventions for patients with chronic low back pain. Their conclusions further supported the initial conclusions of Morley et al.[13] and Van Tulder et al.,[14] reporting that psychological interventions can reduce self-reported pain levels, pain-related interference, depression, and disability and can increase health-related quality of life for patients with chronic low back pain.

In addition to information regarding behavior therapy, CBT, relaxation training, and biofeedback is empirical research supporting the efficacy of positive psychology for patients with chronic pain. Rasmussen, Scheier, and Sieier[16] conducted a meta-analysis reviewing how optimism affected the outcome measures used in the the original research. In all domains, optimisim had positive predictive capabilities with regard to health outcomes, offering additional support to the argument that chronic pain should be addressed with a multimodal approach.

Despite the fact that few empirical data come from a patient population with chronic pain secondary to peripheral neuropathy, reviewed collectively, the body of literature supporting psychotherapeutic intervention for patients with chronic pain offers a strong argument for clinicians working with these patients regardless of the etiology of the pain. Similarly, that these psychotherapeutic interventions should be viewed as dynamic as opposed to static is implied by the reviewed literature. As much of the literature implies, there is no clear-cut, straightforward approach to working with a patient experiencing chronic pain. As a result, the best approach to intervention is to start with one approach keeping in mind applications for other approaches throughout the treatment. Using appropriate outcome measures can be beneficial in helping to direct the course of treatment, as can a thorough assessment and reassessment process. Invariably the patient and the patient's pain experiences must direct the interventions and treatment planning.

Although the research used to support the practice of psychotherapeutic interventions with patients experiencing chronic pain is generally based on patient populations without peripheral neuropathy, the evidence is compelling and is difficult to refute, even for this specific population. The systematic reviews and meta-analyses all support the use of some sort of psychological approach. The pain literature has advanced to encompass the idea of the "pain experience" for individuals with chronic pain, including physical, emotional, and cognitive elements. Even without the support of empirically based research, heuristically it is easy to identify and understand how managing chronic pain and the range of symptoms that come with it would be best done with a multimodal approach.

Despite the overwhelming support of psychological intervention, some people argue against its use. These arguments come from an inability to standardize the psychotherapeutic intervention and the idea that not everyone will benefit from the same type of intervention. In this chapter, we discuss many different approaches to inform professionals who are working with this patient population. As the controversy demonstrates, one approach is not going to work with all patients. Instead, the professionals managing the care of individuals with chronic pain are responsible for knowing what alternatives there are and understanding the differences and distinctions between them—most likely using several approaches with one patient.

The chronic pain experience is multidimensional, and it is the clinician's responsibility to understand these dimensions and intervene with appropriate strategies. In deciding which strategies to use with a patient with chronic pain, it is essential to perform a thorough history and initial assessment. This is a critical part of the care of all patients, particularly patients with challenging diagnoses such as chronic pain. This first step in the process is key to successful treatment planning and should be valued as such. During this initial assessment, the clinician can use his or her knowledge of different models of pain processing to interpret which intervention is most appropriate. The initial assessment also gives the clinician an opportunity to build trust and a relationship with the patient as well as the opportunity to explain the process of psychotherapeutic interventions. Building and maintaining trust is an essential component to working with patients with chronic pain.

CASE STUDY

Mary is an 82-year-old woman with chronic mid-back pain. She was diagnosed with osteoporosis 5 years ago, and she fell last year with a resultant compression fracture of T12. Mary remains in chronic pain despite two courses of physical therapy and two attempts at vertebroplasty. She estimates her pain to be 6/10 at rest and 9/10 with ambulation. She walks functional distances (i.e., 30 feet) with a rolling walker. She requires moderate assistance with dressing and bathing because of her pain. She can no longer travel to visit her children and has all but eliminated going out socially with her husband. She spends most of her day in a recliner watching television. She is unable to take anti-inflammatory medications because of her anticoagulant therapy. She uses a topical narcotic patch over her back that affords "a bit of relief."

Case Study Questions

1. Mary's husband is encouraging Mary to return to physical therapy for a supervised exercise program. Based on the literature, exercise may benefit a patient with chronic pain for which of the following reasons?
   a. Exercise may prevent disuse atrophy of postural muscles.
   b. Exercise may assist with pain control through the expression of endorphins.
   c. Exercise has a direct relationship to the quality of sleep.
   d. All of the above

2. For patients with chronic pain, operant therapy is best defined as which of the following?
   a. Operant therapy is an approach designed to address the gross motor and cognitive/subjective responses to clinical pain.
   b. Operant therapy is a behavioral therapy used to improve risk factor modification.
   c. Operant therapy is a cognitive therapy to improve knowledge of the etiology of pain.
   d. None of the above

3. Examples of manipulating the environment to decrease chronic pain include which of the following?
   a. Maintaining the home at a comfortable temperature
   b. Limiting ambient noise such as turning down the telephone ringer and the television
   c. Purchasing a stair lift rather than ascending steps by crawling
   d. All of the above

4. The depression and anxiety associated with chronic pain may be effectively treated with which of the following modalities?
   a. Exercise
   b. Medication
   c. Talk therapy
   d. All of the above

5. The aberrant learned pain behaviors of people with chronic pain are reinforced by which of the following?
   a. The hardwiring of these behaviors into the cerebral cortex
   b. The behavior of the family
   c. Medication
   d. Behavioral therapy

References

1. Lebovits AH. Psychological interventions with pain patients: evidence for their effectiveness. *Semin Pain Med*. 2003;1(2): 25–37.
2. Banks SM, Kerns RD. Explaining high rates of depression in chronic pain: a diathesis-stress framework. *Psychol Bull*. 1996; 119(1):95–110.
3. Grant LD, Haverkamp BE. A cognitive-behavioral approach to chronic pain management. *J Couns Dev*. 1995;74:25–32.
4. Sanders SH. Operant therapy with pain patients: evidence for its effectiveness. *Semin Pain Med*. 2003;1(2):90–98.
5. Benjamin S. Psychological treatment of chronic pain: a selective review. *J Psychosom Res*. 1989;33(2):121–131.
6. Lewandowski W, Morris R, Burke Draucker C, Risko J. Chronic pain and the family: theory-driven treatment approaches. *Issues Ment Health Nurs*. 2007;28:1019–1044.
7. Farrugia D, Fetter H. Chronic pain: biological understanding and treatment suggestions for mental health counselors. *J Ment Health Couns*. 2009;31(3):189–200.
8. Aspinwall LG, Tedeschi RG. The value of positive psychology for health psychology: progress and pitfalls in examining the relation of positive phenomena to health. *Ann Behav Med*. 2010;39:4–15.
9. Seligman ME, Rashid T, Parks AC. Positive psychotherapy. *Am Psychol*. 2006;61:774–788.
10. Arthur AR, Edwards C. An evaluation of support groups for patients with long-term chronic pain and complex psychosocial difficulties. *European Journal of Psychotherapy, Counselling and Health*. 2005;7(3):169–180.
11. Grant M, Threlfo C. EMDR in the treatment of chronic pain. *J Clin Psychol*. 2002;58(12):1505–1520.
12. Arena JG. Chronic pain: psychological approaches for the front-line clinician. *J Clin Psychol*. 2002;58(11):1385–1396.
13. Morley S, Eccleston C, Williams A. Systematic review and meta-analysis of randomized controlled trials of cognitive behavior therapy and behavior therapy for chronic pain in adults, excluding headache. *Pain*. 1999;80(1–2):1–13.
14. Van Tulder MW, Ostelo R, Vlaeyen JW, Linton SJ, Assendelft WJ. Behavioral treatment for chronic low back pain: a systematic review within the framework of the Cochrane Back Review Group. *Spine (Phila Pa 1976)*. 2001; 26(3):270–281.
15. Hoffman BM, Papas RK, Chatkoff DK, Kerns RD. Meta-analysis of psychological interventions for chronic low back pain. *Health Psychol*. 2007;26(1):1–9.
16. Rasmussen H, Scheier MF, Greenhouse J. Optimism and physical health: A meta-analytic review. *Ann Behav Med*. 2009;37:239–256.

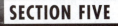
Special Considerations

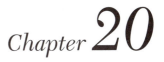

Chapter **20**

Guillain-Barré Syndrome

Megan Mulderig, PT, DPT, NCS

"Through my illness I learned rejection. I was written off. That was the moment I thought, okay, game on. No prisoners. Everybody's going down."

—Lance Armstrong (1971–)

Objectives

On completion of this chapter, the student/practitioner will be able to:

- Discuss possible etiologies of Guillain-Barré syndrome (GBS).
- Discuss the clinical presentation and variations of GBS.
- Develop an evaluative algorithm for individuals with GBS.
- Discuss treatment options for individuals with GBS.

Key Terms

- Guillain-Barré syndrome
- Inflammatory demyelinating polyradiculopathy

Introduction

Guillain-Barré syndrome (GBS) is a relatively common acute form of peripheral neuropathy in which the body's immune system suddenly and rapidly attacks the peripheral nervous system. More specifically, the pathology is an **inflammatory demyelinating polyradiculopathy,** a consequence of inflammation of peripheral nerves and spinal nerve roots. GBS most commonly affects the myelin sheaths, but in severe cases, the axons are also damaged.[1] The exact mechanism by which the immune system is attacked is unclear; however, the pathology of GBS is understood, and effective treatment methods are available.

GBS is an autoimmune disease that typically is preceded by an acute bacterial or viral infection. Although the exact cause is unknown, GBS has been shown to be preceded frequently by a respiratory infection or stomach virus. In rare cases, GBS may manifest in a patient after receiving certain vaccinations. GBS can be identified by various degrees of ascending weakness, sensory abnormalities, diminished or absent reflexes, and autonomic dysfunction, all of which occur symmetrically and evolve rapidly. GBS often emanates in the legs, and the associated pain, weakness, and paresthesia can spread quickly to the arms and face depending on the severity of the disease in a particular patient. On average, the disease achieves its most severe neurological state (i.e., its nadir) within 8 days; however, the nadir must occur during a period of less than 4 weeks to satisfy the diagnostic criteria of acute GBS.[2] In the event that symptoms continue to progress beyond a 4-week period, the diagnostic focus shifts from acute GBS to a more chronic form of inflammatory neuropathy known as chronic inflammatory demyelinating polyneuropathy (CIDP). GBS requires hospitalization for early recognition and treatment.

The diagnosis of GBS is clinically based; however, the diagnosis is typically supported by laboratory and electrophysiological testing to rule out more esoteric neuropathies. Specific criteria have been established for the diagnosis of GBS.[3] It is a syndrome divided into several subtypes. Consideration of motor, sensory, cranial nerve, and autonomic involvement is important in differentiating between other neurological diagnoses and the following GBS subtypes[2,3]:

- Acute inflammatory demyelinating polyradiculoneuropathy
  - Most common—85% of cases
  - Characterized by primary demyelination of sensory and motor nerves
- Acute axonal motor neuropathy and acute axonal motor and sensory neuropathy
  - 5% to 10% of cases
  - Axonal degeneration with motor or motor and sensory involvement
  - Poorer prognosis with motor and sensory symptoms
  - Increased frequency of respiratory and bulbar symptoms
- Miller-Fisher syndrome
  - 5% of cases
  - Rare, more focal form of GBS
  - Characterized by areflexia, ataxia, and ophthalmoplegia
  - Symptoms also may include facial weakness, bulbar signs, ptosis, and pupillary defect

GBS is the most common cause of acute nontraumatic neuromuscular paralysis in the world and is a leading cause of disability in the United States.[2,4] It often results in residual effects that influence quality of life, such as pain, fatigue, and emotional disturbances for 3 to 6 years after diagnosis.[5] The introduction of treatment via immunotherapy has affected how the disease is managed and has had a positive influence on the functional outcomes of patients with GBS.

Rehabilitation of a patient with GBS can be influenced positively by a clinician who is educated about the pathology, effects, and complications of the disease. Overall, the clinician plays an important role in the management of symptoms and rehabilitation of a patient with GBS so that the patient can achieve optimal functional ability and return to his or her premorbid quality of life. A patient with GBS presents myriad challenges to a clinician because of the comprehensive effect of GBS on body structure and function, activity limitations, participation restrictions, environmental factors, and the patient's quality of life. A coordinated approach by all members of the health care team providing treatment to the patient is essential to ensuring that the patient achieves a full functional recovery.

Epidemiology

The annual incidence of GBS is about 1 to 2 per 100,000 persons and is equally dispersed worldwide.[6] Lower rates have been reported in children younger than 16 years old, about 0.6/100,000 per year.[6] GBS does not affect a particular race or socioeconomic class more frequently, and its occurrence has not changed significantly over many years.[48] It affects persons of all ages, although a literature review published in 2009 noted that GBS was most common in elderly adults.[6] Another study reported that GBS is more common among adults between 30 and 50 years old.[7] Men and women are equally affected.[8] No genetic predisposition to GBS has been found, and there is no suggestion that the disease is communicable.[9] Age at onset affects morbidity and the setting to which the patient is discharged after an acute care stay.[5] When GBS is diagnosed in individuals younger than age 50, these individuals are most often discharged to home; individuals between 51 and 75 with a new diagnosis of GBS are most often discharged to a rehabilitation setting or skilled nursing facility. Of patients, 80% are ambulatory 6 months after diagnosis.[5] Mortality rates are 3% to 10%, and mortality is most prevalent when GBS is diagnosed in individuals older than age 75.[5]

Approximately two thirds (40% to 70%) of patients with GBS have a preceding infection, which is often experienced about 4 to 6 weeks before diagnosis.[6,11] The most common preceding infection (up to 70%) is an upper respiratory infection, followed by inflammation of the stomach or intestines (6% to 26%).[6] A preceding infection occurs more frequently in children who develop GBS, with a 67% to 85% incidence rate; upper respiratory infection is most common, followed by gastrointestinal infection.[6] In a literature review, no significant incidence was found with regard to seasonal occurrence.[6] Viruses associated with development of GBS are cytomegalovirus and Epstein-Barr virus.[6] Flu vaccines and HIV have been implicated more recently.[12] Less than 2% to 3% of individuals who develop GBS recently underwent surgery or experienced trauma.[2]

The reason why some individuals develop GBS and others do not is unknown, as is the reason why the severity of the disease varies among individuals. There has been discussion about a connection between vaccines and GBS in susceptible individuals.[11] It is understood that vaccines influence the immune system to produce immunity. Although the etiology of GBS is unknown, it is possible that a vaccine may stimulate the immune system in a way that triggers an autoimmune-like disease process. There is not sufficient evidence at the present time to conclude that vaccines are a cause of GBS.[13] The discussion arose as a result of a slight, but statistically significant, increase in the incidence of GBS after the H1N1 (swine flu) vaccines in 1976.[11,14] Since 1976, studies of vaccines for influenza have found little to no risk for GBS.[11,14] Preliminary examination of data by the U.S. Centers for Disease Control and Prevention after H1N1 vaccination in 2009 showed risk similar to that after seasonal influenza vaccination (<1 case of GBS per 1 million vaccinations) and incidence much less than the incidence after the H1N1 vaccination in 1976.[15] Vaccines aid in preventing the spread of disease and improving disease survival rate across the world, and the benefits of them far outweigh the small risk for developing GBS. It is recommended that patients in the acute phase of GBS and for up to 1 year after onset not receive vaccinations.[13] Patients with a history of GBS should be evaluated on an individual basis and caution should be exercised when determining whether a future vaccine is necessary.[15] Additional, more definitive research is needed in this area.[13]

Clinical Presentation and Diagnosis

According to most resources, GBS is classified as a syndrome, rather than a disease, because there is no evidence of GBS having a specific cause. A syndrome is characterized by a group of clinically based symptoms and laboratory test results without an identifiable cause. Arriving at a diagnosis of GBS is difficult because of variability of presenting signs and symptoms. To make an accurate diagnosis, physicians rely on signs and symptoms along with results of electrophysiological and laboratory tests. A thorough history and evaluation should include length of time that symptoms have been present and discussion of any previous infections. Laboratory testing includes an evaluation of cerebrospinal fluid via lumbar puncture. Typically, testing shows that individuals with GBS have elevated protein in the cerebrospinal fluid.

Two specific features are required for diagnosis of GBS—areflexia and progressive motor weakness of one limb.[3,16] The motor weakness can vary from a mild form in the lower extremities to complete paralysis of all four extremities and the trunk as well as the facial and respiratory muscles.[3,16] Typically, areflexia is widespread throughout the limbs; however, mild forms

Table 20-1 Clinical Diagnostic Indicators for Guillain-Barré Syndrome

Weakness	Progressive motor weakness in more than one limb Symmetrical weakness pattern Areflexia
Progression of Symptoms	May continue for 2–4 weeks
Electrodiagnostic Features	Nerve conduction slowing or block Reduced conduction velocity in two or more nerves
Cerebrospinal Fluid	Elevated protein

Adapted from Asbury AK, Arnason B, Karp HR, McFarlin DE. Criteria for diagnosis of Guillain Barré Syndrome. *Ann Neurol.* 1978;3: 565–566.

Table 20-2 Clinical Diagnostic Indicators Supporting a Diagnosis Other Than Guillain-Barré Syndrome

Weakness	Nonprogressive acute motor weakness Asymmetrical weakness pattern Hyperreflexia
Upper Motor Signs	Positive Babinski or clonus Spasticity
Bowel and Bladder	Dysfunction of bowel or bladder
Sensory	Symptoms exclusive to sensory impairment

Adapted from Asbury AK, Arnason B, Karp HR, McFarlin DE. Criteria for diagnosis of Guillain Barre Syndrome. *Ann Neurol.* 1978;3: 565–566.

may reveal distinct hyporeflexia instead (Tables 20-1 and 20-2).[3]

A complete electrodiagnostic examination is critical to establish the pathology of GBS and to understand the degree of axonal damage.[3] Nerve conduction velocity (NCV) studies are most supportive of the diagnosis of GBS, especially in the initial stages, because they detect demyelination early in the disease process.[4] Electromyography ascertains the integrity of the motor units. The motor portion of the NCV test is found to be abnormal in 90% of patients with GBS approximately 2 weeks after symptom onset and is indicative of an evolving manifestation of the syndrome.[3] In the first 2 to 3 weeks after onset of the most common form of GBS, acute inflammatory demyelinating polyradiculoneuropathy, demyelinating polyneuropathy is the prevalent finding, and axonal degeneration is secondary.[3] NCV studies, specifically motor NCV, are the most reliable predictor of prognosis when done 4 to 6 weeks after symptom onset because the features of the syndrome are clearer at this time.[3,4] Common features for confirming the diagnosis of GBS include reduced conduction velocity, conduction block, abnormal temporal dispersion, prolonged distal latencies, and prolonged or absent F waves and H reflexes.[3] The conduction block and temporal dispersion frequently occur at sites of entrapment—in the peroneal nerve between the ankle and fibular head, median nerve between wrist and elbow, or ulnar nerve between wrist and elbow.[3] In the primary axonal form of GBS, the primary finding is decreased muscle action unit potential of a distally stimulated nerve, excluding all the aforementioned findings of a demyelinated nerve.[4]

Medical Management and Treatment

After GBS is diagnosed, immediate medical management in an acute care hospital is crucial because of the risk of symptom progression to a life-threatening degree. The care of patients with GBS requires the expertise of physicians, nurses, and rehabilitation specialists because morbidity and mortality are closely related to the quality of medical management that occurs early in the disease process. Treatment of primary symptoms and prevention of secondary complications is the main focus in the acute phase. Three phases of GBS typically occur: First, worsening of symptoms to the point of nadir; second, a plateau phase where function remains the same; and third, improvement of function and recovery. Respiratory and circulatory problems are the most frequently seen acute complications. Patients are commonly admitted to the intensive care unit (ICU) in the early phase for monitoring of respiration and vital signs in the event that mechanical ventilation is needed. Because relapses may occur in patients with a more severe course of the disease, it is crucial for regular neurological evaluations to be done in acute care as well as in the inpatient rehabilitation setting.[2]

There is no cure for GBS. Medical management focuses on reducing symptoms and attempting to attenuate the patient's period of recovery to the extent possible.[16] Pharmacological interventions have been found to be effective in accelerating recovery and reversing nerve damage compared with supportive treatments alone.[17] The most popular pharmacological treatments are plasmapheresis and intravenous immunoglobulin (IVIG) therapy. Corticosteroids previously were thought to be useful; however, there is little evidence to support this, and their use is no longer a standard of practice for GBS treatment.

Plasmapheresis, or plasma exchange (PE), was the first treatment known to be effective in the management of GBS. PE is a process that involves removing blood from the body, separating plasma from blood cells for treatment to remove disease-causing antibodies, and returning blood to the body along with a replacement for plasma and a small concentration of albumin to replace protein that may have been lost.[17] The process is performed on consecutive days for a period typically not greater than 5 days.[17] A 2010 Cochrane review concluded that PE is more effective than no treatment and should be started within 2 weeks of symptom onset.[17] In mild, moderate, and severe cases of GBS, up to four sessions of PE have resulted in a meaningful reduction in the length of time between nadir and a patient's recovery of ambulation without an assistive device.[17] These same plasma treatments also have shown a diminishment in the length of time between nadir and a patient's full recovery of strength.[17] Research supports the use of PE to lessen the time patients spend on artificial ventilation and to minimize the residual effects 1 year after diagnosis.[17] However, the complex process involved in PE poses a risk for patients who are hemodynamically unstable; for that reason, medical professionals looked for another, safer treatment option.

IVIG therapy is a medical treatment commonly used to treat autoimmune diseases such as GBS, pediatric HIV, and CIDP. It consists of intravenous administration of purified antibodies (immunoglobulins) taken from third-party human blood specimens to replace antibodies that a patient's compromised autoimmune system is unable to produce.[1] The immunoglobulins are administered intravenously in high doses for 5 days.[1] The goal of the treatment is to fight and prevent further infection.[1] IVIG has been shown to speed recovery as effectively as PE when initiated within 2 weeks of onset of motor symptoms.[1] One study showed added benefit when IVIG was combined with corticosteroids; additional research is necessary to establish the benefit of these therapies when combined.[1] A combination of IVIG and PE has been explored as a treatment option for GBS, but it has been determined that there is no added benefit.[1] When compared with PE, IVIG was determined to be safer, easier to administer, and associated with fewer complications, and so IVIG is usually the first treatment, as determined by physicians, used after GBS is diagnosed.[1]

The initial theory behind treatment with corticosteroids is that they reduce overall inflammation and decrease nerve damage. A 2010 Cochrane review found moderate evidence that treatment with steroids alone does not influence recovery and does not affect the future long-term functional outcome.[18] Evidence of poor quality suggests that oral corticosteroids may postpone recovery.[18] Because corticosteroids have not been shown to have a beneficial effect, they are not currently used to treat GBS.[18]

Clinical Implications

Patients with GBS may experience multiple complications. These complications contribute to prolonged recovery time; extended time needed in rehabilitation; and increased restrictions placed on participation in family, work, and societal roles.[19] Medical and rehabilitative management of typical complications are discussed here.

Cardiovascular and Respiratory Compromise

As a result of the loss of peripheral innervation to the muscles of respiration as well as problems with supporting the airway because of bulbar weakness, one third of patients with GBS experience difficulty breathing independently and respiratory restriction.[2,8] Respiratory complications, most commonly pneumonia, are associated with morbidity and mortality.[20] Artificial ventilation is needed in about 50% of cases, typically more severe cases of GBS, to maintain a properly functioning airway.[8] The need for ventilatory support is correlated with cranial nerve dysfunction, autonomic dysfunction, prolonged immobility, and longer lengths of stay in the acute care and rehabilitation settings.[2] It is also closely associated with morbidity and mortality. The risk for aspiration increases in patients with cranial nerve involvement secondary to weakness of swallowing muscles. Patients are weaned from ventilation when strength and lung function have improved.

Assessment and intervention by physical therapists is an important part of the recovery for the cardiorespiratory system. Goals of physical therapy are to stimulate clearance of pulmonary secretions, optimize oxygenation, and reduce the energy expenditure of breathing. These goals are accomplished with postural drainage, chest percussion techniques, cough stimulation, cough assistance, and inspiratory training.[2] Overfatiguing of respiratory muscles should be avoided because this may induce respiratory failure.[2] Respiratory rate and oxygen saturation should be closely monitored during exertion and upright activity, especially in the acute care setting while the ventilator is being weaned and in the rehabilitation setting when exercise tolerance is progressing.

Autonomic Dysfunction

Dysautonomia reportedly occurs in about 60% to 70% of patients with GBS.[21] Clinically, dysautonomia can manifest as a minor disruption or as a life-threatening complication related to morbidity and mortality. Patients who present with a more severe form of GBS (up to 20% of patients) and require mechanical ventilation are at higher risk for developing severe dysautonomia.[2] Dysautonomia most often manifests as tachycardia, but symptoms may also include blood pressure instability such as orthostatic hypotension,

cardiac arrhythmias, diaphoresis, and gastrointestinal difficulties.[21-23] Symptoms can last throughout the acute care as well as the rehabilitation stay; it is important for vital signs to be closely monitored and for any abnormalities to be communicated immediately to the physician.[2] Bowel and bladder dysfunction (e.g., constipation) is addressed by the physician and improves with a consistent continence program; these symptoms resolve early in the recovery process.[19] Monitoring of autonomic dysfunction occurs in the ICU and acute care settings; however, in the rehabilitation and outpatient settings, physical therapists are responsible for monitoring blood pressure and heart rate regularly. This monitoring is especially important during changes of position from supine to sit and sit to stand as well as after static or dynamic upright activity, such as walking and activities of daily living (ADLs). Orthostatic hypotension is a common complication secondary to autonomic dysfunction and decreased muscle tone of the lower extremities. There is conflicting evidence about orthostatic hypotension and whether it completely resolves during recovery or remains as part of residual disability; however, more research is needed in this area.[17,18] When a patient with GBS presents with dysautonomia, rehabilitative goals should include education of the patient and family on effective ways to manage the process, including the reason for use of compression garments (abdominal binder and antiembolism compression stockings) and the importance of maintaining sufficient hydration.[19] To improve tolerance to the upright position gradually and to assess the response from the respiratory, cardiovascular, and autonomic systems after prolonged immobility, physical therapists use a tilt table during treatment sessions.[19]

Muscle Weakness

Individuals with GBS often present with weakness and flaccid or hypotonic extremities and trunk.[2] Weakness, leading to immobility, is one of the most disabling symptoms of GBS. Very little research exists to determine the effect of muscle strength training in patients with GBS, and there is no evidence to compare and contrast interventions or to support an effective course of physical therapy. Assumptions have been made based on strength and conditioning research done on patients with other polyneuropathies as well as normal subjects. The main precaution to be discussed here involves avoiding overworking muscles to prevent or reduce recurrence or worsening of symptoms.

Strengthening exercises should avoid overworking the muscles to the point of fatigue.[19] Evidence exists to support the theory that overworking the motor unit may delay recovery.[2] There is anecdotal evidence to support the belief that overworking muscles may lead to relapse of weakness and delayed recovery.[23] It is believed that intact motor units are at risk for being overworked.

The effect produced by GBS on the peripheral nerves leads to an impairment of the ability of the motor unit to distribute signals and engage muscle fibers to produce a force and a muscle contraction.[23] Because of injury to the myelin or axons or both, weakness occurs that results from the accessibility of smaller numbers of muscle fibers.[23] During muscle activity or exercise, the available muscle fibers, which are few, are at risk for being overworked.

The literature has established parameters to guide treatment planning and exercise program development by the physical therapist.[23] Before the point of nadir is reached, the role of the physical therapist is to maintain passive range of motion. Specific exercise parameters include refraining from overworking the patient to the point of fatigue, avoiding eccentric contractions because these increase the likelihood of injury, and not emphasizing strength training until muscles are able to achieve full active motion against gravity.[23] Small studies in patients with neuromuscular disease suggest that a high-resistance exercise regimen increases the probability for a loss of muscle strength.[23] A submaximal exercise program is recommended to avoid regression of symptoms.

Strength returns in a descending pattern as nerves regenerate.[24] Recovery of strength and other symptoms occur quickly during the first 6 months after nadir.[24] Clinicians should consider results of electrophysiological testing to determine the severity of damage to the myelin and axons when considering an exercise prescription.[23] The presence and severity of axonal damage are indicative of long-term strength and functional deficits.[20,23] Manual muscle testing and handheld dynamometry are reliable and valid ways of assessing strength. Gains in strength have been documented during the recovery process for 18 months after symptom onset.[30] This should serve as a guide to the exercise prescription and the need for long-term follow-up of the patient with GBS.

In the beginning of the recovery stage, passive range of motion and application of resting splints are important to maintain flexibility to ease return of functional mobility when the patient is able. When the recovery stage begins, assessment of strength and tolerance for upright activity may be initiated. Aerobic exercise is a crucial part of the exercise prescription to ensure the patient returns to a premorbid level of function and endurance; however, vital signs must be closely monitored in case of autonomic dysfunction, and a low to moderate exertion level must be maintained.[23] Strengthening should occur within the limits of functional activities with emphasis on low repetitions. Eccentric contractions are safe at a submaximal level and should ideally be performed during functional activities.[23] The exercise parameters discussed here should be used as a guideline for exercise prescription in patients with GBS. Additional research is necessary to guide our understanding of the effect of exercise on this pathological state.

Pain and Sensory Dysfunction (Dysesthesia)

Most patients with GBS report pain as a disabling symptom. It is often the first symptom experienced by individuals with GBS, before onset of weakness or sensory changes.[2] Pain most commonly begins in the proximal musculature, specifically the low back and upper part of the legs, and is most frequently reported in these areas during the acute and recovery phases of GBS for up to 1 year.[31] The pathogenesis of GBS pain syndromes is unknown. More than three quarters of patients with GBS report pain in the acute phase, and one third experience pain 2 years after diagnosis.[32,33] The severity of pain does not appear to be correlated with functional recovery but is linked with involvement of sensory nerve fibers.[31,33] Moulin et al.[33] discussed three variations of pain as described by patients with GBS. The most frequently reported was throbbing and aching pain in the low back that radiated to the legs. Second, patients described dysesthetic pain, noted to be burning or tingling in the extremities. Less commonly, patients with GBS reported pain related to joint aches and stiffness. The visual analog scale is a reliable and valid assessment of patients' experience and perception of their pain. Pain is primarily managed through pharmacology, specifically with nonsteroidal anti-inflammatory medications or, for patients with disabling pain, narcotics. The best course of pharmacological treatment for each individual patient is determined by the physician.

Although pain and functional recovery are not linked, pain should be assessed and managed in the rehabilitation setting to ensure patient comfort and full participation in the therapy sessions. Because of varying degrees of weakness and immobility of the trunk and extremities, pain can be caused by an imbalance of strength and flexibility or malalignment of spinal joints. Rehabilitation specialists can address pain in the early stages with attention to positioning in the bed and wheelchair. Range of motion exercises are important to maintain flexibility and prevent joint contractures; however, it has been suggested that lengthening of nerve roots, by means of stretching, may induce additional discomfort.[2] Pain-relieving modalities, such as transcutaneous electrical nerve stimulation, and patient education help to relieve symptoms. Referral to a physician who specializes in chronic pain may be necessary if pain persists after strength and endurance deficits have resolved.

Fatigue

Fatigue is a common complaint of patients with acute GBS and is a major contributor to long-term disability. It is seen in up to 80% of patients with immune-mediated polyneuropathies, CIDP, and GBS.[34] Merkies et al.[34] reported that patients describe fatigue as one of the three most disabling symptoms that affects their quality of life. The risk for fatigue doubles in patients with muscular weakness and is closely associated with pain.[35] Fatigue in GBS has been correlated with age but is not related to preceding infection, the severity of symptoms at onset, or the severity of residual neurological deficits.[36] At the onset of GBS, peripheral fatigue appears to have a significant influence on complaints of fatigue. After resolution of neurological symptoms, psychosocial dysfunction and dysautonomia contribute to persistent fatigue.[36] Despite good recovery of physical strength and mobility, fatigue is frequently a long-term effect of GBS that may interfere with overall daily function and social life.[36]

The causes of fatigue in patients with GBS are numerous and may be related to central and peripheral factors. de Vries et al.[36] described different causes of fatigue in patients with GBS—fatigue that is perceived and felt by the patient (experienced fatigue) and fatigue that is related to decreased muscle endurance and force production (peripheral fatigue). The Fatigue Severity Scale is a valid assessment tool for experienced fatigue, with good test-retest reliability and good internal consistency. Muscle capacity in peripheral fatigue can be measured by electrophysiological testing.[36] Physical therapists can use measures of endurance and activity tolerance, such as the 2-Minute Walk Test or 6-Minute Walk Test, and manual muscle testing as assessment tools for this impairment.

Treatment of fatigue should focus on underlying symptoms and discussion of psychosocial causative factors. Exercise prescribed by a physical therapist can have a positive impact on fatigue levels. A small study of a custom-designed low-impact treatment program completed by patients recovered from GBS who experienced persistent fatigue found that patients reported fatigue diminished by 20% in addition to overall improvement of "physical fitness, function and quality of life"; this progress was maintained at 2-year follow-up.[37] In light of the fact that consistent exercise improves physical conditioning and muscle strength, one can deduce that a rehabilitation exercise program would positively influence the degree of fatigue experienced by patients with GBS.[38]

Medications are used to manage fatigue in other demyelinating disorders; however, there is very little evidence for their use in patients with GBS.[36] One randomized controlled trial found that amantadine, a drug that has many purposes but is commonly used to improve arousal in patients with neurological impairments, had no effect on severe fatigue in patients with GBS.[39]

Gait

As a result of the presence of weakness and imbalance that varies from tetraparesis to symmetrical leg weakness, the gait pattern is often affected. In the initial stages of recovery, ambulatory aids such as a walker, crutches, or a cane may be needed. Strength and endurance training should include functional standing and walking activities, taking into consideration the need to avoid overfatiguing the muscles. Persistent lower extremity weakness can lead to difficulty with foot clearance (footdrop) in one leg or both, necessitating the need for an orthosis. One study of 69 patients who were admitted for inpatient rehabilitation found that two thirds of patients required an orthosis at one point during rehabilitation, and one third needed an orthosis 1 year after diagnosis.[17] A case study found neurodevelopmental sequencing to be an effective treatment technique for a geriatric patient with GBS.[40] The use of partial body weight support locomotor training was investigated in a limited fashion.[19] Research to support the efficacy of physical therapy interventions on gait and functional recovery is needed.

Integument

Patients with severe weakness and prolonged immobility are at risk for skin breakdown at areas of bony prominence. Regular skin checks, pressure relief, and patient and caregiver education are imperative for prevention of breakdown.[41]

Swallowing and Speech

Patients whose cranial nerves are affected experience difficulties with swallowing and motor speech. A speech and language pathologist should be consulted for proper assessment and treatment. In rare instances, supplementary feeding methods may be required short-term, such as a nasogastric feeding tube or a percutaneous endoscopic gastrostomy tube.

Deep Vein Thrombosis

Roughly 80% to 90% of patients with GBS are non-ambulatory at one point in the disease process. Because of this prolonged immobility, patients with GBS are at risk for developing deep vein thrombosis or pulmonary embolism.[2] The treating clinician should be mindful of the signs and symptoms of this complication. It is unclear what percentage of patients experience this complication because that has not been studied.[2] Prophylactic measures routinely used include compressive stockings, pneumatic stockings, ankle exercises, early ambulation, and antiplatelet therapies such as low-molecular-weight heparin.

Heterotopic Ossification

Heterotopic ossification (HO) is a complication that occurs infrequently in patients with GBS. HO is the formation of bone in soft tissue in the periarticular space. It typically occurs in patients after trauma to the central nervous system. In a prospective study of outcomes in patients with GBS, a very small percentage of patients were found to have developed HO in the hip region (6%), typically patients with a more severe course who are admitted to the ICU. HO has been reported only in the hip joints.[42]

Psychosocial Implications

Because of the rapid onset of weakness and immobility that is experienced by patients of all ages who have GBS, psychosocial function is significantly affected throughout the acute and rehabilitative phases. The most frequently experienced issues are anxiety, depression, and pain as well as feeling undereducated about their symptoms.[43] The rate and level of physical recovery appear to be related to the level of psychological stress that is present 1 year after diagnosis.[43] Cognitive issues may be present after prolonged mechanical ventilation.[19] It is the health care provider's responsibility to educate the patient and family about symptoms as well as to assist their understanding of what to expect during the course of recovery. An evaluation in the rehabilitation setting should include an assessment of the patient's perception of function and disability as well as education about the effect of GBS on psychological health; a reliable and valid tool is the Short Form-41 (SF-36).[43] If symptoms of depression persist 1 to 2 years after diagnosis, the primary physician should be alerted; extended depression occurs most commonly in patients who have not returned to their premorbid level of physical function. Persistent pain and fatigue can contribute significantly to emotional stress, and these symptoms should be addressed by the physician and rehabilitation clinician. Psychological stress may persist 1 to 2 years after diagnosis because of social limitations such as inability to go to work or attend social functions.[43] Understanding that patients with GBS may experience lingering physical and psychological deficits years after the acute phase will contribute to improved quality of care by health care professionals. More research is needed on the psychological and social outcomes after GBS.

Support groups in the United States and around the world are beneficial to patients with GBS and their families. Such groups allow exchange of emotional support and coping strategies. Support groups also help patients to develop a sense of community, while providing education and promoting advocacy. The GBS/CIDP Foundation International is a nonprofit volunteer organization that provides a forum for networking and education for patients, families, caregivers, and health care professionals.

Rehabilitative Care

Rehabilitation is an integral component in the recovery of premorbid strength, functional mobility, and quality of life; however, very little evidence exists to support physical therapy as an adjunct to medical care. The length of time spent under rehabilitative care has been positively correlated with fewer limitations on long-term functional activity and participation restrictions.[1] Because the speed and degree of recovery vary from person to person, persistent physical and psychological deficits may contribute to decreased overall physical and psychological functioning years after diagnosis.[39] For this reason, rehabilitation should be provided in an adequate time frame to ensure optimal recovery.

Physical therapy should begin during the acute stages to assist in the prevention of decubitus ulcers, prevention of contractures, and monitoring of cardiorespiratory issues during strengthening and functional activity.[2] Education about the length of time and process for recovery is critical.[9] Based on evidence from research on other neuromuscular diseases, exercise and rehabilitation have a positive influence on strength, endurance, functional activities, ADLs, and the prominent residual symptoms of fatigue and pain (Box 20-1).[44-46]

Classification of Signs and Symptoms

The International Classification of Functioning, Disability and Health (ICF) model was established by the

---

BOX 20-1

Physical Therapy Assessment for an Individual With Guillain-Barré Syndrome

History of present illness
Premorbid functional status
Past medical and surgical history
Medications
Review of laboratory, electrodiagnostic, and
　radiographic data
Social status including home support
Vital signs in supine, sitting, and standing before and
　after activity
Visual acuity, depth perception, hearing
Speech
Cognition
Swallowing
Activity tolerance
Integument
Muscle strength, tone, and coordination
Articular and axial range of motion
Reflexes
Bowel and bladder
Balance
Sensory testing
Functional assessment: Bed mobility, transfers,
　ambulation, wheelchair mobility

World Health Organization to create universal domains of assessment associated with the functioning of patients with different conditions.[47] As discussed, GBS has the potential to affect multiple systems throughout the body, which translates to dysfunction on many levels. The signs, symptoms, and clinical effects of GBS can be categorized into different levels according to the ICF[19,47]:

- Body structure and function: Decreased respiratory capacity, fatigue, pain, muscle weakness, decreased range of motion, autonomic dysfunction, dysphagia
- Activity limitations: Transfers, mobility on level surfaces and stairs, speech and communication disorders, ADLs
- Participation restrictions: Difficulty returning to social and family roles and functions, inability to work

Examples of Physical Therapy Goals for Rehabilitation

Short-Term Goals

- Improve activity tolerance (3 hours of therapy in acute rehabilitation)
- Independence with bed mobility
- Independence with mobility at the wheelchair level
- Independence with transfers, toileting, dressing, and bathing
- Maximize articular and axial range of motion to allow performance of ADLs
- Complete patient and family education
- Maximize muscle strength to permit functional activities
- Promote a safe and acceptable gait pattern with or without assistive devices

Long-Term Goals

- Independence with ADLs
- Independent mobility on level and uneven surfaces at premorbid level in the home and community settings
- Return to work

Assessment and Outcome Measures

More research is needed to evaluate the effect of GBS on activity limitations, functional mobility, strength, gait, and participation in life roles. Following is a list of suggested outcome measures that may be beneficial during evaluation and reporting of progress according to the domains of the ICF.[47] To our knowledge, none of these measures have been tested or validated in patients with GBS.

- Activity limitations: Berg Balance Scale, Tinetti Assessment Tool, Functional Independence Measure, 10-Meter Walk Test, 6-Minute Walk Test, Modified Rankin Scale, Modified Barthel Index
- Participation restrictions: Fatigue Impact Scale, Fatigue Severity Scale, GBS disability scale, Short Form-36, Positive Affect Negative Affect Scale, Hughes Disability Scale, Modified Fatigue Impact Scale, Disability Grading Scale for GBS, Erasmus GBS outcome score[7]

Prognosis, Recovery of Function, and Quality of Life

The outlook for most patients with a diagnosis of GBS is positive from a long-term perspective; however, more severe cases may be associated with lasting disability and residual deficits.[17] Older age, presence of comorbidity, onset of autonomic dysfunction, disease severity (specifically the degree of weakness and need for intubation for ventilatory support), and duration of the plateau phase are suggestive of worse overall outcome and are related to morbidity and mortality.[1,10,18] Clinical symptoms are typically more severe in patients with preceding gastrointestinal infection.[2] Approximately 40% of patients who are admitted to the hospital require inpatient rehabilitation after their acute care stay to ensure safe discharge to home.[2] Patients admitted for inpatient rehabilitation have typically experienced medical complications such as respiratory failure, cranial nerve dysfunction, and autonomic dysfunction.[2]

Most patients recover functional mobility and return to their premorbid level of activity participation and quality of life after receiving timely medical treatment and suitable supportive rehabilitative care. Residual disability is present in 20% to 50% of patients, sometimes for 3 to 6 years after diagnosis.[5,9,48] Residual disability is often characterized by pain, fatigue, or weakness, which negatively affect a person in various aspects of life.[19] Individuals with persistent weakness may benefit from ambulation with an orthosis or assistive device.[17] However, most patients are able to resume normal family, work, and social activities within a 2-year period. The amount of time it takes to recover depends on the severity of the disease at its nadir.[21]

Patients with GBS score lower than normal on quality-of-life outcome measures.[45] Following research on self-reported residual deficits from patients with neuromuscular diseases, Rekand et al.[35] concluded that these diseases and syndromes, including GBS, "cause long-lasting disability and interfere with the quality of life." Up to 50% of patients may experience difficulty participating in social and leisure activities for 3 to 6 years after diagnosis.[48] In general, evidence has shown that most patients make a good recovery and return to functional ambulation within 6 months. Notwithstanding such gains in basic strength and mobility, a patient's recovery from GBS may entail longer term deficits in quality of life and activities of functional independence, such as a return to premorbid levels of participation in leisure and work activities. Despite the evidence for potential recovery, the condition is multifaceted and complex, and a cure continues to elude the medical field. It is essential that an integrated health care approach be undertaken, with prolonged medical and rehabilitative care, to ensure proper management of the pathological process and subsequent recovery.

CASE STUDY

While on a business trip to Europe, Bill developed a severe upper respiratory infection. On the flight home, he began to experience numbness and tingling of his toes bilaterally. On leaving the airplane, he had difficulty walking to his car, he noticed his right knee buckling by the time he approached his car. When he arrived home and told his wife about his symptoms, she immediately drove him to the emergency department of a local hospital.

Blood work screening was normal, but based on the history, Bill was admitted to the ICU with suspected GBS. In the ICU, his condition rapidly deteriorated, and within 24 hours of admission, he was placed on a ventilator.

Case Study Questions

1. Which two physical examination criteria are necessary for a diagnosis of GBS?
a. Areflexia and progressive weakness
b. Hyperreflexia and posturing
c. Spasticity and urinary retention
d. Hyporeflexia and a positive Babinski test

2. Which of the following is the "gold standard" test for GBS?
a. Magnetic resonance imaging of the brain
b. Electroneuromyogram
c. Computed tomography scan of the spine
d. Hemoglobin and hematocrit

3. Which of the following therapies are the most effective for the treatment of GBS?
a. Antibiotics
b. Corticosteroids
c. Plasmapheresis and IVIG therapy
d. Radiation therapy

4. Common complications of GBS in the acute stage include which of the following?
a. Respiratory compromise
b. Autonomic dysfunction
c. Muscle weakness
d. All of the above

5. _____ has been reported by more than 50% of patients with GBS 2 years after diagnosis.
a. Pain
b. Paresthesia
c. Dizziness
d. Inability to walk

References

1. Hughes RA, Swan AV, van Doorn PA. Intravenous immunoglobulin for Guillain-Barré syndrome. *Cochrane Database Syst Rev.* 2010;(6):CD002063.
2. Meythaler JM. Rehabilitation of Guillain Barré syndrome. *Arch Phys Med Rehabil.* 1997;78:872–879.
3. Asbury AK, Cornblath DR. Assessment of current diagnostic criteria for Guillain Barré syndrome. *Ann Neurol.* 1990; 27(suppl):S21–24.
4. van Doorn PA. Treatment of Guillain Barré syndrome and CIDP. *J Peripher Nerv Syst.* 2005;10:113–127.
5. van Doorn P, Ruts L, Jacobs B. Clinical features, pathogenesis, and treatment of Guillain-Barré syndrome. *Lancet Neurol.* 2008;7(10):939–950.
6. McGrogan A, Gemma CM, Seaman HE, de Vries CS. The epidemiology of Guillain-Barré syndrome worldwide: a systematic literature review. *Neuroepidemiology.* 2009;32: 150–163.
7. Lunn MP, Willison HJ. Diagnosis and treatment in inflammatory neuropathies. *J Neurol Neurosurg Psychiatry.* 2009;80(3):249–258.
8. Burns TE. Guillain Barré syndrome. *Semin Neurol.* 2008;28: 152–167.
9. Pritchard J. What's new with Guillain Barré syndrome? *Pract Neurol.* 2006;6:208–217.
10. Alshekhlee A, Hussain Z, Sultan B, Katirji B. Guillain-Barré syndrome incidence and mortality rates in US hospitals. *Neurology.* 2008;70:1608–1613.
11. Hughes RA, Cornblath DR. Guillain-Barré syndrome. *Lancet.* 2005;366:1653–1666.
12. Souayah N, Nasar A, Suri MFK, Qureshi AI. Guillain-Barré syndrome after vaccination in United States: data from the Centers for Disease Control and Prevention/Food and Drug Administration Vaccine Adverse Event Reporting System (1990–2005). *J Clin Neuromuscul Dis.* 2009;11:1–6.
13. Haber P, Sejvar J, Mikaeloff Y, DeStefano F. Vaccines and Guillain-Barré syndrome. *Drug Saf* 2009;32(4):309–323.
14. Lehmann HC, Hartung HP, Kieseier BC, Hughes RA. Guillain-Barré syndrome after exposure to influenza virus. *Lancet Infect Dis* 2010;10:643–651.
15. Centers for Disease Control and Prevention (CDC). Preliminary results: surveillance for Guillain-Barré Syndrome After Receipt of Influenza A (H1N1) 2009 Monovalent Vaccine—United States, 2009–2010. *MMWR Morb Mortal Wkly Rep.* 2010;59(21):657–661.
16. Pithadia AB, Kakadia N. Guillain Barré syndrome (GBS). *Pharmacol Rep.* 2010;64:220–232.
17. Asbury AK, Arnason BG, Karp HR, McFarlin DE. Criteria for diagnosis of Guillain-Barré syndrome. *Ann Neurol.* 1978; 3:565–566.

18. Hughes RA, Swan AV, van Doorn PA. Corticosteroids for Guillain-Barré syndrome. *Cochrane Database Syst Rev.* 2010;(2):CD001446.

19. Gupta A, Taly AB, Srivastava A, Murali T. Guillain-Barré syndrome—rehabilitation outcome, residual deficits and requirement of lower limb orthosis for locomotion at 1 year follow-up. *Disabil Rehabil.* 2010;32(23):1897–1902.

20. Nicholas R, Playford ED, Thompson AJ. A retrospective analysis of outcome in severe Guillain-Barré syndrome following combined neurological and rehabilitation management. *Disabil Rehabil.* 2000; 22(10):451–455.

21. Keoppen S, Kraywinkel K, Wessendorf TE, et al. Long term outcome of Guillain Barré syndrome. *Neurocrit Care.* 2006;5:235–242.

22. World Health Organization. *The International Classification of Functioning, Disability and Health (ICF).* Geneva: WHO; 2001.

23. Rekand T, Gramstad A, Vedeler CA. Fatigue, pain and muscle weakness are frequent after Guillain-Barré syndrome and poliomyelitis. *J Neurol.* 2009;256:349–354.

24. Moulin DE, Hagen N, Feasby TE, Amireh R, Hahn A. Pain in Guillain-Barré syndrome. *Neurology.* 1997;48:328–331.

25. Dhar R, Stitt L, Hahn AF. The morbidity and outcome of patients with Guillain-Barré syndrome admitted to the intensive care unit. *J Neurol Sci.* 2008;264:121–128.

26. Raphael JC, Chevret S, Hughes RAC, Annane D. Plasma exchange for Guillain Barré syndrome. *Cochrane Database Syst Rev.* 2012;(7):CD001798.

27. Karavatas SG. The role of neurodevelopmental sequencing in the physical therapy management of a geriatric patient with Guillain-Barre syndrome. *Top Geriatr Rehabil.* 2005;21(2):133–135.

28. Ruts L, Drenthen J, Jongen JL, et al. Pain in Guillain-Barré syndrome: a long-term follow-up study. *Neurology.* 2010;75:1–9.

29. El Mhandi L, Calmels P, Camdessanche JP, Gautheron V, Feasson L: Muscle strength recovery in treated Guillain-Barré syndrome: a prospective study for the first 18 months after onset. *Am J Phys Med Rehabil.* 2007;86:716–724.

30. Khan F, Ng L. Guillain-Barré syndrome: an update in rehabilitation. *Int J Ther Rehabil.* 2009;16(8):451–460.

31. Flachenecker P. Autonomic dysfunction in Guillain-Barré syndrome and multiple sclerosis. *J Neurol.* 2007;254(suppl 2):II196–II101.

32. Forsberg A, Press R, Einarsson U, de Pedro-Cuesta J, Holmqvist L. Impairment in Guillain-Barré syndrome during the first 2 years after onset: a prospective study. *J Neurol Sci.* 2004;227:131–138.

33. Moulin DE, Hagen N, Feasby TE, Amireh R, Hahn A. Pain in Guillain-Barré syndrome. *Neurology.* 1997;48(2):328–331.

34. Merkies IS, Schmitz PI, Samijn JP, van der Meché FG, van Doorn PA. Fatigue in immune-mediated polyneuropathies. *Neurology.* 1999;53:1648–1664.

35. Rekand T, Gramstad A, Vedeler CA. Fatigue, pain and muscle weakness are frequent after Guillain-Barré syndrome and poliomyelitis. *J Neurol.* 2009;256:349–354.

36. de Vries JM, Hagemans ML, Bussmann JB, van der Ploeg AT, van Doorn PA. Fatigue in neuromuscular disorders: focus on Guillain Barré syndrome and Pompe disease. *Cell Mol Life Sci.* 2010;67:701–713.

37. Garssen MP, Bussmann JB, Schmitz PI, et al. Physical training and fatigue, fitness, and quality of life in Guillain-Barré syndrome and CIDP. *Neurology.* 2004;63:2393–2395.

38. Hughes RA, Wijdicks EF, Benson E, et al. Supportive care for patients with Guillain-Barré syndrome. *Arch Neurol.* 2005;62:1194–1198.

39. Bowyer HR, Glover M. Guillain Barré syndrome: management and treatment options for patients with moderate to severe progression. *J Neurosci Nurs.* 2010;42(5):288–293.

40. Bassile CC. Guillain Barré syndrome and exercise guidelines. *Neurol Rep.* 1996;20(2):31–36.

41. Rudolph T, Larsen JP, Farbu E. The long-term functional status in patients with Guillain-Barré syndrome. *Eur J Neurol.* 2008;15:1332–1337.

42. Garssen MP, Schmitz PI, Merkies IS, et al. Amantadine for treatment of fatigue in Guillain-Barré syndrome: a randomised, double blind, placebo controlled, crossover trial. *J Neurol Neurosurg Psychiatry.* 2006;77:61–65.

43. Zeilig G, Weingarden HP, Levy R, Peer I, Ohry A, Blumen N. Heterotopic ossification in Guillain-Barré syndrome: incidence and effects on functional outcome with long-term follow-up. *Arch Phys Med Rehabil.* 2006;87:92–95.

44. Flachenecker P, Wermuth P, Hartung HP, Reiners K. Quantitative assessment of cardiovascular autonomic function in Guillain-Barré syndrome. *Ann Neurol.* 1997;42:171–179.

45. Parry GJ, Steinberg JS. *Guillain-Barré Syndrome: From Diagnosis to Recovery.* Saint Paul, MN: AAN Enterprises, Inc; 2007.

46. Bernsen RA, de Jager AE, Kuijer W, van der Meche FG, Suurmeijer TP. Psychosocial dysfunction in the first year after Guillain Barré syndrome. *Muscle Nerve.* 2010;41:533–539.

47. Eldar R, Marincek C. Physical activity for elderly persons with neurological impairment: a review. *Scand J Rehabil Med.* 2000;32:99–103.

48. Tiffreau V, Rapin A, Serafi R, et al. Post-polio syndrome and rehabilitation. *Ann Phys Rehabil Med.* 2010;53(1):42–50.

Chapter 21

Peripheral Nerve Injury in the Athlete

STEPHEN J. CARP, PT, PHD, GCS

"Do not let what you cannot do interfere with what you can do."

—JOHN WOODEN

Objectives

On completion of this chapter, the student/practitioner will be able to:

- Identify common peripheral neuropathies associated with sports.
- Relate specific neuropathy to a specific sport.
- Identify the biomechanical etiologies of sports-related neuropathies.

Key Terms

- Burner
- Inflammation
- Neuropathy
- Repetitive and overuse athletic movements

Introduction

The last three decades have witnessed a tremendous increase in sports participation at all levels. However, increased sports participation has also increased the numbers, and perhaps the incidence, of sport-related injuries. Injuries can be due to either acute trauma or overuse. Acute injuries are defined as a high-force, low-repetition tissue stress resulting in a wide spectrum of injury severity—from a simple strain or sprain to trauma affecting multiple body systems—the complications of which may include shock, respiratory failure, or death. Overuse injuries may be defined as a low-force, high-repetition tissue stress that subsequently leads to an inflammatory cascade–initiated impairment in tissue reparative mechanisms. Peripheral nerve injury may result from high-force, low-repetition and low-force, high-repetition athletic injuries.

In recent years, a rich literature has significantly contributed to the understanding of the etiologies, types, assessment, intervention, and prevention of peripheral nerve injury related to athletic participation.

This chapter reviews the most frequent peripheral nerve injuries encountered by athletes. For organizational purposes and ease of reader understanding, we discuss the possible neural injuries in the context specific to types of athletic participation and, to a lesser extent, gender, age, and psychological variables that may affect injury.

Background

The pathophysiology of nerve injuries can be initiated by mechanical events involving **repetitive and overuse athletic movements,** such as overhead throwing, running, and jumping, or through direct blunt trauma.[1] The tensile or compressive forces exerted on the nerve stimulate the vasa nervorum, resulting in disruption of the microvasculature and the deformation of the connective tissue. Irritation potentiates a transient inflammatory response (i.e., macrophage/monocyte activity) that can induce chemosensitive and immunosensitive reactions with prolonged exposure producing a noxious response.[2] The edema produced is a consequence of compromised microcirculation at the endoneural level and may lead to hypoxia, local pain, angiogenesis, scarring, and restricted axoplasmic flow.[3] Endoneural edema accumulation is compounded by the lack of lymph tissue present at this level of the nerve to facilitate flow of fluids.[4] Continued mechanical exposure—in these athletic cases continued participation in the etiologic activity—potentiates the increased nerve mechanosensitivity, propagating inflammatory responses inflicting chemosensitivity to the nerve and the surrounding musculature.[5] The trauma may result in signs and symptoms such as dysesthesia, hyperesthesia, hypoesthesia, paresis (hypotonia), and paresthesia.[3,4] Clinical presentations include dysfunction, fatigability, loss of coordination, and disability.[3-5] Postural dysfunction—primarily muscular, capsular, and ligamentous tightness—also occurs as a result of excessive fibrosis, neural budding, and reflexive muscle tone initiated to protect the injured nerve from further damage.[5] Therapeutic management involves eliminating any irritating mechanical stimuli that are present; decreasing the **inflammation;** and maintaining muscle, nerve, and ligamentous range of motion.

Four categories have been reported in the literature to describe the underlying pathophysiology of acute or traumatic peripheral nerve injury. The first category consists of patients with underlying systemic or autoimmune diseases who are thought to have a higher risk for connective tissue and neural injury as a result of the impact of the primary disease on collagen structures. Diagnoses that fit this category include lupus erythematosus, psoriatic arthritis, rheumatoid disease, diabetes mellitus, chronic kidney disease, and hyperparathyroidism. These conditions are thought to cause downstream inflammatory changes that alter the structure of the tendon, muscle, ligament, and peripheral nerve. Histological examination of the nerves of these patients has demonstrated chronic inflammation, ischemia, and amyloid deposition.[6] The additional forces and stresses of athletic competition in patients with these diagnoses may add to the risk of **neuropathy.**

The second category includes athletes with single or multiple dosing of oral or injectable corticosteroids, which are thought to have an association with tendon rupture and possibly neuropathy. It is believed that the steroids affect collagen synthesis and compromise blood supply, weakening the tendon and the neural connective tissue and placing the athlete at risk for injury.[7]

Patients in the third category exhibit inflammatory and degenerative changes on histological studies attributed to microtrauma from chronic overuse. The serial body of work by Barr, Barbe, Safadi, Amin, Carp, and others[2-4] in a rat model of high-frequency, low-force repetitive strain tasks and later with translation to human populations revealed repetition-induced

tendinopathies with documented paratendon inflammation and cellular proliferation, increased production of matrix compounds, tendon degeneration, and functional loss. Histological studies of median nerves of rats trained in high-repetition, low-force reaching tasks exhibited increased numbers of ED1+ inflammatory macrophages in the involved limb and signs of epineural and perineural fibrosis. Conduction testing revealed a slight but significant slowing of nerve conduction velocity in the reach limb, which was consistent with similar studies indicating histological changes occurring before functional change.[3,4,8] Biopsy specimens of rat median nerves involved in high-frequency, low-force task repetitive strain showed ED1+ macrophages in portions of the median nerve located within and adjacent to the site of strain. Increases in these cells were found in the perineural and epineural layers and in association with the axons. Infiltration of the ED1+ macrophages is finely graded to the degree of injury as measured by nerve conduction velocity and the degeneration of nerve fibers and myelin. The rat nerves showed an increase in collagen type I immunoreactivity in the epineurium of the median nerve at the wrist in the trained animals. Progressive thickening of the internal and external epineurium as well as thickening of the perineurium was also seen.[3,4]

Athletes in the fourth category undergo a high-force, low-repetition strain resulting in microinjury and perhaps macroinjury to bone, tendon, muscle, ligament, and nerve. The cascade of the inflammatory reaction is similar to that which occurs secondary to high-repetition, low-force injuries but with the added variables of acute instability and pain, weakness, or loss of neural input or output.

Athletics-induced neural injury differs greatly from contractile tissue and ligamentous tissue injury. Peripheral nerve injury has a length-dependent response to repair; the more proximal the injury, the longer the time for repair. Axonotmetic and neurotmetic injuries often require surgical intervention, such as neurolysis and gap repair. Along with target loss of function, there is also a concurrent afferent and autonomic loss. Proprioceptive, kinesthetic, and tactile loss can be especially devastating to a competitive athlete. The quality and quantity of pain with neural injury differ from most musculoskeletal pain syndromes because of the radicular nature of the presentation. Along with local pain resulting from local nerve inflammation, the associated pain often travels distally along the axis of dermatomal and myotomal innervations, expanding the area of pain perception and, often in the case of nerves, a region of negative or positive symptoms of nerve injury. Often immobilization or limited excursion is required for healing of neural injuries, whereas many musculoskeletal injuries allow for a scaffolding of activity. As the nerve heals, passive insufficiency of a damaged nerve is always a serious concern that must be addressed with neural glide/slide rehabilitation techniques.

Football

Football has been played competitively at the collegiate level in the United States for more than 100 years. Long recognized as a high-risk activity and at the urging of President Theodore Roosevelt, representatives from Princeton, Harvard, and Yale met at the White House in 1905 to "save" football from its inherent violence. In his opening statements, President Roosevelt noted that "18 collegiate deaths" occurred as a result of football in 1904 and requested rule changes to improve safety and "save the game." Ultimately, the colleges banded together to form the predecessor to the National Collegiate Athletic Association (NCAA) with the goal of reforming the sport to limit injuries and fatalities. However, even with ongoing and evidence-based regulation directed at equipment—primarily helmets, safety rules, and the elimination of many techniques such as the "flying wedge"—football remains a very high-risk sport for injury to the participants.[9]

Football is a high-velocity, high-force collision sport in which injuries are expected to occur. Football athletes, many of whom weigh more than 300 pounds and can run the 40-yard dash in less than 5 seconds, collide with enormous quantities of force. Football, of all the common major sports played in the United States, has the highest number and incidence of injuries.[10] Game injury rates in collegiate football average 3.6 per 100 players per game (Table 21-1). Injury rate during practice is 1 per 100 players per practice. Musculoskeletal injuries are the most common football injury reported, with knee derangement and ankle sprains having the greatest frequency of occurrence. Except for the shoulder and knee, current studies are limited in identifying types of football injuries associated with body part (Table 21-2).[10,11] No current references are available delineating the number of peripheral nerve injuries and the locations associated with football.

The "**burner,**" sometimes referred to as "stinger syndrome," is one of the most common peripheral nerve injuries seen in football.[11,12] Frequently underreported by athletes, stingers have been found to affect 65% of college football athletes at least once during their collegiate career.[12] Burner symptoms typically include a burning or stinging pain that radiates down one of the upper limbs with or without associated paresthesias and weakness. In most cases, symptoms are transient and self-limiting. However, recurrences are common, and subtle neurological deficits may persist without being detected. Symptoms of burner syndrome that persist may indicate a more serious neurological injury.[13]

Table 21-1	Frequency Rate of All Specific Musculoneuroskeletal Injuries Occurring in Collegiate Football Games
Injury	Frequency Rate of Injury per Game (per 100 Athletes Participating)
Knee internal derangements	0.617
Ankle ligament sprains	0.539
Concussions	0.234
Neck nerve injury	0.180
Upper leg contusions	0.127
Upper leg strain	0.124
Acromioclavicular joint sprains	0.098
Shoulder ligament strain	0.091
Lower leg contusion	0.063
Foot ligament strain	0.011
Hand fracture	0.010

Data compiled from Albright JP, McAuley E, Martin RK, Crowley ET, Foster DT. Head and neck injuries in college football: an eight-year analysis. *Am J Sports Med.* 1985;13:147–152; Warren RF. Neurologic injuries in football. In: Jordan BD, Tsairis P, Warren RF, eds. *Sports Neurology.* Rockville, MD: Aspen; 1989:235–237; Poindexter DP, Johnson EW. Football shoulder and neck injury: a study of the "stinger." *Arch Phys Med Rehabil.* 1984;65:601–602; and Feinberg JH, Radecki J, Wolfe SW, Strauss L, Mintz DN. Brachial plexopathy/nerve root avulsion in a football player; the role of electrodiagnostics. *HSS J.* 2008;4:87–95.

Table 21-2	Frequency Rate of All Specific Musculoneuroskeletal Shoulder Injuries Occurring in Collegiate Football Games
Shoulder Injury	Frequency Rate of Injury per Game (per 100 Athletes Participating)
Acromioclavicular sprain	0.110
Anterior ligament sprain	0.107
Glenohumeral dislocation	0.101
Contusion	0.068
Muscle/tendon strain	0.064
Nerve injury	0.026

Data compiled from Albright JP, McAuley E, Martin RK, Crowley ET, Foster DT. Head and neck injuries in college football: an eight-year analysis. *Am J Sports Med.* 1985;13:147–152; Warren RF. Neurologic injuries in football. In: Jordan BD, Tsairis P, Warren RF, eds. *Sports Neurology.* Rockville, MD: Aspen; 1989:235–237; Poindexter DP, Johnson EW. Football shoulder and neck injury: a study of the "stinger." *Arch Phys Med Rehabil.* 1984;65:601–602; and Feinberg JH, Radecki J, Wolfe SW, Strauss L, Mintz DN. Brachial plexopathy/nerve root avulsion in a football player; the role of electrodiagnostics. *HSS J.* 2008;4:87–95.

Burners typically result from an upper cervical root (C5–C6) or upper brachial plexus injury. Controversy exists whether these injuries commonly involve the cervical roots, the brachial plexus, or a combination of the two.[13] Burners result from nerve traction or direct compression of the involved nerve fibers. Rare, but catastrophic, sequelae of severe traumatic upper cervical nerve root injury has been reported and may result in permanent nerve root injury—nerve root avulsion. These injuries are usually limited to high-velocity impacts, such as motorcycle collisions, and have been documented in the literature pertaining to football injury.[14]

Burner lexicon defines the injury as a grade 1, 2, or 3 peripheral nerve injury. Grade 1, which constitutes most burner injuries, is neurapraxia, which is a disruption of nerve action potential involving partial demyelinization. Axonal integrity is preserved, and remyelinization occurs within days to 3 weeks. A grade 2 injury is axonotmesis, which entails actual axonal damage and wallerian degeneration. A grade 3 injury is neurotmesis, which often results in permanent nerve damage.[14]

Three mechanisms of burners have been described in the literature.[13–15] The first mechanism is a traction injury to the brachial plexus and nerve roots. Traction injury occurs when any combination of the following movements occurs: The ipsilateral shoulder and scapular are depressed; the ipsilateral shoulder is horizontally abducted past midline; the neck is forced into contralateral lateral flexion. The second mechanism involves a direct blow to the supraclavicular fossa—this causes a percussive injury to the upper trunk. The third mechanism is nerve compression by a combination of neck hyperextension and ipsilateral lateral flexion. Biomechanically, this position mimics the Spurling maneuver, which tests for foraminal stenosis. The third mechanism may, along with brachial plexus injury, injure the nerve roots. One investigator observed that the most persistent and severe symptoms from burners occurred with this mechanism of injury (Fig. 21-1).[14]

Most burner injuries occur with tackling.[15] Shoulder and scapular depression and neck lateral flexion can occur as the tackler drives his shoulder into the ball carrier's body, especially into a thigh or knee. Shoulder horizontal abduction typically occurs with arm tackling lateral to the tackler's torso. The ball carrier's momentum exceeds the strength of the tackler's horizontal adductor muscle groups, forcing the shoulder into an abnormal horizontal abduction position that stretches the plexus. Additionally, direct compression of the brachial plexus can occur from contact with the ball carrier's elbow, knee, or shoulder.

Initial symptoms after injury are paresthesias in any combination of the C5 to T1 dermatomes, acute subclavicular pain, and generalized weakness. In most cases, the symptoms resolve within minutes to hours.

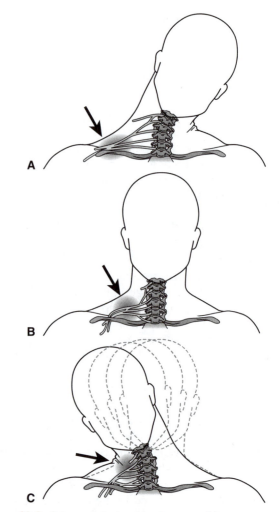

Figure 21-1 Stinger injuries may be caused by (A) contralateral flexion resulting in an ipsilateral tension injury to the plexus, (B) direct trauma to the plexus, and (C) contralateral flexion of the neck with contralateral compressive injury to the plexus.

Symptoms lasting longer than minutes to hours or symptoms that progressively worsen may be indicative of an axonotmetic lesion or additional structural damage in the thoracic outlet. Immediate paralysis requires emergent treatment owing to possible nerve root avulsion or cord injury. Electroneuromyogram testing is unreliable for at least 3 weeks after injury.[14]

There have been reports in the literature of cervical nerve root avulsion in football when severe forces laterally flex the neck, depress the scapula, and horizontally abduct the glenohumeral joint.[16] This etiology has also been well established in other high-velocity impacts that may occur with skiing or motorcycle riding.[17] Feinberg et al.[18] reported the case of a 30-year-old semiprofessional football player who sustained a cervical nerve root avulsion injury. He felt an immediate "frostbite" sensation in his right arm and hand. Subsequent electrodiagnostic and imaging studies revealed a complete avulsion of the C6 and C7 nerve roots from the spinal cord. A nerve graft was eventually performed to bridge the neural gap.

Burners frequently recur. One study reported an 87% chance of recurrence.[11] In another study, 36 upper level athletes who missed playing time secondary to a burner injury had a 42% chance of having another neck injury that results in loss of playing time.[14] The only valid predictor of burner injury is having a previous burner.[18] Players with a history of burners are often fitted with collars (e.g., the Cowboy Collar) that assist with the prevention of severe lateral neck flexion. The effectiveness of these adaptations has not been thoroughly studied.

Axillary nerve injuries most commonly occur after anterior glenohumeral dislocation. Glenohumeral dislocations typically occur in one of two ways: falling backward on an outstretched, extended arm, resulting in an anterior displacement of the humerus from its resting glenoid position, or forced lateral rotation of the humerus. The exact incidence of nerve palsy after acute dislocations of the shoulder ranges from 9% to 18%.[19–21] Inferior dislocations, although rarer than anterior dislocations, have an even higher rate of axillary nerve palsy—reported as high as 60%.[22] Blunt trauma to the anterior aspect of the shoulder without dislocation has been implicated in axillary nerve trauma in sports such as football, wrestling, and gymnastics.[21] Acute axillary neuropathy has also been associated with backpacking, usually in inexperienced hikers.[23] The cause of axillary nerve injury in "rucksack palsy" is thought to be traction caused by depression of the shoulder from the excessively weighted backpack.[24]

Musculocutaneous nerve palsy manifests with wasting of the biceps, coracobrachialis, and brachialis muscles; loss of the biceps reflex; and weakness of elbow flexion and supination. The athlete reports a variable loss of sensation along the lateral aspect of the forearm but generally does not complain of any significant pain. Clinical examination reveals atrophy of the biceps and brachialis muscles and decreased muscle tone in patients with partial nerve injury. Elbow flexion is weak but may be possible using the brachioradialis muscle, which is innervated by the radial nerve. Direct trauma to the anterior shoulder, fractures of the humerus and clavicle, and anterior shoulder dislocations[25] are common etiologies of musculocutaneous nerve injury. Tensile forces through the nerve can occur with prolonged overhead throwing as the nerve stretches over the anterior shoulder and coracoids. Musculocutaneous nerve injuries in weight lifters and rowers have been attributed to engorgement of the coracobrachialis muscle.[25] Forceful extension of the elbow against resistance, such as when a runner attempts to prevent the football being torn from his grasp by a defender, has also been implicated in musculocutaneous nerve palsy. Anterior shoulder surgery, especially for instability in athletes, has been associated with

musculocutaneous nerve palsy. The nerve is at risk with open and with arthroscopic procedures and can be stretched by retractor placement on the coracobrachialis muscle for exposure.[26]

The differential diagnosis for musculocutaneous nerve injury includes rupture of the distal biceps tendon at the elbow and more diffuse brachial plexus injuries. Distal biceps tendon rupture is associated with a loss of the contour of the muscle belly and superior retraction. The athlete can still contract the muscle, although a loss of contour is obvious.[26]

The long thoracic nerve is a pure motor nerve to the serratus anterior muscle, originating directly from the spinal roots of C5, C6, and C7. The long thoracic nerve passes along the anterior lateral aspect of the chest wall, supplying branches to all of the digitations of the serratus anterior muscle. The long thoracic nerve is well protected throughout its proximal course along the superior chest down to the level of the inferior portion of the pectoralis major. The nerve is susceptible to traction injury between its two points of relative fixation: at the medial scalene muscle at the base of the neck and at the superior aspect of the serratus anterior muscle. In general, injuries to the long thoracic nerve occur secondary to asynchronous motion of the arm and scapula, which can occur with a missed shot in golf, handball, or tennis or in contact sports in which the arm is jerked into an abnormal position, such as with football tackling.[27] A direct blow to the shoulder more often results in a diffuse brachial plexus injury than an isolated injury of the long thoracic nerve because of the protected position of the long thoracic nerve along the chest wall.[28] Long thoracic nerve traction injuries have been reported secondary to repetitive motions such as swimming, tennis, and prolonged positioning of the arm while shooting a rifle.[24] Fatigue of the parascapular muscles, as seen in ancillary football exercises such as rope skipping, upper body ergometer workouts, and weight lifting, can allow abnormal scapular motion on the chest wall, resulting in a traction injury to the long thoracic nerve. Weight lifting exercises most commonly associated with long thoracic nerve palsy include behind-the-neck French curls and the bench press. All of these exercises can result in marked translation of the scapula on the chest wall, producing a traction injury to the long thoracic nerve (Box 21-1).[24]

Peroneal nerve compromise has been reported in the football literature.[29] Etiologies include trauma and insidious origins. Traumatic causes of peroneal nerve neuropathy occur in association with musculoskeletal injury or with isolated nerve traction, compression, or laceration. Insidious causes include mass lesions, toxic neuropathies, and metabolic syndromes. The peroneal nerve is easily injured because of its subcutaneous location at the fibular head, the fact that it is tethered by the tendinous origin of the peroneus longus as it winds around the fibular head and passes through the

Box 21-1

Sports Implicated in Long Thoracic Nerve Injury

Archery	Discus
Hockey	Squash
Backpacking	Football
Rope skipping	Swimming
Ballet	Golf
Shooting	Tennis
Skiing	Gymnastics
Bowling	Weight lifting
Basketball	Handball
Skiing	Racquetball
Bowling	Wrestling
Soccer	

Data compiled from Duralde, XA. Neurological injuries to the athlete's shoulder. *J Athl Train.* 2000;35:316–328; McIlveen SJ, Duralde XA, D'Alessandro DF, Bigliani LU. Isolated nerve injuries about the shoulder. *Clin Orthop Relat Res.* 1994;306:54–63; Goodman CE. Unusual nerve injuries in recreational activities. *Am J Sports Med.* 1983;11:224–227; and McIlveen SJ, Duralde XA. Isolated nerve injuries about the shoulder. In: Bigliani LU, ed. *Complications of Shoulder Surgery.* New York: Williams & Wilkins; 1993:64–68.

peroneal tunnel to divide over the fibular neck, and its location on the lateral aspect of the knee and leg making it susceptible to traction forces as the knee or ankle is forced into varus.[29] Peroneal nerve injury results in weakness of ankle dorsiflexion and eversion and weakness of great and lesser toe extension.

At the hip, nerve fibers that terminate in the peroneal nerve may be injured.[18] The lateral fibers of the sciatic nerve are the most susceptible to injury. These fibers form the common peroneal nerve at the knee. The lateral location of the nerve fibers within the nerve trunk, tethering at the fibular head, and the larger size of the funiculi are likely to be responsible for this susceptibility.[29] Acute dislocation, acetabular fracture, proximal and midshaft femoral fracture, or operative repair of these fractures jeopardizes these nerve fibers. The incidence of peroneal nerve compromise secondary to osseous injury and surgical repair of the hip complex ranges from 6% to 33%. The most commonly reported complication of hip osteotomy is sciatic nerve paresis.[18]

The common peroneal nerve may be injured at the knee with a fracture of the distal femur, proximal tibia, or proximal fibula.[29] There is an approximately 1% incidence of peroneal nerve injury with tibial plateau fracture.[30] Peroneal nerve injury also can occur with realignment of the knee extensor mechanism and arthroscopic meniscal repair—common procedures among football players. Stretch injury of the peroneal nerve can occur during reduction treatment of a knee flexion contracture.[31] Using a posterolateral incision and placing a retractor to protect the nerve from traction can help to prevent common peroneal nerve injury during arthroscopic knee surgery.[31]

Peroneal neuropathy at the knee has been reported with ligamentous knee injury.[32] In a series of 31 lower extremity sports injuries, 17 were peroneal nerve injuries indicating the relative commonality of such an injury. Eight of these traumatic injuries were associated with ligamentous injury of the knee. Most of these involved anterior cruciate ligament rupture; this often occurred in conjunction with injury to the medial collateral and posterior cruciate ligaments. Three of the peroneal neuropathies in this series were associated with ankle injuries (attributed to traction injuries associated with severe inversion).[30]

Ligamentous or bony injury of the ankle may lead to peroneal neuropathy. However, nerve damage results more often from treatment of ankle fracture than from the fracture itself. Treatment of ankle injuries with a below-knee splint or cast can damage the peroneal nerve by additive pressure over the fibular head. Associated lower extremity edema, especially immediately postimmobilization, can exacerbate this complication. Cast-induced or splint-induced edema can often be avoided by padding the cast or splint in the area of the fibular head, keeping the superior aspect of the cast at least 1 inch inferior to the fibular head, avoiding prolonged pressure on the lateral knee (as can occur during bed rest with lateral rotation of the leg), performing frequent neurological checks, avoiding dependency, and maintaining elevation.[33]

Ankle sprain is a common cause of morbidity in the general population, and it is the most commonly injured joint complex among athletes.[30] The mechanism of injury in ankle sprain commonly involves inversion of a plantar flexed ankle. This position applies mechanical traction to the peroneal nerve at the fibular head.[33] Peroneal nerve injury after ankle sprain was first described by Hyslop in 1941 in a case series of three patients.[33] The mechanism of injury was proposed as a traction injury of the nerve in the posterolateral knee from a sudden force with the patient's foot in plantar flexion and inversion. Concurrent ankle sprain and peroneal neuropathy at the fibular head may be easily misdiagnosed. Patients with ankle sprain often experience lateral ankle pain and eversion weakness from the primary ligamentous injury. In a series of 66 patients with ankle sprain, electroneuromyographic studies indicated that 86% of patients with grade III sprains and 17% of patients with grade II sprains had evidence of peroneal nerve injury on needle examination.[33]

Trampoline

With increasing popularity of trampolines has come an increased number of injuries.[34] It is unknown whether there is an actual increase in the risk associated with trampoline use for the same number of hours of exposure or simply more injuries because of an increased number of participants. There is some indication that the number of trampoline injures may be due to increased recreational (i.e., backyard) and other creative methods of use. Smith[35] studied the epidemiology of trampoline-related injuries among children and concluded that they were so common that children should not use trampolines. Furnival et al.[36] and Woodward et al.[37] found dramatically increasing numbers of trampoline injuries and recommended a ban of the recreational use of trampolines. In 2000, Brown and Lee[38] reported that trampolines were responsible for more than 6,500 pediatric cervical spine injuries in the United States and supported a ban of the use of trampolines by children.

In a 2006 study, Nysted and Drogset[34] described trampoline-related injures seen at St. Olav's University Hospital in Norway from March 2001 to October 2004. Their study included 556 patients (56% male and 44% female). The mean age was 11 years (range, 1 to 62 years). A lateral ligament injury of the ankle was the most often reported diagnosis (20%), followed by an overstretching of ligaments in the neck (8%) and a fracture of the elbow (7%) (Tables 21-3 and 21-4). The authors observed significantly more fractures and dislocations in the upper extremity than in the lower extremity ($P < 0.001$). Soft tissue injury accounted for almost 30% of injuries in the upper extremity compared with 74% of injuries in the lower extremity ($P < 0.001$). Of the patients, 46 (8%) had a cervical injury—of which 43 were minor overstretching of ligaments with mild to moderate radicular neural signs, 2 were cervical fractures, and 1 was an atlantoaxial subluxation without injury to the spinal cord. Of the patients, 49

(9%) had an injury to the head area—28 were lacerations, and 20 were scalp contusions. None of the patients were assigned a Glasgow Coma Scale score less than 15. A severe injury, as defined by an Abbreviated Injury Scale value greater than 3, was present in 63 of 556 (11%) patients. Patients injured on the mat had a relative risk of 0.07 of a severe injury compared with 0.29 if falling off the trampoline. A total of 70 (13%) patients were hospitalized for a mean of 2.2 days (range, 1 to 8 days). The most common site of injury among the hospitalized patients was the elbow (27 of 70), followed by a fracture of the forearm (14 of 70). There were 23 patients who sustained a supracondylar fracture of the humerus, and 3 of these patients reported an ulnar nerve neuropathy in association with the fracture. None of the four patients with elbow dislocations reported a nerve injury, but one patient sustained an injury to the brachial artery. The artery was repaired with a vein graft. Two patients with supracondylar fractures had diminished radial pulse immediately after the accident; however, angiography was normal.

Cheerleading

Cheerleading injuries in the United States are increasing and present a significant source of injury to

Table 21-3 Main Cause of Trampoline Injury[33–36]

Mechanism of Injury	Number (%)
Awkward landing on the trampoline	292 (53)
Fall off the trampoline	122 (22)
Collision with another person	73 (13)
Performing a somersault	59 (11)
Other	5 (1)
Unknown	5 (1)
Total	551 (100)

Data compiled from Nysted M, Drogset JO. Trampoline injuries. *Br J Sports Med.* 2006;40:984–987; Smith GA. Injuries to children in the United States related to trampolines, 1990–1995. *Pediatrics.* 1998;101:406–412; Furnival RA, Street KA, Schunk JE. Too many trampoline injuries. *Pediatrics.* 1999;103:1020–1025; and Woodward GA, Furnival R, Schunk JE. Trampolines revisited: a review of 114 pediatric recreational trampoline injuries. *Pediatrics.* 1992;89: 849–854.

Table 21-4 Location of Trampoline Injury

Body Part	Number (%)
Head	49 (9)
Neck including radiculopathy	46 (8)
Trunk/back including radiculopathy	24 (4)
Shoulder	8 (1)
Upper arm including plexopathy	8 (1)
Elbow	62 (11)
Forearm	36 (7)
Wrist/hand	77 (14)
Hip/thigh	10 (2)
Knee	49 (9)
Leg	15 (3)
Ankle	141 (25)
Foot	31 (6)
Total	556 (100)

Data compiled from Nysted M, Drogset JO. Trampoline injuries. *Br J Sports Med.* 2006;40:984–987; Smith GA. Injuries to children in the United States related to trampolines, 1990–1995. *Pediatrics.* 1998;101:406–412; Furnival RA, Street KA, Schunk JE. Too many trampoline injuries. *Pediatrics.* 1999;103:1020–1025; and Woodward GA, Furnival R, Schunk JE. Trampolines revisited: a review of 114 pediatric recreational trampoline injuries. *Pediatrics.* 1992;89: 849–854.

participants, most of whom are female.[39,40] According to one study,[39] the number of cheerleading-related injuries sustained by children 5 to 18 years old and treated in U.S. hospital emergency departments more than doubled from an estimated 10,900 injuries in 1990 to an estimated 22,900 injuries in 2002. Cheerleading was a relatively sedentary, ground-based sport 30 years ago with routines consisting primarily of toe-touch jumps, splits, and claps.[40] Today, cheerleading routines incorporate gymnastic tumbling runs and partner stunts consisting of human pyramids, lifts, catches, and tosses. The increasing number of cheerleading injuries may be associated with this change to more gymnastic-style cheerleading routines.[40] An increase in the number of cheerleading participants may also be a factor. Although the actual number of cheerleading participants is unknown, American Sports Data Inc.[41] reported that the number of U.S. cheerleading participants 6 years old and older increased from 3,039,000 in 1990 to 3,579,000 in 2003.

Compared with injuries in other sports, cheerleading injuries have not received the same amount of concern in the literature with regard to tracking, severity, type, and reportability. Few epidemiological studies of cheerleading injuries exist in the literature, and none of the existing studies describe the epidemiology of cheerleading injuries by type of cheerleading team (college, high school, middle school, elementary school, or recreation league) or type of cheerleading event (practice, pep rallies, athletic events, or cheerleading competitions).

Shields and Smith[39] were the first to report cheerleading injury rates based on actual exposure data by type of team and event. A cohort of 9,022 cheerleaders on 412 U.S. cheerleading teams participated in the study. During the 1-year data-collection period, 567 cheerleading injuries were reported: 83% (467 of 565) occurred during practice, 52% (296 of 565) occurred while the cheerleader was attempting a stunt, and 24% (132 of 563) occurred while the cheerleader was basing or spotting one or more cheerleaders. Lower extremity injuries (30%; 168 of 565) and strains and sprains (53%; 302 of 565) were most common. Collegiate cheerleaders were more likely to sustain a concussion ($P = 0.01$, rate ratio [RR] = 2.98, 95% confidence interval [CI] = 1.34, 6.59), and All Star cheerleaders were more likely to sustain a fracture or dislocation ($P = 0.01$, RR = 1.76, 95% CI = 1.16, 2.66) than cheerleaders on other types of teams. Overall injury rates for practices, pep rallies, athletic events, and cheerleading competitions were 1.0, 0.6, 0.6, and 1.4 injuries per 1,000 athlete-exposures.

From a peripheral nerve injury standpoint, the discussion of the type of injury reported is not of sufficient depth to discern if nerve injury occurred with the orthopedic-described pathology. It is certainly possible that a plexus injury may result with a dislocated shoulder or that a median nerve injury may accompany a severe wrist fracture. Additional epidemiological work is required to assess the number and severity of nerve injuries associated with cheerleading.

In a study by Shields and Smith,[39] concussions represented only 4% of all cheerleading injuries. A similar study conducted by Schulz et al.[42] concluded that concussions account for 6% of cheerleading-related injuries. Concussions, if undetected, can expose a cheerleader to the potential for repetitive traumatic brain injury. Repetitive traumatic brain injury occurs after an individual sustains an initial head injury (usually a concussion), followed by a second head injury before symptoms associated with the first have fully cleared. The second blow may be minor and could result in brain swelling. Although repetitive traumatic brain injury is most common in contact and collision sports such as ice hockey, boxing, and football, it may also be sustained when cheerleaders collide with other cheerleaders. However, data do not currently exist to confirm this. Cheerleaders, their parents, cheerleading coaches, athletic trainers, and health care providers should be aware of the signs and symptoms of concussions and the potential for repetitive traumatic brain injury.

Baseball

Most peripheral nerve injuries occurring in baseball are seen with pitchers. The number of pitches thrown in a given day (as many as 200 including warm-up and actual game pitches) over the course of a full 8-month season; the angular velocity of the pitcher's arm (measured as high as 7,500 degrees per second); and the torque produced at the shoulder, elbow, and wrist with throwing curve balls, sliders, and cutters all have been implicated in the relatively high incidence of nerve injury in pitchers.[43] In baseball pitchers, nerve injury has been cited in the literature to account for approximately 2% of all diagnosed shoulder injuries.[43]

Quadrilateral space syndrome represents a chronic compression syndrome of the axillary nerve in throwing athletes. Axillary nerve entrapment occurs insidiously in the quadrilateral space without history of trauma. Fibrous bands at the inferior edge of the teres minor have been implicated, as have randomly oriented fibrous bands found in the quadrilateral space. Both the axillary nerve and the posterior humeral circumflex artery are compressed in the quadrilateral space when the arm is placed in the abducted, externally rotated, or throwing position.[24]

Posterior interosseous neuropathy (PIN) is a peripheral nerve injury commonly characterized by a sensation of a deep ache in the posterior forearm, which can be accompanied by weakness of the forearm extensors and brachioradialis, sensory alterations, or a combination of both. PIN occurs with less frequency in the upper extremity than median and ulnar mononeuropathies.[44] Among athletes, the incidence of PIN is unknown. Mechanical soft tissue injuries can manifest in a self-limiting manner and with symptoms (pain and weakness) similar to a peripheral neuropathy, which can make differentiating each condition a challenge. The proposed mechanism for injury in this case is the mechanics during the late stages of the throwing motion—the follow-through. The follow-through is defined as the progression of motion from maximal shoulder internal rotation to a balanced fielding position after the ball has been released. This is the phase of throwing that exhibits high levels of eccentric loading at the forearm along with repeated supination-pronation as a potential effect that places stress to the soft tissues of the throwing arm.

The muscles involved with the deceleration phase of the follow-through are the rotator cuff muscles, deltoid, triceps brachii, brachialis, supinator, and forearm extensor muscles. These muscles undergo eccentric loading that can theoretically compress or apply excessive tensile loading along the course of the radial nerve. This theory has not been substantiated in the literature.

Upper extremity deep venous thrombosis (UEDVT) is also known as thrombosis of the axillary-subclavian vein or Paget-Schroetter syndrome.[45] It is considered a relatively infrequent disorder that occurs predominantly in young, otherwise healthy individuals who participate in repetitive upper extremity activities that result in subclavian vein irritation.[46] From an epidemiological perspective, the general incidence of UEDVT remains low (approximately 2 per 100,000 persons per year), even though it is regarded as the most common vascular condition among athletes.[47] Symptoms are nonspecific, are variable, range in severity, and may be position dependent. Occasionally, patients may be asymptomatic. However, most commonly, patient complaints include initial "heaviness" in the affected arm and a dull ache and pain in the neck, shoulder, or axilla of the involved limb. The differential diagnosis is complex because patients with UEDVT typically display compressive signs usually associated with thoracic outlet syndrome, contributing to the likelihood that a structure compressing the subclavian vein may also compress the brachial plexus.[48] Other more dramatic signs of UEDVT may include ecchymosis and nonedematous swelling of the shoulder, arm, and hand; functional impairment; discoloration and mottled skin; and distention of the cutaneous veins of the involved upper extremity.[49] Conservative treatment including exercise and anticoagulation medication is often ineffective. Patients with UEDVT commonly require surgical intervention, including the removal of the first rib or scalene muscles. Arterial thoracic syndrome results from the compression of the subclavian artery within the thoracic outlet. Compression may occur as a result of a congenital anomaly, such as a cervical rib or a prefixed plexus; repetitive motion; posture; or muscle hypertrophy. Symptoms include arm and forearm weakness and pallor, loss of distal pulses, and occasionally sensory loss within the C5–T1 dermatomes, owing to the proximity of the plexus to the artery. Exercise including neural glides and soft tissue stretching is often effective. However, many cases progress to conditions that may require surgical neurolysis, scalenectomy, or first rib resection.

Following carpal tunnel syndrome, cubital tunnel syndrome is the second most common peripheral nerve entrapment syndrome in the human body. When appropriately diagnosed in a timely fashion, this condition may be treated by conservative and operative means with little or no resultant loss of function. The cubital tunnel is formed by the cubital tunnel retinaculum, which straddles a gap of about 4 mm between the medial epicondyle and the olecranon. The floor of the tunnel is formed by the capsule and the posterior band of the medial collateral ligament of the elbow joint. It contains several structures, the most important of which is the ulnar nerve. The ulnar nerve is the terminal branch of the medial cord of the brachial plexus and contains fibers from the C8 and T1 spinal nerve roots. It descends the arm just anterior to the medial intermuscular septum and later pierces this septum in the final third of its length. Progressing underneath the septum and adjacent to the triceps muscle, it traverses the cubital tunnel to enter the forearm, where it passes between the two heads of the flexor carpi ulnaris muscle.

This anatomical arrangement has two implications for the nerve. First, the ulnar nerve follows a relatively constrained, nonundulating path,[50] and second, it lies some distance from the axis of rotation of the elbow joint.[51] Movement of the elbow requires the nerve to stretch and slide through the cubital tunnel. Sliding has the greatest role in this process, although the nerve itself can stretch up to 5 mm.[50] The unusual anatomy of the cubital tunnel and the well-recognized increase in intraneural pressure associated with elbow flexion are believed to be key issues in the pathogenesis of cubital tunnel syndrome.[51] In addition, the shape of the tunnel changes from an oval to an ellipse with elbow flexion. This maneuver narrows the canal by 55%.[52]

The American and Japanese literature places a heavy emphasis on the susceptibility of baseball throwers to cubital tunnel syndrome. Ulnar nerve symptoms during the part of the throwing cycle that involves extreme flexion (late cocking, valgus stress, early acceleration) are strongly suggestive of the biomechanical etiology of cubital tunnel syndrome.[53]

Initial treatment for cubital tunnel syndrome is rest and avoidance of the etiological behavior. If rest fails to improve symptoms or if the needle examination becomes positive for distal denervation, surgical exploration is indicated. Neurolysis and transposition anteriorly are two common procedures.

Volleyball

The NCAA conducted its first women's volleyball championship in 1981. In the 1988–1989 academic year, 721 schools sponsored varsity women's volleyball teams comprising 9,486 participants. By 2003–2004, the number of varsity teams had increased 36% to 982, involving 310 participants.[54] Participation growth during this time has been apparent in all three divisions of college sport, but particularly in Divisions II and III.[54]

Agel et al.[55] published an excellent monograph on the epidemiology of volleyball injuries in women. In games, ankle ligament sprains (44.1%), knee internal derangements (14.1%), shoulder muscle strains (5.2%), and low back muscle strains (4.8%) accounted for most injuries. In practices, ankle ligament sprains accounted for 29.4% of all reported injuries, whereas other common injuries were upper leg muscle-tendon strains (12.3%), low back muscle-tendon strains (7.9%), and knee internal derangements (7.8%). A participant had twice the risk of sustaining a knee internal derangement in a game (0.46 vs. 0.22 per 1,000 A-Es; RR = 2.1, 95% CI = 1.8, 2.5) than in a practice. Female volleyball players also had almost twice the risk of sustaining an ankle sprain in a game than during a practice (1.44 vs. 0.83 per 1000 A-Es; RR = 1.7, 95% CI = 1.6, 1.9). The rate of ankle sprains has decreased on average per year by 1.8% ($P = 0.15$) in games and 3.0% ($P = 0.04$) in practices over the 16 years of this study. The specific structures injured most frequently during games and practices combined were the menisci and collateral ligaments. The authors' data did not include concurrent nerve injuries with the reported musculoskeletal injuries, although nerve injury is a common complication of all the diagnoses reported.[55]

Tennis

The ligamentous, osseous, musculotendinous, and neural structures at the posteromedial side of the elbow are at risk for various injuries during overhead athletics. Tennis, in particular, subjects an individual to the combination of valgus and extension overloading. Motions such as an overhead serve result in tensile forces along the medial stabilizing structures, with compression on the lateral compartment and shear stress posteriorly. The combination of tensile forces medially and shear forces posteriorly can result in ulnar collateral ligament (UCL) tears, tendinopathies and tendinoses, flexor-pronator mass injuries, neuritis of the ulnar nerve, posterior impingement, and olecranon stress fractures.[56] Tennis places the ligamentous, osseous, musculotendinous, and neural structures of the elbow at increased risk for various injuries. Proper training and preventive exercise based on sound biomechanical research can result in decrease of loads across the elbow in tennis players.

Knowledge of the kinetic chain of the tennis service and stroke should be taken into account by tennis athletic trainers, physical therapists, and instructors. For example, biomechanical analyses of tennis players indicated that with more effective knee flexion-extension during the service action, there was less valgus strain and loading at the elbow.[57] The exact impact of this finding is as yet unknown and needs to be studied further.

Internal rotation of the upper arm at the shoulder during the overhead service and forehand is of utmost importance—decrease of internal rotation in the shoulder can increase rotatory stress on the elbow. Internal rotation of the upper arm and pronation of the forearm during the early phase of the follow-through of the service most likely reduces the forces on the elbow. Grip size does not seem to play a role in elbow injuries; playing with a "Western grip" can possibly increase valgus stress on the elbow, especially during acceleration.[58]

The primary peripheral nerve injury associated with tennis is cubital tunnel syndrome. Ulnar neuritis around the elbow can be the result of compression or traction from valgus stress and can be seen as an isolated injury or in combination with UCL insufficiency or chronic flexor-pronator mass tendinosis. Compression can occur as a result of a tight cubital tunnel, osteophytes from the ulnohumeral joint, muscle hypertrophy, or subluxation of the nerve. In tennis players, the initial presentation of ulnar neuritis can be pain along the medial joint line associated with dysesthesias, paresthesias, or even anesthesia in the small and ulnar half of the ring finger. The degree of sensory and motor changes can vary depending on the severity and duration of ulnar nerve compression. Functionally, players lose the ability to grasp the racket properly and lose tactile and proprioception sensation in the hand. Surgical intervention is indicated in cases of progressive muscle weakness, persistent muscle weakness for more than 4 months, chronic neuropathy, or failure of a nonsurgical regimen.[59]

In a cadaver study, the movement of the ulnar nerve at the proximal aspect of the cubital tunnel was significantly increased during all service phases with increased elbow flexion ($P < 0.05$). A mean (standard deviation) maximum movement of 12.4 (± 2.4) mm was recorded during the wind-up phase with maximum elbow flexion. The maximum strain on the ulnar nerve during the acceleration phase was found to be close to the elastic and circulatory limits of the nerve.[60] The ulnar nerve is subjected to longitudinal strain in the cubital tunnel during the service motion, and this longitudinal strain is increased as the elbow is in greater flexion.[61]

Suprascapular nerve injuries have also been reported with tennis players. Symptoms of suprascapular nerve palsy generally have an insidious onset and are poorly localized. Athletes with suprascapular neuropathy typically have vague posterior shoulder pain, weakness of abduction and external rotation, and atrophy of the infraspinatus or supraspinatus (or both) muscle bellies. Pain may radiate down the radial axis of the arm. When entrapment of the suprascapular nerve occurs at the spinoglenoid area, pain is an inconsistent finding. Because the suprascapular nerve has no dermal distribution, pain is poorly localized and commonly leads to a delay in diagnosis (on average 12 months). Physical examination of suprascapular nerve entrapment syndrome can follow repetitive motions, prolonged positioning, or single acute events. Entrapment can also occur more distally at the spinoglenoid notch, which is more commonly seen in athletes whose sports require rapid forceful external rotation movements such as volleyball.[58] The cocking motion for the serve results in rapid external rotation of the shoulder. This rapid motion of the infraspinatus muscle is thought to pull the suprascapular nerve against the base of the scapular spine, resulting in nerve injury at this level. Injury to nerves in the spinoglenoid area has also been noted secondary to ganglion cysts. Ganglion cysts in athletes appear to be related to posterior labral injuries and may be associated with posterior instability. Posterior shoulder instability may also result in traction injury of the suprascapular nerve without ganglion cyst formation.[62]

Golf

The effective execution of the golf swing not only requires rapid movement of the extremities but also substantial strength and power of the trunk muscles. The torso rotates away from the target (to the right for a right-handed player; to the left for a left-handed player) at approximately 85 degrees/second on the backswing, and the powerful downswing involves trunk rotational velocities approaching 200 degrees/second.[63] Pink et al.[63] demonstrated relatively high and constant activity in the abdominal oblique muscles throughout most parts of the golf swing of skilled amateur players. In a similar study using professional golfers, Lindsay et al.[64] measured muscle activity in the erector spinae, abdominal oblique, and rectus abdominis. These authors established that all trunk muscles were relatively active during the acceleration phase of the golf swing with the trail-side abdominal oblique muscles showing the highest level of activity.

Because this powerful movement is repeated throughout the game or practice session, decreased endurance or weak muscles could lead to premature fatigue and increased injury risk to the trunk region. McGill[65] discussed and advocated the importance of trunk endurance in preventing low back pain (LBP). Lindsay et al.[64] found associations in a population of golfers between poor static trunk extensor endurance and increased quadriceps inhibition. Quadriceps inhibition was postulated to be reflective of irritation to the lumbar structures. Clinical ramifications from the present study suggest that muscular endurance exercises focusing on rotation of the trunk should be an important component of rehabilitation programs targeting golfers with LPB and as prophylaxis in preventing LBP.

Injuries to the lower back are one of the most common golf-related problems. The incidence of golf-related lower back injury ranges from 15% to 34% in amateur golfers and 22% to 24% in professional golfers.[65] Collectively, the incidence of lower back pain in male golfers is 25% to 36% and 22% to 27% in female golfers.[64] Despite the high participation rate and the large financial support of the golf industry, current data on golf-related injury epidemiology that could specifically direct practitioners in the management of these problems are limited.[66] McGill[65] described the play characteristics of golfers who had an injury to their lower back in the course of play or practice in the previous year (12 months). In addition, common injury mechanisms for the back injury were sought to determine if factors such as age, sex, and amount of play or practice affected the back injury rate. Finally, the study aimed to report the practitioner utilization or back injury management among the golfers surveyed.

McGill[65] reported that of 1,634 Australian amateur golfers surveyed, 17.6% of golfers sustained at least one injury in the previous year. The lower back accounted for 25% of all golf-related injuries in the previous year, making the lower back the most common site of injury. A golfer with a golf-related lower back injury was likely to have a previous history of lower back injury as well. The follow-through phase of the golf swing was reported to be associated with the greatest likelihood of injury compared with other phases of the swing. Most of the injured golfers received treatment of their injury with a general practitioner (69%), a physical therapist (49%), or a chiropractor (40%).

Practitioners treating golfers with a history of lower back injury should evaluate trunk muscle strength and evaluate the golf swing—especially the follow-through—to identify potential causes of aggravation to the lower back. Targeted measures, such as spinal manipulative therapy, soft tissue and back exercise, and conditioning programs to assist the strength and mobility of the golfer, could then be implemented.

Ice Hockey

The common peroneal nerve separates from the sciatic nerve in the upper popliteal fossa. It then passes downward and laterally through the popliteal fossa, lies behind the head of the fibula, winds obliquely around the neck of the fibula, and pierces the superficial head of the long peroneal muscle to enter the anterior compartment of the leg. During its course around the fibula, the nerve is quite superficial and is easily damaged by trauma. In ice hockey, the two most common etiologies for common peroneal nerve injury are direct trauma secondary to "boarding," falls, or being hit by the puck or stick and laceration from an ice skate.[67]

CASE STUDY

Bill is a Division I baseball pitcher who has been averaging 100 pitches per game. He is scheduled to pitch every fifth day. Late in the season, Bill estimates that he has started 18 games over the past 3 months. Bill presents now to the outpatient orthopedic clinic with a "tired arm." He feels his velocity is down compared with early in the year, and he has noticed what he feels is "atrophy" of his pitching shoulder. The quality of his pitching as measured statistically has decreased over his last two starts. He also complains of an "ache" in his pitching shoulder at night that interrupts his sleeping. Bill is quite anxious; he feels he is worsening instead of getting better.

On examination, there is mild atrophy of the involved shoulder. Pulses in all positions are +2. There is mild sensory loss over the involved deltoid. Isokinetic testing reveals an 18% reduction of torque in the involved anterior deltoid compared with the uninvolved side. Altogether, muscle groups test within 5% of the contralateral limb. Deep tendon reflexes are preserved. A cervical spine screen reveals no abnormalities. Volumetric studies reveal no upper extremity edema.

Case Study Questions

1. Based on the information documented in the case study, the best action for you to take as the primary therapist is which of the following?
   a. Instruct Bill to "pitch through the pain" and things will soon get better
   b. Begin Bill on a general strengthening regimen directed at the shoulder and scapular musculature
   c. Refer Bill for further testing with a tentative diagnosis of axillary nerve injury
   d. Prescribe a sling and rest with follow-up in 1 week

2. Bill returns to the clinic 3 days later after having magnetic resonance imaging (MRI) of the shoulder and electrodiagnostic studies. MRI was "normal," but the needle portion of the electroneuromyogram revealed an axonotmetic lesion of the right axial nerve with evidence of mild denervation of the involved deltoid. Your recommendation would be which of the following?
   a. Continue to pitch through the pain
   b. Continue to pitch through the pain and begin shoulder strengthening exercises
   c. Stop pitching and rest
   d. Stop pitching and begin shoulder strengthening exercise

3. If the therapist had noted edema in the involved upper extremity along with the nerve lesion, a possible diagnosis would be which of the following?
   a. Venous thoracic outlet syndrome (Pagett-Schroetter syndrome)
   b. Brachial plexopathy
   c. Arterial thoracic outlet syndrome
   d. Carpal tunnel syndrome

4. Possible etiologies for Bill's problem include which of the following?
   a. Overuse
   b. Intrinsic scapular weakness
   c. Poor pitching technique
   d. All of the above

5. Weakness of which muscle would most likely rule out a simple axillary nerve injury?
   a. Anterior deltoid
   b. Posterior deltoid
   c. Biceps
   d. Teres minor

References

1. Albright JP, McAuley E, Martin RK, Crowley ET, Foster DT. Head and neck injuries in college football: an eight-year analysis. *Am J Sports Med.* 1985;13:147–152.
2. Barbe MF, Safadi FF, Rivera-Nieves EI, Montara TE, Popoff SN, Barr AE. Expression of ED1, ED2, IL-1 and COX2 in bone and in the rat model of cumulative trauma disorder (CTD). Paper presented at: American Society for Bone Mineral Research 21st Annual Meeting; September 30–October 4, 1999; St. Louis, MO.
3. Barr AE, Barbe MF. Inflammation reduces physiological tissue tolerance in the development of work-related musculoskeletal disorders. *J Electromyogr Kinesiol.* 2004;14:77–85.
4. Carp SJ, Barbe MF, Winter KA, Amin M, Barr AE. Inflammatory biomarkers increase with severity of upper-extremity overuse disorders. *Clin Sci (Lond).* 2007;112;305–314.
5. Carp SJ, Barbe MF, Barr AE. Serum biomarkers as signals for risk and severity of work-related musculoskeletal injury. *Biomark Med.* 2008;2:67–79.

6. DiBennedetto M, Markey K. Electrodiagnostic localization of traumatic upper trunk brachial plexopathy. *Arch Phys Med Rehabil.* 1984;65:15.

7. Kepatnas G. The effect of local corticosteroids on healing and biomechanical activity in partially injured tendon sheaths. *Clin Orthop Relat Res.* 1982;163:160–179.

8. Mackinnon SE, Hudson AR, Falk RE, Kline D, Hunter D. Peripheral nerve allograft: an assessment of regeneration across pretreated nerve allografts. *Neurosurgery.* 1984;15: 690–693.

9. Buford K. *Native American: The Life and Sporting Legend of Jim Thorpe.* New York: Alfred A Knopf; 2010:62–64.

10. Warren RF. Neurologic injuries in football. In: Jordan BD, Tsairis P, Warren RF, eds. *Sports Neurology.* Rockville, MD: Aspen; 1989:235–237.

11. Sallis RE, Jones K, Knopp W. Burners: offensive strategy for an underreported injury. *Phys Sportsmed.* 1992;20:47–55.

12. Speer KP, Bassett FJ III. The prolonged burner syndrome. *Am J Sports Med.* 1990;18:591–594.

13. Levitz CL, Reilly PJ, Torg JS. The pathomechanics of chronic, recurrent cervical nerve root neurapraxia. The chronic burner syndrome. *Am J Sports Med.* 1997;25:73–76.

14. Poindexter DP, Johnson EW. Football shoulder and neck injury: a study of the "stinger." *Arch Phys Med Rehabil.* 1984; 65:601–602.

15. Markey KL, Di Benedetto M, Curl WW. Upper trunk brachial plexopathy. The stinger syndrome. *Am J Sports Med.* 1993;21:650–655.

16. Warren RF. Neurological injuries in football. In: Jordan BD, Tsairis P, Warren RF, eds. *Sports Neurology.* Rockville, MD: Aspen; 1989:235–237.

17. Hershman EV. Brachial plexus injuries. *Clin Sports Med.* 1990;9:311–329.

18. Feinberg JH, Radecki J, Wolfe SW, Strauss L, Mintz DN. Brachial plexopathy/nerve root avulsion in a football player; the role of electrodiagnostics. *HSS J.* 2008;4:87–95.

19. Archembault JL. Brachial plexus stretch injuries. *J Am Coll Health.* 1983;31:256–260.

20. Blom S, Dahlback LO. Nerve injuries in dislocations of the shoulder joint and fractures of the neck of the humerus: A clinical and electromyographical study. *Act Chir Scand.* 1970; 136:461–466.

21. Pasila M, Jaroma H, Kiviluoto O, Sundholm A. Early complications of primary shoulder dislocations. *Acta Orthop Scand.* 1978;49(3):260–263.

22. Meister K. Injuries to the shoulder in the throwing athlete: part two: evaluation/treatment. *Am J Sports Med.* 2000;28: 587–601.

23. Katzman BM, Bozentka DJ. Peripheral nerve injuries secondary to missiles. *Hand Clin.* 1999;15(2):233–244.

24. Duralde XA. Neurological injuries to the athlete's shoulder. *J Athl Train.* 2000;35:316–328.

25. McIlveen SJ, Duralde XA, D'Alessandro DF, Bigliani LU. Isolated nerve injuries about the shoulder. *Clin Orthop Relat Res.* 1994;306:54–63.

26. Goodman CE. Unusual nerve injuries in recreational activities. *Am J Sports Med.* 1983;11:224–227.

27. McIlveen SJ, Duralde XA. Isolated nerve injuries about the shoulder. In: Bigliani LU, ed. *Complications of Shoulder Surgery.* New York: Williams & Wilkins; 1993:64–68.

28. Burge PD, Rushworth G, Watson NA. Patterns of injury to the terminal branches of the brachial plexus: the place for early exploration. *J Bone Joint Surg Br.* 1985;67:630–634.

29. McCrory P, Bell S, Bradshaw C. Nerve entrapments of the lower leg. *Sports Med.* 2002;32(6):371–391.

30. Katirji MB, Wilbourn AJ. Common peroneal mononeuropathy: a clinical and electrophysiologic study of 116 lesions. *Neurology.* 1988;38:1723–1728.

31. Fukuda H. Bilateral peroneal nerve palsy caused by intermittent pneumatic compression. *Intern Med.* 2006;45(2): 93–94.

32. Fetzer GB, Prather H, Gelberman RH, Clohisy JC. Progressive peroneal nerve palsy in a varus arthritic knee. *J Bone Joint Surg Am.* 2004;86(7):1538–1540.

33. Langenhove M, Pollefliet A, Vanderstraeten G. A retrospective electrodiagnostic evaluation of footdrop in 303 patients. *Electromyogr Clin Neurophysiol.* 1989;29:145–152.

34. Nysted M, Drogset JO. Trampoline injuries. *Br J Sports Med.* 2006;40:984–987.

35. Smith GA. Injuries to children in the United States related to trampolines, 1990–1995. *Pediatrics.* 1998;101:406–412.

36. Furnival RA, Street KA, Schunk JE. Too many trampoline injuries. *Pediatrics.* 1999;103:1020–1025.

37. Woodward GA, Furnival R, Schunk JE. Trampolines revisited: a review of 114 pediatric recreational trampoline injuries. *Pediatrics.* 1992;89:849–854.

38. Brown PG, Lee M. Trampoline injuries of the cervical spine. *Pediatr Neurosurg.* 2000;32(4):170–175.

39. Shields BJ, Smith GA. Cheerleading-related injuries to children 5 to 18 years of age: United States, 1990–2002. *Pediatrics.* 2006;117(1):122–129.

40. Hutchinson MR. Cheerleading injuries: patterns, prevention, case reports. *Physician Sportsmed.* 1997;25(9):83–96.

41. American Sports Data Inc. *The Superstudy of Sports Participation: Volume II. Recreational Sports 2003.* Hartsdale, NY: American Sports Data Inc; 2004.

42. Schulz MR, Marshall SW, Yang J, Mueller FO, Weaver NL, Bowling JM. A prospective cohort study of injury incidence and risk factors in North Carolina high school competitive cheerleaders. *Am J Sports Med.* 2004;32(2):396–405.

43. Cumming C, Schneider D. Peripheral nerve injuries in baseball players. *Neurol Clin.* 2008;26:195–215.

44. Robb A, Sajko S. Conservative management of posterior interosseous neuropathy in an elite baseball pitcher's return to play: a case report and review of the literature. *J Can Chiropr Assoc.* 2009;53:300–310.

45. Dunant JH. Effort thrombosis, a complication of thoracic outlet syndrome. *Vasa.* 1981;10:322–324.

46. Medler RG, McQueen DA. Effort thrombosis in a young wrestler, a case report. *J Bone Joint Surg Am.* 1993;75: 1071–1073.

47. Urschel HC, Razzuk MA. Paget Shroetter syndrome: what is the best management? *Ann Thorac Surg.* 2000;69: 1663–1668.

48. Joffe HV, Goldhaver SZ. Upper-extremity deep vein thrombosis. *Circulation.* 2002;106:1874–1880.

49. Hurley B, Comins SA, Green RM, Canizzaro J. Atraumatic subclavian vein thrombosis in a collegiate baseball player: a case report. *J Athl Train.* 2006;41:198–200.

50. Kanazawa S, Fujioka H, Kanatani T, et al. The relation between cubital tunnel syndrome and the elbow alignment. *Kobe J Med Sci.* 1994;40:155–163.

51. Descatha A, Leclerc A, Chastang JF, et al. Incidence of ulnar nerve entrapment at the elbow in repetitive work. *Scand J Work Environ Health.* 2004;30:234–240.

52. Kakosy T. Tunnel syndromes of the upper extremities in workers using hand-operated vibrating tools. *Med Lav.* 1994; 85:474–480.

53. Aoki M, Kanaya K, Aiki H, et al. Cubital tunnel syndrome in adolescent base ball players: a report of 6 cases with 3 to 5 year follow up. *Arthroscopy.* 2005;21:758.

54. *1981/1982–2004/2005 NCAA Sports Sponsorship and Participation Rates Report.* Indianapolis, IN: NCAA; 2006.

55. Agel J, Palmieri-Smith RM, Dick R, Wojtys EM, Marshall SW. Descriptive epidemiology of collegiate woman's volleyball injuries: National Collegiate Athletic Association

Injury Surveillance System, 1988–1989 through 2003–2004. *J Athl Train.* 2007;42:295–302.

56. Elliott B, Fleisig G, Nicholls R. Technique effects on upper limb loading in the tennis serve. *J Sci Med Sport.* 2004;6: 76–87.

57. Hatch GF 3rd, Pink MM, Mohr KJ, et al. The effect of tennis racket grip size on forearm muscle firing patterns. *Am J Sports Med.* 2006;34:177–183.

58. Eygendaal D, Rahussen FTG, Diercks RL. Biomechanics of the elbow joint in tennis player related to pathology. *Br J Sports Med.* 2007;41(11):820–823.

59. Posner MA. Compressive ulnar neuropathies at the elbow. II. Treatment. *J Am Acad Orthop Surg* 1998;6:289–297.

60. Aoki M, Takasaki H, Muraki T, Uchiyama E, Murakami G, Yamashita T. Strain on the ulnar nerve at the elbow and wrist during throwing motion. *J Bone Joint Surg Am.* 2005;87: 2508–2514.

61. Eisen A, Danon J. The mild cubital tunnel syndrome. Its natural history and indication for surgical intervention. *Neurology.* 1974;24:608–613.

62. Ferretti A, Cerullo G, Russo G. Suprascapular neuropathy in volleyball players. *J Bone Joint Surg Am.* 1987;69:260–263.

63. Pink M, Perry J, Jobe FW. Electromyographic analysis of the trunk in golfers. *Am J Sport Med.* 1993;21:385–388.

64. Lindsay DM, Horton JF, Paley RD. Trunk motion of male professional golfers using two different golf clubs. *J Appl Biomech.* 2002;18:366–373.

65. McGill SM. Low back exercises: evidence for improving exercise regimens. *Phys Ther.* 1999;78:754–765.

66. Gosheger G, Liem D, Ludwig K, et al. Injuries and overuse syndromes in golf. *Am J Sports Med.* 2003;31(3):438–443.

67. Shevell MI, Steward JD. Laceration of the common peroneal nerve by a skate blade. *Can Med Assoc J.* 1988;139: 311–312.

Effects of Peripheral Neuropathy on Posture and Balance

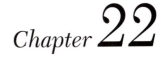

EMILY A. KESHNER, PT, EdD, AND JILL C. SLABODA, PhD

*"Life is like riding a bicycle. In order to keep your balance
you must keep moving."*

—ALBERT EINSTEIN (1879–1955)

Objectives

On completion of this chapter, the student/practitioner will be able to:

- Discuss the relationship of afferent and efferent peripheral nerve contributions to normal balance and postural control.
- Discuss the functional relationship of loss of balance-related sensory pathways.
- Identify the positional and functional impact of diabetic sensory neuropathy.
- Explain the relationship between falls and neuropathy.

Key Terms

- Balance
- Postural compensation
- Postural control

Introduction

Falls resulting in significant injury are a major health issue for older adults. Instability that results in a fall is the leading cause of injury-related death and of nonfatal injury in the United States.[1-3] The probability that an adult will experience a fall increases with age and with age-related disease. It has been reported that individuals with diabetes mellitus experience subjective feelings of instability, and the risk of falling is increased by a factor of 15 in patients with diabetic neuropathy compared with healthy individuals.[4,5] The dynamic process of maintaining an upright posture is vital to the health and independent functioning of the aging population. However, the mechanisms that are necessary for the maintenance of upright posture are exactly the ones impacted by the presence of peripheral neuropathy.

Postural control is the result of a continuous integration of information from the convergence of multiple sensory receptors. Proprioceptive, vestibular, and visual signals have been most frequently identified as the primary contributors to postural control, but corrective postural responses can also be influenced by other somatosensory feedback (e.g., tactile) as well as feedforward (e.g., prediction of a slippery surface) mechanisms. Because there are so many possible pathways that could signal the beginning of a fall, one would think that even if any single input were lost, the other pathways would provide sufficient detail for the postural response to be appropriate to the task demands. However, each sensory pathway has well-defined sensitivities to environmental stimuli.

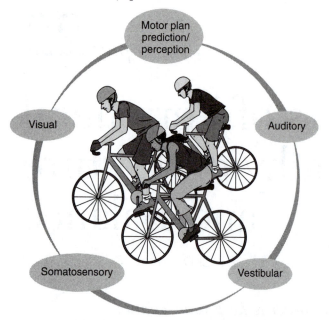

Figure 22-1 Multiple contributions need to be processed by the central nervous system during activities in a natural environment.

For example, imagine the cyclists in Figure 22-1. Do they rely more heavily on their motor plan for advancing beyond the other cyclists or reacting to what they see and hear the others doing? Or do they pay more attention to their muscle and joint receptors telling them how fast they are pedaling or how fatigued they are getting? With all of this continuous feedback, when do they focus on the vestibular information that may be telling them they are starting to tilt? Sensitivities of the pathways for sensory information completely overlap,[6–8] and experimental studies have been able to exclude any single input (i.e., proprioceptive,[9] visual,[10] vestibular,[11] or plantar cutaneous[12]) as the primary trigger for the automatic postural reactions. Instead, the specialized characteristics of each pathway determine whether that pathway more or less modulates the delivery of information about the environmental circumstances encountered during an active lifestyle. To produce a healthy postural response that aligns the body with respect to earth vertical and various body parts with respect to each other across a wide variety of task demands, convergence of information from all of the sensory systems (vestibular, somatosensory, and visual) is preferable.[13]

A large body of evidence demonstrates that the loss of peripheral somatosensory information produces severe consequences on human **balance** and locomotion.[4,14–17] This chapter presents current opinions about the role of three primary sensory pathways for postural control. Modifications in static posture and dynamic balance following the loss of any of these inputs secondary to aging or disease are described. Finally, some emerging treatment approaches for instability resulting from peripheral neuropathy associated with diabetes are presented.

Peripheral Nerve Contributions to Posture Control

Somatosensory Signals

The somatosensory system, including proprioception, touch, pressure, and vibration, is important for precise detection of body position. It is commonly believed that automatic postural responses are triggered by proprioceptive inputs in the lower limb.[18–20] Many studies on automatic postural responses to stance perturbations have shown stereotypical patterns to occur in the leg muscles after displacement of the base of support. These patterns consist of activation of the ankle muscles followed by the upper leg muscles to bring the center of mass (COM) back to its initial position. The automatic postural responses of the leg muscles to base of support translations were shown to be specific to the direction of platform perturbation—that is, reactive to the direction of ankle rotation. These responses were termed "functional stretch reflexes." It was observed that both horizontal translations and up/down rotations of the base of support rotate the ankle joint but with different magnitudes of body sway; yet they trigger similar patterns of postural response in the leg muscles. It was hypothesized that the initiation of these responses was primarily dependent on the ankle proprioceptive inputs elicited by the platform movement.[18] Removal of visual inputs had little effect on the latencies or organization of these leg muscle responses[21] further supporting this hypothesis of proprioceptive control.

The determination of whether it is solely ankle proprioception that generates the postural responses depends greatly on the actual task. When the muscles along both the anterior and the posterior aspects of the body were recorded from ankle to neck,[22] a descending pattern starting from the neck muscles and reorienting the head and trunk to vertical was observed simultaneously with the ascending pattern from the lower limb muscles. The absence of a time delay between the earliest response in the neck and the ankle was strongly indicative that inputs other than lower limb proprioceptors were initiating upper body postural responses. Two possible pathways are the vestibular and the visual systems.

Vestibular Signals

The vestibular system has an ambiguous role in the control of posture. Although the vestibular system is not responsible for initiating automatic postural reactions, it is responsible for establishing orientation in space.[23-29] The somatosensory system provides information about the position and motion of the body with respect to the support surface and body segments with respect to each other, whereas the vestibular system provides information with respect to gravity and other inertial forces.

Otolith function is relatively more resistant to damage than horizontal and vertical canal function and often remains intact even after injury to the semicircular canals. The vestibular otoliths, which detect linear forces acting on the head, are believed to be responsible for identifying vertical orientation through sensitivity to the gravity vector. In addition, reflex responses related to dynamic stimulation of the otolith organs are more robust than reflex responses related to static stimulation of the otolith organs. However, even if the otoliths remain intact with labyrinthine loss, the ability to identify an upright orientation may be impaired.[30] Lateral head oscillations that were not correlated with eye movements during locomotion suggested that oscillopsia was an inability to detect spatial orientation during head or body movements rather than a mere blurring of vision.[31] It was also observed that subjects with bilateral labyrinthine loss standing on a rotating platform were progressively unable to regain an upright posture even though they were repositioned in vertical after each trial.[10] This observation suggests an inability to create or maintain an internal vertical reference in the absence of labyrinthine inputs.

Visual Signals

When vision is removed in a healthy adult, there is no effect on balance other than some increased sway.[10,21,32] It was generally believed that this lack of effect on balance indicated that visual information was unnecessary for the control of balance. However, visual inputs have a strong impact on the maintenance of balance and orientation in space if the parameters of the visual field do not match the velocity of the physical motion parameters.[21,32-37] Motion of the visual field induces body motion,[37-40] and the presence of a stable focal image in the visual field helps diminish body motion.[41-43] However, during a visual tracking task, inappropriate peripheral visual inputs increased the amplitude of postural sway, whereas appropriate peripheral visual inputs decreased postural sway[44] revealing that the stabilizing effect of an object in the central visual field was reduced when there was a conflict in the peripheral visual region. These response characteristics demonstrate that the central nervous system (CNS) does not suppress the effects of inappropriate visual motion even when the visual field motion does not match the actual physical motion feedback.

During quiet stance, motion of the peripheral visual field was found to induce body sway.[33,37,45,46] Postural instability was caused by changes in the velocity and frequency of the visual field motion[47,48] and the direction of gaze.[49] Instability as a result of viewing distance has been reported only for static visual stimuli.[50,51] When spatial orientation and static postural sway were examined in the presence of a looming visual environment,[52-54] it was found that visual inputs dominated the response in the lower (0.1 Hz) frequency range.[7] When there is some unexpected circumstance, such as a tilting room, individuals cannot distinguish between full visual field motion and motion of the body.[24,55] These conflicts often lead to visual illusions that may be exacerbated when vestibular information is lost or unreliable.

Studies of locomotion with combined central and peripheral radial flow demonstrated that central and peripheral regions of the visual field are sensitive to optic flow and differentially influence postural stability in healthy subjects and patients with vestibular disorders.[56-58] Current findings contradict prior assumptions that visual information is redundant to the postural control system unless both vestibular and somatosensory inputs were lost.[59] Both the quality and the location of the visual information evidently influence quiet stance and active motion.

Postural Adaptation to Loss of a Sensory Pathway

Sensory Reweighting

The sensory weighting hypothesis[2] suggests that the CNS multiplies each sensory input by some weight depending on the importance of that input to the task.[60] The weighted variables are summed to produce a response modulated to the relevancy of the incoming afferents (Fig. 22-2). If this is correct and the CNS is using a weighted sum of all inputs in the production of postural behaviors, when one sensory cue is absent or inappropriate, other, more reliable cues would be expected to become more heavily weighted.[61-64] The situation might arise in which an individual relies on slower sensory feedback (e.g., vision) to produce postural stabilization if faster, more direct feedback (e.g., proprioception) has become distorted or diminished.[65] If a sensory pathway is damaged or lost, we might expect that through adaptation to this impairment, the CNS would weight the remaining inputs more heavily and rely on those signals to generate motor responses. For example, an individual with a bilateral labyrinthine deficit would weight visual and somatosensory inputs more heavily to maintain postural orientation in space.

There is evidence that reliance between the available sensory inputs shifts during postural tasks. There is also evidence that, in healthy subjects, this dependence may be due to an individual's perceptual choice or a sampling between the modalities rather than exist solely an adaptation to sensory dysfunction.[66] In complex

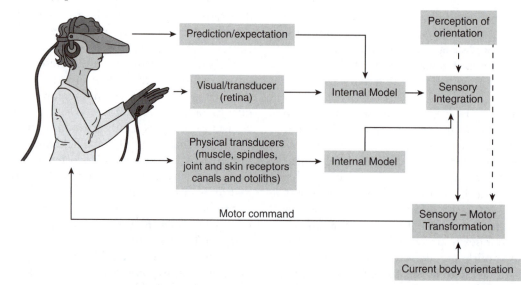

Figure 22-2 Block diagram of the processes involved in producing postural orientation in a natural environment. The individual receives external (visual) and internal (somatosensory and vestibular) information about the position of the body relative to the environment. This information is matched to the internal model of body orientation formed by past experience. The difference between where the individual is and where the individual expected to be is calculated, and the difference is transformed into a motor correction from the current body orientation to the desired body orientation in space.

tasks, healthy and elderly adults exposed to both visual and base of support disturbances simultaneously incorporated specific parameters from each input, rather than diminishing responses to either of them as would be expected with sensory weighting.[67] When healthy young adults stood on a reduced base of support in front of a visual field that translated sinusoidally in the anterior-posterior direction, many of them could not maintain a continuous stance and needed to take a step to stabilize themselves.[68,69] The effect was greatest on their head and whole body COM values (Fig. 22-3). Greater spectral power at the frequency of the visual stimulus in these individuals, combined with whole body delays in the motion of the COM, suggested greater visual field dependency of the steppers. These results imply that the thresholds for shifting from a reliance on visual information to somatosensory information can differ even within a healthy population and strongly point to a role of visual perception in the successful organization of a postural response.

The measure of visual field dependence with a Rod and Frame test has been shown to be a good predictor of a subject's reliance on visual reafference for stabilizing posture.[70–75] In this test, subjects are instructed to ignore the tilted box (frame) that encloses the rod and to attempt to align the rod either to pure horizontal or to pure vertical (Fig. 22-4). Visual field–dependent subjects primarily use visual cues for estimating subjective vertical and body orientation; visual field–independent subjects relied on egocentric or

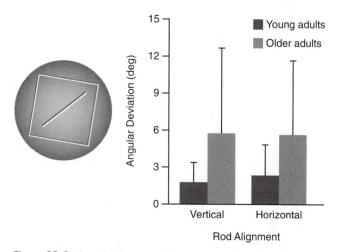

Figure 22-3 (Left) Picture of the projected rod within a tilted frame. (Right) Bar graph showing mean angular deviations (with standard deviations) from pure vertical and horizontal in young and elderly adults.

gravitational cues.[75] Elderly individuals with a history of falling and patients who have had a stroke have been found to be significantly more visual field dependent than healthy young adults.[76] Labyrinthine-deficient individuals who, it is assumed, become more sensitive to visual inputs secondary to the loss of vestibular suppression[77–82] have been shown to increase their visual field dependence and their postural deviation when faced with a tilted visual frame of reference.[83]

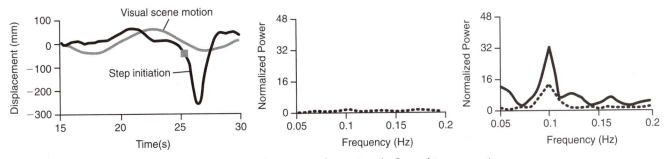

Figure 22-4 (Left) Example of displacement of the center of mass just before taking a step in a healthy young adult standing on a reduced base of support during anterior-posterior translation of the visual field. (Center) Power of the center of mass in adults who did not take a step is negligible at all frequencies. (Right) Center of mass responses match the frequency of visual field motion in adults needing to take a step on both a wide (dashed line) and a narrowed (solid line) platform.

When a specific input is lost or unreliable, shifting dependence (or sensory reweighting) to the more reliable inputs seems to occur.

Loss of Individual Inputs

Loss of either vestibular or somatosensory inputs does not result in delayed or disorganized postural responses. However, both types of sensory deficits alter the type of postural response selected. Somatosensory loss resulted in an increased hip strategy[84] for postural correction, similar to the movement strategy used by control subjects while standing on a shortened surface.[85] Vestibular loss resulted in a normal ankle strategy with absence of a hip strategy, even when required for the task of maintaining equilibrium on a shortened surface.[86,87] Patients who lost vestibular function in infancy did not show normal early hip torque patterns, suggesting that in the absence of vestibular information these individuals select movement patterns that reduce the motion of their upper body.

Loss of vestibular information can occur with destruction of the labyrinths through disease, trauma, or chemical intervention. Vertigo, dizziness, and instability are frequently the result. Some of these impairments are not easily compensated for, and disorientation when moving in a dynamic moving environment, such as walking along a crowded street[88] or driving,[89] is common. Although kinematic adaptations of lower limb postural reactions have been observed in patients with labyrinthine deficit,[90–92] these individuals still evidence a great deal of instability. Adaptation to support surface inputs alone is not an effective compensatory process.

Individuals who had congenital total blindness were examined for the effects of the absence of vision from birth on automatic postural responses to platform displacements during stance.[93] Postural disturbances included forward and backward translations and toe up and down rotations of the base of support. Although the gastrocnemius muscle response amplitudes in the individuals with blindness were smaller than those of sighted subjects with eyes closed, no significant onset latency differences were found between blind and sighted adults. Also, there were no significant differences in the amplitudes of postural sway between blind and sighted subjects with eyes open or closed. These results suggest that the automatic postural response system is unaffected by the absence of vision from birth and that long-term absence of visual information does need to be substituted by other sensory inputs during rapid, transient postural disturbances.[94]

Intramodal Dependencies

During daily activities, we receive continuously varying signals from multiple sensory channels that must be integrated by the CNS. The outcome is our individual perception of self-motion and spatial orientation,[95] which is used for planning subsequent motor actions (see Fig. 22-2). Although we could orient our body posture to a visual, somatosensory, or vestibular reference, the inputs to which we respond most strongly often depend on the particular task and behavioral goals. We also work from an internal estimate of our current body orientation with respect to the environment, incorporating the expected multisensory inputs with our postural reactions for each task.[96,97] Results from studies in a virtual environment demonstrated that converging inputs organized the postural orientation during rotations of the visual scene in pitch and roll.[98] The head and trunk were linked in magnitude and phase, whereas the ankle produced small compensations that were largely out of phase with the upper body. The authors concluded that the upper body was controlled by visual-vestibular signals, whereas the ankle responded to proprioception and changes in ground reaction forces, which is suggestive of the dual ascending and descending systems of postural organization control mentioned previously.[99,100]

If all of an individual's sensory pathways have been operating effectively, a sudden loss or dysfunction of any one pathway would have an impact on the calculation of where the individual is in space and how to move toward the next motor goal. When the relevant inputs are signaling similar circumstances, the movement is not likely to be affected greatly by an absence of a single pathway. For example, adults who are blind stood in a room that could be moved around them. A sound source moved with the room, simulating the acoustic consequences of body sway. Body sway was greater when the room moved than when it was stationary, suggesting that acoustic feedback may have been used to control stance.[101] In another study, when the support surface was stable and visual information matched the performer's expectation (i.e., visual motion feedback was the same as physical motion feedback), the visuo-ocular signals fully substituted for lost vestibular inputs.[102] When healthy young and elderly adults received fore-aft translations of the immersive, wide field-of-view visual environment that did not match amplitude or frequency of the anterior-posterior translations of the support surface, the response to the visual input was strongly potentiated by the addition of the physical motion (Fig. 22-5). With only support surface translation, segmental responses were small and mostly opposed the direction of sled translation. When only the visual scene was moving, segmental responses were negligible in the young adults, but the elderly adults and labyrinthine-deficient subjects were clearly responsive. When the inputs were presented coincidentally, response amplitudes were significantly increased for all subjects. Intramodal dependencies were observed when two conflicting inputs were combined.[67–103]

These results support therapeutic interventions that train patients to cope with other modal inputs to adapt to some sensory loss. When the task requires that the CNS calculate differences between conflicting signals to determine the appropriate response, the responses shaped to fit a single input often do not completely meet the demands of the task.

Neuropathic Effects on Balance

Automatic Postural Reactions

Although postural orientation, or the final calculation of one's position in space, depends on the integration of somatosensory inputs with vestibular feedback,[63,104–106] the importance of direct ankle angle information to postural control cannot be ignored. Disruption of ankle angle feedback has been shown to be more destabilizing than disruption of COM or center of pressure (COP) feedback in healthy subjects and in patients with diabetic peripheral neuropathy who stood on a rotating platform.[107] All subjects showed the greatest amount of sway when surface rotation was rotated in proportion to ankle angle, and patients with somatosensory loss had higher sway velocities in all conditions than healthy subjects. Even when the vision and vestibular systems were intact, altered or reduced somatosensory information[46,59,87] produced delayed compensatory responses and increased instability. These results suggest that the nervous system relies heavily on ankle position to control posture and that pressure sensation in the

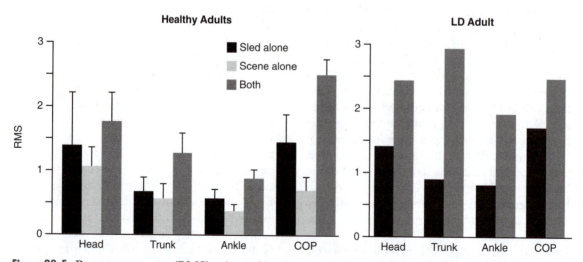

Figure 22-5 Root mean square (RMS) values of head, trunk, ankle, and center of pressure (COP) displacement in healthy young adults (left) and a labyrinthine-deficient (LD) patient (right) when standing on a platform (sled) that was translating in the anterior-posterior direction at 0.25 Hz, in front of a visual scene translating at 0.1 Hz, or with both combined. The patient had no responses to motion of the visual scene alone.

feet, which was absent in the patients with diabetic neuropathy, also contributes to postural orientation.

The extent to which automatic postural responses are triggered by lower leg proprioception has been examined in the lower limbs of patients with diabetic polyneuropathy.[9,108,109] Varying combinations of base of support translations and rotations were used to determine the contribution of lower leg proprioception to the automatic postural responses. The expectation was that healthy subjects would modulate their responses to these conditions, whereas responses in patients with polyneuropathy would be absent.

Patients with neuropathy exhibited the same distal-to-proximal muscle activation patterns as normal subjects. However, the timing and amplitude of the compensatory responses were diminished and delayed. Increased background muscle activity levels and decreased trunk flexibility and lateral instability were also observed in the patients compared with a healthy population.[110,111] The automatic postural response could be triggered by somatosensory receptors located at the knee, hip, or trunk as well as the ankle. Patients also demonstrated an impaired ability to scale the magnitude of ankle torque to the velocity and the amplitude of surface translations, suggesting that somatosensory information from the legs may be necessary for producing the correct response magnitudes of automatic postural responses.[109]

There is also evidence[112-114] that correct alignment of the head with the trunk and with the gravitoinertial vertical requires that the vestibular system receive somatosensory inputs. Postural responses to sinusoidal platform perturbations in patients with bilateral horizontal canal dysfunction were unable to stabilize the trunk in space, and the patients lost balance during high-frequency oscillations of the base of support when their eyes were closed.[115] Most likely to align the body with respect to earth vertical, a convergence of sensory information from the vestibular and somatosensory systems is needed. Patients with bilateral vestibular loss did not use a hip strategy to control posture when on an altered support surface. However, when translated on a normal support surface, patients with adult-onset vestibular loss exhibited normal abdominal muscle activation latencies and early patterns of hip torque indicating that they could initiate a hip strategy when the support surface was unaltered. These results indicate that somatosensory information is critical if the vestibular system is to stabilize the trunk on an unstable platform and that vestibulospinal inputs contribute to the compensatory responses of patients with polyneuropathy.[10,99]

Anticipatory Postural Compensation

Anticipatory postural adjustments maintain postural stability by compensating for expected destabilizations as a result of movement of the limbs or body. They are centrally initiated responses that create the inertial forces necessary to counterbalance an oncoming balance disturbance.[116-118] If the pathways that generate these responses are damaged, it has been demonstrated that new anticipatory responses can be learned through practice to compensate for predictable postural disturbances.[119] Although patients with peripheral neuropathy lacked a particular compensatory trunk motion that was present in healthy subjects, they were able to adapt their motion to platform movement by increasing the distance they traveled and producing earlier anticipatory muscular activity in the lower limb.[120]

Visual information also may strengthen and shape the anticipatory control of balance because of the many cues in the visual flow field that can be used in anticipatory processing. Although visual information is processed too slowly to have a direct impact on the triggered automatic postural reactions appearing within 150 msec of a base of support disturbance, compensatory behaviors following these automatic reactions are greatly modified by visual flow.[121] Healthy subjects were observed to overshoot their initial vertical orientation toward the direction of visual motion with amplitudes that increased as visual velocity increased, exhibiting a direct relationship between orientation in space and motion of the visual world.[122] Postural sway can be reduced by focusing on a stationary visual target or by having prior knowledge of a forthcoming visual displacement.[123]

Assessing the Risk of Falls With Peripheral Neuropathy

Polyneuropathy is a neurological disorder that occurs when many peripheral nerves throughout the body malfunction simultaneously. Patients may experience unusual sensations (paresthesias), numbness, and pain in their hands and feet. In addition, there may be weakness of the muscles in the feet and hands and balance problems that appear as difficulty when walking on uneven surfaces or in the dark. Symptoms of dizziness and instability can also occur because of diminished sensitivity of joint receptors combined with decreased sensitivity of the vestibular labyrinths.[124]

Two systematic reviews identified neuropathy, particularly peripheral neuropathy, as the primary factor causing increased postural instability in individuals with diabetes.[125,126] Patients with diabetes mellitus who did not exhibit strong clinical measures of neuropathy were still identified as having a high risk of falls.[127-129] Acceleration measures of the lumbar spine and ankle during quiet stance revealed that diabetic patients with peripheral neuropathy had higher acceleration values than healthy individuals and diabetic patients without peripheral neuropathy.[130]

Quantitative measures of postural sway during quiet stance are generally believed to be useful as a

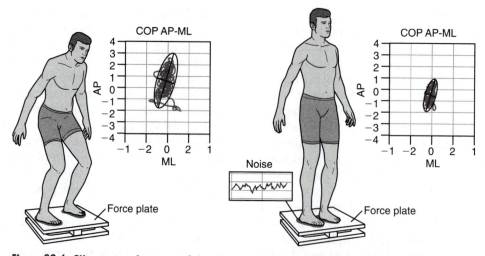

Figure 22-6 Illustrative diagram of the change of center of pressure in both the anterior-posterior and the lateral directions in a healthy young adult standing on a force platform with eyes open. A noisy vibration signal at the soles of the feet produces reduced center of pressure displacements in both directions and improved postural stability.

longitudinal measure of the risk of falling (Fig. 22-6).[131] However, a review of 28 research studies of patients with diabetic neuropathy does not support this point of view and instead argues that no single test effectively explains the relationship between peripheral neuropathy and postural dyscontrol.[125] These authors report that there is insufficient evidence to conclude that postural differences with neuropathy arise from differences in postural strategies.

In 19 of the 28 articles, participants performed quiet standing, and the other 9 articles involved perturbations of upright standing or other movements in addition to upright standing. The predictive capacity of subjective sensory discrimination measures versus objective neural responsiveness measures were clearly dependent on the task. Sensory discrimination was more accurate during quiet stance, and neural responsiveness was more accurate during dynamic tasks. For example, when neuropathy was characterized objectively through an electrophysiological assessment and subjectively by assessing the threshold of vibration perception, neither healthy individuals nor individuals with diabetes exhibited any significant correlation between neural responsiveness and COP indices of postural sway on either a firm or a foam base of support.[132] Neuropathy assessed with subjective sensory testing revealed large fluctuations in the COP path length in patients with diabetic neuropathy.[133] Neural responsiveness did not correlate with changes in the COP, but age was a significant factor in all sensory discrimination measures.

Despite inconsistencies in the reports about how postural behaviors are best assessed, certain differences in the amount of postural sway of patients with neuropathy compared with healthy individuals are consistently reported. Larger measures of COP and trunk velocity have been observed, especially on a foam surface.[134] The time lag between the head and feet was also found to be significantly greater in patients with diabetic neuropathy than in healthy individuals when standing on a sinusoidal moving platform.[119] A comparison of patients with diabetes and healthy adults revealed that all subjects increased their postural sway with their eyes closed. However, the difference in the sway of the patient group with eyes closed or open was greater, especially in the lateral plane.[135] The severity of peripheral neuropathy correlated with the amplitude of the postural sway along the anterior-posterior and lateral planes.[136]

Because nonspecific aspects of diabetes (e.g., high blood pressure, loss of hearing) may affect balance, one must be cautious about attributing instability strictly to peripheral neuropathy. Other factors associated with diabetes that are not directly related to sensory loss can also affect balance. Body mass index, aging, and loss of muscle strength in the lower extremities[137,138] have been cited as the primary factors contributing to an increase in falls. Among women with diabetes, the presence of musculoskeletal pain, high body mass index, and reduced strength in the lower extremities were independently associated with an increased likelihood of recurrent falls.[139,140] Up to 10% of patients with diabetes have orthostatic hypotension, possibly secondary to autonomic neuropathy, reduced baroreflex sensitivity, or hypotensive medication, which correlates with an increased risk of falls.[141] Finally, a strong and significant correlation between dorsiflexion muscle strength and gait velocity was observed in individuals with diabetes older than 55 years old.[142] Logistic regression analysis determined that walking velocity, strength of ankle dorsiflexors, and degree of neuropathy accurately predicted 75% of the self-reported "fallers" in this group.

New Treatments and Interventions for Instability Caused by Neuropathy

Cutaneous mechanoreceptors in the foot and proprioceptive signals from the muscles and joints of the lower limbs provide important information on pressure distributions and joint position that are essential for maintaining balance.[143–145] In a study that anesthetized the feet of healthy adults and exposed them to unexpected platform translations, afferents in the foot were found to be responsible for sensing the limits of the COM, sensing foot contact and weight transfer, and controlling stability during single limb support.[12] Similar studies revealed that gait patterns were more cautious and motion was modified in multiple lower limb segments[146] when the feet were anesthetized in healthy adults. Shifts in the compensatory torque responses from the ankle to the hip during postural translations were also observed.[147,148] Body sway increased and longer latencies of adaptation to the galvanic stimulation were found when galvanic stimulation of the vestibular system was combined with anesthetized feet.[149,150]

Vibrating Insoles and Whole Body Vibration

In patients with neuropathy, cutaneous and proprioceptive information in the foot can deteriorate as a result of disease or the combination of disease and aging, which results in greater postural instability and a greater risk for falls. More recent treatment interventions that focus on simulating receptors in the foot demonstrate promising results. One such intervention is based on the theory of stochastic resonance[151–153] suggesting that subthreshold, random noise (via vibration inputs) to the feet of adults with neuropathy increases somatosensory information and decreases postural instability.[154–157]

The premise guiding this treatment is that an increased risk of falls is believed to be associated with weakened somatosensory signals in individuals with neuropathy, in particular, diminished detection and feedback of pressure changes in the feet. The lack of signal detection may indicate a decrease in the number of mechanoreceptors in the feet of patients with neuropathy resulting in increased tactile thresholds on the plantar side of the feet compared with healthy individuals. A consequence of this increased tactile sensation threshold is that weaker signals are ignored, ultimately leading to a loss in signal transmission to the CNS, which may increase the likelihood that balance corrective responses will not occur. Mechanical

noise added to the foot for a 60-minute period resulted in decreases in the threshold of vibration perception (or increased sensitivity to the vibration inputs) when measured immediately after the application of a noisy signal to the feet in individuals with neuropathy secondary to diabetes.[158] The addition of noisy vibration has been shown to strengthen the recognition of signals that would not normally be detected.[156,159–161]

Several different researchers have developed shoe insoles that deliver random vibrations to the heel and ball of the foot at varying bandwidths of frequencies.[160–162] An application of constant vibration to the ball or the heel of the foot results in compensatory sway responses in the direction opposite the applied stimulation (i.e., vibration on the heel produces a forward shift of the COP).[163–165] The amplitude of the vibration typically chosen is below the threshold for perception of the input or at amplitudes that correspond to 90% of the level that the person reports just feeling the vibration. When random vibration signals were applied to the feet, reductions in postural sway were found during quiet stance and during dual tasking in individuals with neuropathy.[154,157] Reductions in stride, swing, and stance time variability during gait were also found when random vibrating insoles were placed on the feet of elderly adult fallers during a task that required them to walk for 6 minutes. The results suggest that this intervention can potentially reduce the factors that lead to falls[166] making it a valuable intervention for postural instability.

Whole body vibration[167–170] has also been proved to be effective for reduction of postural sway with and without vision in patients who have had a stroke, patients with diabetic neuropathy, and elderly adults. Interventions that used whole body vibration required quiet stance on a stable platform while it vibrated at a frequency of about 20 Hz[171] or standing on a platform tilting side to side while vibrating at 15 to 25 Hz.[172,173] A single session of whole body vibration reduced gait variability in elderly adults who had a history of falls[166] and increased knee extensor torque and muscle activation in patients with stroke.[167,168] Improvements in functional measures such as the Timed Up and Go test and rising from a chair were also found in elderly adults after a 6-week intervention that included whole body vibration 3 days a week. Although vibration does not shorten the time to react to instability, it can decrease the amplitude of fluctuation between the controlled body segment and the unstable surface increasing the likelihood that a corrective response will be effective.[174] Longer term studies on the effectiveness of the vibration interventions and the amount of dosage required to reduce instability are needed.

Rocker Shoes

In some patients with neuropathy, particularly related to diabetes, ulcers or sores are a major concern to the health of their feet and can limit their ability to ambulate or maintain balance. Therapeutic shoes such as rocker shoes have been largely successful in reducing pressure on high-risk areas on the foot by redistributing the pressure in the foot[175,176] without adversely impacting gait.[177] The purpose of rocker shoes is to rock the foot from heel strike to toe off during gait without requiring that the shoe bend.[177] Various rocker shoes have been developed, including heel negative, double rocker, and toe-only rocker.[178] The design of the shoe has an impact on the pressure distribution and can shift the COP while standing and during gait.[179]

The concept of the rocker shoe goes back at least to 1981 when an article was published on the use of the rocker shoe as a walking aid for patients with multiple sclerosis.[180] The authors found that these shoes allowed for normal velocity and stride characteristics combined with a marked decrease in energy cost. However, the impact of rocker shoes on gait and postural stability in healthy adults showed mixed results. Only small changes in kinematics and little to no change in walking speed were found in healthy young adults.[181] Healthy young adults were also greatly destabilized during an unexpected backward translation of a support surface when wearing rocker shoes.[182]

Kinematic changes in gait are found at the ankle with all types of rocker shoes,[183] but modifications at the hip and knees were also found with double rocker and toe-only rocker shoes.[184,185] Reports about changes in the hip or knee with heel-negative rocker shoes are contradictory.[186,187] Toe-only rocker shoes result in increased cadence and decreased stride length,[181] whereas the heel-negative shoes produced no increase in stride length but increased cadence.[187] Decreases in double limb support and increases in heel strike in double rocker shoes were found compared with regular athletic shoes, but no changes in cadence, velocity, single limb support, or swing-stance ratios emerged.[188] The evidence seems to support that rocker shoes are effective for reducing pressure in the foot but have a limited impact on gait kinematics.

Limiting Lateral Motion

When the limit of stability is reached during gait, the cutaneous mechanoreceptors are stimulated by indenting the skin on the foot, which should lead to a balance correction.[189] If the receptors are not functioning properly, lateral instability increases. Typically, reducing lateral instability involves assistive devices such as canes or ankle orthoses, but these devices also alter the body mechanics and might produce long-term postural misalignments. Insoles with a raised ridge around the outside of the foot were developed more recently to decrease lateral instability.[189] This insole was developed as an alternative to vibrating insoles because the vibrating insoles require a large amount of power that may not be feasible for use in everyday life. Decreases in

lateral stability were found in elderly adults with sensory loss unrelated to neuropathy, and this benefit continued at assessment after 12 weeks of wearing the insoles.[189]

There is little doubt that individuals with peripheral neuropathy are at a high risk for postural instability and falling. Symptoms of instability are exacerbated when vision is obstructed, with decreased visual acuity, or when approaching and having to compensate gait around uneven ground and obstacles. New understanding about how individuals might be trained to shift their reliance to other sensory pathways to compensate for impaired inputs offers potential for new therapeutic interventions. In addition, new technologies that directly modify the feedback from the lower limbs during functional activities demonstrate great promise in reducing instability and consequently protecting individuals with neuropathy from the risk of greater injury through falls.

CASE STUDY

Over the past 5 years, Carolyn's retinopathy, which is related to diabetes mellitus, has worsened to the point where she is functionally blind. She can see "shadows" and "figures" but cannot identify faces, objects, curbs, or stairs. She uses a cane for ambulation. Carolyn works as a counselor at a drug rehabilitation facility. She uses public transportation to travel to and from work. She lives alone in a two-story home.

Case Study Questions

1. If Carolyn, with her limited visual acuity, were to walk on a spongy surface such as a shag carpet with high nap (mimicking proprioceptive negative feet), what result would this have on her dynamic ambulation balance?
   a. None
   b. Minimal
   c. Severe
   d. Unable to tell from the information provided

2. Which of the following is the primary cause of postural instability in persons with diabetes?
   a. Blindness
   b. Afferent peripheral neuropathy
   c. Elevated blood sugar
   d. Loss of proximal muscle mass

3. Anticipatory postural adjustments maintain postural stability by compensating for which of the following?
   a. Expected destabilizations as a result of movement of the body limbs
   b. External sounds
   c. Orthopedic maladies such as arthritis
   d. Unexpected ground perturbations

4. Persons with neuropathy exhibit which type of aberrant compensation to external variables impacting balance?

a. Timing of compensatory activities

b. Amplitude of compensatory activities

c. Lateral trunk instability

d. All of the above

5. Research has shown that the primary impact of Carolyn's blindness on her posture is which of the following?

a. Increased lateral sway during quiet stance

b. Decreased step length

c. Ataxia

d. Tremor

References

1. Alexander BH, Rivara FP, Wolf ME. The cost and frequency of hospitalization for fall-related injuries in older adults. *Am J Public Health*. 1992;82(7):1020–1023.

2. Gryfe CI, Amies A, Ashley MJ. A longitudinal study of falls in an elderly population: I. incidence and morbidity. *Age Ageing*. 1977;6(4):201–210.

3. Talbot LA, Musiol RJ, Witham EK, Metter EJ. Falls in young, middle-aged and older community dwelling adults: perceived cause, environmental factors and injury. *BMC Public Health*. 2005;5:86.

4. Cavanagh PR, Derr JA, Ulbrecht JS, Maser RE, Orchard TJ. Problems with gait and posture in neuropathic patients with insulin-dependent diabetes mellitus. *Diabet Med*. 1992;9(5):469–474.

5. Greene DA, Sima AF, Pfeifer MA, Albers JW. Diabetic neuropathy. *Annu Rev Med*. 1990;41:303–317.

6. Kuo AD. An optimal state estimation model of sensory integration in human postural balance. *J Neural Eng*. 2005;2(3):S235–249.

7. Dichgans J, Mauritz KH, Allum JH, Brandt T. Postural sway in normals and atactic patients: analysis of the stabilising and destabilizing effects of vision. *Agressologie*. 1976;17(C spec no):15–24.

8. Peterson BW, Goldberg J, Bilotto G, Fuller JH. Cervicocollic reflex: its dynamic properties and interaction with vestibular reflexes. *J Neurophysiol*. 1985;54(1):90–109.

9. Bloem BR, Allum JH, Carpenter MG, Verschuuren JJ, Honegger F. Triggering of balance corrections and compensatory strategies in a patient with total leg proprioceptive loss. *Exp Brain Res*. 2002;142(1):91–107.

10. Keshner EA, Allum JH, Pfaltz CR. Postural coactivation and adaptation in the sway stabilizing responses of normals and patients with bilateral vestibular deficit. *Exp Brain Res*. 1987;69(1):77–92.

11. Carpenter MG, Allum JH, Honegger F. Vestibular influences on human postural control in combinations of pitch and roll planes reveal differences in spatiotemporal processing. *Exp Brain Res*. 2001;140(1):95–111.

12. Perry SD, McIlroy WE, Maki BE. The role of plantar cutaneous mechanoreceptors in the control of compensatory stepping reactions evoked by unpredictable, multi-directional perturbation. *Brain Res*. 2000;877(2):401–406.

13. Horak FB, Macpherson JM. Postural orientation and equilibrium. In: Rowel JL, Shepard J, eds. *Handbook of Physiology*. New York: Oxford University Press; 1996:255–292.

14. Dingwell JB, Cusumano JP, Sternad D, Cavanagh PR. Slower speeds in patients with diabetic neuropathy lead to improved local dynamic stability of continuous overground walking. *J Biomech*. 2000;33(10):1269–1277.

15. Griffin JW, Cornblath DR, Alexander E, et al. Ataxic sensory neuropathy and dorsal root ganglionitis associated with Sjogren's syndrome. *Ann Neurol*. 1990;27(3):304–315.

16. Katoulis EC, Ebdon-Parry M, Lanshammar H, Vileikyte L, Kulkarni J, Boulton AJ. Gait abnormalities in diabetic neuropathy. *Diabetes Care*. 1997;20(12):1904–1907.

17. Koski K, Luukinen H, Laippala P, Kivela SL. Risk factors for major injurious falls among the home-dwelling elderly by functional abilities. A prospective population-based study. *Gerontology*. 1998;44(4):232–238.

18. Nashner LM. Adapting reflexes controlling the human posture. *Exp Brain Res*. 1976;26(1):59–72.

19. Nashner LM. Fixed patterns of rapid postural responses among leg muscles during stance. *Exp Brain Res*. 1977;30(1):13–24.

20. Nashner LM, Woollacott M, Tuma G. Organization of rapid responses to postural and locomotor-like perturbations of standing man. *Exp Brain Res*. 1979;36(3):463–476.

21. Nashner L, Berthoz A. Visual contribution to rapid motor responses during postural control. *Brain Res*. 1978;150(2):403–407.

22. Keshner EA, Woollacott MH, Debu B. Neck, trunk and limb muscle responses during postural perturbations in humans. *Exp Brain Res*. 1988;71(3):455–466.

23. Dichgans J, Brandt T, Held R. The role of vision in gravitational orientation. *Fortschr Zool*. 1975;23(1):255–263.

24. Dichgans J, Held R, Young LR, Brandt T. Moving visual scenes influence the apparent direction of gravity. *Science*. 1972;178(66):1217–1219.

25. Barmack NH, Yakhnitsa V. Vestibular signals in the parasolitary nucleus. *J Neurophysiol*. 2000;83(6):3559–3569.

26. Guedry FE. Perception of motion and position relative to the earth. An overview. *Ann N Y Acad Sci*. 1992;656:315–328.

27. Guedry FE, Rupert AH, McGrath BJ, Oman CM. The dynamics of spatial orientation during complex and changing linear and angular acceleration. *J Vestib Res*. 1992;2(4):259–283.

28. Wright W, Horak F. Perception of verticality during dynamic postural tasks in healthy and vestibular loss subjects [abstract]. *Soc Neurosci*. 2005;168:19.

29. Young LR, Jackson DK, Groleau N, Modestino S. Multisensory integration in microgravity. *Ann N Y Acad Sci*. 1992;656:340–353.

30. Halmagyi GM, Curthoys IS. Otolith function tests. In: Herdman SJ, ed. *Vestibular Rehabilitation*. 2nd ed. Philadelphia: FA Davis; 2000:195–214.

31. Takahashi M, Okada Y, Saito A, et al. Roles of head, gaze, and spatial orientation in the production of oscillopsia. *J Vestib Res*. 1990;1(3):215–222.

32. Vidal PP, Berthoz A, Millanvoye M. Difference between eye closure and visual stabilization in the control of posture in man. *Aviat Space Environ Med*. 1982;53(2):166–170.

33. Dokka K, Kenyon RV, Keshner EA. Influence of visual scene velocity on segmental kinematics during stance. *Gait Posture*. 2009;30(2):211–216.

34. Guerraz M, Bronstein AM. Mechanisms underlying visually induced body sway. *Neurosci Lett*. 2008;443(1):12–16.

35. Keshner EA, Kenyon RV, Dhaher Y. Postural research and rehabilitation in an immersive virtual environment. *Conf Proc IEEE Eng Med Biol Soc*. 2004;7:4862–4865.

36. Previc FH. The effects of dynamic visual stimulation on perception and motor control. *J Vestib Res*. 1992;2(4):285–295.

37. Previc FH, Kenyon RV, Boer ER, Johnson BH. The effects of background visual roll stimulation on postural and manual control and self-motion perception. *Percept Psychophys*. 1993;54(1):93–107.

38. Ferman L, Collewijn H, Jansen TC, Van den Berg AV. Human gaze stability in the horizontal, vertical and torsional direction during voluntary head movements, evaluated with a three-dimensional scleral induction coil technique. *Vision Res*. 1987;27(5):811–828.

39. Kotaka S, Okubo J, Watanabe I. The influence of eye movements and tactile information on postural sway in patients with peripheral vestibular lesions. *Auris Nasus Larynx*. 1986;13(suppl 2):S153–S159.

40. Previc FH, Donnelly M. The effects of visual depth and eccentricity on manual bias, induced motion, and vection. *Perception*. 1993;22(8):929–945.

41. Bronstein AM, Buckwell D. Automatic control of postural sway by visual motion parallax. *Exp Brain Res*. 1997;113(2): 243–248.

42. Crane BT, Demer JL. Gaze stabilization during dynamic posturography in normal and vestibulopathic humans. *Exp Brain Res*. 1998;122(2):235–246.

43. Jahn K, Strupp M, Brandt T. Both actual and imagined locomotion suppress spontaneous vestibular nystagmus. *Neuroreport*. 2002;13(16):2125–2128.

44. Keshner E, Kenyon RV, Dhaher YY, Streepey JW. Employing a virtual environment in postural research and rehabilitation to reveal the impact of visual information. Paper presented at: International Conference on Disability, Virtual Reality, and Associated Technologies; September 20–22, 2004; Oxford, UK.

45. Black FO, Nashner LM. Postural disturbance in patients with benign paroxysmal positional nystagmus. *Ann Otol Rhinol Laryngol*. 1984;93(6 pt 1):595–599.

46. Black FO, Wall C 3rd, Nashner LM. Effects of visual and support surface orientation references upon postural control in vestibular deficient subjects. *Acta Otolaryngol*. 1983; 95(3–4):199–201.

47. Dijkstra TM, Schoner G, Gielen CC. Temporal stability of the action-perception cycle for postural control in a moving visual environment. *Exp Brain Res*. 1994;97(3):477–486.

48. Masson G, Mestre DR, Pailhous J. Effects of the spatio-temporal structure of optical flow on postural readjustments in man. *Exp Brain Res*. 1995;103(1):137–150.

49. Gielen CC, van Asten WN. Postural responses to simulated moving environments are not invariant for the direction of gaze. *Exp Brain Res*. 1990;79(1):167–174.

50. Dijkstra TM, Gielen CC, Melis BJ. Postural responses to stationary and moving scenes as a function of distance to the scene. *Hum Mov Sci*. 1992;11:195–203.

51. Paulus W, Straube A, Krafczyk S, Brandt T. Differential effects of retinal target displacement, changing size and changing disparity in the control of anterior/posterior and lateral body sway. *Exp Brain Res*. 1989;78(2):243–252.

52. Brooks JN, Sherrick MF. Induced motion and the visual vertical: effects of frame size. *Percept Mot Skills*. 1994; 79(3 pt 2):1443–1450.

53. Howard IP, Childerson L. The contribution of motion, the visual frame, and visual polarity to sensations of body tilt. *Perception*. 1994;23(7):753–762.

54. Lestienne F, Soechting J, Berthoz A. Postural readjustments induced by linear motion of visual scenes. *Exp Brain Res*. 1977;28(3–4):363–384.

55. Lackner JR, DiZio P. Visual stimulation affects the perception of voluntary leg movements during walking. *Perception*. 1988;17(1):71–80.

56. Straube A, Krafczyk S, Paulus W, Brandt T. Dependence of visual stabilization of postural sway on the cortical magnification factor of restricted visual fields. *Exp Brain Res*. 1994;99(3):501–506.

57. Redfern MS, Furman JM. Postural sway of patients with vestibular disorders during optic flow. *J Vestib Res*. 1994;4(3): 221–230.

58. Bardy BG, Warren WH Jr, Kay BA. The role of central and peripheral vision in postural control during walking. *Percept Psychophys*. 1999;61(7):1356–1368.

59. Dichgans J, Mauritz KH. Patterns and mechanisms of postural instability in patients with cerebellar lesions. *Adv Neurol*. 1983;39:633–643.

60. Peterka RJ. Sensorimotor integration in human postural control. *J Neurophysiol*. 2002;88(3):1097–1118.

61. Ravaioli E, Oie KS, Kiemel T, Chiari L, Jeka JJ. Nonlinear postural control in response to visual translation. *Exp Brain Res*. 2005;160(4):450–459.

62. Cenciarini M, Peterka RJ. Stimulus-dependent changes in the vestibular contribution to human postural control. *J Neurophysiol*. 2006;95(5):2733–2750.

63. Mergner T, Maurer C, Peterka RJ. A multisensory posture control model of human upright stance. *Prog Brain Res*. 2003;142:189–201.

64. Carver S, Kiemel T, Jeka JJ. Modeling the dynamics of sensory reweighting. *Biol Cybern*. 2006;95(2):123–134.

65. Speers RA, Kuo AD, Horak FB. Contributions of altered sensation and feedback responses to changes in coordination of postural control due to aging. *Gait Posture*. 2002;16(1): 20–30.

66. Lambrey S, Viaud-Delmon I, Berthoz A. Influence of a sensorimotor conflict on the memorization of a path traveled in virtual reality. *Brain Res Cogn Brain Res*. 2002;14(1):177–186.

67. Keshner EA, Kenyon RV, Langston J. Postural responses exhibit multisensory dependencies with discordant visual and support surface motion. *J Vestib Res*. 2004;14(4): 307–319.

68. Streepey JW, Kenyon RV, Keshner EA. Visual motion combined with base of support width reveals variable field dependency in healthy young adults. *Exp Brain Res*. 2007; 176(1):182–187.

69. Streepey JW, Kenyon RV, Keshner EA. Field of view and base of support width influence postural responses to visual stimuli during quiet stance. *Gait Posture*. 2007;25(1): 49–55.

70. Asch SE, Witkin HA. Studies in space orientation; perception of the upright with displaced visual fields and with body tilted. *J Exp Psychol*. 1948;38(4):455–477.

71. Asch SE, Witkin HA. Studies in space orientation. II. Perception of the upright with displaced visual fields and with body tilted. *J Exp Psychol Gen*. 1992;121(4):407–418; discussion 404–406.

72. Isableu B, Ohlmann T, Cremieux J, Amblard B. Selection of spatial frame of reference and postural control variability. *Exp Brain Res*. 1997;114(3):584–589.

73. Isableu B, Ohlmann T, Cremieux J, Vuillerme N, Amblard B, Gresty MA. Individual differences in the ability to identify, select and use appropriate frames of reference for perceptuo-motor control. *Neuroscience*. 2010;169(3): 1199–1215.

74. Isableu B, Ohlmann T, Cremieux J, Amblard B. Differential approach to strategies of segmental stabilisation in postural control. *Exp Brain Res*. 2003;150(2):208–221.

75. Luyat M, Ohlmann T, Barraud PA. Subjective vertical and postural activity. *Acta Psychol (Amst)*. 1997;95(2): 181–193.

76. Lord SR, Webster IW. Visual field dependence in elderly fallers and non-fallers. *Int J Aging Hum Dev*. 1990;31(4): 267–277.

77. Bronstein AM. Visual vertigo syndrome: clinical and posturography findings. *J Neurol Neurosurg Psychiatry.* 1995;59(5):472–476.

78. Bronstein AM. The visual vertigo syndrome. *Acta Otolaryngol.* 1995;520(pt 1):45–48.

79. Furman JM, Jacob RG. A clinical taxonomy of dizziness and anxiety in the otoneurological setting. *J Anxiety Disord.* 2001;15(1–2):9–26.

80. Guerraz M, Yardley L, Bertholon P, et al. Visual vertigo: symptom assessment, spatial orientation and postural control. *Brain.* 2001;124(pt 8):1646–1656.

81. Peterka RJ. Simple model of sensory interaction in human postural control. In: Mergner T, Hlavacka F, eds. *Multisensory Control of Posture.* New York: Plenum Press; 1995:282–288.

82. Peterka RJ, Benolken MS. Role of somatosensory and vestibular cues in attenuating visually induced human postural sway. *Exp Brain Res.* 1995;105(1):101–110.

83. Oltman PK. A portable rod-and-frame apparatus. *Percept Motor Skills.* 1968;26(2):503–506.

84. Horak FB, Hlavacka F. Somatosensory loss increases vestibulospinal sensitivity. *J Neurophysiol.* 2001;86(2):575–585.

85. Horak FB, Nashner LM. Central programming of postural movements: adaptation to altered support-surface configurations. *J Neurophysiol.* 1986;55(6):1369–1381.

86. Diener HC, Dichgans J, Guschlbauer B, Bacher M, Rapp H, Langenbach P. Associated postural adjustments with body movement in normal subjects and patients with parkinsonism and cerebellar disease. *Rev Neurol (Paris).* 1990;146(10):555–563.

87. Horak FB, Nashner LM, Diener HC. Postural strategies associated with somatosensory and vestibular loss. *Exp Brain Res.* 1990;82(1):167–177.

88. Cohen HS. Vestibular disorders and impaired path integration along a linear trajectory. *J Vestib Res.* 2000;10(1):7–15.

89. Page NG, Gresty MA. Motorist's vestibular disorientation syndrome. *J Neurol Neurosurg Psychiatry.* 1985;48(8):729–735.

90. Allum JH, Honegger F, Pfaltz CR. The role of stretch and vestibulo-spinal reflexes in the generation of human equilibrating reactions. *Progr Brain Res.* 1989;80:399–409; discussion 395–397.

91. Allum JH, Pfaltz CR. Visual and vestibular contributions to pitch sway stabilization in the ankle muscles of normals and patients with bilateral peripheral vestibular deficits. *Exp Brain Res.* 1985;58(1):82–94.

92. Curthoys IS, Halmagyi GM. Clinical changes in vestibular function with time after unilateral vestibular loss. In: Herdman SJ, ed. *Vestibular Rehabilitation.* 2nd ed. Philadelphia: FA Davis; 2000:172–194.

93. Nakata H, Yabe K. Automatic postural response systems in individuals with congenital total blindness. *Gait Posture.* 2001;14(1):36–43.

94. Schmid M, Nardone A, De Nunzio AM, Schieppati M. Equilibrium during static and dynamic tasks in blind subjects: no evidence of cross-modal plasticity. *Brain.* 2007;130(pt 8):2097–2107.

95. Wright WG, Schneider E, Glasauer S. Compensatory manual motor responses while object wielding during combined linear visual and physical roll tilt stimulation. *Exp Brain Res.* 2009;192(4):683–694.

96. Gurfinkel VS, Ivanenko Yu P, Levik Yu S, Babakova IA. Kinesthetic reference for human orthograde posture. *Neuroscience.* 1995;68(1):229–243.

97. Massion J. Postural control system. *Curr Opin Neurobiol.* 1994;4(6):877–887.

98. Keshner EA, Kenyon RV. The influence of an immersive virtual environment on the segmental organization of postural stabilizing responses. *J Vestib Res.* 2000;10(4–5):207–219.

99. Buchanan JJ, Horak FB. Emergence of postural patterns as a function of vision and translation frequency. *J Neurophysiol.* 1999;81(5):2325–2339.

100. Keshner EA, Peterson BW. Motor control strategies underlying head stabilization and voluntary head movements in humans and cats. *Progr Brain Res.* 1988;76:329–339.

101. Stoffregen TA, Villard S, Kim C, Ito K, Bardy BG. Coupling of head and body movement with motion of the audible environment. *J Exp Psychol.* 2009;35(4):1221–1231.

102. Schweigart G, Heimbrand S, Mergner T, Becker W. Perception of horizontal head and trunk rotation: modification of neck input following loss of vestibular function. *Exp Brain Res.* 1993;95(3):533–546.

103. Bugnariu N, Fung J. Aging and selective sensorimotor strategies in the regulation of upright balance. *J Neuroeng Rehabil.* 2007;4:19.

104. Mergner T, Huber W, Becker W. Vestibular-neck interaction and transformation of sensory coordinates. *J Vestib Res.* 1997;7(4):347–367.

105. Mergner T, Nardi GL, Becker W, Deecke L. The role of canal-neck interaction for the perception of horizontal trunk and head rotation. *Exp Brain Res.* 1983;49(2):198–208.

106. Mergner T, Rosemeier T. Interaction of vestibular, somatosensory and visual signals for postural control and motion perception under terrestrial and microgravity conditions—a conceptual model. *Brain Res Brain Res Rev.* 1998;28(1–2):118–135.

107. Horak FB, Dickstein R, Peterka RJ. Diabetic neuropathy and surface sway-referencing disrupt somatosensory information for postural stability in stance. *Somatosens Mot Res.* 2002;19(4):316–326.

108. Inglis JT, Kennedy PM, Wells C, Chua R. The role of cutaneous receptors in the foot. *Adv Exp Med Biol.* 2002;508:111–117.

109. Inglis JT, Horak FB, Shupert CL, Jones-Rycewicz C. The importance of somatosensory information in triggering and scaling automatic postural responses in humans. *Exp Brain Res.* 1994;101(1):159–164.

110. Horlings CG, van Engelen BG, Allum JH, Bloem BR. A weak balance: the contribution of muscle weakness to postural instability and falls. *Nat Clin Pract.* 2008;4(9):504–515.

111. Van de Warrenburg BP, Bakker M, Kremer BP, Bloem BR, Allum JH. Trunk sway in patients with spinocerebellar ataxia. *Mov Disord.* 2005;20(8):1006–1013.

112. Gdowski GT, Boyle R, McCrea RA. Sensory processing in the vestibular nuclei during active head movements. *Arch Ital Biol.* 2000;138(1):15–28.

113. Gdowski GT, McCrea RA. Neck proprioceptive inputs to primate vestibular nucleus neurons. *Exp Brain Res.* 2000;135(4):511–526.

114. Imai T, Moore ST, Raphan T, Cohen B. Interaction of the body, head, and eyes during walking and turning. *Exp Brain Res.* 2001;136(1):1–18.

115. Buchanan JJ, Horak FB. Vestibular loss disrupts control of head and trunk on a sinusoidally moving platform. *J Vestib Res.* 2001;11(6):371–389.

116. Bouisset S, Zattara M. A sequence of postural movements precedes voluntary movement. *Neurosci Lett.* 1981;22:263–270.

117. Jeannerod M. The contribution of open-loop and closed-loop control modes in prehension movements. In: Kornblum

S, Requin J, eds. *Preparatory States and Processes.* Hillsdale, NJ: Lawrence Erlbaum Associates; 1984:323–338.

118. Layne CS, Abraham LD. Interactions between automatic postural adjustments and anticipatory postural patterns accompanying voluntary movement. *Int J Neurosci.* 1991; 61(3–4):241–254.

119. Nardone A, Grasso M, Schieppati M. Balance control in peripheral neuropathy: are patients equally unstable under static and dynamic conditions? *Gait Posture.* 2006;23(3): 364–373.

120. Bunday KL, Bronstein AM. Locomotor adaptation and aftereffects in patients with reduced somatosensory input due to peripheral neuropathy. *J Neurophysiol.* 2009;102(6): 3119–3128.

121. Keshner EA, Dhaher Y. Characterizing head motion in three planes during combined visual and base of support disturbances in healthy and visually sensitive subjects. *Gait Posture.*2008;28(1):127–134.

122. Wang Y, Kenyon RV, Keshner EA. Identifying the control of physically and perceptually evoked sway responses with coincident visual scene velocities and tilt of the base of support. *Exp Brain Res.* 2010;201(4):663–672.

123. Guerraz M, Gianna CC, Burchill PM, Gresty MA, Bronstein AM. Effect of visual surrounding motion on body sway in a three-dimensional environment. *Percept Psychophys.* 2001;63(1):47–58.

124. Agrawal Y, Carey JP, Della Santina CC, Schubert MC, Minor LB. Diabetes, vestibular dysfunction, and falls: analyses from the National Health and Nutrition Examination Survey. *Otol Neurotol.* 2010;31(9):1445–1450.

125. Bonnet C, Carello C, Turvey MT. Diabetes and postural stability: review and hypotheses. *J Mot Behav.* 2009;41(2): 172–190.

126. Kars HJ, Hijmans JM, Geertzen JH, Zijlstra W. The effect of reduced somatosensation on standing balance: a systematic review. *J Diabetes Sci Technol.* 2009;3(4):931–943.

127. Liu MW, Hsu WC, Lu TW, Chen HL, Liu HC. Patients with type II diabetes mellitus display reduced toe-obstacle clearance with altered gait patterns during obstacle-crossing. *Gait Posture.* 2010;31(1):93–99.

128. Sawacha Z, Cristoferi G, Guarneri G, et al. Characterizing multisegment foot kinematics during gait in diabetic foot patients. *J Neuroeng Rehabil.* 2009;6:37.

129. Sawacha Z, Gabriella G, Cristoferi G, Guiotto A, Avogaro A, Cobelli C. Diabetic gait and posture abnormalities: a biomechanical investigation through three dimensional gait analysis. *Clin Biomech (Bristol, Avon).* 2009;24(9):722–728.

130. Turcot K, Allet L, Golay A, Hoffmeyer P, Armand S. Investigation of standing balance in diabetic patients with and without peripheral neuropathy using accelerometers. *Clin Biomech (Bristol, Avon).* 2009;24(9):716–721.

131. Schilling RJ, Bollt EM, Fulk GD, Skufca JD, Al-Ajlouni AF, Robinson CJ. A quiet standing index for testing the postural sway of healthy and diabetic adults across a range of ages. *IEEE Trans Biomed Eng.* 2009;56(2):292–302.

132. Bergin PS, Bronstein AM, Murray NM, Sancovic S, Zeppenfeld DK. Body sway and vibration perception thresholds in normal aging and in patients with polyneuropathy. *J Neurol Neurosurg Psychiatry.* 1995;58(3): 335–340.

133. Simoneau GG, Ulbrecht JS, Derr JA, Becker MB, Cavanagh PR. Postural instability in patients with diabetic sensory neuropathy. *Diabetes Care.* 1994;17(12):1411–1421.

134. Dickstein R, Shupert CL, Horak FB. Fingertip touch improves postural stability in patients with peripheral neuropathy. *Gait Posture.* 2001;14(3):238–247.

135. Ahmmed AU, Mackenzie IJ. Posture changes in diabetes mellitus. *J Laryngol Otol.* 2003;117(5):358–364.

136. Corriveau H, Prince F, Hebert R, et al. Evaluation of postural stability in elderly with diabetic neuropathy. *Diabetes Care.* 2000;23(8):1187–1191.

137. Gutierrez EM, Helber MD, Dealva D, Ashton-Miller JA, Richardson JK. Mild diabetic neuropathy affects ankle motor function. *Clin Biomech (Bristol, Avon).* 2001;16(6):522–528.

138. van Sloten TT, Savelberg HH, Duimel-Peeters IG, et al. Peripheral neuropathy, decreased muscle strength and obesity are strongly associated with walking in persons with type 2 diabetes without manifest mobility limitations. *Diabetes Res Clin Pract.* 2911;91(1):32–39.

139. Schwartz AV, Hillier TA, Sellmeyer DE, et al. Older women with diabetes have a higher risk of falls: a prospective study. *Diabetes Care.* 2002;25(10):1749–1754.

140. Volpato S, Leveille SG, Blaum C, Fried LP, Guralnik JM. Risk factors for falls in older disabled women with diabetes: the Women's Health and Aging Study. *J Gerontol.* 2005; 60(12):1539–1545.

141. Mayne D, Stout NR, Aspray TJ. Diabetes, falls and fractures. *Age Ageing.* 2010;39(5):522–525.

142. Macgilchrist C, Paul L, Ellis BM, Howe TE, Kennon B, Godwin J. Lower-limb risk factors for falls in people with diabetes mellitus. *Diabet Med.* 2010;27(2):162–168.

143. Schlee G, Milani TL, Sterzing T, Oriwol D. Short-time lower leg ischemia reduces plantar foot sensitivity. *Neurosci Lett.* 2009;462(3):286–288.

144. Thompson C, Belanger M, Fung J. Effects of plantar cutaneo-muscular and tendon vibration on posture and balance during quiet and perturbed stance. *Hum Mov Sci.* 2011;30(2):153–171.

145. Roll R, Kavounoudias A, Roll JP. Cutaneous afferents from human plantar sole contribute to body posture awareness. *Neuroreport.* 2002;13(15):1957–1961.

146. Eils E, Behrens S, Mers O, Thorwesten L, Volker K, Rosenbaum D. Reduced plantar sensation causes a cautious walking pattern. *Gait Posture.* 2004;20(1):54–60.

147. Meyer PF, Oddsson LI, De Luca CJ. Reduced plantar sensitivity alters postural responses to lateral perturbations of balance. *Exp Brain Res.* 2004;157(4):526–536.

148. Meyer PF, Oddsson LI, De Luca CJ. The role of plantar cutaneous sensation in unperturbed stance. *Exp Brain Res.* 2004;156(4):505–512.

149. Magnusson M, Enbom H, Johansson R, Pyykko I. Significance of pressor input from the human feet in anterior-posterior postural control. The effect of hypothermia on vibration-induced body-sway. *Acta Otolaryngol.* 1990;110(3–4):182–188.

150. Magnusson M, Johansson R, Wiklund J. Galvanically induced body sway in the anterior-posterior plane. *Acta Otolaryngol.* 1990;110(1–2):11–17.

151. Collins JJ, Chow CC, Capela AC, Imhoff TT. Aperiodic stochastic resonance. *Phys Rev E Stat Phys Plasmas Fluids Relat Interdiscip Topics.* 1996;54(5):5575–5584.

152. Collins JJ, Imhoff TT, Grigg P. Noise-enhanced information transmission in rat SA1 cutaneous mechanoreceptors via aperiodic stochastic resonance. *J Neurophysiol.* 1996;76(1): 642–645.

153. Priplata A, Niemi J, Salen M, Harry J, Lipsitz LA, Collins JJ. Noise-enhanced human balance control. *Phys Rev Lett.* 2002;89(23):238101.

154. Hijmans JM, Geertzen JH, Zijlstra W, Hof AL, Postema K. Effects of vibrating insoles on standing balance in diabetic neuropathy. *J Rehabil Res Dev.* 2008;45(9):1441–1449.

155. Hijmans JM, Geertzen JH, Dijkstra PU, Postema K. A systematic review of the effects of shoes and other ankle or foot appliances on balance in older people and people with peripheral nervous system disorders. *Gait Posture.* 2007;25(2):316–323.

156. Khaodhiar L, Niemi JB, Earnest R, Lima C, Harry JD, Veves A. Enhancing sensation in diabetic neuropathic foot with mechanical noise. *Diabetes Care.* 2003;26(12): 3280–3283.

157. Priplata AA, Patritti BL, Niemi JB, et al. Noise-enhanced balance control in patients with diabetes and patients with stroke. *Ann Neurol.* 2006;59(1):4–12.

158. Cloutier R, Horr S, Niemi JB, et al. Prolonged mechanical noise restores tactile sense in diabetic neuropathic patients. *Int J Low Extrem Wounds.* 2010;8:6–10.

159. Richardson KA, Imhoff TT, Grigg P, Collins JJ. Using electrical noise to enhance the ability of humans to detect subthreshold mechanical cutaneous stimuli. *Chaos.* 1998; 8(3):599–603.

160. Gravelle DC, Laughton CA, Dhruv NT, et al. Noise-enhanced balance control in older adults. *Neuroreport.* 2002; 13(15):1853–1856.

161. Dhruv NT, Niemi JB, Harry JD, Lipsitz LA, Collins JJ. Enhancing tactile sensation in older adults with electrical noise stimulation. *Neuroreport.* 2002;13(5):597–600.

162. Priplata AA, Niemi JB, Harry JD, Lipsitz LA, Collins JJ. Vibrating insoles and balance control in elderly people. *Lancet.* 2003;362(9390):1123–1124.

163. Kavounoudias A, Roll R, Roll JP. The plantar sole is a 'dynamometric map' for human balance control. *Neuroreport.* 1998;9(14):3247–3252.

164. Kavounoudias A, Roll R, Roll JP. Specific whole-body shifts induced by frequency-modulated vibrations of human plantar soles. *Neurosci Lett.* 1999;266(3):181–184.

165. Kavounoudias A, Roll R, Roll JP. Foot sole and ankle muscle inputs contribute jointly to human erect posture regulation. *J Physiol.* 2001;532(pt 3):869–878.

166. Galica AM, Kang HG, Priplata AA, et al. Subsensory vibrations to the feet reduce gait variability in elderly fallers. *Gait Posture.* 2009;30(3):383–387.

167. Tihanyi TK, Horvath M, Fazekas G, Hortobagyi T, Tihanyi J. One session of whole body vibration increases voluntary muscle strength transiently in patients with stroke. *Clin Rehabil.* 2007;21(9):782–793.

168. van Nes IJ, Geurts AC, Hendricks HT, Duysens J. Short-term effects of whole-body vibration on postural control in unilateral chronic stroke patients: preliminary evidence. *Am J Phys Med Rehabil.* 2004;83(11):867–873.

169. van Nes IJ, Latour H, Schils F, Meijer R, van Kuijk A, Geurts AC. Long-term effects of 6-week whole-body vibration on balance recovery and activities of daily living in the postacute phase of stroke: a randomized, controlled trial. *Stroke.* 2006;37(9):2331–2335.

170. Rees SS, Murphy AJ, Watsford ML. Effects of whole body vibration on postural steadiness in an older population. *J Sci Med Sport.* 2009;12(4):440–444.

171. Cheung WH, Mok HW, Qin L, Sze PC, Lee KM, Leung KS. High-frequency whole-body vibration improves balancing ability in elderly women. *Arch Phys Med Rehabil.* 2007;88(7):852–857.

172. Furness TP, Maschette WE. Influence of whole body vibration platform frequency on neuromuscular performance of community-dwelling older adults. *J Strength Cond Res.* 2009;23(5):1508–1513.

173. Rittweger J. Vibration as an exercise modality: how it may work, and what its potential might be. *Eur J Appl Physiol.* 2010;108(5):877–904.

174. Milton JG, Small SS, Solodkin A. On the road to automatic: dynamic aspects in the development of expertise. *J Clin Neurophysiol.* 2004;21(3):134–143.

175. Bus SA, Ulbrecht JS, Cavanagh PR. Pressure relief and load redistribution by custom-made insoles in diabetic patients with neuropathy and foot deformity. *Clin Biomech (Bristol, Avon).* 2004;19(6):629–638.

176. Frykberg RG, Bailey LF, Matz A, Panthel LA, Ruesch G. Offloading properties of a rocker insole. A preliminary study. *J Am Podiatr Med Assoc.* 2002;92(1):48–53.

177. Janisse DJ, Janisse E. Shoe modification and the use of orthoses in the treatment of foot and ankle pathology. *J Am Acad Orthop Surg.* 2008;16(3):152–158.

178. Brown D, Wertsch JJ, Harris GF, Klein J, Janisse D. Effect of rocker soles on plantar pressures. *Arch Phys Med Rehabil.* 2004;85(1):81–86.

179. Xu H, Akai M, Kakurai S, Yokota K, Kaneko H. Effect of shoe modifications on center of pressure and in-shoe plantar pressures. *Am J Phys Med Rehabil.* 1999;78(6):516–524.

180. Perry J, Gronley JK, Lunsford T. Rocker shoe as walking aid in multiple sclerosis. *Arch Phys Med Rehabil.* 1981;62(2):59–65.

181. Van Bogart JJ, Long JT, Klein JP, Wertsch JJ, Janisse DJ, Harris GF. Effects of the toe-only rocker on gait kinematics and kinetics in able-bodied persons. *IEEE Trans Neural Syst Rehabil Eng.* 2005;13(4):542–550.

182. Albright BC, Woodhull-Smith WM. Rocker bottom soles alter the postural response to backward translation during stance. *Gait Posture.* 2009;30(1):45–49.

183. Wang CC, Hansen AH. Response of able-bodied persons to changes in shoe rocker radius during walking: changes in ankle kinematics to maintain a consistent roll-over shape. *J Biomech.* 2010;43(12):2288–2293.

184. Long JT, Sirota N, Klein JP, Wertsch JJ, Janisse D, Harris GF. Biomechanics of the double rocker sole shoe: gait kinematics and kinetics. *Conf Proc IEEE Eng Med Biol Soc.* 2004;7:5107–5110.

185. Long JT, Klein JP, Sirota NM, Wertsch JJ, Janisse D, Harris GF. Biomechanics of the double rocker sole shoe: gait kinematics and kinetics. *J Biomech.* 2007;40(13):2882–2890.

186. Boyer KA, Andriacchi TP. Changes in running kinematics and kinetics in response to a rockered shoe intervention. *Clin Biomech (Bristol, Avon).* 2009;24(10):872–876.

187. Myers KA, Long JT, Klein JP, Wertsch JJ, Janisse D, Harris GF. Biomechanical implications of the negative heel rocker sole shoe: gait kinematics and kinetics. *Gait Posture.* 2006; 24(3):323–330.

188. Peterson MJ, Perry J, Montgomery J. Walking patterns of healthy subjects wearing rocker shoes. *Phys Ther.* 1985;65(10):1483–1489.

189. Perry SD, Radtke A, McIlroy WE, Fernie GR, Maki BE. Efficacy and effectiveness of a balance-enhancing insole. *J Gerontol.* 2008;63(6):595–602.

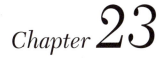

Chapter 23

Brachial Plexopathies

Steven Whitenack, MD, PhD

"Do you not see how necessary a world of pains and troubles is to school an intelligence and make it a soul?"

—John Keats (1795–1821)

Objectives

On completion of this chapter, the student/practitioner will be able to:

- From a historical perspective, discuss the origin of the various terms related to thoracic outlet syndrome and the surgical and conservative interventions used to treat this condition.
- Explain the relationship of the structures within the thoracic outlet to the etiology of the various types of thoracic outlet syndrome.
- Relate the signs and symptoms to the etiological anatomical structures.
- Differentiate between arterial, venous, and neurological thoracic outlet syndrome.

Key Terms

- Scalene muscle
- Subclavian vessels
- Thoracic outlet syndrome

Introduction

Brachial plexopathy can be divided into the same variety of nerve pathologies as other nerve "syndromes." These pathologies may be caused by acute or chronic compression, stretch injury, ischemic injury, electrical injury, radiation injury, and various direct injuries. The management of brachial plexopathies theoretically does not differ from management of other nerve injuries. However, brachial plexopathy is more difficult to understand and treat. This difficulty is largely due to the variation in manifestations caused by the more complex anatomy of the plexus than, for instance, the median nerve at the wrist; the extensive range of motion of the shoulder; and the complex anatomy of the other associated structures intimately related to the brachial plexus. Most patients presenting with brachial plexopathy fit the entity known as **thoracic outlet syndrome** (TOS).

The term *thoracic outlet syndrome* encompasses various clinical entities involving structures around the shoulder girdle. Symptoms can include pain, numbness, paresthesias, headaches, weakness of the arm and hand, ischemia, and arm swelling. The term engenders a great deal of controversy in the literature, especially neurology, because of the difficulty in defining it. TOS may be viewed as a clinical complex that includes four parts: neuropathy of the brachial plexus, compression vasculopathy of the **subclavian vessels,** complex regional pain syndrome (CRPS) or reflex sympathetic dystrophy (RSD), and cervicothoracic and brachial myofasciitis. Conversely, some authors would choose to limit the use of the term TOS to problems involving only the lower portions of the plexus—the C8 and T1 nerve roots, lower trunk, and medial cord.

Manifestations of compromise of the neurological elements associated with the thoracic outlet differ from the manifestations seen in compromise of the vascular elements of the thoracic outlet. However, because the term TOS is so well entrenched in the literature, this chapter attempts to broaden the understanding of the various manifestations of TOS rather than use an entirely new nomenclature. This broader understanding should improve the diagnosis and treatment of this difficult entity.

The variability in presentation of TOS, which causes great debate and misunderstanding, can be explained rationally if time is taken to comprehend fully the complex anatomy of the thoracic outlet region. The variation in mechanism of injury and variation in anatomy of the structures surrounding the brachial plexus cause the lack of a "typical clinical profile" desired by many neurologists. There are many typical profiles, which can be explained and thoroughly understood when these anatomical variations are studied. TOS is also a dynamic entity. Alterations in posture and activity can profoundly affect the clinical picture.

Historical Background

Many different and distinct entities have been grouped together under the term TOS. Rob is generally credited with coining the term "thoracic outlet compression syndrome."[1] Peet et al.[2] first grouped cervical rib syndrome, scalenus-anticus syndrome, subcoracoid-pectoralis minor syndrome, costoclavicular syndrome, and first thoracic rib syndrome into the TOS. Other authors have added the scalenus medius syndrome, Paget-Schroetter syndrome (effort thrombosis of subclavian vein), rucksack palsy, droopy shoulder syndrome, and hyperabduction syndrome. Although including these separate etiologies under one heading can obscure the important differences in diagnosis and treatment, such a grouping is more likely to aid in understanding TOS.

The history of TOS has been well documented in many prior excellent reviews. The first recognition of cervical ribs dates to Galen (Fig. 23-1) and Vesalius. Willshire is generally credited as the first to make the diagnosis of "cervical rib syndrome."[3] Coote[4] reported the first successful cervical rib resection in 1861. W.W. Keen[5] and Halsted[6] wrote extensive reviews and described surgical results.

Patients later were described with similar or identical symptoms in the absence of a cervical rib. In 1910, Murphy[7] was the first to resect a normal first rib and achieve relief of symptoms. In 1927, Brickner[8] was the first to describe resection of the normal first rib in the American literature. Also in 1927, Adson and Coffey[1] initiated a shift in thinking with their belief that the symptoms were related to the relationship of the anterior scalene to the cervical rib and not the rib itself. Adson was "convinced that it was not necessary to remove cervical ribs routinely, and that the chief etiological element was the scalenus anticus muscle."[1] This belief was based on operative findings, surgical results, and the fact that most cervical ribs were asymptomatic. Adson's operative procedure consisted of section of the anterior scalene, removal of any tendinous bands, and occasionally removal of the cervical rib. Adson's sign was described at that time.[1]

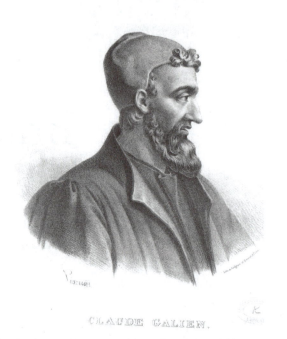

Figure 23-1 Aelius Galenus (A.D. 129–200), commonly known as Galen, was a prominent physician, philosopher, and surgeon of Greek ethnicity. Galen contributed greatly to the understanding and appreciation of numerous disciplines including anatomy, pathology, physiology, and neurology. Courtesy of the National Library of Medicine.

The next step in surgical thinking led to the resection of the anterior scalene in the absence of a cervical rib. Scalenus-anticus syndrome, as credited to Naffziger by Ochsner et al.,[9] became a common diagnosis, and scalenotomy became a common procedure. Over time, the failures in treatment in patients with "Naffziger's syndrome" led to disenchantment with scalenotomy. However, other upper extremity pain syndromes had not yet been described, and many failures may have been in diagnosis rather than procedure. Cervical radiculopathy was described in 1943 by Semmes and Murphy.[10] It was not until 1950 that Phalen[11] described carpal tunnel syndrome or until 1953 that Kremer et al.[12] defined the nerve conduction abnormalities at the carpal tunnel.

Other etiological factors were also described to explain the symptoms being attributed to scalenus anticus syndrome. in 1934, Lewis and Pickering[13] implicated compression of the neurovascular bundle between the clavicle and the first rib as the cause of the symptoms. This condition was later termed the "costoclavicular compression syndrome" by Falconer and Weddell.[14] In 1945, Wright[15] added the concept of hyperabduction of the arms causing neurovascular compression at two levels. In addition to the similarly described costoclavicular compression, he added the concept of compression by the posterior border of the pectoralis minor against the anterior border of the upper ribs. Wright's test was also described at that time.[15]

In 1953, Lord added the concept of resection of the clavicle for relief of the costoclavicular compression syndrome.[16] Scalenotomy remained the preferred procedure, but because of disenchantment with results as described by Raaf,[17] scalenotomy fell into disfavor. Falconer and Li[14] were the first to support direct resection of the first rib in 1962. Later that same year, Clagett[18] solidified the importance of the first rib as the common denominator in the pathophysiology of TOS during the presidential address before the American Association for Thoracic Surgery. Clagett's approach was a posterior, thoracoplasty-type resection of the first rib, befitting a thoracic surgeon trained in tuberculosis surgery.

A major advancement in the surgical approach to TOS was reported by Roos[19] in 1966. The transaxillary first rib resection that he described rapidly became the standard procedure for patients with TOS. The 93% improvement rate reported by Roos was reaffirmed by other authors, including Urschel et al.[20] and Sanders.[21] Roos[22–25] also was primarily responsible for redirecting attention away from the vascular compression and to the brachial plexus compression. In addition, Roos[24] carefully classified the many different types of congenital bands that contribute to TOS.

Nerve compression has remained the central concept for the etiology of symptoms of TOS by most authors. Scar fixation of the nerves causing traction and fixation of the brachial plexus rather than compression as the primary pathological process is the latest concept to aid understanding of this complex problem. Sunderland[26] attempted to help define the difference between nerve compressive problems and nerve entrapment and wrote "the key to the pathogenesis of the entrapment nerve lesion is the local inflammatory reaction that occurs in response to repeated mechanical irritation during limb movements." Simple "decompressive" procedures may be inadequate to relieve the pathological process found in many of these complex cases.

Vascular Syndromes

Vascular manifestations of TOS are rare. Of reported cases of TOC, 3% to 5% are vascular, with only 1% being arterial. These percentages are probably overstated, as the recognition of neurogenic TOS involving the upper plexus has increased. The misunderstanding of the relationship between the vascular diagnostic signs and the neurological manifestations of TOS is one of many aspects of this problem that create the controversy that surrounds this diagnosis. Vascular syndromes are divided into arterial and venous types. Pure lymphatic disorders have not been described.

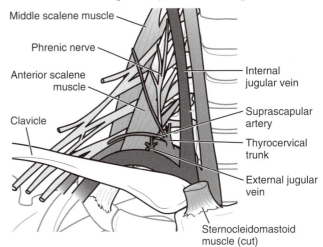

Figure 23-2 The intimate relationship between the subclavian vasculature and the elements of the brachial plexus.

Arterial Thoracic Outlet Syndrome

Symptomatic arterial manifestations of TOS are representative of either acute or chronic compression (Fig. 23-2). Chronic compression of the subclavian artery can cause both occlusive and aneurysmal disease. Aneurysms and arterial occlusive disease are relatively rare. Dense fascial bands running forward and inferiorly from a cervical rib or elongated transverse process of C7 are the usual structural anomalies that predispose to arterial manifestations of TOS. These bands may create positional compression with motion of the arm. The Adson, Wright, and Halstead maneuvers are used to demonstrate arterial compression. However, the presence of the capacity to obliterate the pulse at the wrist with arm motion does not in itself define TOS. Many completely asymptomatic individuals are able to shut off their pulse, particularly at the extremes of range of motion of the shoulder.

The symptoms of arterial compression are generally described as having a "dead arm" or fatigue with use. The symptoms may be positional and may interfere with occupations requiring overhead arm use. The absence of pulses with a completely abducted arm is likely to cause fatigue when trying to perform overhead activity. With appropriate accommodation, many of these types of activities may be continued without creating undue risk of repetitive trauma to the artery. For example, use of extension devices can allow continued productive work to be accomplished.

The sequelae of repetitive trauma to the artery are intimal damage to the vessel, leading to thrombosis, occlusive disease with poststenotic dilation, or occasionally aneurysm formation.[27] The initial symptoms of subclavian artery occlusion depend on the rapidity of the occlusion. A slowly progressive occlusion may allow time for adequate collateral circulation to develop. In this situation, the patient may have complaints only when the arm is used excessively. A more rapid occlusion, representing acute thrombosis, causes the patient to have symptoms of arm claudication, with muscle cramping after minimal use or at rest. Before complete occlusion occurs, examination reveals diminished to absent pulses in the involved arm and a bruit in the infraclavicular space.

The presenting symptoms of aneurysmal disease[28] are usually related to distal embolization to the arm, hand, or fingers. This embolization is caused by fragments of the clotted material within the aneurysm breaking loose and lodging in the distal vessels. The symptoms may vary from acute ischemia of the arm with pain, pallor, paresthesias, and pulselessness to fingertip necrosis suggestive of Raynaud's phenomenon. The presence of a pulsatile mass in the supraclavicular fossa should raise the question of a subclavian aneurysm. Neurogenic symptoms infrequently may be caused by pressure from the aneurysm. An ultrasound study can usually confirm the presence of an aneurysm.

Venous Thoracic Outlet Syndrome

Acute venous occlusion of the subclavian vein results in sudden painful swelling of the arm, often with a bluish discoloration. Most commonly, this subclavian venous thrombosis is the result of sudden maximal arm use and is known as effort thrombosis or Paget-Schroetter syndrome. If the thrombosis is more insidious in onset, the sudden painful swelling does not occur, but rather swelling with significant use occurs. Other etiologies of intravascular thrombosis must be considered, including factor V (Leiden), antithrombin III or anticardiolipin antibodies, and protein C and protein S abnormalities.[29] Spontaneous development of any venous thrombosis without obvious cause should also raise the question of occult malignancy. Subclavian venous catheters for intravenous access and particularly dialysis are the most common etiology of subclavian thrombosis or stenosis at the present time.

Treatment of Vascular Thoracic Outlet Syndrome

The treatment of vascular manifestations of TOS can be divided into immediate and long-term therapy. In the presence of distal arterial embolization, heparin therapy is instituted rapidly. If the embolus is in the larger vessels, embolectomy is indicated. Subsequent thoracic outlet decompression and repair of the arterial pathology with a vein graft or patch should soon follow.[30]

Venous thrombectomy can be effective if performed in the first few days after onset of symptoms. Thrombolysis with streptokinase or urokinase infusion is more likely to be beneficial if the diagnosis is delayed.[30] When operative thrombectomy is performed, rib resection, resection of abnormal bands, and possible scalenectomy should be done at the same time. Rib resection can be delayed 2 to 3 months after thrombolysis is performed, maintaining the patient on anticoagulation until surgery. A residual stricture in the vein after resection of the compressive bands sometimes responds to balloon dilation. There is a high failure rate if angioplasty of the vein is done before decompression. Intraluminal stent placement should be avoided if the etiology of the venous occlusion is external compression.[31]

Short-term anticoagulation should be considered for all forms of vascular TOS.[30] Warfarin (Coumadin) therapy for a minimum of 3 months provides a lower incidence of post-thrombotic complications and should be used unless there is a clear contraindication (e.g., bleeding diathesis, active ulcer disease).

Neurological Thoracic Outlet Syndromes

Most thinking on TOS originally centered on lower plexus pathology resulting in ulnar mediated complaints in the arm and hand. These symptoms are generally more clear-cut and easily defined than with other types of symptoms and consequently have been more accepted over time. At the present time, most patients with TOS have been involved in some type of significant trauma, particularly with a flexion-extension component. The delayed onset of symptoms 1 to 3 months after this type of injury should be expected if the natural consequences of scar contraction and fibrosis are considered and the anatomical abnormalities described later in this chapter are understood. The use of the term "whiplash" carries many of the same negative connotations as TOS, a position it does not deserve. More recent observations will perhaps elevate the understanding of both of these complex problems.[30,31]

The neurology literature has been characterized by an aggressive attack on thoracic outlet diagnoses.[32,33] The neurologist's bias has been made clear by using the terms "true neurogenic" and "disputed" to differentiate types of TOS. One can also consider the more commonly accepted definitions of TOS in the surgical literature as "classic" TOS.

"True Neurogenic" Thoracic Outlet Syndrome

The most clearly defined subset of TOS has been labeled by Wilbourn and Porter[34] as "true neurogenic" TOS. These patients have atrophy of the ulnar intrinsic hand muscles (particularly the thenar eminence and first dorsal interosseous muscles), numbness and paresthesias in the ulnar distribution, and clear peripheral electromyography evidence of neuron loss, always associated with the presence of a cervical rib. The rib itself or a tight musculotendinous band emanating from the end of the rib causes the compressive neuropathy. Pain is often remarkably absent in this variation of TOS, perhaps because of the selective compression of only the C8 nerve root. This syndrome variety is also called "motor type" neurogenic TOS, and because it was first electrically defined accurately by Gilliat in 1970, this type of TOS is also called Gilliat's disease.[35]

Because of the symptoms of hand weakness, carpal tunnel syndrome commonly is mistakenly diagnosed in these cases. Any time the diagnosis of carpal tunnel syndrome is made in a teenager who has thenar wasting, it is imperative to rule out TOS (usually related to a cervical rib) before proceeding with carpal tunnel surgery. It must be reemphasized that the fine motor intrinsic function of the hand is mediated more via the ulnar nerve than the median.

The "true neurogenic" variation is rare in its most narrow form in most reported series as well as our own. In my experience, the C8 nerve root compression seen at surgery has been extreme in these cases, to the point that the nerve has a gelatinous appearance from demyelination when observed at surgery. The onset of symptoms is usually in the late teens or early 20s, presumably secondary to the decreasing bony flexibility and angulation of the cervical rib. The compression seen in these cases is severe, and electromyography and other nerve studies can easily make the diagnosis.

Classic Thoracic Outlet Syndrome

Cases of TOS that do not fulfill the restrictive criteria of "true neurogenic" TOS have been labeled "disputed" TOS. The central issue in these arguments is the variability in symptoms in patients who do not fit precisely into the "true neurogenic" category. A corollary argument centers on the lack of "uniform" criteria for the physical examination. When a full understanding of the anatomical basis for TOS is reached, the concerns of the detractors can be put aside. There is no dispute if the pathophysiology is understood. Figure 23-2 shows the full distribution of the nerves that ultimately derive from the brachial plexus. Compromise at any level of the plexus creates a symptom complex in the anatomical distribution of the involved nerve. Descriptions of symptoms being on a "nonanatomical" basis usually indicate a lack of understanding of the brachial plexus anatomy.

The extensive anatomical studies of Roos and others[21–26] documented the variety of muscle anomalies and fibrous bands found in these patients. The nearly infinite minor variations in the location, path, severity of compression, and density of these muscles and bands are responsible for the differences in symptoms from one patient to another. Fascial bands leading from the C7 transverse process to the pleura and first rib may compress the C8 or T1 nerve roots either separately or together and anywhere from immediately distal to the

foramen to the junction of the anterior and posterior divisions. The symptoms mirror the point of entrapment, and the expression of the upper extremity complaints can be manifest in any of the peripheral nerves of the shoulder girdle and arm that ultimately arise from these nerves.

Mackinnnon[36,37] continued the work of Sunderland[26] and showed that the response of nerves to compression passes through many stages. Initially, there is periodic ischemia related to interruption of local blood flow. Microscopically, there is subperineural edema. More chronic ischemia results in reactive thickening of the perineural tissues. The most external nerve fascicles alone initially show degeneration, whereas the central fibers remain intact. The implications of these findings are not to be underestimated. There can be variation in the peripheral manifestations of more proximal nerve compression based on local anatomical factors.

The arguments of Wilbourn[32] requiring a fixed set of criteria in all patients that can be uniformly reproduced indicate a lack of appreciation for clinical evaluation of patients. In entities such as appendicitis, it is well recognized that the entire picture of the patient including history, physical examination, and laboratory studies must be considered together to establish a diagnosis. Not all patients with appendicitis have identical presentations. It seems unrealistic to expect all patients with TOS to have fixed criteria for diagnosis. Nelems[38] developed a set of subjective criteria that are divided into "must have, may have, and can't have" criteria. This is a useful methodology when approaching nearly all pain-mediated syndromes.

Patient complaints in cases of TOS can be broadly grouped into upper and lower plexus components. They have become clearly separable in our evaluations, along with other secondarily associated manifestations brought about by misuse of the arm and shoulder girdle. The anatomy of the brachial plexus must be repeatedly studied to comprehend the various nerve symptoms that are possible. The distribution of symptoms can follow any of the nerves derived from all branches of the brachial plexus. It is most important to understand that the symptoms caused by proximal plexus compression and entrapment can be distributed to multiple sites distally.

Lower Brachial Plexus Syndromes (Lower Thoracic Outlet Syndrome)

The symptoms of lower trunk plexus involvement involve various combinations of pain and other sensory disturbances in the arm and hand and mild weakness of the hand and arm. In the so-called true neurogenic variety, pain is remarkably absent, and motor symptoms predominate. Pain is the central feature of the remainder of TOS cases that involve the lower plexus.

The pain of lower plexus TOS is often described as beginning at the base of the neck and supraclavicular fossa and heading to the area just inferomedial to the deltopectoral groove, which is the path of the nerve after passing under the acromion. The pain then extends variably down the arm in the ulnar distribution. Usually numbness and paresthesias extending into the fourth and fifth fingers are more prominent distally. Elevation of the arm laterally and above the head places traction on the lower plexus and almost always reproduces the patient's symptoms. Careful history and sensory testing show that the numbness generally involves the ulnar aspect of the middle finger.[39]; this is helpful in differentiating TOS from pure ulnar nerve compression.

Sunderland[26] believed that the usual descriptions of the peripheral sensory distribution of the nerve roots of the brachial plexus were misrepresented in the forearm. The usual presentation of nerve root sensory distribution shows C6 supplying the index and thumb. Sunderland's view shows C6 to have almost no sensory distribution distal to the wrist, with C7 supplying the index and thumb. The distribution in the radial forearm is described as C5–6 (upper trunk) and in the ulnar forearm and hand as C8–T1 (lower trunk), rather than as separate nerve roots. This description fits more clearly the distribution of sensory complaints in these patients. In our experience, the lower trunk seems to split the long finger in patients with lower trunk sensory complaints,[40] rather than involve the whole finger as described by Sunderland.[26]

Variations in the ulnar and median nerves must be understood when differentiating plexus-level from distal neuropathies.[22,25] Absence of thenar wasting with a distal injury to the median nerve at the wrist can occur if both a Martin-Gruber and a Riche-Cannieu anastomosis are present. These communications generally contain motor neurons only. The Martin-Gruber anastomosis occurs distal to the elbow. The sensory findings in the hand should still correlate appropriately with the other findings of plexus-level pathology.

The motor complaints of lower trunk TOS are usually described as fatigue of the hand, loss of penmanship, or loss of the ability to write for lengthy periods. Wasting of the ulnar intrinsic and thenar muscles seldom occurs but must be watched for carefully in patients who are being followed in a therapy program. Development of atrophy is an indication for immediate surgical intervention.

Upper Brachial Plexus Syndromes (Upper Thoracic Outlet Syndrome)

There are many recognizable forms of upper plexus involvement with TOS that fall into repeatable patterns of complaint. To decipher these complaints, one must evaluate all aspects of the history, including the exact mechanism of injury, history of prior injuries, the precise nature of prior treatment and therapy, details of the conditions of the workplace, and other similar details.

The most common constellation of complaints in upper plexus cases involves pain along the trapezius ridge, into the suprascapular notch, and along the medial scapular border. There is also pain running posteriorly up the back of the neck to the occipital protuberance and headaches that pass from the back of the skull forward toward the eye. Pain into the pectoral region that is often burning in quality is also commonly found. Pain along the distribution of the long thoracic nerve, with winging of the scapula, is seen less often.

In many long-standing cases, patients have facial pain that is interpreted as a "TMJ" (temporomandibular joint) symptom. They may also develop what appear to be sympathetic mediated swelling of the unilateral face, occasional lid droop, and eye pain. This group of patients also commonly complains of difficulty with night vision.

To the skeptics of upper plexus–type TOS, these multiple manifestations of nerve compromise are ignored; discarded; or placed into diagnostic categories such as fibromyositis, migraine equivalent, and any variety of shoulder pathology. If one clearly and dispassionately reviews the anatomy of the brachial plexus, it becomes apparent that all of the aforementioned complaints are in the ultimate distribution of C5, C6, and the upper trunk or portions of the cervical plexus involved by scalene spasm and scarring. The pectoral symptoms come from the medial and lateral pectoral nerves, the periscapular symptoms come from the suprascapular and long thoracic nerves, and the radial sensory and first through third finger symptoms more obviously come from the final peripheral nerve distribution of the lateral cord.

The occipital pain can be mediated through the irritation of the greater occipital nerve as it passes through the posterior musculature of the neck, which may be secondarily in spasm.[41] Although often referred to as "migraine" headaches, there is usually no aura preceding the headache, and nausea and vomiting seldom occur. In Britain, these types of post-traumatic headaches have been labeled "footballer's migraine."[42] There also appears to be a referred pain aspect to these complaints mediated through communications with the cervical plexus. Known subcortical crossover pathways may explain the origin of contralateral pain in some instances. These pathways at the spinal and mid-brain level may also explain the complaints of ipsilateral pain or numbness in equivalent fingers and toes that are occasionally reported. In the teaching of acupressure techniques for relief of these posterior headaches, pressure is placed alternately over the occipital protuberance and the web space of the thumb with excellent result.

Mixed Plexus Syndromes

As understanding of the complexities of the brachial plexus improves, it is increasingly evident that the upper and lower plexus symptoms become intertwined.

Patients with diffuse arm and shoulder symptoms must not be written off as having "nonanatomical" complaints. The anatomical abnormalities described by Roos[22] that are repeatedly confirmed at surgery make it clear that the distribution of complaints depends on the mixture of anamolies found in any given individual, particularly with alteration of arm position. There is marked variability in the involvement of C7 and the middle trunk with either the upper or the lower trunk, symptomatically as well as anatomically. Considering that injury is usually the basis of modern plexopathy, it is well to consider that with lower plexus injury C7 may be involved in dense scar fixation to the lower trunk. A "sausage casing" type of material can envelope the middle and lower trunk. The symptoms may overlap in the median nerve distribution. In upper plexus injuries, C5 and C6 may be bound with C7, or the middle trunk, to create symptoms and findings overlapping the median nerve with the upper plexus, lateral cord distribution. The "prefixed" plexus, which has contribution from C4, and the "postfixed" plexus, which has contribution from T2, create further variability in the "usual" manifestations of TOS.[22] With a prefixed or postfixed plexus, nerve roots and trunks do not conform to the same ultimate distribution, and the symptoms may be variable.

Parsonage-Turner Syndrome

A rare type of brachial plexopathy that most commonly involves the upper plexus has become known as Parsonage-Turner syndrome.[43] It has also been called neuralgic amyotrophy, patchwork amyotrophy, shoulder-girdle syndrome, and numerous terms using the name of the muscle involved with pain and wasting.[44] Parsonage-Turner syndrome often begins as a sudden pain in the shoulder girdle region lasting 10 to 14 days before weakness and then atrophy of the muscles of the particular nerve involved occur. The pain usually decreases as the atrophy begins. Recovery takes several months to years and is generally good.

The etiology of Parsonage-Turner syndrome is believed to be immune and inflammatory related often following a viral or bacterial illness, vaccinations, or systemic illness. There is no specific treatment other than supportive to prevent limitation of shoulder motion or secondary injury as a result of the muscle weakness. Involvement of the phrenic nerve is worrisome in individuals with severe chronic obstructive pulmonary disease.[44]

Associated Musculoskeletal Problems

Numerous musculoskeletal complaints are common in patients with TOS and require further elucidation. The importance of understanding the interrelationship between TOS and these other associated problems cannot be understated. Many major orthopedic texts do not have even cursory mention of TOS, which further adds to the lack of understanding and recognition of a patient with TOS.

Impingement Syndrome (Rotator Cuff Tear)

The diagnosis of rotator cuff tear has been made and surgery performed in many patients who eventually are referred for unrelenting arm and hand symptoms.[45] The suprascapular nerve as it comes off the upper trunk is the site of significant fibrous fixation in patients with upper plexus TOS. This fibrous fixation can lead to dysfunction of the supraspinatus and infraspinatus muscles and laxity of the rotator cuff. The sensory branches supply the articular surfaces of the shoulder joint. Impingement also occurs in patients with TOS because of the forward displacement of the scapulothoracic articulation at the shoulder. As a result of this forward displacement, the structures in the suprahumeral space (the tendon of the long head of the biceps, the supraspinatus tendon, the subacromial bursa, and the superior aspect of the joint capsule) may become impinged between the greater tuberosity of the humerus and the acromion as the arm is abducted. Typically, the signs of impingement include pain referred within the C5 dermatome, a classic "painful arc," and loss of range of motion at the glenohumeral joint.[46]

Appropriate shoulder posture and strengthening of the rotator cuff muscle group, particularly the supraspinatus muscle, can rapidly improve this entity. There are multiple causes of rotator cuff injuries not related to TOS. Patients who do have TOS must be recognized because surgery on the rotator cuff is unsuccessful in most cases until the underlying upper plexus pathology is appropriately treated.

Trapezius Spasm

The trapezius is innervated by the C11 (spinal accessory) nerve and plexus pathology cannot be directly implicated in the sometimes severe pain in the trapezial ridge. The forward-sloping shoulder causes an imbalance in the shoulder girdle muscles. When the shoulder is elevated in a shrugging motion, the trapezius works alone if the shoulder is forward. The rhomboids and levator scapulae do not adequately assist the trapezius. The trapezius fatigues and tends to spasm. Appropriate posture, massage, and deep heat often relieve this problem over time.

Biceps Tendonitis

Similar to the previous discussion, biceps tendonitis occurs as the tendon partially subluxes out of the groove when the arms are used laterally and the shoulder is again positioned forward. This entity responds quickly to anti-inflammatory agents in concert with proper shoulder positioning. When tendonitis is very severe, steroids may be used, but repetitive injections should be avoided. The more proximal biceps tendon can also be involved in shoulder impingement.

Trigger Points

Patients who have the other ancillary manifestations almost always have painful areas along the medial scapular border, along the posterior neck, and in the trapezial insertion into the scapula. These points of irritation are areas of periosteal inflammation at muscle insertions or areas of chronic muscle tension from either spasm or improper use of the muscle caused by poor posturing of the shoulder girdle; this may also be manifest as motor end plate sensitivity that becomes involved in a circus reflex within the spinal column. With improvement in the overall position of the shoulder girdle, the tender areas gradually improve.[46] Moist heat, ultrasound, and massage may be beneficial. Resistant areas can be injected with local anesthetic and steroids, but this should not be repeated often.

Lateral Epicondylitis

Symptoms at the lateral elbow are commonly associated with TOS. Chronic use of the extremity in abnormal posture with the shoulders forward causes the patient to use the extensor muscles of the forearm inappropriately. Chronic improper use of these muscles causes irritation at the muscle insertion into the lateral epicondyle. Treatment consists of retraining of shoulder posture and appropriate use of the arms in lifting and with repetitive actions. Anti-inflammatory agents and local modalities sometimes are needed. Surgery should be avoidable with proper preventive measures. Symptoms referable to radial nerve entrapment in the proximal forearm are often confused with lateral epicondylitis. The radial nerve is exquisitely tender at the border of the extensor carpi radialis.

Pathophysiology

To understand TOS is to understand the various anatomical abnormalities and pathophysiological changes that are a consequence of these abnormalities. In a study of the thoracic outlet, Roos[47] compared the anatomy of cadaver specimens with the anatomy at surgery in patients with TOS. This study helped define the numerous findings at surgery. However, Roos' study underestimated the abnormalities found at surgery, particularly at the level of the upper plexus. The interdigitating fibers of the anterior scalene between the C5, C6, and C7 nerve roots found in cases of upper plexus TOS that we have explored have been severely underestimated.

Numerous structures are at risk of compromise in the thoracic outlet, including the brachial plexus, the subclavian artery, and the subclavian vein. The etiology of the resultant brachial plexus compression neuropathies is multifactorial, but certain risk factors predispose to this entity. Three broad categories of risk factors are congenital-structural, post-traumatic structural, and post-traumatic postural. When an inciting event occurs, a clinically significant compromise of the brachial plexus can result. The degree of congenital predisposition and the nature of the inciting event determine the severity and the clinical course of the neuropathy or vasculopathy.

When there has been significant trauma to the neck, particularly flexion-hyperextension type, resulting in tearing of the **scalene muscle** bundles, two potential problems occur that directly affect the nerves of the plexus. First, contraction and fibrosis of the muscle bundles can increasingly compress the nerve roots and trunks. Because scar is an active tissue and undergoes progressive contraction for 18 to 24 months, it is understandable that symptom progression often begins and continues many months after an injury.

Even more poorly understood is the fixation of the nerves to the muscle fascia of the scalene anomalies. This fixation is extremely common and occurs at all levels of the plexus. It is most likely caused by bleeding from the torn muscle and epineural connective tissue causing adherence of the muscle fascia to the epineural tissues. This adherence interferes with the basic need for the roots and trunks to have separate and free mobility with arm shoulder and neck motion that allow the shoulder to function in a 360-degree arc. Repetitive traction injury causes anatomical deformity of the plexus and results in inflammatory repair, adhesion, and progression of the painful neuropathy. This scarring also is likely to progress over time.

Machleder et al.[48] reported significant abnormal histological patterns of the anterior and middle scalene in patients with traumatic TOS. Sanders et al.[49] found atrophy of type II fibers and increase in the average number of type I fibers. Also, the percentage of connective tissue was increased by a mean of 36%. The importance of these findings should not be underestimated. The fibrous tissue content of the scalene muscles is often clinically apparent at the time of surgery as the muscle is transected.

Embryology

During the embryonic development of the upper extremity, numerous changes occur as the limb bud forms that ultimately may become manifest in the problems encountered in patients with TOS. The scalene muscles form as one confluent muscle mass. This scalene muscle mass becomes separated into specific muscles only as the neurovascular structures penetrate it. Some argument remains whether the scalenus minimus variant arises from this original scalene mass. The muscle abnormalities found at surgery represent the variable fragmentation of the scalene mass as the structures of the limb bud pass through it.[50]

A C7 rib also forms in the early embryo and then regresses variably. The residual cervical rib may vary from a complete rib to an elongated C7 transverse process. There may be a dense fibrous band left in the place of the supernumerary rib. Some authors believe that the presence of a cervical rib also signals the presence of a prefixed type of plexus (small T1 nerve and major contribution to the plexus from C4). My operative findings support this finding only occasionally.

Anterior Scalene Anomalies

The many abnormal origins and insertions of the anterior scalene muscle are the "linchpin" on which the remaining plexus anomalies are built. The anterior scalene is described in every textbook of anatomy to take origin from the anterior tubercles of the third through sixth cervical vertebrae and lies in its entirety anterior to the plexus. The insertion is on the scalene tubercle of the first rib. The scalene muscles assist in flexion and lateral flexion of the neck. The function of the scalene as an accessory muscle of respiration has been questioned. The nerve supply to the scalene muscles is from the cervical plexus.

Abnormalities of the anterior scalene can affect the low plexus or the high plexus. The low plexus anomalies have been well described since the beginning of the understanding of TOS.[1,16] The importance of the upper plexus muscle anomalies has been recognized only more recently as has the variability of symptoms related to minor variations in the exact nature of the compression.

The insertion of the anterior scalene may be anomalously attached posteriorly and laterally on the first rib or onto the pleura (actually Sibson's fascia). This attachment serves to fix the lower plexus posteriorly and is more of an inciting factor when there are other structures posterior to the plexus that force it anteriorly. The insertion may be split, with a portion of the muscle posterior to the artery, which also fixes the plexus posteriorly.

Anomalies of the muscle origin superiorly are extremely common. The most frequent anomaly is a splitting of fibers around the C5 nerve root; this can vary from a tiny slip of tendinous tissue to a large mass of muscle. The muscle origins may also pass beneath C6 (Fig. 23-3) and affect the proximal C5, C6, or C7 nerve roots. The fibrous fixation of these proximal anomalies also may extend superiorly and create fixation to the nerves of the cervical plexus. The fusion of the muscle bundles to the C5 and C6 nerve roots may be congenital or may be related to injury with scar fixation. The fibrous tethering restricts nerve gliding. The layer of fascia that invests the anterior scalene extends upward in the neck and may tether portions of the cervical plexus to create the neck and facial symptoms often found with upper plexus TOS cases. Roos[47] found this type of abnormality in 76% of dissections in patients with TOS.

Perhaps the most important anomaly to recognize is the complete posterior position (Fig. 23-4) of the anterior scalene, which places the C5 and C6 nerve roots in jeopardy for injury by an inexperienced surgeon during anterior approaches to the plexus.[51] We have seen many cases in which nerve roots were transected when this anatomical variation was not recognized by the prior surgeon.

There are occasionally unusual medial origins of the anterior scalene. The most inferior of these may compress the subclavian artery.

Middle Scalene Anomalies

Middle scalene anomalies are less well recognized than anterior anomalies but are equally important.[52] The insertion commonly extends well forward on the first rib, occasionally forward of the anterior scalene insertion. This extension may throw the entire plexus forward, into anterior scalene abnormalities, and even against the clavicle. With the arms abducted and supinated, any motion of the arms in a plane posterior to the midline causes the nerves of the plexus to be stretched taut over the forward-placed middle scalene. These abnormalities are particularly important when the anterior border of the muscle is fibrous and sharply demarcated—the so-called middle scalene band. There may be slips of the middle scalene origin that arise anterior to the plane of the lower portions of the plexus and trap the lower plexus against the anterior scalene.

Congenital Fibromuscular Bands

Roos[47] described and categorized 10 types of tissue bands that contribute to the compromise of the nerves of the brachial plexus. *Type 1* passes from the tip of a short cervical rib to the first rib. *Type 2* is a dense band that passes in the position of a cervical rib from the tip of an elongated transverse process of C7. *Type 3* is a rib-to-rib band that passes from the posterior to anterior first rib, elevating the lower trunk or T1 nerve root. Roos believed that type 3 was the most common anomaly he encountered. *Type 4* is the above-mentioned forward abnormal middle scalene attachment to the first rib. *Types 5* and *6* are the scalenus minimus anomalies. *Type 7* is a thin tendinous band that passes from the middle scalene muscle to the sternum under the subclavian vessels. *Type 8* is similar and arises from the anterior scalene. *Type 9* is a dense broad band of tissue that is like a drumhead through which the T1 nerve root must pass; this is what Sunderland[26] believed was the extension of Sibson's fascia. *Type 10* is similar to type 3 but extends to the back of the sternum or costal cartilage.

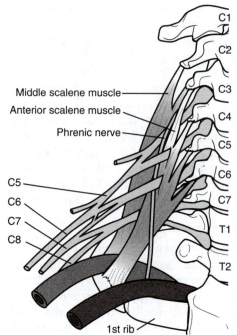

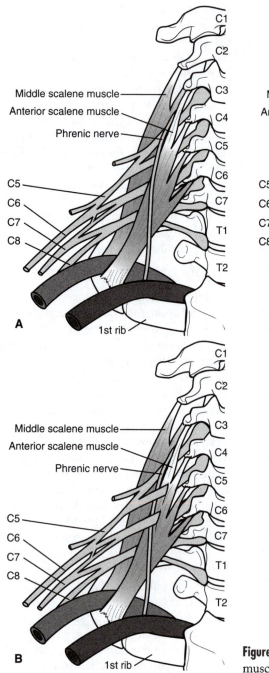

Figure 23-3 Typical anatomy of the scalene muscles within the thoracic outlet.

Scalenus Minimus and Pleuralis

Scalenus minimus and scalenus pleuralis are muscles that arise from the anterior transverse processes of C7 and occasionally C6 and insert onto either the first rib (Fig. 23-5) or the pleura. These muscles, also known as the Albinus muscles, are variably present, unrelated to the presence of any of the other described anomalies. The scalenus minimus muscle passes anterior to the lower trunk or the C8 and T1 nerve roots to insert onto the first rib. A scalenus pleuralis variation may be identical except for inserting onto the pleura anteriorly. Occasionally, there is a double insertion onto rib and pleura. Uncommonly, the scalenus pleuralis variant may pass between the C8 and T1 nerve roots, in which case the lower trunk is not formed until the roots pass beyond the first rib. These muscles vary greatly in their mass, angle of origin and insertion, and fibrous content. The exact nature and position of the lower plexus entrapment may vary significantly.

Axillary Arch Muscles

The axillary arch muscle of Langer and the sternalis muscle are two muscles of the lateral chest that can cause peripheral nerve compression lateral to the

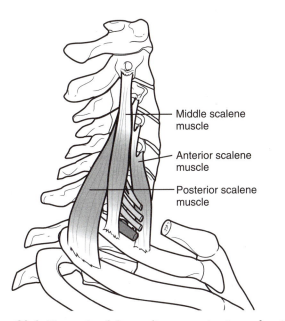

Figure 23-4 The path of the median nerve is pictured as it enters the forearm and hand.

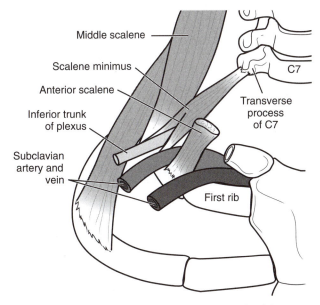

Figure 23-5 The scalenus minimus and pleuralis (also known as the Albinus muscles) arise primarily from the transverse processes of C7 and insert on the first rib or occasionally the pleura and are variably present. These muscles vary greatly in their insertion, angle of origin, and fibrous content.

"thoracic outlet."[53] The muscle of Langer is a broad flat muscle that originates from the tendon of the latissimus and passes anteriorly to insert anterior to the bicipital groove next to the pectoralis major insertion. It may trap the ulnar and median nerves high in the axilla just distal to the plexus and cause symptoms similar to lower trunk or medial cord entrapment. Supposedly present in 2% to 3% of the population, the muscle of Langer was found only twice in our series and has seldom been described in modern texts. The presence of this anomaly should be considered in patients with immediate treatment failures after supraclavicular plexus dissections.

Radiation Fibrosis

Radiation therapy is a well-known cause of scarring and fibrosis. The plexus may be included in the radiation field in the treatment of breast cancer and in the treatment of the mediastinum in lung cancer and lymphomas. Acute radiation injury to the plexus is uncommon in the modern era. The delayed scarring that occurs after radiation therapy progresses slowly over time. There is danger in dissection of the plexus after radiation therapy from interference with the blood supply within the nerves, which may result in severely compromised nerve function.[54]

Other Fibrous Anomalies

Fixation of C7 and C8 in a dense fibrous sheath that appears almost like sausage casing is frequently found.[25,33,47] This type of anomaly may extend out to fuse the entire middle and lower trunks. Similarly, the upper plexus can be entrapped in this dense matting. Based on its location, we have labeled this tissue mesoepineural fibrosis. This mesoepineural fixation is due to trauma, where hemorrhage and oxidative reaction results in fixed scarring. These types of fixation are extremely important in patients with symptoms associated with arm motion. When the arm is abducted, the nerves of the lower plexus are required to move differential distances similar to the reins of a team of horses. When the nerve roots and trunks are fixed together, significant traction on the nerves occurs with motion. These fibrous sheaths also create significant compression when placed under traction, similar to the tightening of a Chinese finger trap.

Clavicle Abnormalities

Clavicular fractures may heal with exuberant callus or may heal improperly with posterior angulation.[55] This posterior angulation can easily cause pressure on the brachial plexus with entrapment against the first rib. First rib resection rather than clavicle resection is generally recommended to relieve the plexus-level compression in active patients.

Cervical Rib Anomalies

Cervical ribs are the most easily understood congenital anomaly and the most easily documented. Anteroposterior and oblique cervical radiographs are the best way to document a cervical rib.[50,56] However, the clinician needs to view the radiographs personally, rather than accept a report of "normal cervical spine." The rib may go unnoticed in a search for more serious acute pathology. A chest x-ray is not optimal for evaluation of cervical rib anomalies because the standard posteroanterior view throws the shoulders forward and may hide the extra rib behind the first rib.

Cervical spine radiographs are much more sensitive at the present time for rib anomalies than computed tomography and magnetic resonance imaging scans. The "slices" viewed on magnetic resonance imaging and computed tomography images make it difficult to reconstruct mentally the presence of these types of rib anomalies in three dimensions. Computer programs that reconstruct the images in three dimensions can enhance the workup of patients with TOS through visualization of these anomalies and the ability to prove more clearly their impact on the surrounding nerves and vessels.

The radiographs of the spine should be obtained in at least four views. The oblique views of the spine are enlightening and often give a much better idea for how far the rib may be angled forward to interfere with the nerves of the plexus (Fig. 23-6). The cervical rib may occasionally be entirely within the substance of the middle scalene and not directly causative of any pathology.

The length of cervical ribs is often discussed relative to the likelihood of the ribs causing symptoms. A short rib that is angled forward is more likely to cause severe deficits than a long rib, which may even be fused to the first rib. The few cases of "true neurogenic" TOS that I have seen have had sharp, forward-pointing ribs that indent the C8 nerve root from behind. All rib anomalies must be considered a significant predisposition to

the development of TOS after some type of inciting event.

Elongated C7 Transverse Process

Cervical spine films should always be carefully inspected for the presence of an elongated transverse process of the C7 vertebra. This process is defined as a projection beyond the plane of the transverse process of T1 and is easily visualized and measured. The importance lies in the anomalous attachments of scalenus minimus, scalenus pleuralis, and fibrous bands, which are commonly found associated with these elongated processes. In the angled cervical spine films, the space-occupying nature of this anomaly can be appreciated.[57]

First Rib Anomalies

Deformity of the first rib is much less common than the presence of a cervical rib.[58,59] However, a surprising number of first rib deformities exist. Fusion of the first to second rib at a point even with the location of the scalene tubercle occurs most commonly. The insertion of the anterior scalene is most obvious, but the middle scalene also may be significantly displaced, and the possibility of pressure on (particularly the lower) plexus may occur. The first rib may also be displaced superiorly, which lessens the already compromised space at the thoracic inlet (outlet); this particularly predisposes the lower plexus to the effects of downward traction of the arm.

Tumors of the first rib as a cause of TOS have been described by Melliere et al.[60] Fracture of the first rib may heal with protuberant callus, which may also compromise the thoracic outlet. First rib fractures are usually associated with severe trauma, and injury to the scalene muscles and direct plexus injury can easily occur.

Postural Abnormalities

Postural abnormalities can contribute significantly to the development of TOS. Most clinicians recognize the concept of the "droopy shoulder syndrome."[61] When the angle of the clavicle is below parallel from the junction with the sternum, the entire shoulder girdle causes traction on the plexus. When there is an underlying congenital structural abnormality, the malpositioned shoulder may in and of itself create the onset of symptoms. Distal injuries in the arm can also contribute greatly to the development of new-onset TOS symptoms. The weight of a heavy forearm cast can create downward forces on the arm.

Fatigue of the scapular elevator muscles in large-breasted women may eventually create drag on the plexus over the first rib. Breast reduction surgery may be warranted in some cases if a trial of physical therapy is unsuccessful at improving the posture and the symptoms. Pregnancy may similarly initiate symptoms in susceptible individuals as the breasts enlarge. Breast

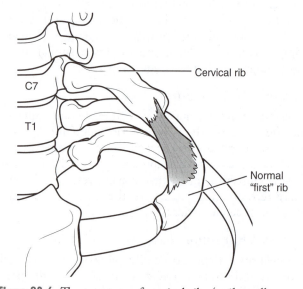

Figure 23-6 The presence of cervical ribs (unilaterally or bilaterally) may predispose an individual to vascular and neurogenic dysfunction within the outlet.

reconstructive surgery can also lead to compromise of the plexus by altering the space at the distal plexus, behind the pectoralis minor.[62,63]

Unusual positioning for long periods can also cause severe problems at the plexus level. There have been many descriptions of lower plexus neurogenic and acute arterial occlusive events occurring after coronary bypass surgery and lateral thoracotomies. The commonly accepted wisdom has been to implicate improper positioning and overzealous sternal retraction causing direct clavicle–to–first rib compression. It is more reasonable to think that the problems arise in individuals who have an anatomical predisposition from one of the many types of tissue bands. Particularly in the lateral thoracotomy position, an axillary roll or beanbag to elevate the chest wall away from the operating table is imperative.

The pivotal concept that unites these various etiologies of TOS is that TOS is often a dynamic problem. Until an event, or series of events, occurs that causes an alteration in the microanatomy of the tissues surrounding the plexus, patients may have no symptoms of any kind.

Traction Plexopathy

The main focus of the TOS type of brachial plexopathy discussed to this point has focused on compressive forces on the nerves. Duchenne[64] described traction brachial palsy in 1872, referring to an obstetrical injury to the upper plexus. Later Erb[65] described injury to the upper plexus in adults secondary to trauma, of which motorcycle accidents are the predominant cause at the present time. These injuries are often generally lumped into "Erb's palsy" or "Erb-Duchenne palsy." Klumpke[66] subsequently described traction injury to the lower plexus. A severe injury may result in avulsion of the nerve root from the spine. The plexus may also rupture within the brachial plexus. Less severe traction or trauma results in a stretch injury, also known as a neurapraxia, from which there can be near-complete recovery. The sequelae of a stretch or neurapraxic injury may result in scarring and fixation of the nerves of the plexus. The same injury may cause a stretch injury of any of the other soft tissue structures near the plexus, causing bleeding, scarring, and fixation of the adjacent nerves. Horsley[67] is credited with the idea that brachial plexus lesions are caused by injuries that tend to spread the head and shoulders apart and to stretch the plexus.

The scarring and fixation of different portions of the plexus are easily seen at surgery and help explain some of the reasons why brachial plexus/TOS is misunderstood. Decompressive-only procedures (first rib resection or scalenotomy), which do not address the scarring and fixation of the nerves, result in continued symptoms with full range of motion of the shoulder. The upper plexus is placed under maximum stretch with the "waiter's tip" position of the arm. Scarring around

the C5, C6 roots, upper trunk, or lateral cord leads to manifestation of symptoms when this position is exaggerated. Similarly, with the arm held laterally at 90° and with the palm extended, the fixation at the C8, T1 roots, lower trunk, and medial cord level results in reproducible symptoms in the appropriate distributions. Close study of the anatomy of the brachial plexus and its terminal nerves enables understanding of the symptoms caused by traction and the resultant scarring or fixation of the various areas of the plexus.

With the contribution that traction and compressive forces and fixation impairments add to the more easily understood concepts of compressive neuropathy of the plexus, one can explore the interaction associated with symptoms originating from the more distal terminal nerves. The concepts of "double crush" and "triple crush" injuries are somewhat disputed. However, if the symptoms caused by variations in posturing as noted earlier are considered, it is easy to understand how injury and subsequent fixation at other points along the peripheral nerves create additive symptoms in different positions.

Complex Regional Pain Syndrome

The International Association for the Study of Pain[68] proposed a new term, *complex regional pain syndrome*, to replace RSD. CRPS is a poorly understood symptom complex that affects a small but important group of patients who have had some type of trauma to the upper extremity. "Shoulder-hand syndrome" and "causalgia" are two of the more common terms used interchangeably with CRPS.[69,70] "Causalgia" is derived from the Greek words *causos* meaning "heat" and *algos* meaning "pain." The term "causalgia" was coined and the first full description was written by Weir Mitchell during the Civil War.[71] Many other terms have been used, which further enforces the misunderstanding (Box 23-1).

BOX 23-1

Common Synonyms Found in the Literature for Complex Regional Pain Syndrome

Reflex sympathetic dystrophy
Sudeck's atrophy, reflex
Reflex neurovascular dystrophy
Shoulder-hand syndrome
Algoneurodystrophy
Causalgia
Vasomotor atrophy
Pseudomotor atrophy
Steinbrocker syndrome
Erythromelalgia
Algodystrophy
Posttraumatic dystrophy

CRPS is further divided into two types.[69] Type 1 represents cases classically referred to as RSD. Type 2 corresponds to causalgia. The essential differentiating feature between the two types using this nomenclature is that causalgia is associated with a major nerve injury. The trauma believed to be associated with RSD is often considered "trivial." There is no definitive test for RSD, causalgia, or CRPS.

It is common for patients to be labeled with the diagnosis of RSD or CRPS because of slight mottling of the hand, unexplained pain, pain with arm motion, edema, sweating, or similar complaints that may be associated with RSD.[72] RSD should be excluded if a more definitive diagnosis can be made, and a diligent search for other causes should be undertaken before allowing this diagnosis of exclusion to be made.

Drucker et al.[73] divided RSD into three stages based on clinical presentation. Stage 1 is a reversible state characterized by hyperhydrosis, warmth, erythema, rapid nail growth, and edema of the hand. Resolution of symptoms may occur after treatment or spontaneously. In stage 2, there is mottling and coldness of the skin associated with brittle nails and increased pain. Osteoporosis is always present. Spontaneous resolution is rare, and response blocks or sympathectomy is less likely to be beneficial. Stage 3 shows a fixed atrophic hand with severe osteoporosis. There is seldom any response to therapy. There is clearly some overlap between the various stages, but this framework serves to divide the syndrome reasonably to allow appropriate expectations from interventions to be forwarded. Schwartzman et al.[74] published an excellent review in 1987.

CRPS remains a series of symptom complex descriptions, not a freestanding diagnosis, in most patients. A patient presenting with CRPS-type symptoms should be thoroughly evaluated for evidence of plexus-level pathology. The relationship between plexus injuries and the development of RSD was recognized in the past but has been understated in more recent literature. To quote from Barnes' 1952 article on causalgia in Seddon's text[75]: "Multiple nerve injuries are commonly present and causalgia may be associated with all. In the upper limb there is always an incomplete lesion of the lower trunk or medial cord of the brachial plexus or the median nerve." Although our practice may see a skewed population, there has been evidence of significant plexus conduction deficits in all cases of "true RSD" that we have studied. The findings at surgery in this group of patients uniformly show extensive fixation of the plexus to the surrounding tissues, particularly at the level of the lower trunk secondary to the presence of a Roos band or scalenus minimus type of anomaly; this fits the type of injury usually seen.

The most confusing aspect of CRPS is that the development and severity of CRPS have not been directly correlated with the severity of the injury.

Classically, development of CRPS follows a traumatic injury to peripheral nerve.[76] The injury frequently is caused by the hand being caught in some type of machinery such as a punch press or roller. A neuroma or peripheral nerve entrapment may precede the development of the RSD symptoms.[69] Careful history of the injury may show that the injury resulted in traction to the brachial plexus as the patient attempted to extract the hand from the machinery. The weight of a cast on the arm may cause traction to the plexus.

Fixation of the C7 nerve root (middle trunk) to the C8 nerve root or lower trunk is also found almost universally in these patients.[72] The traction or fixation signs that are elicited by the provocative postures on examination have profound implications. It is probably safe to say that these signs do not develop unless the patient has more than one point of traction and fixation along the length of the nerve (i.e., the "double crush" phenomenon).

Other authors have clinically implicated sympathetic dysfunction as a significant problem in patients with TOS. Urschel and Kourlis[77] performed a sympathectomy in all patients during transaxillary rib resection. This adjunct to surgery was found to be of limited value early in my experience and was ended in 1983. The residual neurological complaints after transaxillary rib resection appear in most cases to be related more to incomplete decompression and failure to release the traction or fixation at areas of the plexus not treated with transaxillary rib resection than the presence of sympathetic dystrophy.

Several issues remain confusing. The severity of injury is not clearly related to the severity of CRPS. The response to therapy is extremely variable. Finally, untreated CRPS usually "burns out" after several years, and the pain eventually begins to subside, although the hand may remain nearly functionless.

Surgery

Failure of conservative therapy is an indication for surgery if the symptoms are severe enough to warrant intervention. There are a few instances in which surgery should be undertaken rapidly, sometimes without a trial of physical therapy. Development of muscle atrophy is an indication for immediate intervention before further loss of motor units ensues rapidly. Immediate surgery is indicated in cases of venous and arterial thrombosis. In these instances, decompression of the vessels should begin soon after clot removal or lysis. We also believe that extremely positive vascular occlusive signs with minimal arm motion should prompt early intervention because of the risk of arterial complications.

The type of procedure recommended is based on many factors. There are presently two major approaches to surgical decompression of the thoracic outlet: transaxillary first rib resection and comprehensive supraclavicular plexus decompression with scalenectomy. Other procedures such as scalenotomy are of historical interest only.

In cases of lower trunk compression only, without a history of significant trauma, the transaxillary approach described by Roos[19] is the approach of choice. When there has been significant trauma of the "whiplash" type, the likelihood of fibrous fixation of the upper plexus makes transaxillary resection of the first rib a poor choice. In this instance, we prefer a supraclavicular approach. A few surgeons prefer performing first rib resections via a posterior approach. These procedures should be performed only by surgeons with specific interest in this field.

Transaxillary First Rib Resection

Roos[19] described the transaxillary approach for resecting the first rib in 1966. Before this time, the posterior thoracotomy approach was favored, similar to rib resection for thoracoplasty for tuberculosis. The transaxillary approach proved to be much easier technically and came into favor by most chest and vascular surgeons. The theory for first rib resection lies in the concept that TOS is a disease of the lower trunk and medial cord of the plexus, caused by numerous anomalous structures that attach to the first rib or pleura and are accessible through this approach.

Roos[19,23,24] described this approach in great detail in many publications and more recently made a videotape of the procedure, which should be reviewed by anyone who plans to use this technique. The written description in Rutherford's *Textbook of Vascular Surgery*[78] is very clearly presented and is recommended for the many technical details of the procedure. Urschel and Razzuk[79] suggested using a videoscope to assist visualization of the nerves and vessels at the apex.

In the hands of experienced surgeons such as Roos, the transaxillary approach is safe, and the risk of nerve injury or vascular injury is minimal. However, for surgeons with less experience with the procedure, the risks are quite high. It is very common to see on follow-up cervical spine films that a long length of first rib has been left in place posteriorly. When this type of radiological evidence is found, one can be sure that an inadequate decompression of the lower plexus has been performed. Other problems encountered with the transaxillary approach are inadequate removal of the myofascial bands and the very annoying incidence of intercostobrachial nerve neuralgia. Patients with fixed adhesions of the upper plexus (traction or fixation injury) may have increased symptoms after transaxillary first rib resections as the scalene muscle retracts superiorly. If this retraction occurs, an early

supraclavicular resection of residual scalene muscle is indicated.

Scalenotomy and Scalenectomy

Division of the anterior scalene or partial resection as practiced for many years as first described by Adson and Coffey[1] relieves symptoms in a moderate number of patients. It is difficult to predict which patients with isolated lower trunk symptoms will respond to scalenectomy alone. As has been well documented by numerous anatomical studies, there are many other structures that can create lower plexus symptoms other than anomalous attachments of the anterior scalene. In patients with only posterior displacement of the scalene attachments to the first rib or pleura, the resection of the scalene should relieve lower plexus compression.

When combined with resection of other anomalous bands, scalenectomy increases the likelihood of satisfactory decompression of the lower plexus. Other problems cannot be resolved by partial lower anterior scalenectomy, which has resulted in development of the concept of total plexus decompression.

Total Brachial Plexus Decompression

Limitations of the transaxillary first rib resection led to reevaluation of scalenectomy. The original scalenotomy procedure of Naffziger and Grant[80] consisted simply of division of the anterior scalene above its attachment to the first rib. When scalenectomy was performed in the past, it was divided from the first rib and resected above the C7 level. Recurrences particularly at the level of the upper plexus were common enough to cause continuing reevaluation of the procedure. The concept of traction and fixation of the lower plexus was clearly understood; however, continuing symptoms from the upper plexus remained an issue. The interdigitating bundles of anterior scalene between the roots of the upper trunk and middle trunk eventually received the attention they warranted.

The patient is placed supine on the operating table. Nonparalyzing general endotracheal anesthesia is administered so that nerves can be tested throughout the procedure. The endotracheal tube should be brought out of the nonoperative side of the mouth to avoid kinking and provide access for the anesthesiologist. The head is tilted away from the operative side approximately 20°, and the chin is elevated. We use a vacuum beanbag to hold the head in place. The entire neck, anterior chest, and arm are prepared and draped. The impervious stockinet that has been placed on the arm is clipped to the chest wall to keep it in place throughout the procedure. Slight downward traction is placed on the arm by clipping a Kling wrap that has been wrapped about the stockinet to the drapes.

The incision, which splits the lateral border of the sternocleidomastoid, is made in the skin line 2 to 3 cm above the clavicle depending on the size of the patient.

The incision is taken through the platysma muscle. Hemostats are obtained with electrocautery. The lateral border of the sternocleidomastoid is mobilized extensively, and the dissection is carried down to the deep cervical investing fascia. The fascia is opened superior to the omohyoid muscle and is widely separated; this exposes the scalene fat pad. An avascular plane is developed either medially or laterally around the fat pad to avoid venous and lymphatic vessels.

The fat pad is retracted in a self-retaining retractor. The anterior scalene can now be seen. The position of the phrenic nerve is immediately carefully noted. At this time, the upper trunk of the plexus can be encountered lying anterior to the scalene, which must be recognized. When the phrenic nerve lies on the anterolateral aspect of the scalene, it must be mobilized with its surrounding fascia over its full length so that it can be carefully kept medial out of harm's way throughout the procedure. When the phrenic nerve originates directly off of the upper trunk, it is quite short, and the dissection must tediously work around it because it cannot be retracted.

The medial and lateral aspects of the lower anterior scalene are freed exposing the subclavian artery. A plane is developed between the artery and the muscle with a large right-angled clamp. A Kocher clamp is placed across the muscle, carefully observing the phrenic nerve. A bipolar cautery is used to detach the anterior scalene from the first rib, and the muscle is retracted superiorly.

There are usually numerous small vessels along the medial aspect of the muscle, which are also divided with the bipolar cautery. Any aberrant portions of the muscle distally are removed with the specimen. As the dissection continues superiorly, the anterior scalene origins from the transverse processes of C4, C5, and C6 almost constantly split and pass between the C5, C6, and C7 nerve roots. These anomalies occur in almost every case of upper plexus TOS. Using blunt and sharp dissection as appropriate, these slips of muscle are dissected away from the upper nerve roots and divided at the origins from the transverse processes. The use of bipolar electrocautery makes this dissection safe and hemostatic. Care is taken to avoid the branches to the long thoracic nerve, which emanate from the posterior aspect of C5, C6, and usually C7.

After the anterior scalene is totally removed, the C7 nerve root/middle trunk is identified and encircled with a vessel loop. Sometimes C7 is fused to C8 with a dense matted epineural fixation that must be dissected away to free the nerves completely. The subclavian artery is encircled with a vessel loop. If there are any branches of the subclavian passing through the lower plexus, they are divided with silk ties.

If a scalenus minimus muscle is present, it is encountered at this time and is resected. Any other anterior Roos bands are resected. The lower trunk is exposed and is also encircled with a vessel loop. Any anomalies of the middle scalene are resected at this time. When the middle scalene has a firm fibrous anterior border, it is partially resected. There are also quite commonly portions of the origins of the middle scalene that pass forward to lie in a plane anterior to the nerve roots. These slips of muscle are also resected.

When a cervical rib is present, it is now resected along with any muscle attachments. The periosteum is removed with the rib to avoid the possibility of regrowth of the rib. Kerrison rongeurs are used to remove the rib proximally so that the nerves can be fully visualized as the rib is removed.

When all of the muscle anomalies have been resected, attention is directed to the nerves themselves. The fusion of C7 to either the upper or the lower trunk is quite common. The mesoepineural fixation of the various trunks must be separated to allow the nerves of the plexus to move through the full ranges of shoulder motion. The need to release this fixation is apparent when the arm is moved during surgery. The tension on the various trunks is assessed at different positions during motion. Nerves that are significantly taut either require further mobilization and relief of the mesoepineural fixation or are fixed at other levels distally. The roots, trunks, and divisions of the plexus can be mobilized without fear of devascularization. There is never any bleeding from the nerves when the dense scar is removed, indicating that the blood supply of the nerves is internal at this level. Equally important is the complete lack of any nerve functional loss when this type of dissection is done. This is not an internal neurolysis.

Assessment of the need for a first rib resection is made. If there is compression of the plexus between the first rib and clavicle or if there is evidence of the lower trunk being pulled tight over the rib with arm motion, a first rib resection is done. The first rib resection can be accomplished safely via this same incision except in extremely muscular individuals. The middle scalene attachments to the first rib are cleared from the superior surface of the rib. Care must be taken to be sure of the position of the long thoracic nerve, which often passes through the substance of the middle scalene. The most posterior aspect of the first rib is transected serially with Kerrison rongeurs. The intercostal muscle is separated from the first rib by dissection with either blunt or sharp scissors. A good view of the anterior rib can be obtained by forward displacement of the shoulder. Using angled duckbill or Kerrison rongeurs, the rib is transected anteriorly and removed. In some cases, piecemeal resection is necessary.

A sympathectomy is easily done from this approach if required. The pleura is bluntly separated from the ribs at the posteromedial rib and retracted forward. Finger palpation easily identifies the sympathetic chain at the level of the second rib. The sympathetic chain is elevated on a right angle clamp and grasped with the right angle. Dissection is the taken distally at least to the fourth rib, and the chain is divided. Through this approach, the stellate ganglion is easily seen. The efferent branch to the T1 nerve root can be seen, and the chain is divided at this level. In theory, there should never be a Horner's syndrome if the sympathetic chain is divided at this level. I have seen several cases in which there were no eye symptoms but there was absence of facial sweating on the operated side and two cases of mild permanent Horner's syndrome despite carefully dividing the sympathetic chain at a level that was clearly below the stellate ganglion.

The wound is drained with a 7-mm silicone drain, which is brought out lateral to the external jugular vein. The scalene fat pad is tacked back in place over the plexus. The platysma is closed with 3-0 absorbable polyglactin suture. The skin is closed with a 4-0 pull-out polypropylene. The drain is left in place until there is minimal drainage over a 24-hour period. Therapy is begun on the first postoperative day. The initial goal of therapy is to maintain full range of motion and proper posture.

Combined Anterior and Transaxillary Procedure

Because of dissatisfaction with the completeness of plexus decompression that could be accomplished with the transaxillary and the anterior approach, the concept of a combined procedure was introduced. Roos[25] continued to recommend the combined procedure, largely because of comfort with the transaxillary approach to rib resection. The first rib can be removed from the anterior approach, but this is technically difficult in heavyset or muscular individuals. When rib resection is deemed necessary, it should be performed by whatever technique with which the surgeon is most comfortable.

Robotic Surgery

Robotic surgery gives remarkable views of the plexus and vessels of the thoracic inlet area. As instrumentation is developed that aids in the proper dissection and protection of the nerves and vessels, the precision allowed will undoubtedly add to the ability of surgeons trained in these techniques to obtain excellent results.

Complications

Numerous postsurgical complications can occur. Most can be avoided with careful attention to surgical detail. Careful hemostasis prevents significant hematoma formation, which increases the likelihood of recurrent scar fixation. Permanent silk ties should be used for ligatures rather than surgical clips. Clips can get caught in the surgical drain and be pulled out when the drain is removed. An infected pseudoaneursym of the subclavian artery resulted in one such case and prompted conversion to ties for all vessels. The thoracic duct on the left and the accessory duct on the right must be avoided at the inferomedial end of the scalene fat pad. If a significant amount of chyle is seen in the drain postoperatively, the incision should be reexplored. The proteinaceous fluid of a chylous leak leaves extremely dense scar around the plexus if not repaired immediately.

Phrenic nerve injury occurs in a few cases despite careful attention to detail and attempts to avoid undue traction by retractors. Diaphragmatic palsy usually recovers over several months. There were only two cases of permanent palsy in our series.

There were two cases of permanent plexus injury in our series. Both occurred in patients who had prior radiation therapy for carcinoma of the breast. Supraclavicular brachial plexus dissection should be undertaken with extreme caution in patients who have undergone prior radiation therapy near the plexus. If possible, radiation therapy ports should be adjusted to avoid the plexus in patients with a diagnosis of TOS. Another patient who had a diagnosis of stage 3 RSD experienced significant motor dysfunction of the entire upper extremity despite conduction studies which showed that function had returned to normal and lack of atrophy. Temporary motor dysfunction occurs occasionally, more likely involving the upper trunk from traction on the nerves as they are dissected from the dense scar tissue. Injury to the long thoracic nerve can easily occur if the nerve is displaced anteriorly within the substance of the middle scalene. Care must be taken to section the muscle serially over a right angle clamp or similar technique to prevent winging of the scapula.

Mild numbness and paresthesias are common from manipulation of the plexus early after plexus decompression, but recovery is rapid. There is sometimes hypersensitivity in the peripheral nerve distribution as the distal signals return.

Pneumothorax from pleural entry should not be problematic if a Jackson-Pratt type of drain that has a one-way valve at the bulb is used. At the time of drain removal, the drain site must be treated like a chest tube and covered with an occlusive dressing.

Horner's syndrome may occur after sympathectomy, even if the division of the sympathetic chain is carefully done below the efferent nerve to the T1 nerve root. Interestingly, with surgical sympathectomy there is often absence of the expected unilateral facial sweating with miosis or lid droop. According to anatomical descriptions, this should not occur. There is more variation in the level of fibers involved in development of a Horner's syndrome than has been appreciated.

Vascular injury is rare but potentially hazardous. If the artery has been severely entrapped by anomalous bands or muscles, it may become fragile to manipulation as in the original description of scalenotomy by Adson and Coffey.[1] Some slight subintimal dissection occurs infrequently and has presented no significant sequelae. Manipulation of the artery should be kept to a minimum. Venous injury most commonly occurs as the anterior scalene is being removed from the first rib in the anterior approach. During transaxillary rib resection, the subclavian vein is at greatest risk during resection of the anterior portion of the rib. Control of the vein when injured during an anterior supraclavicular approach usually requires a subclavicular counterincision. There has been only one significant venous injury in our series.

Results

The success of surgical procedures for TOS can be divided into short-term and long-term results. The success rate has been shown to deteriorate over time through the first 2 years because of numerous factors.[30] Recurrent injury and failure to conform to the therapy program are the most common causes of failure. Rear-end automobile collisions are the leading cause of TOS as well as the leading cause of treatment failure.[33] Although the concept that postoperative therapy is equally important as the surgery is stressed from the initial consultation, one of the most frustrating problems we see are patients who stop the daily exercise program after 3, 4, or 5 months because they are "feeling fine."

Successful surgical results depend on the definition used for determination of success. Several points must be stressed. Complete relief of symptoms is unlikely except in nontraumatic cases limited to the lower plexus. In this instance, a transaxillary rib resection can achieve superior results that are likely to be permanent. Recurrent scarring about the upper plexus is unlikely, and the likelihood of new-onset upper plexus symptoms secondary to muscle abnormalities is low. When there are upper plexus symptoms, there are muscle abnormalities. These cases, in which transaxillary rib resection is recommended, manifest in a more straightforward manner and tend to have fewer of the ancillary manifestations described in this chapter. Cases related to post-traumatic and repetitive injuries are more likely to have other associated problems, be of a more chronic nature, and have more significant perineural traction and fixation.

If return to prior levels of activity is required for inclusion as a good or excellent result, a large number of patients would be eliminated. Demands that patients resume such occupations as assembly line work, heavy construction, or overhead activities cannot often be met without significant likelihood of recurrence. When there is willingness on the part of insurance companies, businesses, and the patients themselves to aid the patient's return to the workplace with appropriate accommodation, rather than limit the patient to the preinjury status, the entire workers' compensation process is improved. It is also incumbent on the patient to accept some responsibility by avoiding avocations that would be likely to cause reinjury.

A small number of patients experience recurrence despite careful follow-up and compliance. In the series by Sanders et al.[33], the delayed poor results occurred equally with transaxillary rib resection, anterior scalenectomy, and supraclavicular rib resection. The immediate improved results showed a 93% cumulative success rate at 3 months, 81% at 1 year, and 74% at 5 years. Our data mirror the report of Sanders et al.[33] if limited to TOS procedures only.

Some of the 1-year failures reported by Roos[23,24] and Sanders et al.[33] represent less a failure of the primary TOS surgery than a failure to recognize the significant associated peripheral neuropathy ("double crush"). Early in my experience, the number of immediate failures from transaxillary rib resection despite a technically satisfactory procedure caused a reevaluation of the approach. It became apparent after study that upper plexus involvement was found in these post-traumatic cases and that transaxillary rib resection alone worsened the upper plexus symptoms in a large number of patients. The nearly constant anterior scalene anomalies at the upper plexus level had not been previously recognized. Marked relief of upper plexus symptoms, headache, and facial pain can be achieved only if completed decompression of the upper plexus is performed.

CASE STUDY

SC is a starting pitcher for his college baseball team. Now 21 years old, SC has been pitching competitively for 15 years. He has averaged 200 innings each of the past 2 years, which is a marked increase over his workload the prior 3 to 5 years. Over the past 6 months, SC has noticed that his right (throwing) hand feels cooler than his left. The right hand sometimes appears blue and mottled after much pitching. There is no swelling of the hand. SC approached the trainer with his concerns and was referred to a vascular specialist. After an extensive physical examination, the vascular surgeon determined the working diagnosis to be arterial TOS secondary to chronic overuse of the upper extremity and possible aberrant congenital fascial bands within the thoracic outlet. Diagnostic imaging tests were ordered. SC was instructed to stop pitching immediately.

Case Study Questions

1. Which of the following arteries is most likely involved in arterial TOC in SC?
   a. Subclavian artery
   b. Brachial artery
   c. Aorta
   d. Radial artery

2. Aberrant congenital bands associated with arterial TOC typically originate on which structures?
   a. First rib and spinous process
   b. First rib and transverse process
   c. Spinous process and transverse process
   d. Transverse process and coracoid process

3. In arterial TOS, which of the following tests would typically be negative?
   a. Halstead
   b. Wright
   c. Adson
   d. Shoulder impingement

4. Arterial TOS is often confused with which of the following conditions?
   a. CRPS
   b. Raynaud's phenomenon
   c. Multiple sclerosis
   d. Venous TOS

5. The presence of which of the following diagnostic signs may lead to a diagnosis of subclavian artery aneurysm?
   a. Hypoactive deep tendon reflexes in the involved arm
   b. A supraclavicular pulsatile mass
   c. Hand and wrist edema
   d. Supraclavicular Tinel's sign

References

1. Adson AW, Coffey JR. Cervical rib: a method of anterior approach for relief of symptoms by division of the scalenus anticus. *Ann Surg.* 1927;85:839–857.
2. Peet RM, Hendriksen JD, Anderson TP, Martin GM. Thoracic outlet syndrome: evaluation of the therapeutic exercise program. *Proc Mayo Clin.* 1956;31:281–287.
3. Borchardt M. Symptomatologie und Therapie der Halsrippen. *Berl Klin Wochenschr.* 1901;38:1265.
4. Coote H. Pressure on the axillary vessels and nerves by an exostosis from a cervical rib; interference with the circulation of the arm; removal of the rib and exostosis, recovery. *Med Times Gaz.* 1861;2:108.
5. Keen WW. The symptomatology, diagnosis and surgical treatment of cervical ribs. *Am J Med Sci.* 1907;133:173–218.
6. Halsted WS. An experimental study of circumscribed dilation of an artery immediately distal to a partially occluding band, and its bearing on the dilation of the subclavian artery observed in certain cases of cervical rib. *J Exp Med.* 1916;24:271–286.
7. Murphy T. Brachial neuritis caused by pressure of first rib. *Aust Med J.* 1910;15:582–585.
8. Brickner WM. Brachial plexus pressure by the normal first rib. *Ann Surg.* 1927;858:1927.
9. Ochsner A, Gage M, DeBakey M. Scalenus anticus (Naffziger) syndrome. *Am J Surg.* 1935;28:699.
10. Semmes RE, Murphy F. The syndrome of unilateral rupture of the 6th cervical intervertebral disc with compression of the seventh cervical nerve root; report of 4 cases simulating coronary artery disease. *JAMA.* 1943;121:1209–1214.
11. Phalen CM. The carpal-tunnel syndrome. Seventeen years' experience in diagnosis and treatment of six hundred fifty-four hands. *J Bone Joint Surg Am.* 1966;48(2):211–228.
12. Kremer M, Gilliat RW, Golding JSR, Wilson TG. Acroparasthesia in the carpal tunnel syndrome. *Lancet.* 1953;2:590–595.
13. Lewis M, Pickering DC. Pressure at the cervicobrachial outlet. *Br Med J.* 1947;3:341–342.
14. Falconer MA, Li FWP. Resection of the first rib in costoclavicular compression of the brachial plexus. *Lancet.* 1962;1:59–63.
15. Wright IS. The neurovascular syndrome produced by hyperabduction of the arm. *Am Heart J.* 1945;29:1–19.
16. Lord JW, Urschel HC Jr. Total claviculectomy. *Surg Rounds.* 1988;11:17–27.
17. Raaf J. Surgery for cervical rib and scalenus anticus syndrome. *JAMA.* 1955;157:219.
18. Clagett OT. Presidential address: Research and prosearch. *J Urol Nephrol (Paris)* 1962;44:153–166.
19. Roos DB. Transaxillary approach for first rib resection to relieve thoracic outlet syndrome. *Ann Surg.* 1966;163(3):354–358.
20. Urschel HC Jr, Razzuk MA, Albers JE, Wood RE, Paulson DL. Reoperation for recurrent thoracic outlet syndrome. *Ann Thorac Surg.* 1976;21(1):19–25.
21. Sanders RJ. *Thoracic Outlet Syndrome: A Common Sequela of Neck Injuries.* Philadelphia: Lippincott; 1991.
22. Roos DB. Congenital anomalies associated with thoracic outlet syndrome. *Am J Surg.* 1976;132:771–778.
23. Roos DB. Thoracic outlet syndromes: update 1987. *Am J Surg.* 1987;154:568–573.
24. Roos DB. The place for scalenectomy and first-rib resection in thoracic outlet syndrome. *Surgery.* 1982;92(6):1077–1085.
25. Roos DB. Historical perspectives and anatomic considerations. Thoracic outlet syndrome. *Semin Thorac Cardiovasc Surg.* 1996;8(2):183–189.
26. Sunderland S. The anatomy and physiology of nerve injury. *Muscle Nerve.* 1990;13:771–784.
27. Adams JT, De Weese JA. "Effort" thrombosis of the axillary and subclavian veins. *J Trauma.* 1971;11(11):923–930.
28. Greenhalgh RM, Powell JT. Endovascular repair of abdominal aortic aneurysm. *N Engl J Med.* 2008;358:494–501.
29. Braverman AC, Thompson RW, Sanchez LA. Diseases of the aorta. In: Bonow RO, Mann DL, Zipes DP, Libby P, eds. *Braunwald's Heart Disease: A Textbook of Cardiovascular Medicine.* 9th ed. Philadelphia: Saunders; 2011.
30. Urschel HC Jr, Razzuk MA. Neurovascular compression in the thoracic outlet: changing management over 50 years. *Ann Surg.* 1998;228(4):609–617.
31. Urschel HC Jr, Razzuk MA. Improved management of the Paget-Schroetter syndrome secondary to thoracic outlet compression. *Ann Thorac Surg.* 1991;52(6):1217–1221.
32. Wilbourn AJ. Thoracic outlet syndrome: a neurologist's perspective. *Chest Surg Clin N Am.* 1999;9:821–839.
33. Sanders RJ, Hammond SL, Rao NM. Thoracic outlet syndrome: a review. *Neurologist.* 2008;14:365–373.
34. Wilburn AJ, Porter JM. Thoracic outlet syndrome. *Spine.* 1988;2:598.
35. Tender GC, Thomas AJ, Thomas N, Kline DG. Gilliatt-Sumner hand revisited: a 25-year experience. *Neurosurgery.* 2004;55(4):883–890.
36. Mackinnon SE. Thoracic outlet syndrome: introduction. *Semin Thorac Cardiovasc Surg.* 1996;8(2):175.
37. Mackinnon SE. Thoracic outlet syndrome. *Chest Surg Clin N Am.* 1999;9:701.
38. Nelems W. On subjectivity. *Can Med Assoc J.* 1994;150:65.

39. Urschel HC Jr, Razzuk MA, Wood RE, Perekh M, Paulson DL. Objective diagnosis (ulnar nerve conduction velocity) and current therapy of the thoracic outlet syndrome. *Ann Thorac Surg.* 1971;12(6):608–620.

40. Jaeger SH, Singer DI, Whitenack SH, Mandel S. Nerve injury complications. Management of neurogenic pain syndromes. *Hand Clin.* 1986;2(1):217–234.

41. Adson AW. Surgical treatment for symptoms produced by cervical ribs and the scalenus anticus muscle. *Clin Orthop Relat Res.* 1986;207:3–12.

42. Mathews WB. Footballer's migraine. *Br Med J.* 1972;5809: 326–327.

43. Spillane JD. Localised neuritis of the shoulder girdle: a report of 46 cases in the MEF. *Lancet.* 1943;242:532–535.

44. Fabero K, Hawkins R, Jones M. Neuralgic amyotrophy. *J Bone Joint Surg Am.* 1987;69:195–198.

45. Brown KE, Stickler L. Shoulder pain and dysfunction secondary to neural injury. *Int J Sports Phys Ther.* 2011;6(3): 224–233.

46. Kirchhoff C, Imhoff AB. Posterosuperior and anterosuperior impingement of the shoulder in overhead athletes—evolving concepts. *Int Orthop.* 2010;34(7):1049–1058.

47. Roos DB. Congenital anomalies associated with thoracic outlet syndrome. Anatomy, symptoms, diagnosis, and treatment. *Am J Surg.* 1976;132(6):771–778.

48. Machleder HI, Moll F, Verity A. The anterior scalene muscle in thoracic outlet compression syndrome. Histochemical and morphometric studies. *Arch Surg.* 1986;212:1141–1144.

49. Sanders RJ, Jackson CG, Banchero N, Pearce WH. Scalene muscle abnormalities in traumatic thoracic outlet syndrome. *Am J Surg.* 1990;159:231–236.

50. Ferrante MA. The thoracic outlet syndromes. *Muscle Nerve.* 2012;45(6):780–795.

51. Wayman J, Miller S, Shanahan D. Anatomical variation of the insertion of scalenus anterior in adult human subjects: implications for clinical practice. *J Anat.* 1993;183(pt 1): 165–167.

52. Thomas GI, Jones TW, Stavney LS, Manhas DR. The middle scalene muscle and its contribution to the thoracic outlet syndrome. *Am J Surg.* 1983;145(5):589–592.

53. Clarys JP, Barbaix E, Van Rompaey H, Caboor D, Van Roy P. The muscular arch of the axilla revisited: its possible role in the thoracic outlet and shoulder instability syndromes. *Man Ther.* 1996;1(3):133–139.

54. Mullins GM, O'Sullivan SS, Neligan A, et al. Non-traumatic brachial plexopathies, clinical, radiological and neurophysiological findings from a tertiary centre. *Clin Neurol Neurosurg.* 2007;109(8):661–666.

55. Skedros JG, Hill BB, Pitts TC. Iatrogenic thoracic outlet syndrome caused by revision surgery for multiple subacute fixation failures of a clavicle fracture: a case report. *J Shoulder Elbow Surg.* 2010;19(1):e18–e23.

56. Brintnall ES, Hyndman OR, Van Alien WM. Costoclavicular compression associated with cervical rib. *Ann Surg.* 1956; 144:921.

57. Le Forestier N, Moulonguet A, Maisonobe T, Léger JM, Bouche P. True neurogenic thoracic outlet syndrome: electrophysiological diagnosis in six cases. *Muscle Nerve.* 1998;21(9):1129–1134.

58. Kirschbaum A, Palade E, Csatari Z, Passlick B. Venous thoracic outlet syndrome caused by a congenital rib malformation. *Interact Cardiovasc Thorac Surg.* 2012;15(2): 328–329.

59. Balakrishnan A, Coates P, Parry CA. Thoracic outlet syndrome caused by pseudoarticulation of a cervical rib

60. Melliere D, Ben Yahia NE, Etienne G, Becquemin JP, de Labareyre H. Thoracic outlet syndrome caused by tumor of the first rib. *J Vasc Surg.* 1991;14(2):235–240.

61. Al-Shekhlee A, Katirji B. Spinal accessory neuropathy, droopy shoulder, and thoracic outlet syndrome. *Muscle Nerve.* 2003; 28(3):383–385.

62. Iwuagwu OC, Bajalan AA, Platt AJ, Stanley PR, Drew PJ. Effects of reduction mammoplasty on upper-limb nerve conduction across the thoracic outlet in women with macromastia: a prospective randomized study. *Ann Plast Surg.* 2005;55(5):445–448.

63. Rubio PA, Rose FA. Thoracic outlet syndrome caused by a latissimus dorsi flap for breast reconstruction. *Chest.* 1990; 97(2):494–495.

64. Duchenne G. De l'électrisation localisée et de son application à la pathologie et la thérapeutique. Paris: JB Ballière et fils; 1872.

65. Erb W. Ueber eine eigenthümliche Localisation von Lähmungen im Plexus brachialis. *Verhandlungen des naturhistorisch-medicinischen Vereins zu Heidelberg.* 1874;2: 130–137.

66. Klumpke A. Contribution a l'etude des paralysies radicularies de plexus brachial. *Rev Med (Paris)* 1885;5:591–790.

67. Horsley V. Brachial plexus injuries. *Practitioner.* 1899; 63:131.

68. Harden NR, Bruehl S, Perez R, et al. Validation of proposed diagnostic criteria (the "Budapest Criteria") for complex regional pain syndrome. *Pain.* 2010;150(2):268–274.

69. de Mos M, de Bruijn AG, Huygen FJ, Dieleman JP, Stricker BH, Sturkenboom MC. The incidence of complex regional pain syndrome: a population-based study. *Pain.* 2007;129:12–20.

70. Ribbers GM, Geurts AC, Stam HJ, Mulder T. Pharmacologic treatment of complex regional pain syndrome I: a conceptual framework. *Arch Phys Med Rehabil.* 2003;84:141–146.

71. Pearce JMS. Silas Weir Mitchell (1829–1914). *J Neurol Neurosurg Psychiatry.* 1992;55:924.

72. Stanton-Hicks M, Baron R, Boas R, et al. Complex regional pain syndromes: guidelines for therapy. *Clin J Pain.* 1998;14: 155–166.

73. Drucker WR, Hubay CA, Holden WD, et al. Pathogenesis of post traumatic sympathetic dystrophy. *Am J Surg.* 1959;97: 454–461.

74. Schwartzman RJ, Liu JE, Smullens SN, Hyslop T, Tahmoush AJ. Long-term outcome following sympathectomy for complex regional pain syndrome type 1 (RSD). *J Neurol Sci.* 1997;150:149–152.

75. Seddon H. *Surgical Disorders of the Peripheral Nerves.* London: Harcourt Brace/Churchill Livingstone; 1972.

76. Wilder RT. Management of pediatric patients with complex regional pain syndrome. *Clin J Pain.* 2006;22: 443–448.

77. Urschel HC, Kourlis H. Thoracic outlet syndrome: a 50-year experience at Baylor University Medical Center. *Proc (Bayl Univ Med Cent).* 2007;20(2):125–135.

78. Cronenwett JL, Johnston W, eds. *Rutherford's Vascular Surgery.* 7th ed. Philadelphia: Saunders; 2010.

79. Urschel HC Jr, Razzuk MA. Neurovascular compression in the thoracic outlet: changing management over 50 years. *Ann Surg.* 1998;228(4):609–617.

80. Naffziger HC, Grant WT. Neuritis of the brachial plexus mechanical in origin: the scalenus syndrome. *Surg Gynecol Obstet.* 1938;67:722–730.

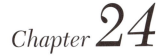

Chapter *24*

Entrapment Neuropathy in the Forearm, Wrist, and Hand

Teri O'Hearn PT, DPT, CHT

"If you can force your nerve, heart and sinew to serve you long after they are gone, and so hold on when there is nothing in you except the will which says to them: 'Hold on!'"

—Rudyard Kipling (1865–1936)

Objectives

On completion of this chapter, the student/practitioner will be able to:

- Describe the anatomical course of each upper extremity peripheral nerve.
- Identify common nerve entrapment sites in the upper extremity.
- Discuss the signs and symptoms of common tunnel syndromes of the upper extremity.
- Discuss the possible functional loss attributed to each neuropathy.

Key Terms

- Compressive neuropathy
- Entrapment
- Tensile neuropathy
- Tunnel syndrome

Introduction

With the undulating course of peripheral nerves from the central nervous system distally to the end organs, nerves pass through bony, fibrous, osteofibrous, and fibromuscular tunnels risking injury from compression, **entrapment,** and tensile forces. Because most peripheral nerves carry motor, sensory, and autonomic fibers, the potential spectrum of impairment is impressive. Careful linking of the presenting signs and symptoms assists the clinician in identifying a list of differential diagnoses that, through examination and testing, can be confirmed, disproved, or added to.

The nomenclature of the etiology of entrapment, **compressive,** and **tensile neuropathies** is diverse. Some syndromes are named after the describing author, such as Kiloh-Nevin syndrome. Some are named after an anatomical area, such as metatarsalgia and thoracic outlet syndrome. The movement producing the symptoms may provide the name, such as glenohumeral hyperabduction syndrome. "Tunnel" is often in the name, such as carpal **tunnel syndrome** (CTS) or tarsal tunnel syndrome. The nerve may be the descriptor, such as ilioinguinal syndrome. Lastly, the etiological structure may be the descriptor, such as pronator teres syndrome.

Although the diagnostic names may vary, all entrapment, compressive, and tensile neuropathies originate from a lesion to the peripheral nerve and associated structural elements in a narrow anatomical space. Neuropathy may be compressive, such as from a hypertrophied muscle, aberrant bone or bone formation, or tumor. Traumatic neuropathy may occur from a missile, laceration, repetitive use, or blunt contact. Metabolic etiologies include diabetes mellitus or hyperthyroidism. Toxic neuropathies occur with lead and mercury intoxication or with some prescriptive medications. Infections may produce space-occupying lesions or neural necrosis via bacteria and viruses. Tensile causes

289

include stretching over or around aberrant anatomy. Anatomical variations may affect nerves, such as a post-fixed brachial plexus or a cervical rib. In this chapter, we concentrate on entrapment, compressive, and tensile neuropathic sites of injury. Other chapters provide more detailed descriptions of the etiology of the neuropathy.

For this chapter, the term "tunnel syndromes" indicates all entrapment, compressive, and tensile neuropathies. Although there are a large number of tunnel syndromes in the upper extremity, this chapter focuses only on the more common syndromes in the upper extremity. This text also includes chapters detailing tunnel syndromes in the lower extremity and thoracic outlet syndrome.

Lundborg[1] stated: "For a peripheral nerve to function properly, two basic requirements must be met: 1, its connection with the mother cells in the central nervous system must remain undisturbed; and 2, it must receive a continuous and adequate supply of oxygen through the intraneural vascular system." Compression or entrapment of a nerve blocks its ability to exchange essential nutrients, resulting initially in dysfunction and ultimately in nerve tissue destruction.

This chapter highlights commonly encountered neuropathies, such as radial tunnel, posterior interosseous nerve, pronator, anterior interosseous nerve, carpal tunnel, cubital tunnel, and Guyon's canal (ulnar tunnel) syndromes. However, entrapment can occur anywhere along the course of the peripheral nerve. Recognition of symptoms helps to locate the site of the lesion, but treatment depends on reversing the mechanism of entrapment and facilitating normal physiological neural function. According to a study by Ochoa[2] conducted in 1972, "the differences in pressures between the compressed and uncompressed nerve generate longitudinal forces that tend to extrude exoplasm like toothpaste from a tube." Axonal flow, designed to be unidirectional, is imperative to nerve function. Nerve entrapment syndromes commonly occur where anatomical restrictions, natural or otherwise, diminish the ability of the nerve to maintain optimal pressure gradients and mobility.[3]

Tissue loading can result in elevated extraneural pressures within minutes or hours, restricting blood flow and axonal transport; this may result in endoneural edema and increased intrafascicular pressure. There is evidence that the amount of endoneural edema is related to the degree of axonal injury.[3]

In addition to the physical aspect of nerve entrapment related to mechanical forces, comorbidities, such as diabetes, increase the risk of development of neuropathy. It is estimated that nearly one third of patients with diabetes are affected with nerve entrapment, although it is difficult to distinguish this from diabetic neuropathy.[4] The rate of progression from initial injury to onset as well as severity of symptoms appears to be accelerated in individuals with diabetes.[4] Appreciating the occurrence of diminished sensation that is common in patients with diabetes, the risk of complications such as ulcerations or other injuries is especially great. Use of diagnostic testing, such as electromyography (EMG) and nerve conduction velocity (NCV) studies, is helpful in distinguishing a nerve compression from diabetic neuropathy and is important in the provision of appropriate treatment. Predictably, recovery rate is often slow compared with individuals without diabetes and is greatly influenced by glycemic control.[4]

Pathogenesis of Tunnel Injuries

Narrowing of the osteofibrous or fibrous neurovascular tunnel is a major risk factor in the development of tunnel syndromes. Intrinsic or extrinsic factors may precipitate tunnel syndromes (Table 24-1). Extrinsic causes are systemic events that happen outside the tunnel; intrinsic causes are systemic events that happen within the tunnel. Many tunnel syndromes are classified as idiopathic. The Seddon classification of severity of tunnel syndrome as related to nerve injury is the most commonly used designation (Table 24-2).

Neurapraxic lesions to nerve are the most common nerve injury and result in the mildest symptoms. Typically, there is only a temporary loss of function, and there is no structural neural disruption. Recovery occurs in minutes to weeks. Axonotmetic lesions result in axonal and sheath disruption with preservation of the

Table 24-1	Intrinsic and Extrinsic Causes of Tunnel Syndrome
Category	**Examples**
External to Tunnel	
Congenital	Cervical rib, post fixed plexus
Trauma	Elbow dislocation, fracture
Infectious	Herpes zoster
Neoplasm	Pancoast tumor, osteogenic sarcoma
Metabolic	Diabetes mellitus, hyperthyroidism
Hormonal	Pregnancy
Toxic	Lead intoxification, some medications
Iatrogenic	Surgical injury, casting, wrapping
Internal to Tunnel	
Congenital	Anomalous scalene muscle
Infectious	Tuberculosis, abscess
Neoplasm	Schwannoma, hemangioma, myeloma
Hormonal	Pregnancy
Toxic	Lead intoxication, some medications
Iatrogenic	Surgical injury

connective and structural elements. Wallerian degeneration occurs distal to the site of injury. Recovery time is related to the distance the neural elements need to regrow to reach the effector organ. Neurotmetic lesions are the most severe and result in a complete anatomical disruption of the nerve and the associated connective structures. There is no spontaneous recovery. Surgical intervention is required.

Clinical Symptoms and Signs

Because most peripheral nerves carry motor, sensory, and autonomic fibers from and to multiple myotomes and dermatomes, the spectrum of presenting signs and symptoms can be quite varied (Table 24-3). The astute clinician can correctly diagnose the syndrome only through a valid and reliable physical examination and aided by radiographic, laboratory, and electrodiagnostic studies.

Diagnosis begins with a thorough document review (i.e., laboratory results, imaging results, consultations) before the patient encounter, history, and physical examination. The document review, history, and physical examination provide clinical scripts to the clinician that assist with building a differential diagnosis list. Further questioning and physical assessment techniques complemented by radiographic, laboratory, and electrodiagnostic tests assist in adding to, removing, or confirming the items on the differential diagnosis list (Figs. 24-1 and 24-2). Eventually, through meticulous

Table 24-2 Seddon Classification of Peripheral Nerve Injuries

Lesion	Definition	Recovery Potential
Neurapraxia	Temporary loss of function; no neural disruption	Excellent without intervention
Axonotmesis	Disruption of axon and sheath; connective sheath intact	Good to excellent with length-dependent variability
Neurotmesis	Complete anatomical disruption of nerve	Poor to fair; requires surgical intervention

Table 24-3 Symptoms and Signs of Peripheral Neuropathy

Type	Symptoms and Signs
Sensory	Loss of tactile discrimination, sharp, dull, vibration, kinesthesia, proprioception, light touch, pain, paresthesia, hyperesthesia, hypoalgesia, pain
Motor	Myalgia, weakness, paralysis, hypoactive deep tendon reflexes, atrophy
Autonomic	Vegetative disturbances, trophic nails, abnormal hair growth, cool or warm skin, erythema, blanching, hyperhidrosis, hypohidrosis

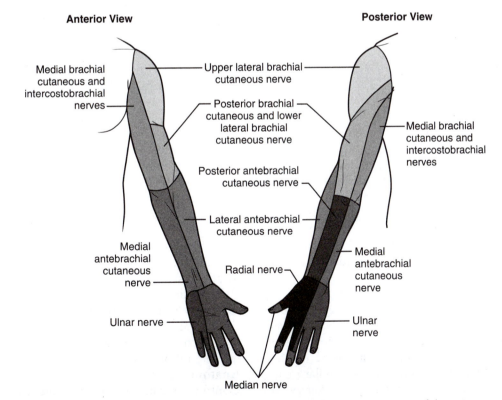

Figure 24-1 Mapping of the peripheral dermatomes of the upper extremity delineating the nerve name and geographic distribution.

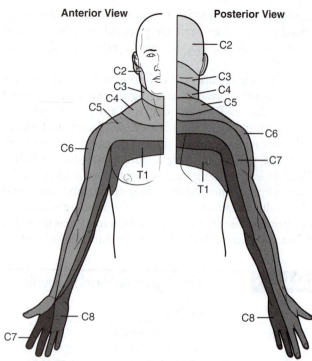

Figure 24-2 Mapping of the segmental dermatomes of the upper extremity delineating the nerve name and geographic distribution.

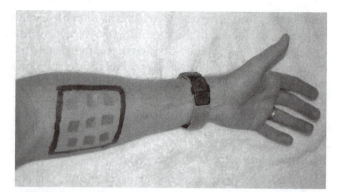

Figure 24-3 Rule-of-nine test. Square grid, proximal aspect is volar elbow flexion crease, with lateral-medial and distal borders of equal length. Nine equal points within the grid are palpated; a subjective report of pain at a specific point or points that correlates with the posterior interosseous nerve indicates a positive test. (Note: Photo is intended to illustrate the test layout and is not meant to be used in actual testing; the bottom of the photo represents the proximal volar left arm.)

evaluation and assessment, the clinician arrives at the correct diagnosis. See Chapter 14 for a specific evaluation algorithm.

Radial Nerve

Radial Tunnel Syndrome

Presentation

Radial tunnel syndrome (RTS) was first described in 1956.[5] The etiology of RTS may include pressure to the radial nerve caused by tumors or other lesions that impose on the space occupied by the nerve, edema and inflammation, or blunt trauma to the proximal forearm. More commonly, the development of RTS appears to be correlated to activity that involves vigorous or repetitive elbow, forearm. and wrist motion.[6] RTS commonly is misdiagnosed as atypical lateral epicondylitis, or tennis elbow, although the two conditions often coexist.[7]

Studies have listed risk factors related to RTS to include occupations that involve maintaining the elbow in extension between 0° and 45°, especially when combined with forearm supination; engagement of the supinator muscle imposes a compressive force on the nerve as it is tensioned across the radiocapitellar joint. Roquelaure et al.[8] reported that factory workers who exerted regular force of at least 1 kg more than 10 times per hour were at risk for development of RTS.[6]

The classic presentation of RTS is reported pain at the lateral aspect of the proximal forearm without motor weakness. The Rule-of-Nine test is a method of identifying radial nerve irritation in the forearm (Fig. 24-3).[9] The patient typically complains of a deep burning ache about 4 to 5 cm distal to the lateral epicondyle over the mobile wad of extensor carpi radialis longus (ECRL), extensor carpi radialis brevis (ECRB), and brachioradialis (BR). Increased pain is commonly reported after activities that include wrist extension combined with forearm supination. Pain at night and at rest may also be reported.[6] This pain may result in limited ability to achieve complete active wrist extension and forearm pronation and often is accompanied by the patient's complaint of needing to modify normal movement or depend more on others to accomplish tasks.[6]

Many publications seem to use the terms RTS and posterior interosseous nerve (PIN) syndrome interchangeably; however, the hallmark difference is that RTS involves pain over the radial aspect of the proximal forearm, whereas PIN syndrome is associated with motor weakness at the wrist and digits (see section on PIN syndrome later).[6–9]

In contrast to PIN compression, radial tunnel compression symptoms typically include forearm pain located distal to the lateral epicondyle of the humerus. PIN syndrome is not always associated with pain; marked weakness of the finger and wrist extensors is the typical presentation.[9] It has been hypothesized that RTS pain is a predecessor to PIN compression, which results in motor deficits.[10]

Anatomy

Continuing from the posterior cord, the radial nerve is the largest terminal branch of the brachial plexus and carries the C5–T1 nerve fibers, directly providing innervation to the triceps, anconeus, BR, and ECRL muscles and possibly innervating the ECRB.[11] The nerve descends behind the axillary and upper brachial arteries and courses in front of the latissimus dorsi and teres major tendons. It crosses from the medial to the lateral aspect of the humerus between the medial and lateral heads of the triceps and continues distally to pierce the lateral intermuscular septum, passing between the brachialis and BR muscles. At the level of the lateral epicondyle of the elbow, the radial nerve divides into deep and superficial branches.[6]

The proximal aspect of the radial tunnel lies near the level of the radiocapitellar joint where the nerve rests on the joint capsule. A surgical capsular release or other trauma at this location may injure the nerve. The medial border of the tunnel is formed by the BR muscle proximally and the biceps tendon distally. The lateral border and roof of the tunnel is provided by the ECRB and ECRL. The tunnel extends to the distal aspect of the supinator muscle.[6]

Compression of the radial nerve may occur anywhere along this pathway. In the forearm, areas of compression may be:

- Most commonly, at the proximal margin of the deep and superficial layers of the supinator muscle.[12]
- At the proximal ECRB at the level of the radiocapitellar joint and may be associated with arthrosis.[9]
- At the fibrous bands at the level of the radial head.[10]
- At the radial recurrent vessels (leash of Henry).[6,12]
- At the ligament/arcade of Frohse or at the distal border of the supinator muscle, or both.[10]

The anatomy of the radial nerve at the forearm is considered to be highly variable, making accurate diagnosis a challenge.[6]

Manual tests for RTS include the following:

- Resisted middle finger[12]
  - Pain is reported at the dorsal forearm over the radial tunnel with resisted middle finger extension; this assists in differential diagnosis of RTS versus resistant tennis elbow (lateral epicondylitis).
- Resisted forearm supination[10]
  - With elbow held in flexion, isometric forearm supination with patient report of pain over the radial tunnel is considered a positive test for RTS.

Posterior Interosseous Nerve Syndrome

Presentation

Patients demonstrating motor deficits and resulting functional impairment of the extensors of the wrist and digits may be affected with compression of the PIN.

Typical reported patient history may include trauma to the lateral forearm, repetitive manual work, and lengthy time spent at the computer, and the condition is highly correlated with rheumatoid arthritis. A common presentation is weakness of finger extension, thumb abduction, and wrist extension. EMG studies often show increased differential latency of the PIN.[10] BR, ECRB, and ECRL, which are innervated by more proximal branches of the radial nerve, are typically spared,[13] resulting in a presentation of active wrist extension combined with radial deviation. The extensor carpi ulnaris and extensor digitorum communis are innervated by the PIN and, with compression of the motor neuron, may become unable to produce adequate force to accomplish active neutral alignment of the wrist. The patient may also report pain at the proximal forearm, but this is more likely related to RTS, which may coincide with PIN compression. PIN syndrome, in itself, is not associated with sensory deficits (see section on Wartenberg's syndrome).[11] Although the PIN is considered to be a motor nerve, it does supply innervation to the dorsal capsule of the wrist, providing proprioceptive and nociceptive sensation. As innervation is supplied to the extensor pollicis longus, a branch to the distal radioulnar joint enters the fourth dorsal extensor compartment and further divides into three or four smaller branches at the dorsal wrist capsule. Patients presenting with symptoms of the deep terminal sensory branch of the PIN complain of a deep, dull ache in the wrist, which may be exacerbated with forcefully resisted wrist extension. The patient may also report pain with deep palpation of the forearm in combination with wrist flexion.[14] A study investigating the possibility of proprioceptive deficits related to PIN neurectomy after surgeries to treat conditions such as carpal instability, distal radius fracture, and distal radioulnar joint pathology concluded there were no significant proprioceptive changes when the surgical population of the study was compared with the healthy, nonsurgical control group.[15]

The loss of active extension of the fingers associated with PIN paralysis may mimic extensor tendon rupture in patient presentation. The use of tenodesis (passive wrist flexion) to elicit digital extension can allow the therapist to rule out rupture of the extensor tendons and validate suspicion of PIN paralysis.

The literature reviewed in this chapter suggests pain related to RTS precedes motor dysfunction related to PIN syndrome, and onset of symptoms is often seen in individuals who engage in repetitive manual upper extremity activity.[10]

Anatomy

Distal to the anconeus muscle, the radial nerve continues to the dorsal forearm, lateral to the radius, and pierces the supinator muscle at the arcade of Frohse. The deep branch of the radial nerve is also referred to as the PIN. A further division results in the medial and lateral branches.

The level of bifurcation of the radial nerve into the posterior (deep) and superficial branches is variable and not entirely reliable when it comes to diagnosing the site of PIN entrapment. The position of the forearm influences the location of the PIN; as the forearm rotates from supination into pronation, the nerve may move 1.0 cm lateral to medial.[12]

The PIN provides motor innervation to the ECRB, supinator, extensor carpi ulnaris, extensor digiti minimi, all extensor digitorum communis, extensor indicis, extensor pollicis brevis, abductor pollicis longus, and extensor pollicis longus muscles. The terminal branch of the PIN supplies pain and proprioceptive innervation to the wrist.

As the PIN continues distally on the interosseous membrane anterior to the extensor pollicis longus and onto the wrist, it provides sensory fibers to the ligaments of the wrist joint.[10] The ECRB may be innervated by the radial nerve or by the PIN.[11]

Entrapment of the PIN may occur:

- Most commonly, at the proximal edge of the supinator muscle.[11]
- Within or at the distal aspect of the supinator muscle.
- As a result of radial head fracture or dislocation.
- Secondary to a mass imposing pressure onto the nerve (e.g., ganglion cyst, lipoma, synovitis).
- As a complication after surgery, such as open reduction with internal fixation of a proximal radius fracture.[13]
- After bifurcation into the medial and lateral branches,
  - Involvement of the medial branch may manifest as paralysis of extensor carpi ulnaris, extensor digiti minimi, and extensor digitorum communis or
  - If the lateral branch is compressed, paralysis may be seen in abductor pollicis longus, extensor pollicis brevis, extensor pollicis longus, and extensor indicis proprius, but compression of both medial and lateral branches is uncommon.[11]

Congenital anatomical anomalies resulting in increased risk of PIN entrapment have been reported. In a study reported by Prakash et al.[16] in 2008, absence of the ECRB was discovered and two tendons extending from the ECRL into the second compartment of the extensor retinaculum deep to the abductor pollicis longus. The authors thought this anomaly further increased the chance of PIN entrapment.

Wartenberg's Syndrome

Entrapment of the superficial branch of the radial nerve (SBRN) is also known as Wartenberg's syndrome. The condition was first described as an inflammation of the SBRN by Wartenberg, a neurologist, in 1932. He suggested the term *cheiralgia paraesthetica*, an obsolete term for pain and paresthesia in the hand.[17,18] SBRN entrapment is also known as handcuff neuritis/neuropathy/neurapraxia and wristlet watch neuritis.[19]

Individuals who wear tight gloves or wristwatches and athletes who use tape, archery guards, or straps with a racquetball racket may present with symptoms of this type of compression. Entrapment of the SBRN may be seen in patients who have had traumatic injury, such as Colles' fracture; repeated exposure to cold; or other external compression at the wrist, such as from a cast.[17] A soft tissue mass, such as a lipoma, or other anatomical variations, such as tight fascial bands, have been reported in association with Wartenberg's syndrome.[17] Athletes who participate in activities such as batting, throwing, or rowing or in contact sports such as football, lacrosse, and hockey may experience nerve injury secondary to direct trauma.[14]

The patient typically reports dorsoradial wrist, hand, thumb, and index finger pain, numbness, and paresthesias.[14] Symptoms are often misdiagnosed as de Quervain's stenosing tendovaginitis, although the two diagnoses are often seen concurrently. The rate of association between the two diagnoses has been reported as 50%.[20] Sensory testing, absence of edema and tenderness at the radial styloid, positive Tinel's sign over the SBRN, or electrodiagnostic studies can distinguish Wartenberg's syndrome from de Quervain's stenosing tendovaginitis.[20]

Anatomy

The SBRN travels deep to the BR tendon, emerging through the fascia that connects the BR and the ECRL tendons at the middle to distal third of the forearm.[20,21] The nerve can become compressed between these tendons, especially during forearm pronation. Dellon et al. described this type of compression as a scissoring effect as the nerve becomes superficial.[14] As the SBRN continues distally after piercing the deep fascia, it further divides into the five dorsal digital nerves.[21]

The SBRN supplies cutaneous innervation to the dorsoradial hand over the first, second, and third rays. The patient typically reports paresthesia and numbness at this region. Sensory disturbance over the first extensor compartment may be associated with overlapping innervation between the SBRN and the lateral cutaneous nerve of the forearm, which is a continuation of the musculocutaneous nerve. Because of the superficial location of the nerves, entrapment neuropathies are common.[19]

Median Nerve

Pronator Syndrome

Presentation

A patient complains of forearm pain and numbness that makes his job as a dental hygienist very difficult.

There is no particular event that seems to have caused these symptoms, which were gradual in onset. Range of motion in the forearm, wrist, and hand is within normal limits but difficult because of pain.

Symptoms of pronator syndrome may mimic CTS, but PS is much less common and is often considered to be a reason patients do not respond as expected after carpal tunnel release (CTR) or may exist in combination with a double crush phenomenon.[22] The diagnostic contrast to CTS is the absence of nocturnal symptoms.

The cardinal signs of PS are:

- Pain in the proximal forearm.
- Paresthesias in the digits.
- Numbness in the palm associated with the palmar cutaneous branch of the median nerve.

Exacerbating activities may include forced or repetitive forearm pronation and supination, repetitive grasping, or direct pressure at the volar forearm. Studies have investigated populations at risk for development of PS, which may include assembly line workers, carpenters, weightlifters, tennis players, forklift drivers, musicians, dentists and dental hygienists, and people who provide child care that involves cradling a baby on the volar forearm.[14] Patients often present with symptoms in the fifth decade, but onset of symptoms may be influenced by the intensity or frequency of the exacerbating activities and medical comorbidities and general health of the individual. Athletes who participate in sports that include repetitive, forceful forearm pronation and gripping may be at increased risk for development of PS. Included in this population are pitchers, weightlifters, archers, tennis players, arm wrestlers, and rowers. Patients typically present with volar forearm pain, which is exacerbated with the activity and is relieved with rest, as well as occasional hand pain.[14]

PS is considered to be a rare condition compared with CTS. It has been reported to be seen more commonly in women than in men.[23]

Compression of the median nerve may occur between the superficial and deep heads of the pronator teres and has been noted between both heads in 4.6% of cases. It has been reported that the deep head of the pronator teres may be absent in 21.7% of the population.[24]

The condition termed "pronator syndrome," as previously described in the medical literature, has been suggested to be nonexistent; rather, the appropriate term for this malady is "median nerve entrapment in the forearm."[25] The clinical presentation includes subtle weakness that may be unnoticed by the patient other than on clinical examination; vague hand pain or numbness in the median nerve distribution that may be intermittent (noticed distally, as opposed to at the compression site at the elbow), commonly seen with concurrent diagnosis of CTS or with demonstration of postural deficits; absence of forearm pain; and EMG findings that may or may not reveal an abnormality.[25] Ericson[25] emphasized the essential component of addressing the entire person, as opposed to focusing on the location of the symptoms, as a CTR may be ineffective in resolution of symptoms because the proximal problem has not been addressed or has not resolved. Ericson[25] attributed the development of median nerve entrapment in the forearm to the following "critical sum" of etiology, which should be considered in appropriate diagnosis and treatment:

- Normal aging process
- Chronic hand pain
- Sustained or repetitive forearm pronation
- Thoracic outlet symptoms
  - Postural deficits increase the amount of hand pain experienced
- Cervical spondylosis/radiculopathy
- Obesity
- Depression
- Ligamentous laxity

Anatomy

The median nerve is formed by lateral (C5–7) and medial (C8–T1) cords of the brachial plexus. Lying anterior to the brachialis, deep to the lacertus fibrosus, the nerve passes between the superficial (humeral) and deep (ulnar) head of the pronator teres in the proximal one third of the forearm. The nerve crosses lateral to the ulnar artery, separated by the deep and superficial heads of the pronator teres muscle. It proceeds posterior to the fibrous arch formed by two heads of the flexor digitorum superficialis (FDS) and emerges in the distal one third of the forearm along the lateral FDS. The median nerve innervates pronator teres, flexor carpi radialis, palmaris longus, and FDS.

The anterior interosseous nerve (AIN) branch of the median nerve originates 5 to 8 cm distal to the medial epicondyle of the elbow, distal to the proximal border of the superficial head of the pronator teres. Together, the AIN and median nerves go through the fibrous arch of the FDS. The palmar cutaneous branch of the median nerve arises from the lateral aspect of the nerve approximately 7 cm proximal to the distal wrist crease and runs deep to the antebrachial fascia close to the medial border of the flexor carpi radialis, innervating the skin over the palm proximal thenar eminence (Fig. 24-4).

The three most common sites for median nerve compression associated with PS are as follows:

- Bicipital aponeurosis, otherwise known as lacertus fibrosus; its fascia is intimately connected with pronator teres[14]
  - This site of compression is most common when the pronator teres origin is especially proximal[14]

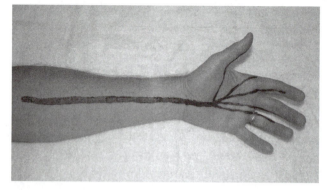

Figure 24-4 Path of the median nerve as it enters the forearm and hand.

- At the site of the pronator teres as the nerve passes between the humeral and ulnar heads
  - This site is often associated with muscle hypertrophy, fibrous bands within the muscle, or anomalous course of the nerve, which has been seen below or piercing the humeral head[14]
- Below thickened fibrous arch of the FDS[14]
- Less commonly, deep to the ligament of Struthers, which spans the supracondylar process and medial epicondyle at the distal humerus
- Persistent median artery
- Rarely, secondary to an enlarged bursa at the bicipital tuberosity[14]

Anterior Interosseous Nerve Syndrome
Presentation

AIN syndrome is associated with loss of flexor pollicis longus (FPL), flexor digitorum profundus (FDP) (index and occasionally middle, ring, and small fingers), and pronator quadratus in severe cases.[26] Forearm pain, often described as "vague" or "aching," which may develop over several hours, leads to weakness and motor dysfunction in the thumb and index finger and potentially affects forearm pronation. Pain may be experienced at rest but is exacerbated with activity.[26] Weakness results in difficulty with handwriting because of inability to achieve functional tip pinch.

- Incomplete syndrome is characterized by loss of FPL or index finger FDP strength.
- Complete syndrome is characterized by weakness of FPL, FDP of index and middle fingers, and pronator quadratus.
  - All FDP muscles may be innervated by the AIN, resulting in weakness in all fingers.[26]
- "Classic attitude" of weak pinch and inability to make "0" sign is associated with late stages of AIN syndrome.[6]
  - With attempted index finger–thumb opposition, the index finger distal interphalangeal joint hyperextends with compensatory proximal interphalangeal joint hyperflexion.
- Hyperextension at the thumb interphalangeal joint is combined with hyperflexion at the metacarpophalangeal joint.[26]

There is no reported paresthesia, which is the key differentiating symptom from CTS. Clinically, AIN is considered a pure motor nerve, but it has sensory branches at distal radioulnar and radiocarpal joints.[26] The development of AIN syndrome may be associated with chronic (repetitive or prolonged) forearm pronation or elbow flexion or acute trauma, such as fracture.[27]

Weakness of the muscles innervated by the AIN, in itself, is rare with incidence reportedly less than 1% of all peripheral neuropathies of the upper extremity.[26,28] There is continued question as to whether AIN syndrome is a neuritis, compression/entrapment neuropathy, or both.[26]

Electrodiagnostic studies may assist in differentiating between main median nerve trunk and AIN entrapment. In a case study of a young Coast Guardsman who had lost functional pinch, motor and sensory conduction assessment was performed to determine the site of neural lesion. An assessment of the median nerve from axilla to wrist revealed normal conduction in the main median nerve trunk, but no evoked action potentials were elicited in the FPL, indicating probable entrapment at the proximal aspect of the AIN. Surgical decompression resulted in resolution of symptoms.[29]

AIN syndrome, although a rare condition, should be considered whenever a patient presents with a history of forearm pain in association with hand or forearm weakness that may be the result of acute trauma.[27] Loss of digital flexion may be the result of tendon rupture related to diagnoses such as rheumatoid arthritis, Kienböck's disease, and scaphoid nonunion. To rule out rupture and validate suspicion of AIN syndrome, passive wrist flexion and extension produce the tenodesis effect of FPL and FDP.[30]

Anatomy

The AIN is the largest branch of the median nerve, which arises about 5 to 8 cm distal to the medial epicondyle of the elbow from the posterior aspect of the median nerve.[26] Lying anterior to the brachialis muscle and deep to lacertus fibrosus, it is crossed by the deep head of the pronator teres in the proximal one third of the forearm. It may lie deep to ulnar collateral vessels, an accessory muscle from the FDS (Gantzner's muscle), and an accessory muscle from the FDS to FPL. As the nerve continues distally, it passes lateral to the ulnar artery and between the FDP and FPL, along the volar surface of the interosseous membrane with the interosseous artery. Continuing distally, it travels posterior to the fibrous arch formed by the two heads of FDS, emerging in the distal third of the forearm. The AIN provides motor innervation to the FDP of the index and middle fingers, FPL, and pronator quadratus muscles.[31]

Possible compression sites of the AIN include, but are not limited to, the following:

- Deep head of pronator teres
- Fibrous tissue arcade of FDS
- Gantzner's muscle (accessory head of FPL), flexor carpi radialis brevis[26]
- Tendinous origin of palmaris profundus
  - Rare anomaly of the forearm, originating from the radial aspect of the common flexor tendons in the proximal forearm and inserting at the palmar aponeurosis[32]
- Accessory lacertus fibrosus
- Direct physical compression of nerve or vascular supply by blood vessel
  - Ulnar recurrent vessels
  - Aberrant radial artery
  - Anomalous median artery
  - Anterior interosseous vessels as they cross the AIN
  - Enlarged bursae, tumors, accessory bicipital aponeurosis[26]

Carpal Tunnel Syndrome

Presentation

CTS is the most common peripheral nerve compressive disorder in the upper extremity.[33–36] CTS is considered to be responsible for the highest rate of work missed by affected employees[37] and, in a report released in 2002, accounted for $2 billion in annual surgical costs.[38] Although CTS is commonly thought of as a work-related condition, the evidence supporting this assumption is lacking.

CTS is defined by the American Academy of Orthopaedic Surgeons as a symptomatic compression neuropathy of the median nerve at the level of the wrist, characterized physiologically by evidence of increased pressure within the carpal tunnel and decreased function of the nerve at that level.[39] The condition affects male and female individuals of varying ages and is not specific to ethnic or occupational factors.[39] Plenty of attention has been paid to this common pest of medical diagnoses, but progress has been slow in developing methods of prevention, diagnosis, and treatment.

Complaints associated with CTS include numbness and tingling in the thumb and index, middle, and radial half of the ring fingers; burning pain at night; and, in advanced cases, distal forearm pain, diminished grip and pinch strength, and loss of sensation. Symptoms may vary from day to day.[35,39] Median nerve irritation associated with position and activity is well documented. Compression on the median nerve within the carpal tunnel compromises oxygen delivery to the nerve and may result in mechanical injury.[40] Increases in pressure within the carpal tunnel have been measured with extremes of wrist flexion and extension and resisted grip,[41] and pressure increases are greater in patients with a diagnosis of CTS compared with healthy control individuals.[42] Although the carpal tunnel has openings at either end, it maintains its unique tissue pressure levels as though it were a closed compartment.[26,43]

The debate regarding the etiology of CTS makes determining the cause of this condition challenging. Authors have attributed risk for development of CTS to vocation, occupation, lifestyle, gender, and genetics. There does not appear to be any direct correlation of cause and effect that has substantiating evidence. Although CTS has historically been a common workers' compensation issue, it is difficult for the physician to declare clearly the relationship of one's occupation to injury in the case of CTS.

Increased risk factors that are not related to vocation include thyroid disease, diabetes mellitus, rheumatoid arthritis, alcoholism, obesity, and pregnancy.[33,44] There appears to be a correlation with greater weight and female gender.[33] Other factors that may compromise the space within the carpal tunnel include, but are not limited to, cysts, tumors, osteophytes, fractures, or hypertrophic synovial tissue. According to a literature review conducted by Falkiner and Myers[38] in 2002, primary risk factors for development of CTS are female gender, menopausal age, obesity or physically unfit, diabetes including family history of diabetes, osteoarthritis of the first carpometacarpal joint, smoking, and alcohol abuse. It was concluded that the disease process was not correlated with work except in cases of cold environments, such as butchery, but was correlated with general health and lifestyle.

The literature suggests three causes of CTS related to compression of the neurovascular structures within the carpal tunnel:

- Compromised oxygen delivery and resulting ischemia
- Decreased longitudinal excursion of the median nerve
- Injury or compression to carpal structures secondary to mechanical influence[26]

Because evidence supporting the reliability of diagnostic evaluation for CTS is lacking, no particular test is considered a gold standard for diagnosis of CTS. EMG and NCV testing are commonly used as an objective augmentation to clinical diagnosis, which may otherwise be based on subjective information (Figs. 24-5 and 24-6).[39]

Manual tests considered to be reliable in screening for CTS include the following:

- Tinel's percussion test[33]
  - The Tinel percussion test was developed by Tinel in 1915. Gingerly tapping over an irritated nerve may produce paresthesia at

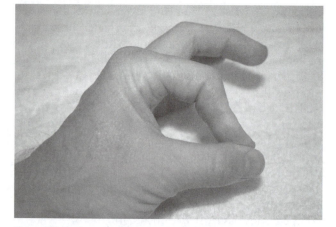

Figure 24-5 In a pure anterior interosseous nerve lesion, there may be weakness of the flexor pollicis longus and the flexor digitorum profundus I and II as revealed by the abnormal posturing associated with a pinch. Classic attitude of a weak pinch: thumb metacarpophalangeal hyperflexion combined with interphalangeal hyperextension, index finger proximal interphalangeal hyperflexion combined with distal interphalangeal hyperextension.

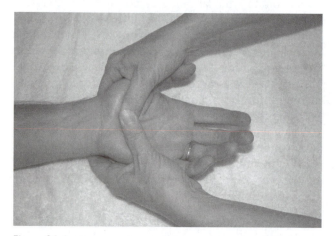

Figure 24-6 Compression test for median neuropathy is performed by pressing on the median nerve at the level of the distal palmar crease. A positive test elicits paresthesia over the dorsal cutaneous distribution of the median nerve. Manual pressure is applied directly over the carpal tunnel flexor retinaculum for up to 1 minute; the test is positive if the subject reports paresthesia or dysesthesia in the median nerve distribution.

the percussion site and in the nerve distribution. This test is not used exclusively to test for CTS and is often used generally to test for nerve irritation.

- Phalen's test[35]
  - Phalen, an American hand surgeon (1966), developed and named this test. Increased carpal tunnel pressure is achieved as the patient is positioned in bilateral wrist hyperflexion by pressing dorsal hands

together for 60 seconds; a positive test result is symptom reproduction in median nerve distribution. (Reverse Phalen test is conducted in "praying hands" fashion, achieving wrist hyperextension.)
- Carpal compression test[40]
  - In 1991, Durkan developed this simple test. It is performed by applying direct pressure on the carpal tunnel for up to 1 minute. The test is considered to be positive if the subject reports paresthesia/dysesthesia in the median nerve distribution.

CTR surgery is considered an effective treatment for CTS. Postoperative complications are infrequent but may pose a frustrating challenge to the patient and the treating therapist. Pillar pain, tenderness superficial to the carpal tunnel, thenar, or hypothenar areas after CTR, is sometimes encountered but poorly understood. The pain is not experienced with activity and may be accompanied by swelling. It is not commonly associated with sensory disturbance.[45] Scar sensitivity, neuromas of cutaneous nerve endings, changes in carpal arch dynamics or thenar and hypothenar muscle origins, and decreased median nerve gliding may be factors in development of pillar pain, which often results in the patient having difficulty returning to work.[45]

Taizo and Hiroyuki[46] studied patients after CTR who experienced pillar pain; spontaneous resolution of symptoms occurred within 1 month in 58% (n = 146 hands), and the pain continued 3 to 9 months in 9% (n = 13 hands). Women recovered more quickly than men, but men were significantly younger and more active. The authors suggested that pillar pain "might be caused by a continuous synovitis by mechanical stimulation" after CTR.[46] (See the section on treatment later for a discussion of the treatment of pillar pain.)

Anatomy

The median nerve arises from the lateral and medial cords of the brachial plexus. After it descends the proximal arm, the nerve crosses the antecubital fossa deep to the biceps aponeurosis between the biceps tendon and pronator teres, lying on the distal brachialis muscle. It continues beneath the two heads of the FDS, emerging between FDS and FDP at the distal forearm. The nerve route becomes ulnar to the flexor carpi radialis and deep to the palmaris longus tendon, entering the carpal tunnel superficial to the flexor tendons.

The floor of the carpal tunnel is formed by the eight carpal bones; the roof of the tunnel is the transverse carpal ligament, a strong fibrous band that is bordered by the hamate and pisiform ulnarly and the scaphoid and trapezium radially. The median nerve and the nine tendons of the FDS, FDP, and FPL muscles are contained within the tunnel. Also to be considered is the often additional presence of the proximal aspects of the lumbrical muscles, which are attached to the FDP tendons. It has been suggested that lumbrical tightness, resulting in proximal migration, contributed significantly to the etiology of CTS and was correlated with occupations that involved repetitive hand motions.[47]

Two separate layers of fascia span the volar carpal canal, the most superficial being the antebrachial fascia proximally and palmar fascia distally; the deep layer is the flexor retinaculum.[26] Superficial to the flexor retinaculum (not within the carpal tunnel) lies the palmaris longus muscle and ulnar nerve, and the radial artery is located lateral to the flexor retinaculum.

The palmaris profundus is a muscle that arises from the lateral edge of the radius, lateral to the FDS and deep to the pronator teres. Its distal tendon passes beneath the flexor retinaculum, broadening in the palm and inserting into the palmar aponeurosis. It has also been termed musculus comitans nervi mediani because the tendon of palmaris profundus and the median nerve are often enveloped in a common sheath. This muscle was first described by Frohse and Fraenkel in 1908 (*Die muskeln des menschlichen Armes*) and may be found with or in the absence of the palmaris longus.[32] Because of its proximity to the median nerve, entrapment at this site is possible and often overlooked, which may result in suboptimal results from CTR.[48]

The deep motor branch of the median nerve emerges within or just distal to the flexor retinaculum and typically provides innervation to the thenar muscles (abductor pollicis brevis, opponens pollicis, superficial and deep heads of the flexor pollicis brevis and adductor pollicis) and the lumbricals of the index and middle fingers. The abductor pollicis brevis has a separate muscle belly, but the opponens pollicis, superficial and deep heads of flexor pollicis brevis, and adductor pollicis are more closely connected as the deep thenar muscle group and receive innervation from branches of the recurrent nerve and accessory recurrent nerve from the median nerve as well as terminal branches of the deep branch of the ulnar nerve.[49] Variations in motor and sensory innervation have been reported, further increasing diagnostic challenges.[26]

The sensory branches of the median nerve supply the thumb; index, middle, and radial aspect of the ring fingers; and radial aspect of the palm of the hand. The palmar cutaneous nerve arises from the median nerve about 5 cm proximal to the wrist crease, coursing separately under the antebrachial fascia between the palmaris longus and flexor carpi radialis tendons, providing sensory innervation to the thenar eminence. As it becomes more superficial, it divides into a radial and one or more ulnar branches and may be encountered in a routine CTR.[26]

The common areas of median nerve compression within the carpal tunnel are as follows:[32,33,44–48]

- Proximal edge of the transverse carpal ligament
  - Exacerbated by wrist flexion, validating Phalen's test

- Adjacent to the hook of the hamate
  - Commonly observed with CTR as hourglass deformity in the nerve
- Space-occupying lesion
  - Flexor tenosynovitis
  - Fracture-dislocation of carpal or radius bones
  - Tumors
  - Ganglia

Edema and vascular sclerosis are seen concurrently with CTS but may be secondary factors rather than primary causes for entrapment neuropathy.[26]

Ulnar Nerve

Cubital Tunnel Syndrome

Presentation

Cubital tunnel syndrome, the entrapment of the ulnar nerve at the elbow, may manifest with motor and sensory impairments in the forearm and hand.[50] It is considered to be the most common ulnar nerve entrapment neuropathy and the second most common entrapment neuropathy in the arm, second to CTS.[50–52] Early in the disease process, the patient typically complains of numbness in the small finger and ulnar aspect of the ring finger, which often is exacerbated by prolonged flexion of the elbow, such as while sleeping, as well as with repeated external pressure over the nerve. Individuals who lean their elbows on hard surfaces, such as desktops, wheelchair arm rests, or an automobile window frame while driving, are at risk. Occupational hazards include prolonged telephone use and operation of vibrating tools.[50] The symptoms progress from being occasional, while the position or activity is taking place, to becoming constant and unrelenting anesthesia.[50] Additionally, patients often report pain at the medial aspect of the elbow, related to extensive wrist flexion, specifically with extensive use of flexor carpi ulnaris (FCU).[50]

Cubital tunnel syndrome is not limited to individuals who commonly assume static postures that impose sustained tension or compression on the ulnar nerve. Athletes who engage in repeated throwing are susceptible to ulnar nerve irritation at the elbow. The literature reports diagnosis and treatment for cubital tunnel syndrome in baseball players ranging from Little League through professional levels. Instability of the elbow secondary to repetitive valgus stress, which has been suggested to contribute to ulnar nerve compression, also is seen in throwing athletes. Repetitive throwing is believed to result in the forward-medial movement of the hypertrophic medial head of the triceps when the elbow is flexed greater than 90°. The triceps imposes pressure on the nerve, increasing compression under the arcuate ligament of Osborne.[51,53,54]

In addition to throwing athletes, individuals at risk for development of cubital tunnel syndrome include assembly line workers; violinists; and individuals with occupations that involve concussive activity such as hammering or shoveling, heavy lifting, and exposure to extensive vibration. In a study by Kakosy[55] of individuals whose occupations involved use of hand-arm vibration tools, it was reported that a significant number of the population studied displayed signs and symptoms of cubital tunnel syndrome, suggesting that use of such tools increased the risk of developing ulnar neuropathy at the elbow.[50]

Bony changes resulting from fractures or other pathologies such as Paget's disease, rheumatoid arthritis, or osteoarthritis can make the ulnar nerve more vulnerable to external pressure. The normally narrow configuration of the cubital tunnel becomes further compromised as the condylar groove space is affected by osteophytes or other deformity. Soft tissue compression on the nerve at the condylar groove may also impair function owing to the presence of ganglia, fibrolipomas, epidermoid cysts, or thickened synovium associated with rheumatoid arthritis, giant cell tumors, synovial cysts, or tophaceous gout.[50]

The cause of cubital tunnel syndrome typically has been attributed to longitudinal traction associated with position or activity resulting in friction force and volar subluxation of the nerve. As the elbow is flexed, the nerve becomes stretched across the bony surface, becoming narrowed and flattened within the condylar groove. Prolonged elbow flexion, such as during immobilization/casting, use of a sling after injury, or repetitively (e.g., while sleeping in a fetal position), has been associated with development of cubital tunnel syndrome.[50] Mechanical compression related to prior trauma, such as supracondylar fracture, and swelling at the medial elbow after injury or surgery may also result in ulnar nerve compression.[51]

Hand weakness secondary to intrinsic muscle impairment and resulting contractures are indications of more advanced stages of ulnar nerve entrapment.[50,51] Muscle atrophy associated with cubital tunnel syndrome is four times as likely to occur compared with atrophy related to CTS.[51] However, muscle impairment without reported paresthesias is more likely to be related to C8–T1 nerve root involvement as opposed to cubital tunnel syndrome.[50] Initially, motor deficits manifest with the patient demonstrating impaired dexterity in the hand and reporting feeling "clumsy." If the compression is not relieved, the patient may eventually lose grip and pinch strength. Froment's sign, the compensatory hyperflexion of the thumb interphalangeal joint with attempted adduction (e.g., holding a pen in the thumb-index finger web space), is the result of adductor pollicis paralysis (Figs. 24-7 and 24-8). Instability at the thumb metacarpophalangeal joint is a common occurrence because of adductor weakness resulting in unopposed thumb extension; unopposed thumb flexors lead to interphalangeal joint

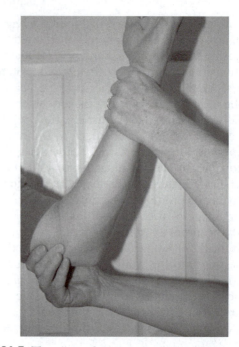

Figure 24-7 The elbow flexion test is a poorly standardized test for cubital tunnel syndrome. The test consists of the examiner passively flexing the elbow with full extension of the wrist and fingers for 3 minutes. A positive test is defined as an indication of one or more of the following symptoms: pain, numbness, or tingling. The elbow is positioned in maximum flexion, with the wrist neutral, while the therapist palpates over the ulnar nerve proximal to the cubital tunnel; this is sustained for 1 minute. The test is considered positive if the patient describes pain or paresthesias in the ulnar nerve distribution.

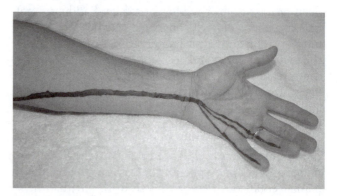

Figure 24-8 Path of the ulnar nerve in the forearm and hand as it courses distally from the cubital tunnel.

hyperflexion deformity (Jeanne's sign). Wartenberg's sign, the patient's inability to adduct the small finger, results from paralysis of the interosseous muscles and ulnar lumbricals and unopposed ulnar insertion of extensor digiti minimi (Fig. 24-9).

Advanced stages of ulnar neuropathy are associated with visible atrophy of the intrinsic hand muscles. Unopposed extensors, owing to paralysis of interosseous

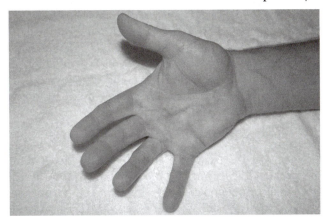

Figure 24-9 To elicit Wartenberg's sign, the patient is directed to extend the fingers; abduction or clawing of the little finger occurs. As the patient attempts to adduct the fingers, the small finger (and, in this case, the ring finger to a degree) remains abducted.

and ulnar lumbrical muscles, manifest as clawhand deformity, also known as benediction posture or *main en griffe,* and inability to form a functional grip.[50]

The four most common sites of ulnar nerve compression and resulting compromise to intraneural microcirculation are the following:[50-56]

- Arcade of Struthers
  - The arcade of Struthers is a thick fascial band located approximately 8 to 10 cm proximal to the medial epicondyle of the elbow, which runs from the medial head of the triceps to the medial intermuscular septum. Entrapment of the ulnar nerve takes place between the muscles and the ligamentous sheath.
- Humeroulnar arcade (cubital tunnel)
  - Traction force caused by hyperflexion of the elbow results in flattening of the ulnar nerve, which has been considered to be the most common cause of cubital tunnel syndrome.
- Ulnar groove
  - The nerve is vulnerable to traumatic impact and pressure as well as bony or soft tissue irregularities, including mass lesions, fibrosis and scarring, abnormalities such as cubitus valgus, and injuries such as radial head anterior dislocation.
- FCU aponeurosis
  - Location of entrapment is approximately 5 to 7 cm distal to the medial epicondyle of the elbow. During elbow flexion, the aponeurosis tightens, constricting the cubital tunnel space and compressing the ulnar nerve.

The elbow flexion test is considered to be reliable in screening for cubital tunnel syndrome. The examiner positions the subject's elbow in full flexion while palpating the ulnar nerve proximal to the cubital tunnel. Pressure and position are sustained for up to 1 minute. The test is considered to be positive if the subject reports pain/paresthesia in the ulnar nerve distribution.[56]

Anatomy

The ulnar nerve originates as a terminal branch of the medial cord of the brachial plexus at the C8 (occasionally C7) to T1 nerve root levels. At the middle to distal third of the proximal arm medial to the axillary artery, the ulnar nerve pierces the intermuscular septum at the brachialis and triceps muscle borders and enters the posterior/extensor compartment. It continues distally between the aponeurosis of the two heads of the FCU, which blend with the arcuate ligament of Osborne, forming the roof of the cubital tunnel as it joins the medial epicondyle of the humerus and olecranon process. This bridge stretches approximately 5 mm for each 45° of elbow flexion, which results in a flattening and narrowing of the nerve in the cubital tunnel.[50] The medial collateral ligament of the elbow provides the floor of the tunnel; as the elbow flexes, the medial collateral ligament becomes slack and bulges into the tunnel, further invading the cubital tunnel space.

The nerve becomes subcutaneous as it emerges from the extensor/posterior compartment of the arm to the flexor compartment of the forearm within the epicondylar groove of the distal humerus. It enters the forearm between the two heads of the FCU and gives off small branches that innervate the FCU and the ulnar half of the FDP muscles. Approximately 5 cm proximal to the pisiform, the nerve emerges at the medial border of the FCU. It bifurcates into the dorsal and palmar cutaneous branches supplying the dorsal ulnar side of the hand and fourth and fifth digits and the ulnar side of the palm. At the level of the wrist, the ulnar nerve, together with and medial to the ulnar artery, continues through the ulnar tunnel, otherwise known as Guyon's canal. The canal is formed by the hamate and pisiform bones of the wrist. Within the canal, the nerve bifurcates into its terminal deep and superficial branches. The superficial branch of the ulnar nerve provides motor innervation to the palmaris brevis and cutaneous innervation over the hypothenar eminence and ultimately divides into digital branches supplying the volar small finger and ulnar ring finger (Fig. 24-10).

The deep branch of the ulnar nerve emerges between the abductor and flexor digiti minimi muscles and provides motor innervation to the hypothenar eminence, ring and small finger lumbricals, interosseous muscles, adductor pollicis, and deep head of the flexor pollicis brevis.[50]

Guyon's Canal Syndrome (Ulnar Tunnel Syndrome)

Presentation

Guyon's canal syndrome, also known as ulnar tunnel syndrome, is a result of entrapment of the ulnar nerve

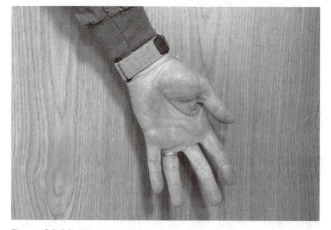

Figure 24-10 The ulnar claw, also known as the claw hand, is an abnormal resting position of the hand that develops secondary to an ulnar nerve lesion. The hand in ulnar claw has the fourth and fifth fingers drawn toward the back of the hand at the metacarpophalangeal joint and flexed at the interphalangeal joints. Classic intrinsic hand wasting is associated with ulnar neuropathy.

at the wrist as it passes through the narrow fibro-osseous opening between the palmar carpal ligament at the pisiform bone and origin of the hypothenar muscles at the level of the hamate bone.[57] This passageway is known as Guyon's canal or the ulnar tunnel. For the sake of simplicity, the term "Guyon's canal" is used henceforth.

Initial symptoms commonly include numbness and tingling and occasionally pain in the ulnar distribution of the palm, the small finger, and ulnar aspect of the ring finger. Sensitivity to cold may also be reported. As muscle function is affected, the hand becomes clumsy, and muscle atrophy may be observed.

At risk for development of Guyon's canal syndrome are individuals who have experienced concussion or compression at the area; hammering (with or without a hammer), forced gripping, and use of crutches may impose trauma to the nerve. Use of power tools that excessively jar or vibrate (e.g., a jackhammer) the area of the hamate and pisiform bones are often associated with the etiology of Guyon's canal syndrome. Also at risk are cyclists who weight-bear on the hands for prolonged periods of time or ride through rough terrain. Acute trauma, such as fracture of the hook of the hamate, may result in the collapse of the tunnel, compromising the narrow space that is occupied by the nerve and artery. Soft tissue compression may result from the presence of tumors/lipomas, ganglia, anomalous muscle bellies of palmaris brevis hypertrophy, thrombosis or aneurysm of the ulnar artery, and, more rarely, arteriovenous malformation.[58–60]

A common mistake the therapist may make is not recognizing contributing factors to Guyon's canal

syndrome, which may exist proximally. A study by Smith et al.[52] suggested concurrent thoracic outlet syndrome in cyclists and altered axonal transport secondary to compression or tension loading of the brachial plexus resulted in increased vulnerability to pressure at the cubital tunnel or Guyon's canal or both. Etiology must be fully considered in diagnosis as well as treatment.

Anatomy

Guyon's canal is triangular in shape and is located at the proximal aspect of the ulnar palm. It is bordered laterally by the hook of the hamate and transverse carpal ligament and medially by the pisiform and attachments of the pisohamate ligament.

The ulnar nerve continues down the forearm between the muscle bellies of the FDS and FDP and enters the canal along with the ulnar artery.[13] The passageway is about 4 cm in length. The proximal border is the transverse carpal ligament, and the distal border is the aponeurotic arch of the hypothenar muscles. The nerve divides into the deep motor and superficial sensory branches at the level of the pisiform bone.[57] The deep motor branch proceeds between the abductor digiti minimi and flexor digiti minimi brevis, pierces the opponens digiti minimi, and continues beneath the flexor tendons into the palmar arch.[57]

About 5 to 6 cm proximal to the wrist, the ulnar nerve contributes to the branch of the dorsal cutaneous nerve, which passes deep to the FCU, pierces through the deep fascia, and continues to the dorsoulnar aspect of the wrist and hand. It divides into two dorsal digital branches, one supplying the ulnar aspect of the small finger and the other providing sensory innervation to the radial aspect of the small finger and ulnar aspect of the ring finger. The radial aspect of the ring finger and ulnar aspect of the ring fingers are mainly supplied by the superficial radial nerve but are assisted by the ulnar digital nerve. The dorsal cutaneous branch of the ulnar nerve does not enter Guyon's canal.

The deep branch provides motor innervation to the muscles of the hypothenar eminence, as follows:

- The abductor digiti minimi is the most superficial.
- The flexor digiti minimi lies lateral to the abductor digiti minimi.
- The opponens digiti minimi lies deep to the abductor digiti minimi and flexor digiti minimi.

Innervation is also provided by the deep branch of the ulnar nerve to all interossei muscles, which abduct and adduct the fingers; third and fourth lumbricals, which flex the fourth and fifth metacarpophalangeal joints; adductor pollicis; and medial head of flexor pollicis brevis. The superficial branch lies deep and medial to the ulnar artery, superficial to the hypothenar fascia, providing sensation to the small finger and ulnar aspect of the ring finger.

Treatment of Entrapment Neuropathies

Manual Therapy

As therapists, we have the gift of our hands to assist our patients in their healing process. Extensive study and practice are required to develop the art and science of manual therapy. Understanding of anatomy, the mechanism of injury, and nerve physiology assists in providing appropriate manual intervention. However, this is not simply a matter of a mechanical influence on neural function; symptoms related to neuropathies have a strong emotional component. Butler[61,62] referred to research that revealed that injured neural tissue expressed more adrenaline-sensitive ion channels, and sympathetic fibers sprouted, resulting in increased adrenaline sensitivity. He stated that two facts must be considered: (1) Ion channels are produced reactively to the brain's response to stress, and (2) stress reduction can rapidly influence the sensitivity of the peripheral nerve as the ion channels degrade and reproduce over a short period of time.[61,62] With this in mind, the therapist must be appreciative of the potential influence of manual therapy on the neural tissue and avoid exacerbation of symptoms, which may result from overly exuberant or otherwise inappropriate delivery of technique. Following are some widely accepted manual strategies for the treatment of entrapment neuropathies of the upper extremity.

Myofascial Release

Fascia, connective tissue that is present throughout the body, covers virtually every corporal structure. Injury secondary to postural changes, inflammation, and trauma may result in alterations in pressure on structures, including neural tissue, resulting in dysfunction of the entrapped nerve or nerves. Mobilization of the fascia is directed at restoring functional mobility and nutrition to the affected structures (Figs. 24-11 through Fig. 24-14).[63]

General contraindications to performing myofascial release:

- Malignancy
- Aneurysm
- Acute rheumatoid arthritis
  Considered regional contraindications:
- Hematoma
- Open wounds
- Healing fracture

Before attempting to perform myofascial release, instruction by a qualified professional is required to provide appropriate treatment to the patient and minimize risk of accidental injury.

Soft tissue mobilization is often used by manual therapists to facilitate tissue extensibility and to relieve

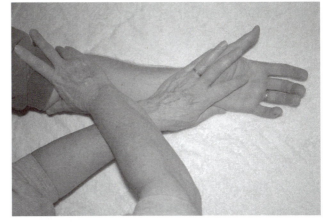

Figure 24-11 Myofascial release is a form of soft tissue therapy used to treat somatic dysfunction and resultant pain, dysesthesia, and limited mobility. The therapist is applying stress across the scar: sustained and combined distal and proximal glide on the flexor surface of the forearm.

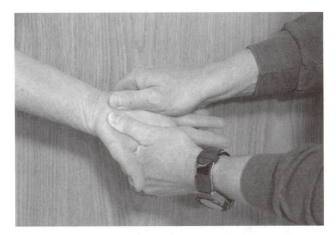

Figure 24-12 A myofascial technique using traction forces across a scar. Light tractioning gently encourages myofascial mobility.

pain. For example, pillar pain after CTR seems to be a mysterious phenomenon that has challenged therapists' abilities; research that supports any particular etiology or intervention is lacking. It has been suggested that tendon and nerve gliding and use of therapeutic modalities intended to decrease peri-incisional inflammation may be helpful in the treatment of pillar pain.[45]

The following online discussion excerpts list certified hand therapists' experiences and techniques in the treatment of pillar pain after CTR. The following entries are not based on published research studies and reflect the online opinions and experiences of various participating hand therapists.[64]

- Vigorous soft tissue mobilization (helps relieve pillar pain): having the patient wear a (scar pad) around the incision site at night for 3 to 4

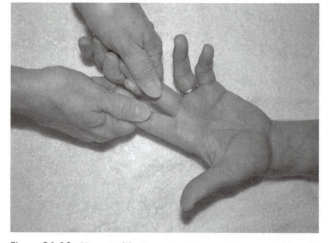

Figure 24-13 Kinesio Taping provides support to impaired joints without affecting circulation or range of motion. Indications include muscular facilitation of inhibition, pain, edema, ligament injury, muscle strain, and prevention of injury. Light tractioning is used to encourage gently myofascial mobility.

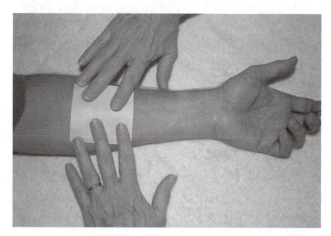

Figure 24-14 Myofascial release technique using tacky fabric. The patient may be instructed to use this technique as a component of home exercise program.

weeks (has resulted in reduction of tenderness and scar firmness).

- Vigorous massage: between 4½ and 5 weeks (postoperatively) decreases pillar pain and scar firmness/tenderness
- One session of vigorous massage between 4½ and 5 weeks (postoperatively) and instruction in "golf ball massage" (included in) home program (four times daily) 5 to 10 minutes: patients have reported quick and lasting results.

Neural Mobilization

Considering the intrinsic structure of the nerve and its inherent dependence on gliding as the body moves to continue metabolic activity, the mobilization of an entrapped nerve is intended to restore optimal function. Normal neural mobility becomes impaired when inflammation results in intraneural edema, producing increased intraneural pressure and interrupting vital blood flow, which provides oxygen and nutrient delivery to the nerve.[65]

In addition to cumulative or acute nerve trauma, iatrogenic injury may occur as a result of tourniquet use during surgery, casting, or splinting. Immobilization during the early remodeling phase after injury has been reported to hinder optimal joint and soft tissue loading, impairing nutrient exchange. Nerve compression from the orthosis secondary to a tightly fitting device or unpadded cast may occur. Neural tension and flattening of the nerve related to positioning, such as immobilization in elbow flexion, has been reported to lead to the development of neuropathy.[65]

Surgical neural mobilization may be indicated in severe cases, but conservative treatment using nerve gliding techniques may facilitate recovery in mild to moderate cases.[35,65] Neural mobilization after surgical intervention is also appropriate to prevent or minimize postsurgical scarring, which may impair normal nerve excursion. Scar mobilization, when intended to facilitate neural gliding, should be performed in one direction at a time to avoid tractioning (tensioning) of the nerve. It is reported that increased neural tension leads to increased intraneural pressure, which impairs nutrient exchange and nerve function.[65,66]

Terms associated with manual neural mobilization include "flossing," "gliding," "neurodynamic mobilization," or "neural sliding," and the actions these terms describe are intended to reduce symptoms related to restricted oxygenation to the nerve by increasing neural excursion and decreasing adhesions.[35,67] Neural mobilization techniques were introduced in the treatment of pain and radiculopathy more than 25 years ago.[67,68] Controversy surrounding nerve gliding techniques perhaps should cause us to rethink the methods we may have been taught in the past.[65] Neural mobilization techniques should focus on the restoration of normal physiological glide, as opposed to tensioning of the nerve through stretch, which results in the lengthening of the structure. Increasing tension on the nerve increases intraneural pressure, which may result in an inflammatory response and increased pain.[67] The goal of neural mobilization is to restore excursion of the nerve during activity of the individual, minimizing (ideally, eliminating) tension, which interrupts neural function.[67] Exercises may be instructed and prescribed for the patient to perform independently as an augmentation to manual techniques performed in the clinic.

A sliding technique involves limiting the combined tension placed on a nerve by reducing the number of joints involved; rather than tensioning the nerve across two or more joints, sliding is accomplished by unloading the nerve across one or more joints. This technique was used in a report by Coppieters et al.[65] with the objective of reducing intraneural and extraneural edema, increasing vascular and neural mobility. It was discovered in a cadaveric study of radial nerve excursion that about 15 mm of unimpeded nerve glide at the elbow and about 10 mm at the wrist is required to perform full motions that involve the shoulder, elbow, wrist, and fingers.[69] If there is an increase in tension greater than approximately 15% of normal, direct mechanical damage to the nerve may result because of ischemia.[69]

In a study by Dilley et al.[70] ultrasound imaging of healthy subjects measured neural strain, nerve trunk and fascicular folding, and excursion of the median nerve. It was discovered the nerve moved proximally as the arm abducted from 10° to 90°, with the greatest excursion in the final 40° to 50°. Median nerve excursion when measured with contralateral cervical flexion was variable among subjects without correlation to age or height; the study found significantly less nerve movement at 30° shoulder abduction compared with 90°. Elbow extension resulted in the nerve moving distally in the upper arm and proximally in the forearm from 90° flexion to full extension with the shoulder abducted at 90°, resulting in no significant strain. Wrist extension resulted in the median nerve gliding distally up to 6 mm. The study determined that with the arm positioned at 90° abduction combined with full elbow extension, the median nerve "behaved like a continuous spring under tension" with stretch occurring throughout the length of the nerve. Unloading of the nerve occurred when the shoulder was positioned at less than 45° abduction in combination with 90° elbow flexion.[70] In a study by Akalin et al.,[71] median nerve and tendon gliding combined with night splinting resulted in improved pinch strength and patient satisfaction for 5 to 11 months after a 4-week study. Although the study had design limitations, the information lends support to the potential benefits of this type of conservative treatment.

Coppieters et al.[65] conducted a study on nerve gliding in conservative treatment of cubital tunnel syndrome and found that a movement-based treatment plan resulted in substantial improvement; there was no recurrence in symptoms within the 10-month follow-up. Illustrating the undesired maximum traction on the ulnar nerve that occurs with the arm positioned in shoulder abduction, elbow hyperflexion, and wrist extension combined with forearm supination, treatment was conducted to avoid this cumulative tension by unloading the nerve at adjacent joints. Nerve gliding with care to minimize loading was accomplished by performing manual passive range of motion and assigning ulnar nerve mobilizations as part of the home exercise program.

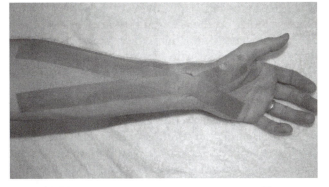

Figure 24-15 Myofascial release technique using Kinesio Taping for carpal tunnel syndrome.

Therapeutic Taping

Products such as KinesioTape and Physiotape may assist in the treatment of nerve compression disorders by improving vascular and lymphatic flow, facilitating neurological function.[72-74] In acute cases, symptom relief is expected soon after application; in chronic cases, prolonged treatment and retaping may be indicated. Consultation with a physician is advised to ensure appropriate management of symptoms relative to compression neuropathy (Fig. 24-15).

Therapeutic Modalities

Applying the principles of wound healing, facilitation of the processes leading to recovery of a tissue may be enhanced by use of therapeutic modalities.[75] However, evidence supporting use of modalities specifically for treatment of entrapment neuropathies is lacking, and more research is needed to provide therapists and other providers with a broader base for sound clinical decision making. Three common treatment modalities are addressed in this section.

Ultrasound

Ultrasound treatment to facilitate tissue regeneration and healing has been studied and found to be a viable augmentation to conservative and nonconservative treatment protocols. Bone stimulation to facilitate fracture healing using ultrasound has been reported to reduce healing time.[76] There appears to be evidence that pulsed ultrasound positively influences nerve regeneration; in animal studies focusing on the effects of ultrasound after sciatic neurotomy, rapid nerve regeneration was observed and attributed to ultrasound treatments.[77,78] Animal studies have been conducted with the hope of establishing safe and effective human treatment parameters using ultrasound for facilitating nerve recovery. Accelerated nerve regeneration was observed in traumatically injured sciatic nerves in rats treated with ultrasound.[77-79] Despite evidence of enhanced tissue healing in these studies, there are no human studies on the use of ultrasound for treatment of entrapment neuropathies. In a study comparing ultrasound treatment with placebo, Oztas et al.[80] concluded outcomes to be comparable and reported suspicion that ultrasound may have a negative effect on motor nerve function. Appropriate treatment parameters must be selected; increasing tissue temperature through use of high or continuous duty cycle and delivery of excess ultrasound energy may result in an inflammatory response as the body attempts to cool the tissues to normal levels.

The effects of nonthermal ultrasound, achieved at intensities of less than 0.3 to 1 W/cm^2, include cavitation and streaming, the formation and flow created by ultrasound energy. These effects have been reported to produce changes in membrane permeability and metabolite perfusion, reducing the time of the inflammatory phase of healing and facilitating the proliferative phase.[75] With this source of clinical reasoning, exploration of the use of ultrasound in treatment of neuropathies has been ongoing.

Mild to moderate idiopathic CTS may respond favorably to ultrasound treatment, inducing biophysical effects that result in decreased tissue inflammation.[81–84] Ebenbichler et al.[81] used treatment parameters of 1 MHz, 1.0 W/cm^2 pulsed at 25% for 15 minutes over the carpal tunnel for 20 sessions; the initial 10 sessions were performed at a frequency of 5 sessions per week, and the final 10 treatments were performed twice weekly for 5 weeks. The study suggested that by controlling inflammation and excess pressure within the carpal tunnel, the healing process and nerve recovery may be facilitated. In response to the study by Ebenbichler et al., alarm was expressed from a hand surgeon's perspective relative to choosing use of ultrasound versus CTR in treatment for CTS. The authors responded by reiterating that the purpose of their study was to explore the efficacy of ultrasound treatment for CTS because research is lacking in this area, not to recommend ultrasound as an alternative to CTR. As stated by Ebenbichler et al.,[81] optimal treatment schedules and parameters have not been reliably established.

In a study by Bakhtiary and Rishidy-Pour[85] published in 2004, ultrasound was compared with low level laser therapy (LLLT) in treatment of CTS with similar parameters used in the study by Ebenbichler et al.[81] and infrared laser parameters of 9 J, 830 nm, each for 15 treatment days. The study concluded that ultrasound was more effective than LLLT in treatment of CTS.[81,85] (Note recommendations regarding selection of laser treatment parameters in the following section on laser therapy.)

In selecting treatment parameters for compression neuropathies, there are no clear recommendations relative to the use of ultrasound. Understanding of the mechanical effects of ultrasound on tissue physiology is necessary to choose this modality.

Laser Therapy

"Low level laser therapy (LLLT) is a light source treatment that generates light of a single wavelength. LLLT emits no heat, sound, or vibration. Instead of producing a thermal effect, LLLT may act via nonthermal or photochemical reactions in the cells, also referred to as photobiology or biostimulation."[86] Also known as cold laser therapy, this treatment modality is theorized to increase mitochondrial activity, resulting in increased cellular oxygen consumption as well as lymphatic flow, resulting in decreased edema, enhancing recovery of damaged nerve tissue.[86,87]

The regeneration and recovery of damaged nerves is one of the most promising indications for use of laser therapy.[87] Reduction in edema through enhancement of lymphatic vessel regeneration has also been reported.[87]

In a study published in 2007 by Evcik et al.,[88] positive effects on hand grip and pinch strengths were achieved using treatment parameters of 7 J of LLLT over the course of 2 minutes five times per week for 2 weeks. Laser therapy for CTS was one of the first indications to receive approval from the U.S. Food and Drug Administration, being limited to "adjunct use" in obtaining temporary pain relief.[87] In selection of laser therapy for compression neuropathies, it is recommended to refer to the individual product manual for guidance because various laser therapy systems are currently on the market.

Electrical Stimulation

Regeneration of injured peripheral nerves may be assisted by use of electrical stimulation modalities, but studies on research in humans are scarce. When edema is suspected to be imposing pressure on a nerve, electrical modalities may be helpful for edema management.

Animal studies have reported positive results relative to edema reduction and nerve regeneration using direct current.[89,90] Human studies on edema management employing high volt pulsed current using negative polarity resulted in reduction in edema compared with using positive polarity; the literature suggested treatment parameters that included 120 pulses per second, and that submotor intensity may result in some improvement in edema and range-of-motion measurements.[91] Although the mechanism that results in edema reduction when high volt pulsed current is used with a negative polarity is not completely understood, it is hypothesized that the conduction of negatively charged electrical current repels the like-charged plasma proteins associated with edema, a phenomenon known as "cataphoresis."[92]

The mechanism of electrical stimulation resulting in edema reduction is not completely understood, but it is speculated that edema formation is retarded because of reduced microvessel permeability to plasma macro-molecules.[93] Further research is needed to understand better and use this treatment modality appropriately.

CASE STUDY

BR is a long distance runner averaging more than 25 miles per week. He has noticed over the past few months that at the 5-mile point of his run his left hand becomes numb. The numbness continues to worsen the longer he runs and extends from his two medial fingers along the outside of his wrist to just below his elbow. When he stops running, the numbness gradually abates after a few hours. He also notes a constant dull ache behind his elbow. He does not perceive any weakness in the hand.

On physical examination, the only "hard" finding uncovered by the therapist is a positive Tinel sign over the olecranon fossae. During the examination, the therapist could not identify any focal weakness, loss of deep tendon reflex, or tactile sensory loss. There was no evidence of upper motor neuron involvement. Cranial nerves were intact.

Case Study Questions

1. Based on the subjective complaints of the patient, the symptoms appear to be associated with which nerve?
   a. Ulnar
   b. Median
   c. Anterior interosseus
   d. Posterior interosseus

2. Which of the following would be a differential diagnosis for this impairment?
   a. Ulnar nerve impingement at the tunnel of Guyon
   b. C8–T1 cervical radiculopathy
   c. Ulnar nerve impingement at the olecranon fossa
   d. All of the above

3. If the correct diagnosis is ulnar nerve impingement at the elbow and if there is muscle weakness related to the impingement, which muscle would have the highest probability of exhibiting weakness?
   a. Flexor carpi radialis
   b. Pronator teres
   c. Abductor digiti minimi
   d. Opponens pollicis

4. If the correct diagnosis is ulnar nerve impingement at the elbow, which behavioral change may be indicated?
   a. Encourage sleeping with the elbow extended
   b. Avoid leaning on the elbow when sitting at a desk
   c. Maintain elbow extension when running
   d. All of the above

5. To quantify the neuropathy based on the Seddon classification, which diagnostic test would be the most helpful?
   a. Phalen's
   b. Electroneuromyogram
   c. Magnetic resonance imaging of the elbow
   d. X-ray of the elbow

References

1. Lundborg G. Structure and function of the intraneural microvessels as related to trauma, edema formation, and nerve function. *J Bone Joint Surg Am.* 1975;57:938–948.
2. Ochoa J. Nerve fiber pathology in acute and chronic compression. In: Omer G, Spinner M, VanBeek A, eds. *Management of Peripheral Nerve Problems.* 2nd ed. Philadelphia: Saunders; 1998:475–483.
3. Rempel D, Dahlin L, Lundborg G. Pathophysiology of nerve compression syndromes: response of peripheral nerves to loading. *J Bone Joint Surg Am.* 1999;81(11):1600–1610.
4. Tapadia M, Mozaffar T, Gupta R. Compressive neuropathies of the upper extremity: update on pathophysiology, classification, and electrodiagnostic findings. *J Hand Surg Am.* 2010;35:668–677.
5. Michele AA, Krueger FJ. Lateral epicondylitis of the elbow treated by fasciotomy. *Surgery.* 1956;39:277–284.
6. Standard of Care: Radial Tunnel Syndrome. Copyright 2007 The Brigham and Women's Hospital, Inc., Department of Rehabilitation Services. All rights reserved.
7. Stanley J. Radial tunnel syndrome: a surgeon's perspective. *J Hand Ther.* 2006;19:180–185.
8. Roquelaure Y, Raimbeau G, Saint-Cast Y, Martin YH, Pelier-Cady MC. Occupational risk factors for radial tunnel syndrome in factory workers. *Chir Main.* 2003;22(6):293–298.
9. Loh YC, Lam WL, Stanley JK, Soames RW. A new clinical test for radial tunnel syndrome—the Rule-of-Nine test: a cadaveric study. *J Orthop Surg.* 2004;12(1):83–86.
10. Tennent TD, Woodgate A. Posterior interosseous nerve dysfunction in the radial tunnel. *Curr Orthop.* 2008;22(3):226–232.
11. Stern M. Radial nerve entrapment. Medscape Web site. http://emedicine.medscape.com/article/1244110-overview. Updated September 2, 2009. Accessed July 12, 2010.
12. Thomas SJ, Yakin DE, Parry BR, Lubahn JD. The anatomical relationship between the posterior interosseous nerve and the supinator muscle. *J Hand Surg Am.* 2000;25:936–941.
13. Wilhelmi B, Naffziger R, Neumeister M. Hand, nerve compression syndromes. Medscape Web site. http://emedicine.medscape.com/article/1285531-overview. Updated May 31, 2009. Accessed July 12, 2010.
14. Dillon AL, Mackinnon SE. Chronic nerve compression model for the double-crush hypothesis. *Am Plast Surg.* 1991;26:259–265.
15. Patterson RW, van Niel M, Shimko P, Pace C, Seitz WH Jr. Proprioception of the wrist following posterior interosseous sensory neurectomy. *J Hand Surg Am.* 2010;35:52–56.
16. Prakash, Rai R, Ranade AV, Prabhu LV, Pai MM, Singh G. Multiple variations of extensor muscles of forearm in relation to the radial nerve: a case report and review. *Int J Morphol.* 2008;26(2):447–449.
17. Tosun N, Tuncay I, Akpinar F. Entrapment of the sensory branch of the radial nerve (Wartenberg's syndrome): an unusual cause. *Tohoku J Exp Med.* 2001;193:251–254.
18. *Stedman's Medical Dictionary.* Baltimore: Lippincott, Williams & Wilkins; 2006.

19. Lanzetta M, Foucher G. Entrapment of the superficial branch of the radial nerve (Wartenberg's syndrome). *Int Orthop.* 1993;17:342–345.

20. Szabo R. Entrapment and compression neuropathies. In: Green DP. Hotchkiss RN, Pederson WC, eds. *Green's Operative Hand Surgery.* Vol 2. 4th ed. Philadelphia: Churchill Livingstone; 1998:1439.

21. Surendran S, Bhat SM, Krishnamurthy A. Compression of radial nerve between the split tendon of brachioradialis muscle: a case report. *Neuroanatomy.* 2006;5:4–5.

22. Pronator syndrome discussion. EHand.com: The Electronic Textbook of Hand Surgery Web site. http://www.eatonhand.com/dis/dis315.htm. Accessed July 22, 2010.

23. Hagert S, Englund J. Pronator syndrome: a retrospective study of median nerve entrapment at the elbow in female machine milkers. *J Agric Saf Health.* 2004;10(4):247–256.

24. Lee M, LaStayo P. Pronator syndrome and other nerve compressions that mimic carpal tunnel syndrome. *J Orthop Sport Phys Ther.* 2004;34:601–609.

25. Ericson WB. Median nerve entrapment in the forearm: diagnosis and treatment. Poster presented at: ASSH March 13–16, 2004, San Francisco, CA.

26. Koo JT, Szabo RM. Compression neuropathies of the median nerve. *Journal of the American Society for Surgery of the Hand.* 2004;4(3):156–175.

27. Collins D, Weber E. Anterior interosseous nerve syndrome. *South Med J.* 1983;76(12):1533–1537.

28. Nigst H, Dick W. Syndromes of compression of the median nerve in the proximal forearm (pronator teres syndrome: anterior interosseous nerve syndrome). *Arch Orthop Trauma Surg.* 1979;93:307–312.

29. Nelson R, Currier D. Anterior interosseous syndrome: a case report. *J Phys Ther.* 1980;60:194.

30. Mody B. Tenodesis effect: a simple clinical test to differentiate rupture of flexor pollicis longus and incomplete anterior interosseous paralysis. *J Hand Surg Br.* 1992; 17:510.

31. Farber J, Bryan R. The anterior interosseous nerve syndrome. *J Bone Joint Surg Am.* 1968;50:521–523.

32. Stark E, Dell M, Wisco J. A case report: a variation of the palmaris profundus muscle. *IJAV.* 2010;3:36–38.

33. Bickel K. Carpal tunnel syndrome. *J Hand Surg Am.* 2010;35: 147–152.

34. Moscony AMB. Common peripheral nerve problems. In: Cooper C, ed. *Fundamentals of Hand Therapy: Clinical Reasoning and Treatment Guidelines for Common Diagnoses of the Upper Extremity.* Philadelphia: Mosby; 2007:201–250.

35. Medina McKeon J, Yancosek K. Neural gliding techniques for the treatment of carpal tunnel syndrome: a systemic review. *J Sport Rehabil.* 2008;17:324–341.

36. Silverstein B, Fine L, Armstrong T. Occupational factors and carpal tunnel syndrome. *Am J Ind Med.* 1987;11(3): 343–358.

37. U.S. Department of Labor. *Occupational Injuries and Illnesses: Counts, Rates, and Characteristics. Bulletin 2538.* Washington, DC: U.S. Bureau of Labor Statistics; 2001.

38. Falkiner S, Myers S. When exactly can carpal tunnel syndrome be considered work-related? *Aust N Z J Surg.* 2002; 72:204–209.

39. American Academy of Orthopaedic Surgeons Work Group Panel. Clinical guidelines on diagnosis of carpal tunnel syndrome. www.aaos.org/research/guidelines/CTS_guideline.pdf. Accessed July 12, 2010.

40. Werner R, Andary M. Carpal tunnel syndrome: pathophysiology and clinical neurophysiology. *Clin Neurophysiol.* 2002;113(9):1373–1381.

41. Seradge H, Parker W, Baer C, Mayfield K, Schall L. Conservative treatment of carpal tunnel syndrome: an outcome study of adjunct exercises. *J Okla State Med Assoc.* ;95(1):7–14.

42. Luchetti R, Schoenhuber R, Nathan P. Correlation of segmental carpal tunnel pressures with changes in hand and wrist positions in patients with carpal tunnel syndrome and controls. *J Hand Surg Eur.* 1998;23(5):598–602.

43. Cobb TK, An Kai-Nan, Cooney W. Externally applied forces to the palm increase carpal tunnel pressure. *J Hand Surg.* 1995;20(2):181–185.

44. Geoghegan JM, Clark DI, Bainbridge LC, Smith C, Hubbard R. Risk factors in carpal tunnel syndrome. *J Hand Surg Eur.* 2004;29(4):315–320.

45. Rodner C, Katarincic J. Open carpal tunnel release. *Tech Orthop.* 2006;21(1):3–11.

46. Taizo K, Hiroyuki H. Clinical analysis of pillar pain after endoscopic carpal tunnel release: the Okutsu method. *J Jpn Soc Surg Hand.* 2005;22(2):6–9.

47. Siegel D, Kuzma G, Eakins D. Anatomic investigation of the role of the lumbrical muscles in carpal tunnel syndrome. *J Hand Surg.* 1995;20(5):860–863.

48. Gwynne D. Bilateral palmaris profundus in association with bifid median nerve as a cause of failed carpal tunnel release. *J Hand Surg.* 2006;31(5):741–743.

49. Homma T, Sakai T. Thenar and hypothenar muscles and their innervation by the ulnar and median nerves in the human hand. *Acta Anat.* 1992;145:44–49.

50. Robertson C, Saratsiotis J. A review of compressive ulnar neuropathy at the elbow. *J Manipulative Physiol Ther.* 2005;28: 345.e18.

51. Palmer B, Hughes T. Cubital tunnel syndrome. *J Hand Surg Am.* 2010;35:153–163.

52. Smith T, Sawyer S, Sizer P, Brismee J. The double crush syndrome: a common occurrence in cyclists with ulnar nerve neuropathy—a case control study. *Clin J Sport Med.* 2008;18: 55–61.

53. Aoki M, Takasaki H, Muraki T, Uchiyama E, Murakami G, Yamashita T. Strain on the ulnar nerve at the elbow and wrist during throwing motion. *J Bone Joint Surg Am.* 2005;87(11): 2508–2514.

54. Aoki M, Kanaya K, Aiki H, Wada T, Yamashita T, Ogiwara N. Cubital tunnel syndrome in adolescent baseball players: a report of six cases with 3- to 5-year follow-up. *Arthroscopy.* 2005;21(6):758e1–758e6.

55. Kakosy T. Tunnel syndromes of the upper extremities in workers using hand-operated vibrating tools. *Med Lav.* 1994; 85:474–480.

56. Gelberman RH, Yamaguchi K, Hollstien S, et al. Changes in interstitial pressure and cross-sectional area of the cubital tunnel and of the ulnar nerve with flexion of the elbow: an experimental study in human cadavera. *J Bone Joint Surg Am.* 1998;80:492–501.

57. Zeiss J, Jakab E, Khimji T, Imbriglia J. Ulnar tunnel at the wrist (Guyon's canal): normal MR anatomy and variants. *AJR Am J Roentgenol.* 1992;158:1081–1085.

58. Chalidis B, Sachinis N, Dimitriou C. Ulnar nerve penetration by a volar ganglion in the Guyon canal. *Plast Reconstr Surg.* 2009;124(5):264e–266e.

59. Sierakowski A, Zweifel CJ, Payne S. Compression of the ulnar nerve in Guyon's canal caused by a large hypothenar cyst. *ePlasty.* 2009;10:32–36.

60. Rohilla S, Yadav R, Dhaulakhandi D. Lipoma of Guyon's canal causing ulnar neuropathy. *J Orthop Traumatol.* 2009;10: 101–103.

61. Butler DS. *The Sensitive Nervous System.* South Australia: Noigroup Publications; 2000.

62. Butler D. Neurodynamics—Physical Neural Health Web site. http://noineurodynamics.blogspot.com. Updated July 23, 2008. Accessed July 12, 2010.

63. Barnes JF. *Myofascial Release: The Search for Excellence. A Comprehensive Evaluatory and Treatment Approach.* Paoli, PA: MFR Seminars; 1990.

64. Fedorczyk J. Online discussion: Clinical treatment issues. Subject: re: Pillar pain (e-mail communication, October 13, 2010).

65. Coppieters M, Bartholomeeusen K, Stappaerts K. Incorporating nerve-gliding techniques in the conservative treatment of cubital tunnel syndrome. *J Manipulative Physiol Ther.* 2004;27:560–568.

66. Wehbe M, Schlegel J. Nerve gliding exercises for thoracic outlet syndrome. *Hand Clin.* 2004;20:51–55.

67. Coppieters M, Hough A, Dilley A. Different nerve-gliding exercises induce different magnitudes of median nerve longitudinal excursion: an in vivo study using dynamic ultrasound imaging. *J Orthop Sports Phys Ther.* 2009;39(3): 164–171.

68. Elvey RL. Treatment of arm pain associated with abnormal brachial plexus tension. *Aust J Physiother.* 1986;32:225–230.

69. Wright T, Glowczewskie F, Cowin D. Radial nerve excursion and strain at the elbow and wrist associated with upper-extremity motion. *J Hand Surg Am.* 2005;30:990–996.

70. Dilley A, Lynn B, Greening J, DeLeon N. Quantitative in vivo studies of median nerve sliding in response to wrist, elbow, shoulder and neck movements. *Clin Biomech.* 2003;18: 899–907.

71. Akalin E, El O, Peker O, et al. Treatment of carpal tunnel syndrome with nerve and tendon gliding exercises. *Am J Phys Med Rehabil.* 2002;81:108–113.

72. Kase K, Hashimoto T, Okane T, Kinesio Taping Association. *Kinesio Taping Perfect Manual: Amazing Taping Therapy to Eliminate Pain and Muscle Disorders.* Boston, MA: Kinesio USA;1998.

73. Thelen MD, Dauber JA, Stoneman PD. The clinical efficacy of Kinesio tape for shoulder pain:A randomized, double blinded, clinical trial. *Journal of Orthop and Sports Physical Therapy.* 2008;38:389–395.

74. Kase K, Hashimoto T. *Changes in the volume of the peripheral blood flow by using Kinesio taping.* San Francisco, CA:Kinesio Taping Association International; 1998.

75. Hess C, Howard M, Atringer C. A review of mechanical adjuncts in wound healing: hydrotherapy, ultrasound, negative pressure therapy, hyperbaric oxygen and electrostimulation. http//hessplasticsurgery.net/pdf/wound-healing.pdf. Accessed July 15, 2010.

76. Kristiansen TK, Ryaby JP, McCabe J, Frey JJ, Roe LR. Accelerated healing of distal radial fractures with the use of low-intensity ultrasound. A multicenter, prospective, randomized specific, double-blind, placebo-controlled study. *J Bone Joint Surg Am.* 1997;79:961–973.

77. Crisci AR, Ferreira AF. Low-intensity pulsed ultrasound accelerates the regeneration of the sciatic nerve after neurotomy in rats. *Ultrasound Med Biol.* 2002;28(10): 1335–1341.

78. Mourad PD, Lazar D, Curra FP, et al. Ultrasound accelerates functional recovery after peripheral nerve damage. *Neurosurgery.* 48:1136–1141, 2001.

79. Chang C-J, Hsu S-H. The effects of low-intensity ultrasound on peripheral nerve regeneration in poly (DL-lactic acid-Co-glyconic acid) conduits seeded with Schwann cells. *Ultrasound Med Biol.* 2004;30(8):1079–1084.

80. Oztas O, Turan B, Bora I, Karakaya MK. Ultrasound therapy effect in carpal tunnel syndrome. *Arch Phys Med Rehabil.* 1998;79(12):1540–1544.

81. Ebenbichler G, Resch K, Nicolakis P, et al. Ultrasound treatment for treating the carpal tunnel syndrome: randomised "sham" controlled trial. *BMJ.* 1998;316:731–735.

82. Barnett SB, Ter Haar GR, Ziskin MC, Nyborg WL, Maeda K, Bang J. Current status of research on biophysical effects of ultrasound. *Ultrasound Med Biol.* 1994;20:205–218.

83. El Hag M, Coghlan K, Christmas P, Harvey W, Harris M. The anti-inflammatory effects of dexamethasone and therapeutic ultrasound in oral surgery. *Br J Oral Maxillofac Surg.* 1985;23:17–23.

84. Dyson M. Mechanisms involved in therapeutic ultrasound. *Physiotherapy.* 1987;73:116–120.

85. Bakhtiary AH, Rashidy-Pour A. Ultrasound and laser therapy in the treatment of carpal tunnel syndrome. *Aust J Physiother.* 2004;50:147–151.

86. Wang G. Low level laser therapy (LLLT) technology assessment. http://www.lni.wa.gov/ClaimsIns/Files/OMD/LLLTTechAssessMay032004.pdf. Updated May 3, 2004. Accessed July 16, 2010.

87. Tuner J, Hode L. *Laser Therapy: Clinical Practice and Scientific Background.* Tallinn, Estonia: UP Print; 2002.

88. Evcik D, Kavuncu V, Cakir T, Subasi V, Yaman M. Laser therapy in the treatment of carpal tunnel syndrome: a randomized controlled trial. *Photomed Laser Surg.* 2007;25(1): 34–39.

89. Mendal FC, Fish DR. New perspectives in edema control via electrical stimulation. *J Athl Train.* 1993;280(1):63–74.

90. Dolan MG, Mendel FC. Clinical application of electrotherapy. *Athl Ther Today.* 2004;9:11–16.

91. Sandoval MC, Ramirez C, Camargo DM, Salvini TF. Effect of high-voltage pulsed current plus conventional treatment on acute ankle sprain. *Rev Bras Fisioter, São Carlos.* 2010;14(3): 193–199.

92. Cosgrove KA, Alon G, Bell SF, *et al.* The electrical effect of two commonly used clinical stimulators on traumatic edema in rats. *Phys Ther.* 1992;72(3):227–233.

93. Reed B. Effect of high voltage pulsed electrical stimulation on microvascular permeability to plasma proteins: a possible mechanism in minimizing edema. *Phys Ther.* 1988;68(4): 491–495.

Chapter 25

Entrapment Neuropathies in the Foot and Ankle

John P. Scanlon, DPM, Crystal N. Gonzalez, DPM,
Benjamin R. Denenberg, DPM, and Krupa J. Trivedi, DPM

"The human foot is a masterpiece of engineering and a work of art."

—Leonardo da Vinci (1452–1519)

Objectives

On completion of this chapter, the student/practitioner will be able to:

- Describe the anatomical pathways of the major peripheral nerves in the lower extremity.
- Identify possible sites of entrapment of the major peripheral nerves in the lower leg.
- Discuss the pathogenesis of peripheral nerve injury.
- Discuss the possible etiologies of lower extremity peripheral nerve entrapment.
- Describe the surgical and conservative interventions for each lower extremity nerve entrapment site.
- Include peripheral nerve entrapment as a potential differential diagnosis for lower extremity impairments during the clinical evaluation.

Key Terms

- Entrapment neuropathy
- Neurolysis
- Neuroma
- Peripheral nerve

Introduction

Symptoms of nerve compression in the lower extremities account for a large percentage of patients visiting their primary physician and being referred to a specialist. Because of the myriad symptoms reported by patients with potential lower extremity neuropathy, the list of potential differential diagnoses is long. Lack of proper diagnostic testing and assessment may lead to inappropriate referral, chronic pain, disability, and surgeries that are not helpful or indicated. Complicating the diagnostic process is that low back pain often accompanies tunnel syndromes in the lower extremity through systemic or multiple nerve involvement or as a direct result of gait compensation secondary to lower extremity antalgia. Lower extremity neuropathic symptoms may also be the indirect result of neoplasm, connective tissue disease, infection, peripheral vascular disease, psychiatric disturbances, hormonal imbalances, toxins, overuse, and metabolic illnesses. The diagnostician must have a good understanding of the anatomy of the lower extremity including the nerve paths. In addition, content knowledge of the endocrine, neural, musculoskeletal, integument, renal, gastrointestinal, and cardiopulmonary systems often is relevant to the diagnosis and interventions associated with lower extremity neurological symptoms.

Anatomy

The lower extremity receives sensory and motor innervation from branches of the sciatic nerve along with the saphenous nerve. The sciatic nerve is the only nerve in the lower extremity arising from the lumbar plexus. Branches of the sciatic nerve include the common peroneal nerve and tibial nerve. The common peroneal nerve branches further to form the superficial peroneal nerve and the deep peroneal nerve. The superficial peroneal nerve provides cutaneous innervation to the anterior and anterolateral aspect of the foot and ankle and provides motor innervation to the muscles in the lateral compartment of the leg. The deep peroneal nerve innervates muscles of the anterior compartment of the leg and intrinsic musculature of the dorsal foot and provides cutaneous innervation to the first interspace. The tibial nerve branches into the sural nerve, medial plantar nerve, lateral plantar nerve, and medial calcaneal nerve. The sural nerve provides cutaneous innervation to the lateral aspect of the foot. The medial plantar nerve innervates the plantar intrinsic musculature of the foot. The lateral plantar nerve innervates the lateral plantar intrinsic musculature of the foot.

The saphenous nerve, the largest cutaneous branch of the femoral nerve, exits from the adductor canal, descends under the sartorius muscle, and winds around the posterior edge of the sartorius muscle at its tendinous portion. The infrapatellar branch pierces the sartorius muscle and crosses anteriorly to the infrapatellar region. The descending branch passes down the medial aspect of the leg and at the lower third of the leg divides into two branches. One of the branches of the descending portion of the nerve courses along the medial border of the tibia and ends at the ankle, whereas the other branch passes anteriorly to the ankle and is distributed to the medial aspect of the foot, reaching the metatarsophalangeal joint of the great toe.

Variables such as anatomical path, location of adjacent structures, tension, superficiality, size, composition, and vascular supply subject the **peripheral nerve** to a spectrum of injury types. Seddon and Sunderland individually developed nomenclature systems for the severity of injury to peripheral nerves. Seddon[1] defined three types of nerve injuries, including neurapraxia, axonotmesis, and neurotmesis. Sunderland[2] described five degrees of nerve injuries, which correlate with Seddon's classification (Box 25-1). With the progression from neurapraxic to axonotmetic to neurotmetic lesions, the mechanism of injury, the severity of the symptoms, and the healing time all tend to escalate. Neurapraxic lesions tend to be the mildest of lesions with transitory sensory symptoms that last from minutes to weeks. Healing is spontaneous. There is no denervation. The hallmark of axonotmetic lesions is axonal injury with frank denervation. Depending on the location of these injuries, recovery, although typically spontaneous, may require months or years. Neurotmetic lesions often require surgical intervention, and the prospect of recovery is guarded.

Box 25-1

Seddon and Sunderland Classifications of Severity of Peripheral Nerve Injury

Seddon's Classification

Neurapraxia: Temporary interruption of conduction without loss of axonal continuity; endoneurium, perineurium, and epineurium are intact.

Axonotmesis: Involves loss of relative continuity of the axon and its covering of myelin, but preservation of the connective tissue framework of the nerve; epineurium and perineurium are preserved. Wallerian degeneration occurs.

Neurotmesis: Total severance or disruption of the entire nerve fiber.

Sunderland's Classification

First degree: Seddon's neurapraxia.

Second degree: Seddon's axonotmesis.

Third degree: Interruption of the nerve fiber with epineurium and perineurium intact. Recovery is possible with surgical intervention.

Fourth degree: Interruption of the nerve fiber with only the epineurium intact. Surgical repair is required.

Fifth degree: Complete transection of the nerve.

Pathology

Entrapment neuropathy is a generalized term frequently used to describe common nerve pathology involving compression of a peripheral nerve; another term often used is "tunnel neuropathy." Although entrapment neuropathy is not directly defined or described by the Seddon and Sunderland classification systems, there is a definite correlation between the severity of the nerve lesion and the mechanism of injury. Entrapment neuropathies tend to develop as a result of external or internal compressive or occlusive factors. Internal factors, such as narrow fibro-osseous tunnels through which the nerves pass and space-occupying lesions such as an osteophyte or tumor may disrupt the nerve and precipitate axonal damage leading to neuropathy. External factors, including nerve damage secondary to trauma, biomechanical factors, toxin ingestion, medication, endocrine disease, and systemic disease (e.g., rheumatoid arthritis, systemic lupus erythematosus, Sjögren's disease), are also relevant contributing features. Systemic diseases may contribute to a pathology described in 1973 by Upton and McComas[3] and later by Osterman[4] known as "double crush syndrome." Double crush occurs when a proximal nerve is compressed altering axonal transport and contributing to a secondary distal entrapment. A concomitant cervical nerve root lesion is found in 70% of patients with symptomatic carpal tunnel or ulnar neuropathy via electroneurophysiological testing.[3] With all individuals with a suspected peripheral nerve lesion, a thorough and comprehensive physical and electrophysiological evaluation must be performed before contemplating any intervention not only to rule out differential diagnoses but also to ascertain if additional sites of entrapment may be present.

Examination

The physical examination begins at first contact with the patient. The practitioner should identify postural or gait abnormalities, which may act as "clinical scripts" to assist with guiding the interview and physical examination.

After establishing a relationship with the patient, the nerve examination should begin with a series of questions to pinpoint the origin of entrapment. The previous medical and surgical history should be documented with special regard to items related to systemic illness or prior neuropathy diagnoses. The medication history should be obtained and should not be limited to current medications. Because medication-related neuropathies are common and may last for a significant period of time or forever, medications taken over the past 5 years should be identified and researched for potential neuropathic complications. The use of over-the-counter, herbal, and illegal medications and drugs should be queried. The practitioner should attempt to identify any behavioral, vocational, occupational, or biomechanical stresses that have an impact on the severity of the neuropathic symptoms.

For lower extremity symptoms, the physical examination begins with a screening manual muscle test. Choosing specific muscles that capture each segmental and peripheral myotome is mandatory. If focal weakness is identified, additional muscles should be tested to confirm the involved myotome. Range-of-motion screening should be performed to identify overt articular and axial abnormalities. Screening can be performed via commands such as "squat down," "raise up," "bend," "straighten up," "stand on your toes," and "stand on your heels."

Next, the physical examination moves to the origin of the peripheral nerve at the spinal cord. Herniated discs or arthritis can be the primary etiology for nerve pain secondary to compression and entrapment of the peripheral nerve roots that stem from the lumbar plexus and innervate the lower extremity. To test for lumbar nerve root entrapment/compression, the straight leg raise or slump test can be performed. Both tests stretch the sciatic nerve to tension eliciting pain. Both tests should elicit a "soft tissue end-feel." Eliciting neurological symptoms such as radicular pain or paresthesias is considered a positive test. The straight leg raise is performed with the patient positioned supine and lifting the leg vertically without flexing the knee. The slump test is performed in three parts. The patient should be seated in a chair and asked to slump the lower back. If this movement does not elicit pain, flexion at the neck may be added to elicit a response. Finally, the addition of extending the knee with concomitant dorsiflexion of the foot may be the final maneuver to elicit sciatic nerve tension.[5]

Palpation of the path of the peripheral nerve should be performed. Typically, nerves, contractile tissues, and noncontractile tissues are not painful to light palpation. Pain may indicate a problem. Particular emphasis should be directed at palpating where the nerve passes into the subcutaneous tissue, is adjacent to a bony structure, or passes through a fibro-osseous tunnel. Following light palpation, the nerve should be percussed, which may elicit various symptoms. A Tinel sign occurs when a nerve is tapped and paresthesias are elicited distal to the area of percussion. Sensation should be tested through multiple modalities, including light touch, pin, and vibration. Balance assessment can be performed by using validated tests such as the Berg, Romberg, or Timed Up and Go.[6] Large-fiber afferent neuropathy, which is a presenting sign of diabetic neuropathy, is often identified by decreased static and dynamic standing balance.

The next area of focus during the examination is the biomechanical and visual component. Range of motion of all the joints distal and proximal to the nerve should be examined for impairment. Alignment should also be noted, especially as related to the back, hip, knee, and foot. Long-term abnormal alignment almost always results in abnormal soft tissue stresses. The joints should also be examined in the weight-bearing position. Misalignment may be present only during weight bearing. In addition, positional change and weight bearing may exacerbate symptoms. The patient should be asked to fan the toes in weight-bearing and non–weight-bearing positioning. The inability to perform this task as well as the presence of digital deformities could indicate weakness of the intrinsic musculature.

The biomechanical examination should include a gait analysis because weakness in the muscles and range of motion of joints can be more clearly identified through the phases of gait. Ambulation should be assessed on level ground, at various speeds, up a ramp, down a ramp, ascending and descending steps, and ascending and descending curbs. Electromyography is another diagnostic tool that is helpful in arriving at a definitive diagnosis of entrapment neuropathy. This test is performed with the insertion of a needle into the muscle innervated by the nerve to assess electrical potentials within the motor unit at rest, with minimal contraction, and with maximal contraction. Nerve conduction velocity testing performed serially with electromyography provides important information regarding conduction time and nerve latency.

These data can be compared with and correlated to the normative values. For practitioners whose state licensing rules permit, a diagnostic block using local anesthetic may be performed to obtain further diagnostic information or to confirm a differential diagnosis.

Intervention Overview

Conservative and surgical treatments may be effective depending on the particular clinical case. Neurapraxic lesions of the common peroneal nerve typically heal with conservative treatment. Conversely, neuropathy associated with long-term poor glycemic control typically has a poor long-term prognosis.

A sound conservative therapeutic regimen involves correction of the biomechanical deformities through the use of physical therapy modalities and prescribed exercises, orthotic devices, and bracing. Because the symptoms of entrapment may not fully resolve with conservative measures alone, surgery may be the next consideration. Surgical options include, but are not limited to, **neurolysis** or a release of the fibro-osseous tunnels and decompression and release of fibrotic adhesions around the nerve.

If conservative intervention is not effective, surgical intervention for the treatment of entrapment neuropathies may be indicated. Several procedures have been described, including decompression, neurolysis, nerve wrapping, and nerve grafting. Decompression often involves careful anatomical dissection and release of adhesions and fascial constraints. Neurolysis refers to the surgical resection of a portion of the fibrosed nerve. Another viable addition to corrective procedures is nerve wrapping. The primary purpose of this procedure is to minimize re-entrapment and prevent fibrosis by providing an autogenous tissue such as a vein or synthetic material to serve as a protective barrier. Other techniques that have been described include fat grafts and rerouting of the nerve, which allow the nerve to heal in an adhesion-free environment.[7]

Entrapment Neuropathy of Specific Lower Extremity Nerves

Sural Nerve

The sural nerve is largely responsible for the cutaneous innervation of the dorsal lateral aspect of the foot and heel and articular innervations to the inferior tibiofibular joint, talocrural joint, and talocalcaneal joints. Measuring approximately 2 cm in diameter, it comprises the medial sural nerve—a branch of the tibial nerve—and the sural communicating nerve, which is a branch of the common peroneal nerve. Originating at the popliteal fossa, the medial sural nerve courses between the

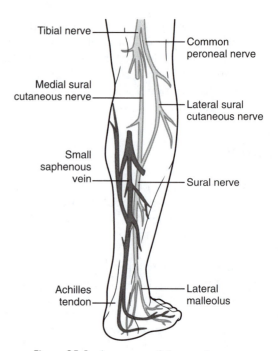

Figure 25-1 Anatomy of the sural nerve.

medial and lateral heads of the gastrocnemius muscle, piercing the deep fascia to anastomose with the sural communicating nerve at the middle of the posterior leg forming the sural nerve. Continuing distally, it traverses along the lateral border of the Achilles tendon to pass along the posterior border of the lateral malleolus approximately where it splits into its two terminal branches, the lateral dorsal cutaneous nerve and the lateral calcaneal nerve (Fig. 25-1).

Entrapment of the sural nerve can occur at any point along its length. Intrinsically, this may be seen along changes in fascial planes or along fibro-osseous tunnels. In our practice, sural nerve compression is common in runners with tight crural fascia presenting with chronic compartment syndrome of the leg. In addition, impingement may occur secondary to trauma where blunt force compresses the nerve against a bony structure.[7,8] Athletes, particularly soccer players who sustain kicks to the posterior aspect of the leg, often experience entrapment of the sural nerve.[9] Plantar flexion inversion injuries with concomitant fifth metatarsal fractures have also been described as an etiology.[9] Recurrent ankle sprains or twisting injuries may lead to fibrosis of the nerve sheath, creating an entrapment.[10] Similar entrapment scenarios are evident with the presence of ganglions of the peroneal sheath or calcaneocuboid joint and Achilles peritendonitis.[11]

The sural nerve should be examined from the popliteal fossa to the toes. Patients may report numbness and paresthesias. Local tenderness along with a positive Tinel sign running along the course of the nerve is characteristic of this syndrome.

Superficial Peroneal Nerve

A branch of the common peroneal nerve, the superficial peroneal nerve provides cutaneous innervations to the dorsal aspect of the foot spanning from the medial aspect of the fifth toe to the medial aspect of the great toe excluding the first interspace. Muscular innervation to the lateral compartment of the leg, including peroneus (fibularis) longus and brevis muscles, is provided by the superficial peroneal nerve. Coursing around the fibular head, the nerve travels in the lateral compartment and pierces the fascia approximately 12 cm above the tip of the lateral malleolus. Extending distally in the subcutaneous layer, it branches into the intermediate and medial dorsal cutaneous nerves, which end in the terminal digital branches.

Common areas of entrapment include at the junction where it egresses from the deep fascia and at locations of fascial defect with muscle herniation. Chronic ankle sprains may predispose to nerve entrapment as repeated ankle sprains stretch the nerve (Fig. 25-2). Entrapment elicits symptomatic pain over the distal calf and dorsum of the foot. Patients may report pain at the distal third of the leg with or without the presence of edema. A significant percentage of patients report numbness or paresthesias along the nerve distribution. Pain is typically exacerbated with physical activities including walking and running. A previous history of trauma, most commonly ankle sprains, is present in 25% of all patients with superficial peroneal nerve entrapment.[12]

A few provocative tests have been described by Styf for the evaluation of this syndrome. First, the patient is asked to actively dorsiflex and evert the foot against resistance while the examiner palpates the nerve impingement site. Then the examiner passively plantar flexes and everts the foot without pressure over the nerve and then with percussion along the length of the nerve.[13]

Deep Peroneal Nerve

The deep peroneal nerve, measuring 1 to 3 mm in diameter, serves as cutaneous innervation to the first interspace and provides motor innervation to the anterior leg compartment muscle group and the common short extensor muscle of the foot. Originating from the common peroneal nerve in the popliteal fossa, the deep peroneal nerve pierces the extensor digitorum longus (EDL) muscle as it courses distally. As it descends the leg, it is found between the EDL and tibialis anterior in the upper third of the leg. Further distally, in the middle third of the leg, it courses between the tibialis anterior and extensor hallucis longus (EHL) and toward the lower third of the leg between the EHL and EDL. At approximately 1 cm above the talocrural joint, it separates into lateral and medial branches. The medial branch extends distally alongside the dorsalis pedis artery underneath the inferior extensor retinaculum. It continues distally between the extensor hallucis brevis and EHL to provide innervation to the first interspace. The lateral branch extends in an anterior-lateral direction penetrating the extensor digitorum brevis muscle, terminating into smaller branches that make up the second and fourth dorsal interosseous nerves, which provide articular innervations to the tarsometatarsal, metatarsophalangeal, and interphalangeal joints of the lesser digits (Fig. 25-3).

The nerve may become compressed and entrapped at the location where the medial branch traverses underneath the inferior extensor retinaculum. This is the most common location for deep peroneal entrapment, and entrapment in this location is often referred to as anterior tarsal tunnel syndrome. Entrapment may

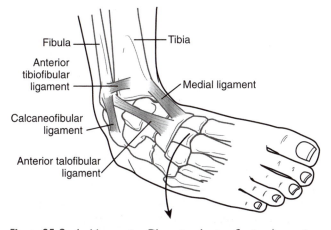

Figure 25-2 Ankle sprain. Chronic plantar flexion/inversion ankle sprains may lead to a tensile neuropathy involving the superficial peroneal nerve.

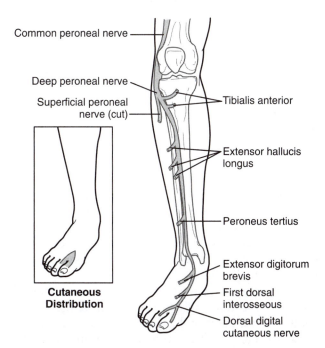

Figure 25-3 Anatomy of the deep peroneal nerve.

also occur where the nerve passes underneath the extensor hallucis brevis. Compression may also occur in areas where underlying bony prominences exist. Dorsal osteophytes of the talonavicular joint or os intermetatarseum between the first and second metatarsals may predispose to the development of this syndrome. Trauma may also contribute to the development of entrapment. Recurrent ankle sprains have been identified as a contributing etiology because as the foot plantar flexes and supinates, the nerve is placed under significant stretch. This repetitive stretch can lead to nerve inflammation and scarring as previously described. External compression is a very important factor to consider in the development of this syndrome and is most commonly seen with athletes. Wearing tight-fitting shoes, ski boots, and running shoes with tight lacing at the area of the nerve and performing certain activities such as push-ups or sit-ups with feet hooked under a rigid weight all contribute to the compression of the nerve and symptomatic presentation.[12]

Patients most often present with a complaint of pain along the dorsum of the foot with possible radiation to the first interspace. The pain is often described to occur during the aforementioned athletic activities and tends to subside with rest and removal of external compression such as shoes. Physical examination may reveal hypoesthesia or loss of sensation to the first interspace. Pain may also be elicited with dorsiflexion and plantar flexion of the foot. Weakness of the EDB may also be noted depending on the area of entrapment.

Posterior Tibial Nerve

Arising from the sciatic nerve, the posterior tibial nerve branches into the lateral sural cutaneous nerve, medial sural cutaneous nerve, medial calcaneal nerve, and medial and lateral plantar nerve. It is responsible for the cutaneous innervation of the posterior aspect of the leg and the plantar and plantar medial aspect of the foot. It provides motor innervation to the superficial and deep posterior muscle compartment of the leg. In the proximal leg, the nerve is situated between the tibialis posterior muscle and flexor hallucis longus muscle in the deep posterior muscle compartment. Distally, it is situated between the flexor hallucis longus and flexor digitorum longus. In the inferior leg, the nerve enters the subcutaneous layer traversing the tarsal tunnel along with the posterior tibial artery and venae comitantes. The tarsal tunnel is formed by the medial and posterior aspect of the calcaneus, the posterior talus, the distal tibia, the medial malleolus, the flexor retinaculum (laciniate ligament), and the abductor hallucis muscle (Fig. 25-4).

As it emerges from the fibro-osseous tarsal tunnel, the posterior tibial nerve separates into the medial plantar nerve, the lateral plantar nerve, and the medial calcaneal nerve.[10] The structures within the tarsal tunnel include the posterior tibial nerve, the posterior

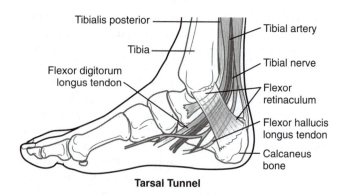

Figure 25-4 Anatomy of the tarsal tunnel.

tibial tendon, the flexor digitorum longus tendon, the flexor hallucis longus tendon, and the posterior tibial artery and vein. A high degree of anatomical variability exists when considering the contents of the tarsal tunnel because the posterior tibial nerve may branch within the tunnel or distally to the tunnel. Because of the narrow structural anatomy of the tarsal tunnel, entrapment of the tibial nerve within the tarsal tunnel is common. More common causes of entrapment include space-occupying lesions, coalitions, biomechanical dysfunction, and bony prominences or exostoses.[14] Patients may present with entrapment symptoms to the areas of distribution for the medial calcaneal, medial plantar, or lateral plantar nerves. Symptoms include hypoesthesias, paresthesias, and symptoms associated with an individual nerve (described in further detail later).[15]

Ganglion cysts are the most common space-occupying lesions to occur in the tarsal tunnel.[15] Many theories exist regarding the development of these lesions, including displacement of synovial tissue during embryogenesis, proliferation of pluripotent mesenchymal cells, degeneration of connective tissue after trauma, and migration of synovial fluid.[16] Ganglion cysts causing entrapment syndrome at the tarsal tunnel may arise from the subtalar joint; ankle joint; or tibialis posterior, flexor digitorum longus, and flexor hallucis longus tendons. Other space-occupying entities causing similar symptoms include, but are not limited to, synovial chondromatosis, schwannomas, and varicose veins.[17] Conservative treatments include rest, NSAIDs, bracing, and icing. However, conservative treatments often fail because the cause is not addressed. Surgical intervention is considered a better option because the actual etiology is addressed. Procedures involve anatomical dissection, ligation of vascular supply, and resection of the impingement-causing lesion.[17] When resecting a ganglion cyst, it is essential to identify the stalk, or the area where the cyst invests in the capsule or tendinous sheath, and carefully ligate it so as to disrupt the synovial flow. Ganglion cysts generally have a high recurrence rate, and as such it is possible to have a recurrent tarsal tunnel syndrome.[17]

Osseous etiological factors, such as coalitions and exostoses, increase compartment pressure by decreasing compartment size, creating an entrapment syndrome. Surgical decompression by resection of the offending exostosis or coalition is a successful treatment modality.

Biomechanical dysfunction is a significant causative factor in the development of tarsal tunnel syndrome.[15] Examples include excessive subtalar and midtarsal joint pronation which result in internal rotation of the tibia, plantar flexion, and adduction of the talus; a decrease in the calcaneal pitch; and a flattening of the medial longitudinal arch of the foot. This biomechanical dysfunction causes increased motion in the foot, which leads to increased stress on all the structures in the foot and leg. Increased stress and strain can cause an increased risk of nerve damage and greater likelihood of nerve entrapment. The goal of treatment in this case is to address excessive motion in the foot and leg by means of reconstructive surgery to correct the overpronatory movement by creating a more rigid lever arm. Bracing and the use of orthoses can also aid in decreasing pronation during gait.

Medial Plantar Nerve

Larger than the lateral plantar nerve, the medial plantar nerve is one of the terminal branches off the posterior tibial nerve. Situated anteriorly, the nerve travels along with the medial plantar artery and passes superior to the lateral plantar artery. The nerve leaves the tarsal tunnel, passing along the intersection of the long flexors in the second muscle compartment of the foot at the master knot of Henry. As it continues distally, the nerve is located in the medial portion of the deep compartment of the foot. It divides into its terminal branches, three common digital nerves, at the level of the first metatarsal base. The medial plantar nerve cutaneously innervates the medial sole of the foot. The muscular branches of the medial plantar nerve supply the abductor hallucis, flexor digitorum brevis, flexor hallucis brevis, and first lumbrical. The nerve provides articular innervation to the talonavicular and cuneonavicular joints and vascular innervations to the medial plantar artery.

Entrapment of the medial plantar nerve is typically thought to occur in joggers and is often referred to as "jogger's foot."[18] This type of entrapment occurs at the location of the master knot of Henry. Most patients presenting with this syndrome tend to run with excessive heel valgus or hyperpronation. The pathology often coincides with a history of previous ankle injury or chronic ankle instability. Excessive abduction or adduction at the talonavicular joint may result in compression of the nerve at the master knot of Henry leading to entrapment syndrome. Arch supports may also aggravate the medial plantar nerve leading to entrapment symptoms.

Patients typically present with pain radiating distally into the medial toes and proximally into the ankle. Pain is reportedly worse when running on flat ground, especially when turning corners and during stair workouts. On examination, tenderness can be noted most typically in the medial plantar arch and in the area of the navicular tuberosity. The examiner may test for symptom reproducibility by everting the heel or by having the patient stand on the ball of the foot. Hypoesthesia and loss of sensation is usually noted after the patient has been jogging. Tinel's sign may also be present.[19]

Lateral Plantar Nerve

The lateral plantar nerve travels in the lower segment of the tarsal tunnel entering the deep central plantar space between the quadratus plantae and flexor digitorum brevis. Traveling forward in an anterior-lateral direction, the nerve passes plantar to the quadratus plantae and along the lateral plantar vessels. At this point, it penetrates the lateral intermuscular septum, and at the level of the fifth metatarsal base it terminates into the deep and superficial end branches. The superficial branch divides into the fourth common digital nerve and the lateral plantar cutaneous nerve of the fifth toe. The deep branch subsequently provides articular branches to the tarsal and tarsometatarsal joints as well as muscular branches to the lateral lumbricales, interossei, and adductor hallucis.

Although not commonly occurring as a single entity, the lateral plantar nerve can become compressed alone or along with the tibial nerve as previously described with tarsal tunnel syndrome. Typically, the patient experiences loss of sensation to the lateral third of the plantar aspect of the foot. Because the lateral plantar nerve innervates the abductor digiti minimi, functional loss of this muscle may also be noted, as is seen with Baxter's neuritis.[20] Baxter's neuritis is a syndrome that is caused by the entrapment of the nerve to the abductor digiti minimi. Symptoms often include heel pain, typically not associated with a heel spur. Entrapment of this nerve is believed to occur between the deep fascia of the abductor hallucis muscle and the medial head of the quadratus plantae muscle. Patients tend to be athletes presenting with tenderness along the anteromedial heel along with inability to abduct the fifth toe. Treatment entails surgical sectioning of the deep fascia to release the entrapment.[20]

Saphenous Nerve

The saphenous nerve, a branch of the femoral nerve, travels in the thigh in the subsartorial canal. It pierces the sartorius muscle and travels in the subcutaneous tissue to innervate the medial knee and leg. It provides sensory innervation from the medial aspect of the knee extending down to the medial aspect of the hallux.[10]

Being so superficial, the saphenous nerve does not have a high tendency to become impinged secondary to internal factors. However, trauma to the surrounding areas, especially in and around the adductor canal, can cause perineural fibrosis, leading to entrapment syndrome. Chief complaints of saphenous nerve entrapment include medial knee or leg pain after prolonged standing or walking in the distribution of the saphenous nerve. Symptoms may also be exacerbated by lower extremity hip adduction or knee extension strengthening exercises. Treatment options are limited to the surgical release of fibrotic tissue and adhesions.

Neuroma

A **neuroma,** also referred to as perineural fibrosis, is hypertrophy of a given common digital plantar nerve as it courses between the condyles of the proximal phalanges (Fig. 25-5). The exact mechanism causing neuromas is unknown. However, many causes have been described. One theory attributes friction and subsequent trauma that occurs when the condyles engage with one another during the gait cycle. Another theory suggests trauma occurring at the nerve as a result of the pressure exerted on the nerve by the deep transverse intermetatarsal ligament during propulsion.[21] Patients often present with complaints of burning, numbness, and tingling in the area of the neuroma. Often patients describe experiencing a sensation in having a pebble in their foot or as though they are walking on a pebble. On physical examination, a Mulder click, which is a palpable click, may be palpated by laterally squeezing the forefoot and manually manipulating the intermetatarsal space. Another indicator of the presence of a neuroma is the presence of Sullivan's sign. Sullivan's sign is a clinical marker that can be seen when the patient is weight bearing and the toes associated with the affected interspace spread.[12] Treatment for neuromas often begins with accommodative devices such as metatarsal pads that serve to keep the metatarsals separated during the gait cycle to decrease the irritation to the nerve. Injections at the site of the neuroma are often considered along with accommodative devices. Practitioners often concoct a combination of a local anesthetic and corticosteroid to inject; the combination of substances that is injected is based on practitioner preference. Another injectable used to treat neuromas that is controversial is an alcohol sclerosing agent. A 4% alcohol solution, usually mixed with a local anesthetic, is injected in small quantities, usually 0.5 to 1 mL per injection for a total of three treatments. Surgical treatment includes resection of the neuroma.

Detailed knowledge of the nerve origin, course, and area of innervation is essential for appropriate diagnosis and understanding of entrapment neuropathies. Understanding the different etiological factors that contribute to the development of symptoms allows the practitioner to diagnose and treat these conditions accurately. Nerve entrapment in the foot and ankle has several presentations, all of which have been described in detail in this chapter. Conservative and surgical treatment options are aimed at correcting or limiting the cause of entrapment and reducing the severity of axonal loss and impairment. With early and accurate diagnosis and appropriate treatment, most patients experience complete resolution of symptoms.

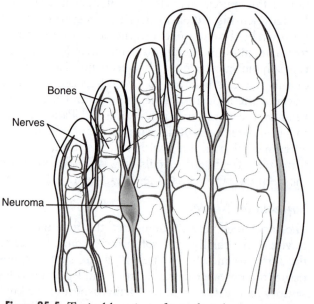

Figure 25-5 Typical location of interdigital neuroma pain.

CASE STUDY

JD, an electrician, presented to the physical therapist with a chief complaint of pain and neuralgic symptoms (tingling, burning, numbness) of his right second and third toes and the space between the toes. JD states that the symptoms have been present for about a year but have increased recently. He can "bring out" the symptoms by passively dorsiflexing his toes. Kneeling is also an issue. As an electrician, he is often kneeling, and this position worsens his symptoms. JD also states that symptoms are exacerbated by standing on his toes on a stepladder. He has self-treated with NSAIDs and aspirin without success.

Case Study Questions

1. From the clinical scripts presented in the history, which diagnosis appears to be the leading differential diagnosis?
   a. L5–S1 radiculopathy
   b. Morton's neuroma
   c. Deep peroneal nerve entrapment
   d. Sural nerve entrapment

2. If the correct diagnosis is an interdigital neuroma, which clinical sign would be present?
   a. Erythema along the second toe
   b. An ulceration of the second toe
   c. A positive Tinel sign between the second and third metatarsal heads
   d. Weakness of the anterior tibialis muscle

3. All the following are appropriate treatments for an interdigital neuroma except:
   a. Orthoses.
   b. Corticosteroid injection.
   c. Sclerosing alcohol injection.
   d. Electrical stimulation.

4. JD is an electrician. Which job-related factors may have contributed to the formation of an interdigital neuroma?
   a. Constant kneeling
   b. The use of a ladder
   c. Standing on toes
   d. All of the above

5. Which of the following is a factor thought to be the cause of women having a higher incidence of interdigital neuroma than men?
   a. Women tend not to participate in contact sports
   b. Women have a higher incidence of age-related osteoporosis than men
   c. Women wear tighter shoes than men
   d. Women often wear high-heeled shoes

References

1. Seddon HJ. Classification of nerve injuries. *BMJ*. 1942;2:237.
2. Sunderland S. A classification of peripheral nerve injury producing loss of function. *Brain*. 1951;74:491–516.
3. Upton AR, McComas AJ. The double crush in nerve entrapment syndromes. *Lancet*. 1973;18:359–362.
4. Osterman AL. The double crush syndrome. *Orthop Clin North Am*. 1988;19:147–155.
5. Johnson EK, Chiarello CM. The slump test: the effects of head and lower extremity position on knee extension. *J Orthop Sports Phys Ther*. 1997;26:310–317.
6. Fiatarone CL, Singh MA, Bundy A, et al. Integration of balance and strength training into daily life activity to reduce rate of falls in older people (the LiFE Study): randomized parallel trial. *BMJ*. 2012;345:4547.
7. Anseimi SJ. Common peroneal nerve compression. *J Am Podiatr Med Assoc*. 2006;5(69):413–417.
8. Gross JA, Hamilton WJ. Isolated mechanical lesions of the sural nerve. *Muscle Nerve*. 1989;3:248–249.
9. Baxter DE: Functional nerve disorders in the athlete's foot, ankle, and leg. *The Lower Extremity in Sports*. 2008;34: 185–194.
10. Lawrence SJ, Bott MJ. The sural nerve in the foot and ankle: an anatomic study with clinical a surgical implications. *Foot Ankle Int*. 1994;15:490–494.
11. Pringle RM, Protheroe K, Mukherjee SK. Entrapment neuropathy of the sural nerve. *J Bone Joint Surg*. 1974;56: 465–468.
12. Lorei MP, Hershman EB. Peripheral nerve injuries in athletes. Treatment and prevention. *Sports Med*. 1993;16: 130–147.
13. Barrett SL, Dellon AL, Rossen GD, Walters L. Superficial peroneal nerve: the clinical implications of anatomic variability. *J Foot Ankle Surg*. 2006;45:174–176.
14. Tsang AM, Mackenney PJ, Adepado AO. Tarsal tunnel syndrome: a literature review. *Foot Ankle Surg*. 2012;18: 149–152.
15. Gould JS. Tarsal tunnel syndrome. *Foot Ankle Clin*. 2011;16:275–286.
16. Ahn JH, Choy WS, Kim HY. Operative treatment for ganglion cysts of the foot and ankle. *J Foot Ankle Surg*. 2010;49:442–445.
17. Spinner RJ, Delton AL, Rosson GD, Anderson SR, Amrami KK. Tibial intraneural ganglion in the tarsal tunnel. *J Foot Ankle Surg*. 2007;46:27–31.
18. Trafton PG. Jogger's foot. *Clin Orthop Relat Res*. 1979;141: 308–309.
19. Beltran LS, Bencardino J, Ghazikhanian V, Beltran J. Entrapment neuropathies in the lower extremity III. *Semin Musculoskelet Radiol*. 2010;14:501–511.
20. Fuhrmann RA, Frober R. Release of the lateral plantar nerve in case of entrapment. *Oper Orthop Traumatol*. 2010;22: 335–343.
21. Title CL, Schon LC. Morton neuroma: primary and secondary neurectomy. *J Am Acad Orthop Surg*. 2008;16: 550–557.

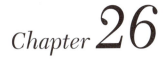

Chapter 26

Fall Risk and Fall Prevention Strategies for Individuals With Peripheral Neuropathy

Roberta A. Newton, PT, PhD, FGSA, and Dennis W. Klima, PT, MS, PhD, GCS, NCS

"Our greatest glory is not in never falling but in rising every time we fall."
—Confucius (551–479 B.C.E.)

Objectives

On completion of this chapter, the student/practitioner will be able to:

- List possible fall etiologies.
- Identify fall risks.
- Discuss the fall risk impact of medications.
- Develop a comprehensive fall prevention program.

Key Terms

- Fall prevention
- Fall prevention program
- Fall risk assessment
- Somatosensation

Introduction

Two of the most important capabilities of an individual, regardless of physical, health, or cognitive status, are the ability to navigate the environment and the ability to perform social roles. Physiological mechanisms supporting these capabilities include postural alignment, balance, and mobility, all of which depend on sensation and strength in the lower extremities. Impairment among these entities resulting from peripheral neuropathy increases the likelihood of an individual experiencing a fall. Unintentional falls in all age groups (excluding ages 15 to 24 years) are the leading cause of nonfatal injuries treated in hospital emergency departments; falls rank as the leading cause of death from injury in adults older than age 65 years. In 2007, greater than 8 million individuals were seen in emergency departments for treatment related to unintentional falls, of which more than 2.6 million were adults 55 years old

and older.[1] The cost of these unintentional falls can be a financial burden on the health care system and the individual and family and a loss of revenue generation.

Balance, mobility impairments, and falls are commonly reported in older adults who have peripheral neuropathy associated with diabetes mellitus.[2-5] However, studies found that not all older women who have diabetes mellitus and peripheral neuropathy fall.[6,7] Although these impairments are typically not reported, they may be secondary consequences for other types of pathologies resulting in peripheral neuropathy. For the purpose of this chapter, a fall is defined as an unexpected event during which the person comes to rest on the ground, floor, or lower level.[8]

The purposes of this chapter are to provide (1) an overview of mechanisms leading to **fall risk** in individuals with lower extremity peripheral nerve dysfunction; (2) guidelines for **assessment** of balance and falls; and (3) guidelines for interventions to maintain or regain balance or strategies to compensate for sensory and motor neuron loss, reducing the risk of falls. Detailed descriptions of pathologies leading to peripheral nervous system dysfunction are not included in this chapter but do appear in Chapters 3 through 13. Table 26-1 provides some examples of peripheral nerve dysfunction and potential mechanisms that increase the likelihood of falling. As is evident from the literature, fall risk is not specifically discussed because falling may be considered a secondary consequence of the medical condition. Inferences regarding fall risk can be made by examining the medical condition and mechanisms contributing to a fall.

Mechanisms Contributing to Falls

In a 6-month span, the absolute risk of falls occurring in individuals with peripheral neuropathy is 55%. Two

Table 26-1	Examples of Impairments Contributing to Fall Risk			
Condition	**Mechanism**	**Sensory**	**Neuromotor**	**Joints and Foot**
Charcot-Marie-Tooth disease or hereditary motor and sensory neuropathy	Peripheral sensory and motor neurons: demyelization and axonal degeneration	Subclass CMT1: decrease or loss in cutaneous sensation and proprioception below knee	Distal, symmetrical muscle weakness evident in dorsiflexors and evertors; atrophy; decreased DTRs	High-arched pes cavus foot deformity; hammertoes
Diabetic mellitus: diabetic neuropathy	Slow, progressive loss of sensory, motor, and autonomic function	Sensory neuropathy: sensations of tingling, burning, numbness; complete loss of sensation in feet; pain owing to alteration of foot biomechanics; ulceration	Bilateral, asymmetrical distal muscle weakness	Foot deformity: flatfoot with valgus of midfoot, claw toes, collapse of longitudinal arch
Guillain-Barré syndrome: variants have differing characteristics	Acute inflammatory demyelinating polyneuropathy	Acute sensory ascending neuropathy exhibits greater sensory changes than muscle weakness	Progressive paralysis and areflexia; proximal to distal recovery	Residual distal weakness may be present following recovery trajectory
HIV (AIDS)	Peripheral nerve damage secondary to HIV, related opportunistic infections (e.g., CMV), or medications	Primarily sensory: distal symmetrical peripheral neuropathies; proprioceptive loss spreads distal to proximal; tingling or burning pain; contact sensitivity	Bilateral symmetrical and motor loss	Residual ankle weakness may lead to muscle imbalance
Pernicious anemia secondary to vitamin B_{12} deficiency	Symmetrical sensory neuropathy beginning in lower extremities and feet	Late manifestation of vitamin B_{12} deficiency: loss of motor function	Sensory loss leads to decreased balance abilities	
Postpolio syndrome	Hypothesized latent aging effects superimposed on reduced alpha motor neuronal pool from initial polio attack	Muscle atrophy; decline in strength, particularly knee extensor strength; decreased endurance and fatigue	Weakness typically asymmetrical, often exacerbating muscle groups affected during initial infection	Resultant contractures from postpolio syndrome or hypermobile joints owing to compensatory strategies
Lumbar radiculopathy	Irritation of nerve roots, particularly affecting lumbar disc disruption	Sensory roots may result in low back pain and radiating pain into one or both legs; sensory decline owing to sensory root at level of rupture and adjacent nerve roots	Motor decline owing to motor roots at level of rupture and adjacent nerve roots	Compensatory mechanisms to relieve pain: postural realignment or more sedentary behavior: both strategies lead to balance instability

CMV, Cytomegalovirus; DTRs, deep tendon reflexes.

studies calculated odds ratios for falls in individuals with peripheral neuropathy as 6.3 and 17.[9] Risk factors, alone or in combination, may be sufficient to produce balance instability and falls. These risk factors are categorized as intrinsic (individual), extrinsic (e.g., medications, footwear), and environmental. A risk factor present in one individual may not be a risk factor for another individual. The impact of a risk factor is viewed in context of the individual's health; the type, severity, and progression of the individual's medical condition; any comorbidities; and the psychological and mental health of the individual.

Peripheral Sensory Declines

Decreased **somatosensation** (e.g., the foot in contact with the floor) and decreased proprioception (joint position and muscle length) decrease the ability of the individual to detect the relationship of the lower extremity to the trunk and to the support surface, reducing the ability to locate the center of mass for postural alignment and balance. Additionally, there is a decreased ability to detect the condition of the support surface (e.g., hard or compliant, slippery or resistive, even or uneven).

Decreased somatosensation as measured by vibratory threshold perception is higher in women with diabetes and a history of falls compared with women with diabetes and no fall history (21.0 volts vs. 17.9 volts). Individuals with diabetic peripheral neuropathy also demonstrate decreased tactile sensitivity[10] and decreased proprioception as measured by ankle and great toe joint movement detection.[11,12]

If sensory loss is gradual, redundant but unique contributions of the other sensory systems (vestibular and vision) compensate for the somatosensory losses. These compensatory strategies may be sufficient until a critical threshold is reached at which time these strategies become insufficient, resulting in balance and dysfunction and increased probability for falls. The use of an assistive device may help compensate for balance dysfunction by increasing the base of support as well as providing additional touch information through the device to provide cues for upright stance.[13] An understanding of the mechanism of sensory decline and the ability of other sensory systems to compensate underlie guidelines for assessment and treatment protocols for fall risk reduction.

Depending on the severity of the condition, loss of sensation predisposes the joints to repeated trauma, and progressive loss of joint proprioception results in Charcot disease or arthropathy, particularly in individuals with diabetes mellitus. Continued joint trauma can cause subluxation of the tarsal and metatarsal joints resulting in a rocker-bottom foot deformity. This alteration in biomechanics of the foot increases joint stress, particularly at the midtarsal and tarsometatarsal joints, and may result in ulceration secondary to the stress of the foot against the shoe. These sensory and biomechanical impairments underlie fall risk.

Neuromotor Dysfunction in the Lower Extremities

Declines in the number of alpha motor axons can result in decreased scaling of force and power as well as decreased timing and sequencing of muscle activity, decreasing the ability to produce coordinated muscle synergies to accomplish a particular task. These declines are evident by decreased muscle strength, dropfoot, instability in balance and gait, trips, and falls. Similar to somatosensation declines, compensatory strategies may offset motor function degradation until a critical threshold is reached and alternative compensatory strategies are needed. If the medical condition results in an abrupt change in peripheral sensory and motor systems, the ability of the individual to respond quickly to perturbations is decreased, causing a potential loss of balance and perhaps falling. In addition to the rate of decline in the peripheral sensorimotor systems, the critical threshold is also based on contributory factors such as age, health, progression of the medical condition, and prescription medications.

Muscle weakness secondary to the medical condition can lead to altered foot biomechanics, impaired balance and postural control, and walking difficulties. Decreased muscle strength linked with decreased range of motion, particularly distally (ankle and foot), limits the individual's ability to adapt to changes in the walking surface. Weakness is due to either a decline in the number of functioning motor units (motor axon and associated muscle cells) or a decreased capability of intact motor units to produce sufficient force to accomplish the same task as a muscle with a normal complement of motor units would.

Depending on the specific condition, muscle weakness may be evident as a symmetrical distal muscle weakness in the dorsiflexors and evertors as observed in clients with Charcot-Marie-Tooth disease, or hereditary motor and sensory neuropathy, the most frequently inherited peripheral neuropathy.[14] Footdrop secondary to muscle weakness of the dorsiflexors decreases the ability of the foot to clear the floor during swing phase of gait, leading to walking difficulties and increased frequency of tripping. Similarly, individuals may be unable to lower the foot during the loading phase of gait and subsequently trip over uneven terrain.

Diabetic peripheral neuropathy has been shown to impair ankle strength, balance, and walking stability.[15] Foot deformity, a consequence of muscle weakness and postural malalignment, leads to secondary conditions such as foot pain and ulceration and results in balance instability and falls. Mauer et al.[16] followed 139 nursing home residents for 299 days and noted that 78% of residents with diabetes fell compared with 30% of residents without diabetes.

Continued declines in the number of motor neurons and their associated muscle cells (motor units) can overburden the remaining motor units and produce fatigue. For example, postpolio syndrome is defined as newly acquired neuromotor weakness in clients with a prior diagnosis of polio.[17] Symptoms include muscle atrophy, decline in the strength of the affected muscles particularly knee extensor strength, decreased endurance, and fatigue with activity, all of which contribute to decreased balance abilities, tripping, and fall risk. Depending on the severity of these symptoms, these individuals may restrict their activity and may use an assistive device (cane or wheelchair).

Lifestyle and Activity Level

Peripheral sensory and motor pathology may result in decreased endurance and fatigue with activity, limiting the mobility of the client and his or her ability to carry out social roles and participate as a productive member of the workforce.[18,19] Compensatory mechanisms to relieve pain (e.g., clients with lumbar radiculopathy) include postural realignment or the assumption of more sedentary behavior. Both of these strategies may lead to balance dysfunction.

More than 60% of clients with a neuromotor condition such as hereditary motor and sensory neuropathy type I, postpolio syndrome, or Guillain-Barré syndrome experience severe fatigue.[20] The peripheral neuromotor pathology as well as the client's psychological state may contribute to fatigue and may lead to a more sedentary lifestyle. The resultant spiral includes the secondary consequences of the medical condition, resulting in increased inactivity; declines in strength, balance, and mobility; and increased fall risk.

Medications

Single medications and medication combinations may result in muscle weakness, dizziness, and balance instability. Certain classes of drugs are known to produce dizziness, balance instability, and falls via different mechanisms. These mechanisms include the metabolism of the individual, which may alter the absorption and half-life of the drug; polypharmacy; and medication scheduling. If an individual is taking a diuretic in the evening, nighttime fall risk increases because the individual may walk to the bathroom in the dark.

In older adults, benzodiazepines, antidepressants (particularly tricyclic antidepressants and selective serotonin reuptake inhibitors), antiepileptics, and antihypertensive medications increase fall risk; taking four or more medications also increases fall risk.[21,22] Combinations of medications taken for HIV management may cause neuropathy and subsequent falls. Antiretroviral medications containing dideoxynucleosides ("d-drugs"), such as didanosine and stavudine, may induce peripheral neuropathy.[23]

Elements of a Fall Prevention Program

The following eight principles provide a guide to implement a **fall prevention program.**

1. The causes of a fall in one individual may not cause a fall in another individual.
2. Falls are generally due to an individual and environmental mismatch where the individual is unable to recover balance, resulting in a movement of the body to a lower surface (chair, bed, floor, or against the wall).
3. Deficits in physiological factors, such as somatosensation, muscle and skeletal strength, balance, and gait, are associated with an increased risk for falling. The risk of falls increases with the number of physiological risk factors, the number of medications, and the number of functional impairments. These factors are important to identify in terms of fall risk and potential fall-related injuries as well as to prevent or reduce the impact of a fall.
4. Falls can lead to a fear of falling and a fear of the inability to get back up after falling.
5. Inactivity is a fall risk behavior and includes the spectrum from prolonged bed rest to a chosen or medical condition–related inactive lifestyle.
6. An individual may not be committed to make the recommended changes in lifestyle or home environment for various social, cultural, financial, or personal reasons.
7. No program can guarantee a reduction in falls if the information is not relevant or the person does not actively take part to reduce his or her risks.
8. A fall prevention program should include a screening component, an education component, and an activity component.[24] Education alone is not sufficient.

Generally, fall prevention programs have been custom-designed for specific settings, and multiple fall prevention programs, rather than a single reliable and valid program, exist. The purpose of any fall prevention program is to inform and motivate adults to make necessary adaptations to their lifestyles and home environment to reduce the risk for falls.

Guidelines for Assessing Individuals at Risk for Falls

To determine appropriate interventions for balance dysfunction and to decrease the risk of falls, a comprehensive assessment of sensory integrity, range of motion, muscle strength, balance, and functional mobility and assessments of physical activity and health-related quality of life are indicated. Depending on the medical and health status of the individual, disease-specific and behavioral assessments are also recommended. Assessment of the home environment is discussed in conjunction with strategies to reduce fall risk in the home. Assessments are briefly outlined in this chapter. Selection of the appropriate assessments depends on the client's status, the practitioner's expertise, and the ability to identify the risk factors that are modifiable.

Fall History and Fear of Falling

Obtaining a fall history starts with simply asking if the person has fallen within the past month, 3 months, or 6 months.[25] The circumstances surrounding the fall or falls should be determined, noting time of day, medication schedule, activity surrounding the fall, and location of the fall inside or outside the house.

A single dichotomous question can be asked, "Do you have a fear of falling?" This question can be followed by the question, "Does this fear restrict your activities?"[26] A more detailed assessment determines the confidence an individual has to perform routine activities. Assessments developed for older adults are the Falls Efficacy Scale,[27] which is used for frail or homebound individuals, and the Activities-specific Balance Confidence Scale, which is used for more active individuals.[28]

Medical and Medication History

Medical history, including acute or chronic conditions and comorbidities, may solely or in combination contribute to falls. The use of a mobility aid such as a cane or walker is also noted. Medication type, dose, and frequency and adherence to taking the medication[29] are documented. Over-the-counter medications are also noted.

Sensory Integrity

Bilateral examination of the lower extremities and foot to obtain baseline measurements is necessary, particularly for individuals with an asymmetrical sensory loss.

- Cutaneous sensation is measured with 5.07g Semmes-Weinstein monofilament. Gradation measures the perception of light touch to loss of protective sensation.[30] Proprioceptive testing includes passive joint movement (yes/no response to movement) or matching joint positions.[31]
- Pain in the lower extremity and foot is measured using a visual analog scale[32] or the McGill Pain Questionnaire.[33]
- Vision acuity is assessed using the Snellen chart,[34] and a vestibular screen, the Dizziness Handicap Inventory, assesses perceived disability secondary to symptoms of unsteadiness or dizziness.[35]

Integumentary and Foot Posture

- Trophic changes include dryness of the skin, distribution of hair growth, and condition of the toenails.
- Pressure areas caused by shoes range from redness to ulceration.
- Foot deformities include hammertoes, fallen arches.

Deep Tendon Reflexes and Electromyographic Examination

Review of findings is performed to determine the extent of peripheral nerve and muscle pathology.

Range of Motion and Muscle Strength

Although range of motion and muscle strength can be tested separately,[36] they can be observed during physical performance testing (balance and gait).

- The Five Times Sit to Stand Test is used in older adults to obtain an indication of lower extremity muscle strength. Performance on this test may be influenced by pain.

Health Status and Measure of Physical Performance and Ability to Accomplish Activities of Daily Living

Self-report of the person's perception of his or her health is obtained by asking the question, "How do you perceive your health?" The rating is excellent, good, fair, or poor.

Functional Mobility and Gait

- The Short Physical Performance Battery (SPPB) test consists of three components: balance (feet together, semitandem, tandem), timed 4-m walk, and five chair stands.[37] The SPPB predicts the loss of ability to walk 400 m.[38]
- The Timed Up and Go test records the time an individual stands from a chair, walks 10 ft (3 m) at his or her preferred speed, returns to the chair, and sits down. The TUG test has established concurrent validity with the Berg Balance Scale (BBS), gait speed, and Barthel Index and excellent reliability (intraclass correlation coefficient = 0.99).[39]
- The Dynamic Gait Index assesses the ability of the individual to walk under different conditions including changes in gait speed and negotiating obstacles.[40]
- The gait stability ratio measures the number of steps per meter and is a measure of stability during walking.[41]

- Gait speed is obtained from timed walk tests ranging from 4- to 10-m distances. The 6 Minute Walk Test[42,43] is used to measure functional endurance.

Balance Assessments

- The Multi-Directional Reach Test (MDRT) measures limits of stability by having the person reach in the forward, right, and left directions and lean backward. The MDRT demonstrates strong test-retest reliability and internal consistency (Cronbach $\alpha = 0.842$), along with concurrent validity with the BBS and TUG.[44]
- The Four Square Step Test measures an individual's ability to negotiate a four-square matrix created by straight canes affixed to the floor.[45] Facing forward through the entire sequence and beginning in the upper left "square," the person enters each of the four quadrants while stepping over the four canes. The sequence is in a clockwise direction and is repeated in the counterclockwise direction. Time scores slower than 15 seconds are indicative of fall risk. The test is particularly challenging for individuals with peripheral neuropathy because of the requisite cane clearance involved with the stepping sequence.
- The BBS assesses balance during performance of 14 in-home and out-of-home tasks.[46] Scoring is on a 5-point scale from 0, unable to perform, to 5, able to meet the criteria independently for the test item. The BBS has a Cronbach α value of 0.96 and excellent interrater (intraclass correlation coefficient = 0.98) and intrarater (intraclass correlation coefficient = 0.99) reliability. In community-dwelling older adults, a score of less than 45 predicts assistive device use.[47]
- The multi-item stance test evaluates the ability of the person to maintain balance under conditions of narrowing the base of support: feet together, semitandem, tandem, and single leg stance. The client assumes and maintains the position for up to 30 seconds. Loss of balance or movement away from the test position warrants termination of the test. Instrumented balance assessment can differentiate postural sway in healthy individuals and individuals with diabetes.[48]

Social, Occupational, Leisure, and Functional Status

- Disease-specific or global assessments of health-related quality of life provide an indication of the impact of the medical condition on the ability of the individual to participate in societal, employment, and recreational activities.[49,50] The 36-Item Short Form Health Survey is a valid tool not specific to any one condition or disease and is considered a generic health-related quality of life scale,[51] whereas the Fear-Avoidance Beliefs Questionnaire focuses on the client's perception about the effect of physical activity and work on low back pain.[52]
- The Borg Rating of Perceived Exertion documents the perceived level of fatigue.[53] This tool can monitor perceived exertion during physical activity programs to reduce fall risk.
- The Physical Activity Scale for the Elderly assesses physical activity including participation in sports, recreational activities, and housework as well as participation in seated activities.[54]
- Prochaska and DiClemente[55] developed the transtheoretical model to explain behavioral change. The stages include precontemplation— no intention to change behavior; contemplation—intention to change; preparation—beginning to make an effort for change within 30 days; action—actively engaged in the activity; and maintenance— sustain activity for at least 6 months. More recently, the transtheoretical model has been applied to fall prevention programs for older adults.[56]

Fall Prevention Strategies

When addressing modifications to an individual's lifestyle or the environment, practitioners should consider the health and medical condition of the individual, the individual's culture, the individual's finances, relevance of behavioral change to the individual, and willingness of the individual to change. Generally, people are more willing to change the environment than change themselves. Evidence-based activity programs exist for older adults; impairment-specific rehabilitative programs, such as for low back pain,[57] incorporating activities designed to improve muscle strength, endurance, function, and mobility can reduce fall risk. Level II evidence was used to confirm the combination of strengthening and aerobic exercise for individuals with peripheral neuropathy.[58] Elements of fall prevention programs are detailed next.

Education and Activity

Sensory Loss and Footwear

- Understand how reduced lower leg sensation, particularly proprioception, can impair balance, particularly when walking on uneven or compliant surfaces.
- Wearing shoes with low heels and firm rubber soles may enhance proprioceptive input from the feet. Studies have investigated the use of vibratory insoles to facilitate foot sensation.[59]

- Areas with reduced sensation are inspected daily to determine pressure areas and potential ulceration.
- Use of an assistive device (e.g., cane or rolling walker) improves stability by creating a wider base of support and enhancing tactile input for balance.

Activity Program

Selecting an activity program is influenced by factors such as age, culture, employment status, and attitudes toward participating in exercise or leisure and recreational activities. The activity program is graded in intensity and frequency to meet the client's goals and to avoid fatigue or exacerbation of symptoms such as pain. Identifying barriers to activity participation and establishing an activity contract monitored by the client and health care professional may facilitate adherence.[60] An activity program can be custom designed and may include rehabilitative interventions such as functional electrical stimulation to facilitate muscle activity, such as the anterior tibialis muscle to decrease footdrop. An activity program may be part of an individual intervention or incorporated into leisure and recreational activities. Activities can include, but are not limited to, the following:[61–65]

- Low-impact exercises including the use of resistive bands,[66] stationary bike, and aquatic exercise[67]
- Stretching activities, particularly at the ankle, to improve balance strategies[68]
- Dancing, gardening, walking, yoga,[69] tai chi chuan,[70–73] and tae kwon do[74]
- Wii or other video games promoting movement or balance[75]
- Borg Scale of Perceived Exertion can be used to monitor effort

How to Get Up From the Floor

Many clients need a strategy to get up after a fall has occurred, particularly if assistance is unavailable or not close by (e.g., phone out of reach). The client can practice in the safety of a clinic setting or with a health care professional in the home setting. Box 26-1 is an instruction sheet used to teach this maneuver in a group setting.

Box 26-1

Teaching Clients to Get Up From the Floor

Following is a general scripted instruction sheet for helping clients get up from the floor after a fall. Personal experience or other hints are encouraged to make the talk appropriate to the audience.

The longer a person remains on the floor after a fall, the greater the chances for secondary complications resulting from lying there. It is a given that everyone falls.

Before the person attempts to get up, determine if someone is available to assist. If the individual is living with someone, it is better to call for assistance, even if it means waking the person up. The fall may have caused an injury or badly shaken the individual. In all cases, the key is to move slowly, remain calm, and run through your mind the next step in getting up.

First, check to see if anything is broken—does the bone feel broken, or does it just really hurt a lot? Generally, broken bones are associated with severe pain. If the person is living alone and believes that something was broken, the person needs to move on the floor to reach a telephone. This is done slowly.

Ask the audience, how they would get up from the floor if they have fallen. If the floor is clean (always bring a floor covering) lie down and have the group problem-solve how you would get up. This way they see the demonstration as well as being actively involved by providing hints. (I find that most groups like this and will provide additional hints.)

The steps include moving along the floor to a sturdy chair that will not move or the sofa or some other fixed support (not a bathroom sink because it could pull away from the wall).

- Moving can occur by pulling oneself along, crawling, or scooting.
- Get into a side-sitting position. Once in this position, pause a second to get your bearings (orient yourself and catch your breath).
- Kneel with support of the chair or sofa. Once in this position, pause a second to get your bearings (orient yourself and catch your breath).
- Use the stronger knee to push yourself onto the chair or sofa. Putting your forearms on the chair or sofa seat also helps to get some leverage. Once in this position, pause a second to get your bearings (orient yourself and catch your breath).

It is important to emphasize doing this slowly and not impulsively because the person is embarrassed that a fall occurred.

Once sitting in a chair or on the sofa, take time to calm down, catch your breath, and decide the next course of action—do I need to call a friend, neighbor, relative, ambulance, or 911 for help? Do I just need to talk to someone for assurance?

For individuals who may be reluctant to learn to get up because of fear, anxiety, or the belief that they do not have the physical capability to get up, other strategies are needed. For example, some individuals may be able to afford some type of alarm system. For all people, recommend a buddy system—that is, have someone call the person at least once a day. Also, recommend placing the telephone in easy reach and not attached to a kitchen wall where one has to stand to use it.

Modified and reprinted with permission from RA Newton, Fall Prevention Project, 1998.

Modifications to the Environment

An individual with peripheral neuropathy may have the capability but may be unable to participate (perform) because of environmental barriers. If the work or residence environment is modified and the person can perform within the limits of his or her health condition, individual participation and performance levels may improve.

Making the interior and exterior of the living area safe can be achieved by doing a room-by-room assessment or examining commonalities (e.g., lighting, support surface, stairs). Willingness to make the modification and financial constraints are potential barriers for making environmental changes. The following list outlines strategies to improve the home environment and potentially to reduce fall risk.

Lighting: Sufficient illumination and location in stairs and frequently traveled areas are considerations.

Support surface: Thick carpet and underpadding decrease the ability of a person with decreased foot sensation to detect the support surface. The carpet can be removed, or the client can use additional support to travel through these areas. Scatter rugs should be removed or firmly secured. Ramps and stairs may pose a problem for individuals with anterior tibialis weakness.

Furniture: Low and soft-cushioned furniture poses difficulty when sitting and standing up. Modifications include higher and more firm-cushioned furniture and tables. Furniture may become an obstacle if it is located in the most frequently traveled path. Tables with glass or clear tops may be difficult to see.

Bathroom: There should be an appropriate number and position of grab bars for the toilet, bathtub, and shower. A sturdy bench seat that extends from inside the bathtub into the bathroom alleviates the need to step over the bathtub to enter or exit.

Frequently used items: These should be located between shoulder and knee height to avoid potential unexpected perturbations when reaching or moving items.

Falls can be a secondary consequence of impairments associated with peripheral neuropathy. Often, the medical status and medical management of clients are the primary focus, and falls tend to be an afterthought. As noted, multiple fall risk factors exist and include impairments, medication management, and environmental factors. A fall prevention program includes assessment, education, physical activity program, and environmental modifications. Such a program not only reduces the risk of falls but also may improve overall strength, endurance, and functional mobility in the client to maintain his or her quality of life.

CASE STUDY

Mary is a 75-year-old woman who has been admitted to the acute care hospital with a urinary tract infection. She has a fever, and her white blood cell count is elevated. Her past medical history is significant for Parkinson disease. She was admitted for administration of intravenous antibiotics for the urinary tract infection. A physical therapy evaluation was also ordered for identification of fall risk. Mary tells the physical therapist that she has been falling "once a week." She lives alone and states that she "walks around the house very unsafely." Her house is one story. An aide helps her with housework, shopping, and meal preparation (she cannot do any of these on her own). She also receives Meals on Wheels from a local volunteer group. Her lawyer handles all financial matters. Mary spends her day watching TV and reading. Functional evaluation by the physical therapist reveals contact guard for transfers and contact guard for ambulation with a cane. Ambulatory distance is 30 feet limited by fatigue. Mary's gait is slow with a marked decreased stride length. The BBS score is 44, markedly worse than the accelerated risk of falling score of 49.

Case Study Questions

1. When performing the physical and functional evaluation, which of the following would you consider to be the most important evaluative data point as a predictor of overall health, well-being, and safety?
   a. Stair-climbing assessment
   b. Deep tendon reflexes
   c. BBS
   d. Upper extremity manual muscle test

2. The assistive device most indicated for Mary to use at home now is:
   a. No device.
   b. Standard walker.
   c. Quad cane.
   d. Wheeled walker.

3. With Mary's diagnosis of Parkinson disease, you most likely would expect to find which of the following on evaluation?
   a. Spasticity, positive Babinski sign, resting tremor
   b. Rigidity, no confusion, resting tremor
   c. Hypotonus, negative Babinski sign, confusion, no resting tremor
   d. Flaccidity, no confusion, no resting tremor

4. As an intervention related to the goal of improving the ankle strategy, the most indicated, safest, and most appropriate for Mary is:
   a. Outdoor distance walking around a track.
   b. Heel-to-toe ambulation.
   c. Catching and tossing a volleyball.
   d. TheraBand for strengthening the anterior tibialis and the gastrocnemius/soleus in the seated position.

5. The score on the BBS was 44 indicating a high risk for fall. Taken at face value and without the performance of other tests and measures, the BBS results indicate to the physical therapist that the fall risk is due to:

a. Age.

b. Musculoskeletal weakness.

c. Parkinson disease.

d. The BBS alone cannot determine the cause of fall risk.

References

1. CDC Center for Injury Prevention and Control. http://www.cdc.gov/injury/index.html. Accessed May 31, 2010.

2. Richardson JK. Factors associated with falls in older patients with diffuse polyneuropathy. *J Am Geriatr Assoc.* 2002;50:1767–1773.

3. Menz HB, Lord SR, St George R, Fitzpatrick RC. Walking stability and sensorimotor function in older people with diabetic peripheral neuropathy. *Arch Phys Med Rehabil.* 2004;85:245–252.

4. Richardson JK, Thies SB, DeMott TK, Ashton-Miller JA. Gait analysis in a challenging environment differentiates between fallers and nonfallers among older patients with peripheral neuropathy. *Arch Phys Med Rehabil.* 2005;86:1539–1544.

5. Patel S, Hyer S, Tweed K, et al. Risk factors for fractures and falls in older women with type 2 diabetes mellitus. *Calcif Tissue Int.* 2008;82:87–91.

6. Volpato S, Leveille SG, Blaum C, Fried LP, Guralnik JM. Risk factors for falls in older disabled women with diabetes: the Women's Health and Aging Study. *J Gerontol A Biol Sci Med Sci.* 2005;60:1539–1545.

7. Franklin GM, Kahn LB, Baxter J, Marshall JA, Hamman RF. Sensory neuropathy in noninsulin dependent diabetes mellitus: the San Luis Valley Diabetes Study. *Am J Epidemiol.* 1990;131:633–643.

8. Hauer K, Lamb SE, Jorstad EC, Todd C, Becker C (on behalf of the ProFane-group). Systematic review of definitions and methods of measuring falls in randomised controlled fall prevention trials: systematic review. *Age Ageing.* 2006;35:5–10.

9. Hurman DJ, Stevens JA, Rao JK. Practice Parameter: Assessing patients in a neurology practice for risk of falls (an evidence-based review): report of the Quality Standards Subcommittee of the American Academy of Neurology. *Neurology.* 2008;70:473–479.

10. Holewski JJ, Stess RM, Graf PM, Grunfeld C. Aesthesiometry: quantification of cutaneous pressure sensation in diabetic peripheral neuropathy. *J Rehabil Res Dev.* 1988;25:1–10.

11. Kars HJ, Hijmans JM, Geertzen JH, Zijlstra W. The effect of reduced somatosensation on standing balance: a systematic review. *J Diabetes Sci Technol.* 2009;3(4):931–943.

12. Simoneau G, Derr J, Ulbrecht J, Becker M, Cavanagh P. Diabetic sensory neuropathy effect on ankle joint movement perception. *Arch Phys Med Rehabil.* 1996;77:453–460.

13. Dickstein R, Shupert CL, Horak FB. Fingertip touch improves postural stability in patients with peripheral neuropathy. *Gait Posture.* 2001;14:238–247.

14. Chetlin RD, Gutmann L, Tarnopolsky M, Ullrich IH, Yeater RA. Resistance training effectiveness in patients with Charcot-Marie-Tooth disease: recommendations for exercise prescription. *Arch Phys Med Rehabil.* 2004;85:1217–1223.

15. Menz HB, Lord SR, St George R, Fitzpatrick RC. Walking stability and sensorimotor function in older people with diabetic peripheral neuropathy. *Arch Phys Med Rehabil.* 2004;85:245–252.

16. Mauer MS, Burcham J, Cheng H. Diabetes mellitus is associated with an increased risk of falls in elderly residents of a long-term care facility. *J Gerontol.* 2005;60A:1157–1162.

17. Stolwijk-Swüste J, Beelen A, Lankhorst J, Nollet F. The course of functional status and muscle strength in patients with late-onset sequelae of poliomyelitis: a systematic review. *Arch Phys Med Rehabil.* 2005;86:1693–1701.

18. Gálvez R, Marsal C, Vidal J, Ruiz M, Rejas J. Cross-sectional evaluation of patient functioning and health-related quality of life in patients with neuropathic pain under standard care conditions. *Eur J Pain.* 2007;11:244–255.

19. Willén C, Thoren-Jönsson A-L, Grimby G, Sunnerhagen KS. Disability in a 4-year follow-up study of people with postpolio syndrome. *J Rehabil Med.* 2007;39:175–180.

20. Zwarts MJ, Bleijenberg G, van Engelen BGM. Clinical neurophysiology of fatigue. *Clin Neurophysiol.* 2008;119(1):2–10.

21. Hartikainen S, Lönnroos E, Louhivuori K. Medication as a risk factor for falls: critical systematic review. *J Gerontol A Biol Sci Med Sci.* 2007;62(10):1172–1181.

22. Berlie HD, Garwood CL. Diabetes medications related to an increased risk of falls and fall-related morbidity in the elderly. *Ann Pharmacother.* 2010;44:712–717.

23. Hung CF, Gibson SA, Letendre SL, et al. Impact of long-term treatment with neurotoxic dideoxynucleoside antiretrovirals: implications for clinical care in resource-limited settings. *HIV Med.* 2008;9:731–737.

24. AGS/BGS Clinical Practice Guideline: Prevention of Falls in Older Persons. 2010. http://www.americangeriatrics.org/health_care_professionals/clinical_practice/clinical_guidelines_recommendations/prevention_of_falls_summary_of_recommendations. Accessed May 31, 2010.

25. Lamb SE, Jorstad-Stein EC, Hauer K, Becker C, on behalf of the Prevention of Falls Network Europe and Outcomes Consensus Group. Development of a common outcome data set for fall injury prevention trials. The Prevention of Falls Network Europe Consensus. *J Am Geriatr Soc.* 2005;53:1618–1622.

26. Jørstad EC, Hauer K, Becker C, Lamb SE; ProFaNe Group. Measuring the psychological outcomes of falling: a systematic review. *J Am Geriatr Soc.* 2005;53:501–510.

27. Tinetti ME, Richman D, Powell L. Falls efficacy as a measure of fear of falling. *J Gerontol.* 1990;45(6):P239–P243.

28. Myers AM, Fletcher PC, Myers AH, Sherk W. Discriminative and evaluative properties of the activities-specific balance confidence (ABC) scale. *J Gerontol A Biol Sci Med Sci.* 1998;53:M287–M294.

29. Berry SD, Quach L, Procter-Gray E, et al. Poor adherence to medications may be associated with falls. *J Gerontol A Biol Sci Med Sci.* 2010;65A(5):553–558.

30. Despande N, Metter J, Ferrucci L. Validity of clinically derived cumulative somatosensory impairment index. *Arch Phys Med Rehabil.* 2010;91:226–232.

31. Deshpande N, Connelly DN, Culham EG, Costigan PA. Reliability and validity of ankle proprioceptive measures. *Arch Phys Med Rehabil.* 2003;84:883–889.

32. Maio RF, Garrison HG, Spaite DW, et al. Emergency Medicine Services Outcomes Project (EMSOP) IV: pain measurement in out-of-hospital outcomes research. *Ann Emerg Med.* 2002;40(2):172–179.

33. Possidente CJ, Tandan R. A survey of treatment practices in diabetic peripheral neuropathy. *Prim Care Diabetes.* 2009;3(4):253–257.

34. Davidson JA, Ciulla TA, McGill JB, Kles KA, Anderson PW. How the diabetic eye loses vision. *Endocrine.* 2007;32(1):107–116.

35. Jacobson GP, Newman CW. The development of the dizziness handicap inventory. *Arch Otolaryngol Head Neck Surg.* 1990;116:424–427.

36. Kendall FP, McCreary EK, Provance PG, Rodgers MM, Romani WA. *Muscles: Testing and Function.* 5th ed. Baltimore, MD: Lippincott Williams & Wilkins; 2005.

37. Guralnik JM, Ferrucci L, Pieper CF, et al. Lower extremity function and subsequent disability: consistency across studies, predictive models, and value of gait speed alone compared with the short physical performance battery. *J Gerontol A Biol Sci Med Sci.* 2000;55:M221– M231.

38. Vasunilashorn S, Coppin AK, Patel KV, et al. Use of the short physical performance battery score to predict loss of ability to walk 400 meters: analysis from the InCHIANTI study. *J Gerontol A Biol Sci Med Sci.* 2009;64(2):223–229.

39. Podsiadlo D, Richardson S. The timed "up and go": a test of basic functional mobility for frail elderly persons. *J Am Geriatr Soc.* 1991;39:142–147.

40. Shumway-Cook A, Baldwin M, Pollisar N, Gruber W. Predicting the probability of falls in community-dwelling adults. *Phys Ther.* 1997;77:812–819.

41. Cromwell RL, Newton RA. Relationship between balance and gait stability in healthy older adults. *J Aging Phys Act.* 2004;12:90–100.

42. Guyatt GH, Thompson PJ, Berman LB, et al. Assessment of respiratory function in patients with chronic obstructive airways disease. *Thorax.* 1979;34:254–258.

43. Rogers HL, Cromwell RL, Newton RA. Association of balance measures and perception of fall risk on gait speed: a multiple regression analysis. *Exp Aging Res.* 2005;31:191–203.

44. Newton RA. Validity of the multi-directional reach test: a practical measure for limits of stability in older adults. *J Gerontol A Biol Sci Med Sci.* 2001;56:M248–M252.

45. Dite W, Temple VA. A clinical test of stepping and change of direction to identify multiple falling older adults. *Arch Phys Med Rehabil.* 2002;83:1566–1571.

46. Berg KO, Wood-Dauphinee SL, Williams KI, Gayton D. Measuring balance in the elderly: preliminary development of an instrument. *Physiother Can.* 1989;41:304–311.

47. Bogle-Thorbahn L, Newton RA. Can Berg's balance test predict falls in the elderly. *Phys Ther.* 1996;76:576–585.

48. Schilling RJ, Bollt EM, Fulk JD, Skufca JD, Al-Ajlouni AF, Robinson CJ. A quiet standing index for testing the postural sway of healthy and diabetic adults across a range of ages. *IEEE Trans Biomed Eng.* 2009;56(2):292–302.

49. McDowell I. *Measuring Health: A Guide to Rating Scales and Questionnaires.* 3rd ed. New York: Oxford University Press; 2006.

50. Huang IC, Hwang CC, Wu MY, et al. Diabetes-specific or generic measures for health-related quality of life? Evidence from psychometric validation of the D-39 and SF36. *Value Health.* 2008;11(3):450–461.

51. Contopoulos-Ioannidis DG, Karvouni A, Kouri I, Ioannidis JPA. Reporting and interpretation of SF-36 outcomes in randomised trials: systematic review. *BMJ.* 2009;338:a3006.

52. Waddell G, Newton M, Henderson I. A Fear-avoidance Beliefs Questionnaire (FAB-Q) and the role of fear-avoidance beliefs in chronic low back pain and disability. *Pain.* 1993;52:157–168.

53. Borg G. Psychological bases of perceived exertion. *Med Sci Sports Exerc.* 1982;14:377–381.

54. Washburn RA, Smith KW, Jette AM, Janney CA. The Physical Activity Scale for the Elderly (PASE): development and evaluation. *J Clin Epidemiol.* 1993;46(2):153–162.

55. Prochaska JO, DiClemente CC. Stages and processes of self-change in smoking: toward an integrative model of change. *J Consult Clin Psychol.* 1983;51:390–395.

56. Snodgrass SJ, Rivett DA, Mackenzie LA. Perceptions of older adults about fall injury prevention and physical activity. *Aust J Ageing.* 2005;24(2):114–118.

57. Hayden JA, van Tulder MW, Tomlinson G. Systematic review: strategies for using exercise therapy to improve outcomes in chronic low back pain. *Ann Intern Med.* 2005;142:776–785.

58. Cup EH, Pieterse AJ, ten Broek-Pastoor JM, et al. Exercise therapy and other types of physical therapy for patients with neuromuscular diseases: a systematic review. *Arch Phys Med Rehabil.* 2007;88:1452–1464.

59. Priplata AA, Niemi JB, Harry JD, Lipsitz LA, Collins JJ. Vibrating insoles and balance control in elderly people. *Lancet.* 2003;362:1123–1124.

60. Robinson L, Dawson P, Newton J. Promoting adherence with exercise-based falls prevention programs. In: Vincent ML, Moreau TM, eds. *Accidental Falls: Causes, Prevention and Intervention.* New York: Nova Science Pub, Inc; 2008:283–298.

61. National Council on Aging. The Creative Practices in Home Safety Assessment and Modification Study and State Coalitions on Fall Prevention: A Compendium of Initiatives. http://www.ncoa.org/news-ncoa-publications/publications/. Accessed May 21, 2010.

62. Sherrington C, Whitney JC, Lord SR, Herbert RD, Cumming RG, Close JC. Effective exercise for the prevention of falls: a systematic review and meta-analysis. *J Am Geriatr Soc.* 2008;56(12):2234–2243.

63. Callahan LF. Physical activity programs for chronic arthritis. *Curr Opin Rheumatol.* 2009;21(2):177–182.

64. White CM, Pritchard J, Turner-Stokes L. Exercise for people with peripheral neuropathy. *Cochrane Database Syst Rev.* 2004;(4):CD003904.

65. Gillespie LD, Gillespie WJ, Robertson MC, et al. Interventions for preventing falls in elderly people. *Cochrane Database Syst Rev.* 2003;(4):CD000340.

66. Ruhland JL, Shields RK. The effects of a home exercise program on impairment and health-related quality of life in persons with chronic peripheral neuropathies. *Phys Ther.* 1997;77(10):1026–1039.

67. Bartels EM, Lund H, Hagen KB, Dagfinrud H, Christensen R, Danneskiold-Samsøe B. Aquatic exercise for the treatment of knee and hip osteoarthritis. *Cochrane Database Syst Rev.* 2007;(4):CD005523.

68. Bird ML, Hill K, Ball M, Williams AD. Effects of resistance and flexibility exercise interventions on balance and related measures in older adults. *J Aging Phys Activity.* 2009;17(4):444–454.

69. Schmid AA, Van Puymbroeck M, Koceja DM. Effect of a 12-week yoga intervention on fear of falling and balance in older adults: a pilot study. *Arch Phys Med Rehabil.* 2010;91(4):576–583.

70. Richerson S, Rosendale K. Does Tai Chi improve plantar sensory ability? A pilot study. *Diabetes Technol Ther.* 2007;9(3):276–286.

71. McCain NL, Gray DP, Elswick RK, et al. A randomized clinical trial of alternative stress management interventions in persons with HIV infection. *J Consult Clin Psychol.* 2008;76(3):431–441.

72. Hall A, Maher C, Latimer J, Ferreira M. The effectiveness of Tai Chi for chronic musculoskeletal pain conditions: a systematic review and meta-analysis. *Arthritis Rheum.* 2009;61(6):717–724.

73. Lelard T, Doutrellot PL, David P, Ahmaidi S. Effects of a 12-week Tai Chi Chuan program versus a balance training program on postural control and walking ability in older people. *Arch Phys Med Rehabil.* 2009;1(1):9–14.

74. Cromwell RL, Meyers PM, Meyers PE, Newton RA. Tae Kwon Do: an effective exercise to improve balance and walking ability in healthy older adults. *J Gerontol A Biol Sci Med Sci.* 2007;62A:641–646.

75. Graves LE, Ridgers ND, Williams K, Stratton G, Atkinson G, Cable NT. The physiologic cost and enjoyment of Wii Fit in adolescents, young adults, and older adults. *J Phys Act Health.* 2010;7(3):393–401.

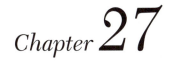

Chapter 27

Peripheral Neuropathies in Individuals With HIV Disease

DAVID M. KIETRYS, PT, PHD, OCS, AND MARY LOU GALANTINO, PT, PHD, MSCE

"The global HIV/AIDS epidemic is an unprecedented crisis that requires an unprecedented response. In particular it requires solidarity—between the healthy and the sick, between rich and poor, and above all, between richer and poorer nations. We have 30 million orphans already. How many more do we have to get, to wake up?"

—KOFI ANON (1938–), GHANIAN DIPLOMAT and FORMER SECRETARY GENERAL
OF THE UNITED NATIONS

Objectives

On completion of this chapter, the student/practitioner will be able to:

- Discuss the role of antiretroviral medication in the treatment of HIV/AIDS.
- List the various neuropathies associated with HIV/AIDS.
- Describe the signs and symptoms of distal symmetrical polyneuropathy associated with HIV/AIDS.
- List the risk factors associated with the development of distal symmetrical polyneuropathy in individuals with HIV/AIDS.
- Discuss the role of complementary and alternative medicines used to treat HIV/AIDS–related polyneuropathy.

Key Terms

- Antiretroviral medications
- Distal symmetrical polyneuropathy
- Highly active antiretroviral therapy
- Human immunodeficiency virus (HIV)

Introduction

Following acute infection with **human immunodeficiency virus (HIV),** people who are untreated gradually progress from a period of being asymptomatic to having advanced HIV disease, or acquired immunodeficiency syndrome (AIDS). This progression may take several months or years. If left untreated, HIV/AIDS eventually leads to death. HIV/AIDS causes catastrophic levels of immunosuppression, increasing the risk of acquiring life-threatening opportunistic infections. Such infections are the leading cause of death in untreated HIV/AIDS. As a result of advances in medications used to treat this disease, people with HIV disease are living longer and leading more active lives. Successful treatment with antiretroviral drugs allows many people to live out their natural life span, but many of the drugs have adverse side effects. As people live longer with the disease, comorbidities may develop that complicate medical management and adversely affect quality of life. Common conditions, injuries, or other problems related to aging might affect long-term survival, especially in cases of advanced disease. Finally, a diagnosis of HIV disease may complicate medical management of preexisting health conditions.

Antiretroviral medications to treat HIV disease have been available since the 1980s. The first antiretroviral drug, AZT (zidovudine), came into widespread use in the United States in 1986. Adverse side effects and toxicities associated with AZT as a monotherapy soon emerged. Later, "cocktails" of at least three different antiretrovirals from at least two different drug classes became the standard of care. Treatment of HIV disease with multiple antiretrovirals is known as **highly active antiretroviral therapy** (HAART). Because of HAART, HIV disease is now a chronic and generally manageable disease, assuming that patients have access to and are adherent to HAART. Although HIV/AIDS is not curable at the present time, pharmaceutical agents for the successful management of this disease continue to evolve and improve.

Overview of HIV/AIDS–Associated Neuropathies

As with other chronic diseases, complications and comorbidities may emerge over time. **Distal symmetrical polyneuropathy** (DSP) is the most common neurological complication of HIV/AIDS[1,2] accounting for approximately 90% of neuropathies seen in patients with HIV/AIDS,[3] and this neuropathy is the focus of this chapter. Other, less common neuropathies are reviewed briefly toward the end of the chapter. The types of neuropathies seen in patients with HIV/AIDS are listed in Box 27-1.

Peripheral neuropathies in patients receiving HAART are challenging to diagnose and treat because of overlap of symptoms with comorbidities. Some patients recently placed on HAART experience immune reconstitution inflammatory syndrome. The risk of this syndrome is highest for patients who start

---

Box 27-1

Types of Peripheral Neuropathy Associated With HIV/AIDS

Distal sensory polyneuropathy

Autonomic neuropathy

Acute inflammatory demyelinating polyneuropathy (Guillain-Barré syndrome)

Chronic inflammatory demyelinating polyneuropathy

Mononeuropathy multiplex or mononeuropathy

Neuropathy associated with diffuse infiltrative lymphomatosis syndrome

Progressive polyneuropathy

Neuropathies associated with opportunistic infections

Progressive polyradiculopathy (associated with cytomegalovirus)

Herpes zoster

HAART with low CD4 counts (<50 to 100 cells/μL) and patients for whom HAART is initiated soon after treatment for an opportunistic infection is begun.[4] Immune reconstitution inflammatory syndrome may further complicate the symptom presentation or be associated with the development of peripheral neuropathies.[5] DSP and other neuropathies also may emerge in patients with untreated disease. In addition, subclinical neuropathy is common in patients with HIV disease; 30% of asymptomatic patients may have clinical signs of DSP.[6,7]

DSP is believed to be related to immunological dysfunction associated with HIV infection or exposure to dideoxynucleosides, nucleoside reverse transcription inhibitor (NRTI) antiretroviral drugs. In addition, other risk factors and mechanisms of interaction with comorbid conditions exist.[8] Reports of prevalence of DSP range from 30%[9] to greater than 50%[10] to 62%[11] in patients with AIDS and between 8% and 30% in all infected individuals.[12] This variation may be explained partly by variance in definitional criteria. Before the emergence of HAART, patients with advanced disease and advanced immunosuppression had a high incidence of DSP.[8] In a study of 1,539 HIV-infected individuals, most of whom were receiving HAART, Ellis et al.[13] found clinical evidence of HIV-associated sensory neuropathy in 57% of patients. Of those, 38% reported neuropathic pain, and 61% reported at least one sensory symptom (pain, paresthesia, or loss of sensation). In this study, pain had a negative effect on quality of life and function. Other studies reported 50% to 60% of patients with DSP experienced pain as a key symptom.[14,15] DSP may affect 34% of children with HIV disease.[16]

Prolonged life expectancies in individuals treated with HAART and occurrences of new HIV infections in older individuals have resulted in increased numbers of older patients with HIV disease. Greater frequency of DSP may occur in older patients with HIV because of greater immune compromise or comorbidities associated with aging.[8] A study of comorbidity prevalence in adults with HIV across each decade of life found that the greatest prevalence of peripheral neuropathy occurred in the oldest cohort (≥60 years old).[17]

Since the advent of HAART, central nervous system complications of the disease have declined, but the incidence and prevalence of peripheral neuropathies, especially DSP, remain high and may be increasing for two main reasons.[18] First, because of HAART, survival rates for individuals infected with HIV have increased and for some individuals may approach normal life expectancy, resulting in prolonged disease duration. Second, certain NRTIs may have a neurotoxic effect. NRTIs have been used in many individuals as part of HIV management. DSP attributable to NRTI toxicity is sometimes referred to antiretroviral toxic neuropathy[19,20] and is sometimes considered as a different pathology than HIV-related DSP. DSP associated with neurotoxic antiretroviral drugs can occur in 21% of individuals receiving dideoxynucleosides as part of their HAART regimen.[21] These two factors (long-term survival and use of potentially neurotoxic drugs) often exist concurrently and help explain why the incidence of peripheral neuropathy is still a major concern in the management of patients with HIV disease. Although disease progression and host factors are associated with increased risk of developing DSP, these same factors may predispose some individuals to the neurotoxic effects of certain HAART medications.[5]

The most disabling component of DSP is pain, which may be either spontaneous or evoked.[22] Neuropathic pain accounts for 25% to 50% of all pain-related clinic visits by patients with HIV disease.[23] Clinically, the signs and symptoms of DSP are similar regardless of whether the pathology is related to HIV disease or NRTI toxicity. Symptoms include bilateral pain, burning, numbness, paresthesias, allodynia, and leg cramping (Box 27-2). Pain may not have a stimulus (i.e., it may occur spontaneously), or it may have a stimulus, with a lowered threshold to noxious stimuli and allodynia.[9]

Weakness in intrinsic muscles of the foot may be seen in severe cases.[10,18] As disease progresses, sleep disturbances and difficulties with activities of daily living may emerge.[9] Symptoms usually occur in lower extremities first, with involvement of upper extremities in later stages.[18]

Pathophysiology and Risk Factors

The pathogenesis of DSP is likely multifactorial, although the precise mechanisms are not well understood.[5] Understanding of the mechanisms that lead to DSP in HIV disease is a matter of ongoing investigation. In general, early initiation of HAART therapy may reduce the risk of developing DSP[24] because it reduces viral load and minimizes long-term exposure to the virus. Small-fiber dysfunction of peripheral nerves sometimes precedes clinical manifestations of DSP.[25] Although DSP symptoms first occur in the distal extremities, peripheral sensitization, central sensitization, and chronic pain emerge as the disease progresses.[22]

It is widely believed that peripheral nerves are not directly infected, and such a mechanism is not the cause of DSP.[3,7] However, HIV replication does occur in macrophages and supporting cells of the dorsal root ganglion (DRG), nerve roots, and peripheral nerves.[25] A relatively direct mechanism is proposed to exist. Nerve cell exposure to an HIV envelope protein, gp120, may have a neurotoxic effect and is associated with allodynia and hyperalgesia.[5] Possible Schwann cell–mediated neurotoxicity from gp120 has been described.[10] The binding of gp120 glycoproteins to receptors on Schwann cell membranes causes release of RANTES (regulated upon activation, normal T-cell expressed, and secreted). Chemokine ligand 5 (CCL5) is a protein that is encoded by a5 gene and then binds to receptors on sensory neurons and induces a tumor necrosis factor alpha–mediated axonal degeneration and apoptotic cell death.[20] The gp120 glycoproteins can also bind directly to receptors on sensory nerves and the DRG,[26] disturbing the regulation of intercellular calcium and inducing upregulation of other proinflammatory cytokines.[27] Other toxic HIV accessory proteins, such as viral protein R (Vpr), also play a role in causing peripheral nervous system injury.[28]

Indirect, or parainfectious, mechanisms associated with chronic infection and inflammation are also believed to play a key role in the development of DSP, via a cascade of events associated with neuroimmune activation.[29] DSP may be due to indirect damage from products of immune activation after HIV infection.[30] These events lead to myelin and axon damage in peripheral nerves, loss of unmyelinated fibers, and macrophage infiltration in peripheral nerve and DRG.[9,31] Macrophages are possibly drawn to peripheral nerves as a result of nutritional deficiencies and axonal damage from infectious agents.[32] Injured nerves demonstrate adverse excitability changes and can evoke spontaneous peripheral ectopic activity leading to spontaneous sensations such as burning.[9] Neural tissue may be injured as a result of the presence perivascular macrophages, satellite cells, Langerhans cells, and proinflammatory cytokines (e.g., tumor necrosis factor alpha, interferon gamma, interleukin-1 and interleukin-6) with resident macrophages in nerve and adjacent to nerve mediating the damage.[9,10,23,30]

The axonal damage/degeneration, or "dying back," of primary afferent fibers occurs in multiple peripheral

---

BOX 27-2

Signs and Symptoms of HIV-Related Distal Sensory Polyneuropathy

Sensory disturbances (paresthesias, numbness; stocking/glove distribution)

Impaired sensation (vibration, pain, light touch, temperature; stocking/glove distribution)

Pain (burning; stocking/glove distribution)

Decreased deep tendon reflexes (Achilles)

Allodynia

Hyperalgesia

Leg cramping

Weakness in intrinsic muscles (in advanced cases)

Sleep disturbances

Difficulty with activities of daily living

Gait dysfunction

Impaired balance

nerves. The first fibers affected are small myelinated and unmyelinated fibers of nociceptive axons,[5,10,27] with larger fibers affected as the disease progresses.[9] In the DRG, the Nageotte nodules that appear are cellular proliferations, consisting mostly of lymphocytes and activated macrophages.[22] Several possible relationships may exist between the DRG and peripheral nerve fibers. Disturbed function of the DRG leads to axon damage/degeneration (dying-back phenomenon) and spinal cord changes characterized by degeneration of the gracile tracts.[27] Conversely, axonal damage can lead to changes in DRG. In addition, some patients with HIV have antisulfatide antibodies to myelin glycolipids.[33] There is also evidence that elevated levels of inflammatory cytokines that occur with HIV infection can injure mitochondria in muscle and nerve, interfering with normal metabolic processes and function of these tissues.[34]

Peripheral and central sensitization occurs via numerous mechanisms. The production of cytokines, chemokines, and surface antigens and upregulation of membrane channels in injured nerve and DRG leads to spontaneous discharge and lower activation thresholds. In addition, the multifocal inflammation and products of macrophage activation result in abnormal spontaneous activity of neighboring uninjured nociceptive fibers (peripheral centralization).[35] Neuron degeneration and macrophage and lymphocyte activation also occur in the DRG[5] and centrally directed extensions of sensory neurons.[27] The sprouting of sympathetic axons around cell bodies also leads to an exaggerated response to discharges. The alterations in neuronal sodium and calcium channel expression in DRG (that contribute to ectopic impulse generation/hyperexcitability) cause central remodeling within the dorsal horn, owing to A-fiber sprouting and synaptic formation with pain fibers in lamina II.[35,36] Second-order neurons in spinal cord fire spontaneously secondary to activation of N-methyl-D-aspartate receptors and subsequent downregulation of gamma-aminobutyric acid receptors.[23] Secondary hyperalgesia, originating in dorsal root ganglia and second-order neurons in the dorsal horn, extends up to brainstem, cortex, periaqueductal gray and rostral ventromedial medulla,[37] ultimately affecting ascending and descending pathways. Increased substance P enhances excitation of spinal interneurons.[23] The perception of pain is facilitated and the analgesia is inhibited as the spinal cord and brain become sensitized.[9] The perpetuation of the cascade of inflammatory events, leading to changes in ascending and descending neural pathways involving the spinal cord and brain, is an important mechanism in the development of chronic pain.[9,38] These central changes may play a role in the propagation of chronic pain secondary to changes in pain processing capabilities or increased sensitivity of sensory nerves. Such spinal cord changes may contribute further to axonal degeneration.[35]

Another possible contributing mechanism to DSP in individuals with HIV disease is side effects of NRTIs, especially "d-drugs" (dideoxynucleoside reverse transcriptase inhibitors) such as didanosine (ddI), zalcitabine, dideoxycytidine (ddC), and stavudine (d4T). Peripheral neuropathy associated with these drugs is known as antiretroviral toxic neuropathy; it is clinically indistinguishable from HIV-related DSP.[22,35] Neurotoxic effects of d-drugs are estimated to occur in 15% to 30% of patients who receive them.[5] Antiretroviral toxic neuropathy appears to be dose dependent, with ddC having the greatest neurotoxic potential.[23] Use of multiple "d-drugs" may have a synergistic neurotoxic effect.[8] In antiretroviral toxic neuropathy, interference with nerve DNA synthesis and mitochondrial dysfunction are believed to be causal factors.[10,31,38] These drugs may interfere with mitochondrial gamma DNA polymerase, leading to impairment of mitochondrial DNA synthesis, mDNA depletion, disruption of cristae, and interference with mitochondrial function.[39,40] Individuals with mitochondrial haplotype T have a greater risk for developing DSP.[41] The adverse effects of d-drugs on mitochondrial function may increase serum lactate concentrations and pose an increased risk of lactic acidosis and other disorders such as myopathy.[34,35] There is conflicting evidence as to whether the use of d-drugs depletes levels of acetyl-L-carnitine, but it is known that depletion of carnitine disrupts mitochondrial metabolism.[41,42]

Differentiation between HIV-related DSP and neurotoxic neuropathy is challenging; the temporal association between the onset of DSP symptoms and the initiation of HAART treatment that includes NRTIs may be helpful.[18,35] For example, rapid onset of DSP symptoms after initiation of NRTIs or clinical improvement in DSP symptoms after cessation of NRTI use may incriminate NRTIs as a causal factor.[3] Some patients demonstrate a transient "coasting effect" (i.e., a temporary worsening of DSP symptoms) after cessation of NRTI; this finding also incriminates NRTIs as a causal factor. Assessment of blood lactate levels (indicative of mitochondrial dysfunction) or serum acetyl-L-carnitine levels may be helpful in determining if DSP in HIV-infected individuals is due to the HIV itself or a side effect of medications because elevated serum lactate levels have been found in patients with DSP prescribed d4T,[1] and decreased levels of acetyl-L-carnitine have been noted in some studies.[11] Toxic neuropathy risk related to d-drugs is magnified in the presence of a high HIV viral load; combination use of d-drugs in patients with advanced disease; hydroxyurea; older age; malnutrition; anemia; or presence of neuropathies from other causes such as alcoholism, vitamin B_{12} deficiency, or diabetes.[3] Although many studies found that use of d-drugs may cause or exacerbate neuropathy, some studies reported that use of d-drugs did not increase the risk for development of neuropathy.[11,43,44] Nonetheless, cases of neuropathy related to d-drug toxicity have been reported. There is evidence that HIV-positive patients with certain mitochondrial haplotypes have a higher risk of d-drug neurotoxic neuropathy,[41] but precise mechanisms explaining variance in susceptibility to developing d-drug–related neuropathy are unclear. The use of d-drugs has been reduced in recent years because of the availability of comparably effective and less toxic agents.

Protease inhibitors, such as indinavir, saquinavir, and ritonavir, have also been associated with neuropathy[2,10] because of their neurotoxic properties and inhibition of mDNA polymerase.[42,44] However, in a multivariate analysis that included other risk factors, neither the duration of protease inhibitor use nor exposure to individual protease inhibitor drugs was associated with DSP.[38]

Generally, long-term survival (and chronicity of the disease) goes hand in hand with HAART. Long-term survival is attributable to successful management of HIV disease with HAART. The emergence of DSP in long-term survivors is potentially related to a combined effect or interaction between chronic HIV infection and neurotoxic effects of some drugs. Long-term HIV infection coupled with long-term use of HAART may make some patients especially vulnerable to DSP.

The risk of development of DSP in a patient with HIV disease may also include a history of very low CD4 counts or high viral loads, although the evidence for this is conflicting. Some studies have reported HIV disease severity (in particular, CD4+ cells counts <50 cells/mm^3 and viral load >10,000 copies/mL) is a predictor of increased risk for DSP,[24,32,45] although findings of other studies had disputed this.[11] The discrepancies may be related to the timing and use of HAART: Subjects from the pre-HAART era showed correlations between HIV disease severity and DSP, whereas correlations in subjects in the current HAART era are not evident.[5,11,44] In general, it is believed that DSP risk is greater with worse disease severity or delayed initiation of HAART.[32]

Drugs other than antiretrovirals are sometimes used to treat comorbidities or infections and may have neurotoxic effects.[23] For example, isoniazid, used to treat tuberculosis, may have neurotoxic effects. Vitamin B$_6$ (pyridoxine) may be used in conjunction to mitigate the neurotoxic effects of isoniazid, but excessively high doses of vitamin B$_6$ (>200 mg/day) may produce a neurotoxic effect. Metronidazole, an antibiotic used in treatment of *Clostridium difficile* may have neurotoxic effects. A complete medical history and list of medications are important in determining if exposure to certain medications may be factors in patients with HIV disease and DSP.

Other risk factors for DSP in general include advancing age, poor nutrition, diabetes, other autoimmune diseases, malignancy, exposure to environmental

---

BOX 27-3

Risk Factors for Distal Sensory Polyneuropathy in Patients With HIV/AIDS

Older age

Nucleoside reverse transcriptase inhibitors (in particular, "d-drugs")

Severity of HIV disease (high viral load and low CD4 counts in pre-HAART era or in untreated individuals)

Diabetes

Elevated triglycerides

Autoimmune diseases

Renal, liver, or thyroid impairment or disease

Abnormal serum hemoglobin or albumin levels

Poor nutrition

Weight loss

Vitamin B$_{12}$ or thiamine deficiency

Alcohol consumption, dependency/abuse

Other neurological abnormalities/diseases

Medications with neurotoxic side effects

Opiate or methamphetamine abuse

Co-infection with hepatitis C (conflicting evidence, but hepatitis C neuropathy manifests with similar signs and symptoms)

Protease inhibitors (unclear; risk is likely small)

HAART, Highly active antiretroviral therapy.

---

toxins, co-infection with hepatitis C or syphilis, impaired glucose tolerance, weight loss, abnormal serum hemoglobin and albumin levels, renal or liver impairment, thyroid dysfunction, other neurological abnormalities, alcohol abuse, and opiate or methamphetamine abuse.[7,10,11,19,24,32,38,39,44,46–51] Box 27-3 summarizes risk factors associated with the development of DSP in patients with HIV disease.

Diagnosis

Clinically, it is difficult to distinguish between DSP associated with HIV disease and NRTI toxicity neuropathy because the symptoms are similar.[18] Distinguishing between these two causal factors was described in the prior section. Although DSP is the most common form of neuropathy in patients with HIV disease, it is important to make a sound differential diagnosis. Other forms of neuropathy, such as uremic neuropathy, diabetic neuropathy, toxic neuropathy, alcoholic neuropathy, or vitamin B$_{12}$ deficiency–associated neuropathy, need to be ruled out or treated accordingly if present. Other forms of HIV-related neuropathies may exist. HIV-related neuropathies other than DSP are described later in this chapter.

DSP is primarily a clinical diagnosis based on subjective complaints of bilateral pain, burning (dysesthesia), numbness, and paresthesias in a stocking/glove distribution (because all peripheral nerves are involved) that begins distally and creeps proximally over time.[10,18] Symptoms typically appear first in the lower extremities, and walking or applying pressure to the feet (e.g., with socks or bed sheets) may aggravate symptoms.[9] Hyperesthesia (increase in contact sensitivity) may become so severe that the patient cannot tolerate wearing shoes or socks.[23] Pain symptoms often increase in the evening.[22] The patient's gait pattern may be antalgic secondary to pain with weight bearing. Pain may or may not depend on a stimulus, and allodynia (painful sensation evoked by nonpainful stimuli) may be present. Pain scales, such as visual analog, numerical, or Wong-Baker scales, should be used on an ongoing basis to document the level of perceived pain. As a measure of pain, Simpson et al.[11] advocated calculating a 7-day median of pain ratings on a 10-cm visual analog scale or the Gracely pain scale used twice a day, separated by 12 hours, for 7 consecutive days.

Typical physical examination findings include decreased sensation for temperature, pain (pinprick), vibration, and pain sensitivity to cold.[10,25] Monofilament testing may also show impairment.[52] Often proprioception is relativity unimpaired.[10] Achilles' jerk reflex is absent or diminished.[10] In addition, a loss of hair and tightness in skin of the lower leg may be observed.[10] Although muscle strength is usually preserved, patients with severe DSP may exhibit weakness in toe flexion, extension, or abduction (owing to weakness in the foot intrinsic); rubor; and pedal edema.[2,10]

The Brief Peripheral Neuropathy Screen[11,53,54] is a validated instrument that includes questions regarding symptoms (pain, aching, burning, paresthesias, or numbness) in legs or feet, great toe vibration sensation testing with a 128-Hz tuning fork, and ankle deep tendon reflex assessment. Ellis et al.[54] used this tool to diagnose DSP in subjects with a history of advanced HIV disease if they demonstrated either a mild loss of vibratory sensation in both great toes or impaired ankle (Achilles jerk) reflexes (relative to the knee/patellar tendon). The Brief Peripheral Neuropathy Screen had a sensitivity of 80% and specificity of 59%. An alternative version of the screening tool required vibration sensation impairment and decreased reflexes; with those criteria, sensitivity was considerably worse (49%), but specificity was much better (88%). Positive findings of vibration sensation and reflex test, along with subjective complaints, are highly suggestive of DSP, but about half of patients with DSP demonstrate false-negative findings when only those criteria are applied. A more sensitive instrument with excellent intrarater and interrater reliability is the Total Neuropathy Score. This instrument includes questions regarding presence of pain, aching, burning, paresthesia, or numbness,

nerve conduction velocity results, and quantitative sensory testing.[55] However, Evans et al.[56] found that a model including only assessment of pain sensitivity, tendon reflexes, and quantitative sensory testing had 85% sensitivity and 80% specificity. They found that the addition of nerve conduction velocity or epidermal nerve fiber density testing did not add significant diagnostic value. Robinson-Papp et al.[57] reported that HIV-infected patients presenting with distal lower extremity neurological symptoms usually have objective evidence of sensory neuropathy on neurological examination or nerve conduction velocity testing, but subjective complaints had only 52% sensitivity for detecting the presence of sensory abnormality.

Nerve conduction velocity and electromyography (EMG) can be used to help diagnose DSP; however, these electrodiagnostic tests have low sensitivity because DSP primarily involves small fibers. When these tests are positive, findings include decreased or absent sensory nerve action potentials and other changes in the distal lower extremity that are indicative of axonal loss.[9,20] The most sensitive finding in patients with HIV-related DSP is reduced or absent sural nerve sensory potential amplitude.[22] In severe cases, abnormal (decreased) motor conduction, late responses on nerve conduction velocity, and denervation of distal muscles on EMG are seen.[5,10] The most robust tools to diagnose DSP might include a combination of subjective symptoms, clinical signs, and electrodiagnostic study results.

Epidermal skin punch biopsy can be used to help diagnose or predict DSP. In patients with DSP, decreased epidermal nerve fiber density is seen,[58] and epidermal nerve fiber density assessment has been correlated with clinical and electrophysiological severity of DSP.[59] Skin biopsy may be helpful for early detection before the onset of symptoms and in evaluating specific types of neuropathy.[31] In asymptomatic patients, nerve fiber density of less than 11 fibers/mm is predictive of developing symptomatic DSP within 6 to 12 months.[7] Nerve biopsy, although not commonly used as a diagnostic test, would likely show axonal degeneration and some demyelination, with greater fiber loss in distal fibers ("dying back"); perivascular infiltration by T lymphocytes and macrophage may also be noted.[9,20]

Medical Management and Pharmacological Interventions

Effective treatment of HIV disease with HAART may slow the progression of DSP in some cases or even lead to improvement, provided that the drugs used in the HAART regimen do not have a neurotoxic effect.[20] Replacement of neurotoxic antiretrovirals with other retroviral drugs should be considered, if feasible. If genotype or phenotype testing of the patient's viral strain suggests that other antiretroviral drugs with less neurotoxicity would be effective (i.e., the virus strains are not resistant to other antiretroviral drugs), a change in the combination therapy may be helpful in averting further progression of the DSP. However, DSP symptoms may persist or transiently worsen for several weeks after cessation of neurotoxic antiretroviral medications; this phenomenon is known as the "coasting effect."[12,60] Patients typically do not return to an asymptomatic state even on cessation of NRTIs.[20] Adjustments in HAART regimens used to minimize DSP must still provide effective virologic control. If DSP symptoms persist beyond several weeks after modification of the HAART regimen and elimination or dose reduction of neurotoxic agents, symptoms are likely related to HIV-associated neuropathy. For patients suspected to have an antiretroviral neurotoxic cause of neuropathy, carnitine supplementation may be helpful.[61]

Reversible causes of DSP should be addressed. For example, effective medical management of diabetes, recovery from alcoholism, or supplementation for nutritional vitamin (vitamin B_{12} or thiamine) deficiencies would be needed if any of those potential causal factors exist. Effective management of such conditions may be beneficial in mitigating the progression of DSP. However, there is no known cure or effective reversal of DSP.[10]

Because direct treatments of DSP are lacking, pharmacological treatment of DSP is geared toward symptom management (i.e., controlling pain, burning, and paresthesias), preservation of physical function, and enhancement of quality of life. Palliative therapy for persistent or worsening symptoms of DSP is often needed, albeit it is sometimes underused because of concerns over addiction or dependency, patient reluctance to report pain, or inefficiencies in the health care system. Neuropathic pain is often underrecognized and undertreated.[3,62] Breitbart et al.[62] reported that greater than 80% of patients with HIV disease–related pain were receiving inadequate analgesia. Despite numerous pharmacological options, drugs used to manage neuropathic pain in patients with HIV disease do not fully ameliorate the pain. Rather, they are used to help control pain to, it is hoped, a tolerable level. Monotherapy generally reduced pain only by 30% to 50%, whereas polypharmacy using different drugs with different mechanisms of action may be more effective.[3] For mild symptoms of DSP, nonopioid analgesics such as acetaminophen or NSAIDs such as ibuprofen may be used. For more chronic, moderate to severe pain, prescription of long-acting opioids such as oxycodone or methadone or transdermal fentanyl, with additional shorter acting agents (e.g., codeine or hydrocodone) for breakthrough pain, may be needed. Stronger opioids such as morphine or fentanyl may be needed for management of severe pain. When opioids are prescribed, tolerance over time often leads to increased dosing and physical dependency.[18] Patients on long-term opioid therapy must also be monitored for side effects such as constipation and respiratory depression. Techniques such as contracts or agreements between the patient and the physician may be needed to minimize aberrant behaviors such as drug abuse or diversion.

Because there are no drugs approved by the U.S. Food and Drug Administration for treatment of HIV-related DSP, several drugs have been used "off label" for treatment of symptoms of DSP. Antiepileptic drugs such as pregabalin (Lyrica) or gabapentin (Neurontin) may benefit patients with HIV-related DSP.[63,64] Common side effects of pregabalin include dizziness and drowsiness, although these side effects may be minimized by reducing the dosage of the drug.[10] Gabapentin, an older drug with similar metabolic pathway, mechanism of action, and common effects as pregabalin, has also been used in patients with HIV DSP.[10] Gabapentin and lamotrigine were found to be more effective than placebo in reducing pain or sleep interference in several trials.[63,65] Other antiepileptic drugs that are less commonly used for HIV-related DSP include phenytoin, carbamazepine, lamotrigine, and valproate. In general, antiepileptic drugs need to be prescribed and monitored carefully because of risk of renal or hepatic stress or interactions with protease inhibitors.[66]

Antidepressant drugs, including tricyclic antidepressants (TCAs) and selective serotonin reuptake inhibitors (SSRIs), are also used "off label" in the treatment of HIV-related DSP. Antidepressants impart an analgesic effect, most likely secondary to enhancement of central descending pain inhibition pathways.[10] Common TCAs such as amitriptyline and nortriptyline have been available for treatment of depression for decades. Common side effects include, but are not limited to, sedation, confusion, orthostatic hypotension, urinary retention, dry mouth, blurred vision, and cardiac arrhythmia.[66] Common SSRIs include duloxetine (Cymbalta), escitalopram (Lexapro), and sertraline (Zoloft). Common side effects of SSRIs include, but are not limited to, apathy, nausea, drowsiness, insomnia, vivid dreams, headache, bruxism, and tinnitus. Prescription and dosing of antidepressant drugs in patients the HIV-related DSP must be carefully administered and monitored, not only to determine effectiveness in management of DSP symptoms but also because of the possibility of less common but more serious side effects and the potential for drug interactions with other medications that the patient may be taking. For example, certain TCAs and SSRIs are metabolized in the liver and have potential interactions with antiretroviral drugs that are metabolized along the same pathway.[10] When used to manage symptoms of HIV-related DSP, antidepressants may be concurrently used to manage depression in these same patients. Referral to a psychiatrist is often indicated.

Topical medications, typically delivered via a cream or patch, may also be used in the treatment of DSP. Topical applications are attractive because the potential for side effects and drug interactions is minimized compared with orally administered drugs. Specific topical agents include lidocaine and high-concentration capsaicin. In general, their effectiveness has not been well established.[18] Simpson et al.[67] reported significant reductions in pain for up to 12 weeks after a one-time dose of a high-concentration capsaicin patch.

Depending on the individual patient's needs and responsiveness to pharmacological therapies, analgesics, antiepileptics, antidepressants, and topical agents may be used in combination for management of symptoms associated with DSP, with the therapeutic goal of sustained analgesia. Multiple drugs from several classes are commonly used to achieve adequate analgesia, although controlled studies to confirm efficacy are lacking.[5] Even with successful long-term analgesia, some individuals experience episodes of transient breakthrough pain, and short-term use of opioids such as oxycodone with acetaminophen (Percocet) or fentanyl may be prescribed to help manage breakthrough pain.[10] Any prescription of opioids must be carefully administered and monitored because of the risk of addiction and physical dependency, especially in patients with a prior history of recreational drug use or addiction issues.

Medical cannabis (marijuana) may be beneficial for HIV-related neuropathy. Smoked cannabis combined with analgesic therapy was found to be effective in controlling refractory pain in patients with HIV-associated DSP.[68-70] In addition, medical cannabis may be helpful in treatment of nausea, stimulation of appetite, management of anxiety, and management of depression.[69] One drawback is that marijuana use has a negative impact on adherence to HAART.[71] Medical cannabis is available by prescription in a limited number of states in the United States. Criticisms of medical cannabis include the potential side effect of altered memory-related brain function and the common method of delivery via smoking. Smoking comes with its own set of risks, including potential for abuse. However, vaporizers, pill forms (dronabinol [Marinol]), and edible forms are also available. Individuals considering the use of medical cannabis for treatment of DSP should ascertain the legality of possession and use of this substance in their state of residence.

Other pharmaceuticals are also under investigation. A 2010 systematic review and meta-analysis of randomized controlled trials of pharmacological treatment of HIV-related DSP found greater efficacy than placebo with smoked cannabis, topical capsaicin (8%),

and recombinant human nerve growth factor, but not with amitriptyline, gabapentin, pregabalin, prosaptide, peptide T, acetyl-L-carnitine, mexiletine, or lamotrigine. Cognitive-behavior therapy or supportive psychotherapy has been shown to have a beneficial effect on pain in patients with HIV-related peripheral neuropathy, but feasibility and acceptability may be an issue for some patients.[71]

Physical Therapy Interventions

There is a paucity of literature regarding effective physical therapy interventions for patients who have HIV-related DSP. Two case reports described favorable outcomes in pain and function using an impairment-based approach and microcurrent electrical stimulation.[72] In a patient with HIV-related DSP, a thorough physical therapy examination is recommended to determine the nature and magnitude of any impairments that may exist. Although DSP is generally considered a progressive disease, some impairments may be reversible. A comprehensive physical therapy program can potentially yield positive results in an individual patient. Table 27-1 lists potential impairments and proposed physical therapy interventions.

Because patients with neuropathic foot pain may self-limit their weight-bearing activities to avoid pain, it is quite plausible that impairments associated with reduced activity, such as heel cord tightness and ankle/foot hypomobility, may exist. Manual therapy procedures and exercises should be used to address any specific impairments in soft tissue and joint mobility that are identified on examination. Examination should also include assessment of balance. The Dynamic Gait Index, or other commonly used balance assessment tests such the Romberg balance test or standing on one leg with eyes open or eyes closed, can be used for this purpose. If balance impairments are identified, the physical therapy program should include balance exercises and activities. Although muscle weakness does not appear in early stages of DSP, in advanced stages, strengthening exercises, particularly for intrinsic musculature of the foot, may be indicated.[10]

Physical therapy modalities and patient education can be an effective adjunct to comprehensive pain management. Such interventions should be administered with knowledge of the patient's current medical and pharmacological treatment of pain, and communication with the patient's physician is important for coordinated care. The patient may need lifestyle modifications or adjustments in activities of daily living, such as avoidance of long periods of walking or standing in unsupportive footwear or avoiding restrictive or tight-fitting shoes. Common recommendations for self-treatment of pain include warm soaks, rest, exercise, elevation, and massage of feet, depending on

Table 27-1 Possible Impairments in Patients With HIV-Related Distal Sensory Polyneuropathy and Proposed Physical Therapy Interventions

Impairments That May Exist in Patients With HIV-Related Distal Sensory Polyneuropathy	Proposed Physical Therapy Interventions
Pain; sensory changes	• Trial of electrical stimulation (various forms) • Patient education in self-management techniques (heat, ice massage, rest, elevation, exercise) • ROM exercises • Neural mobilization/gliding exercises • Massage • Lower extremity night splint
Hypersensitivity or allodynia	• Desensitization (e.g., brushing skin with terrycloth towel after a warm soak)
Heel cord tightness or other impairments in flexibility	• Soft tissue mobilization • Stretching exercises
Joint hypomobility (talocrural, subtalar, mid-tarsal, tarsal-metatarsal, intertarsal, metatarsophalangeal)	• Joint mobilization/manipulation • ROM exercises and activities
Excessive pronation; compromised dynamic arch support associated with intrinsic muscle weakness	• Taping • Arch supports • Orthoses
Weakness	• Strengthening exercises • Functional activities
Balance impairments	• Balance exercises and activities
Impaired endurance	• Reconditioning exercises (with consideration of patient tolerance for weight bearing)
Gait dysfunction	• Address soft tissue, joint, and biomechanical issues that may be affecting gait • Gait training • Assistive device use (if needed)
Impaired function or activities of daily living	• Functional training • Activity modification as needed

ROM, Range of motion.

patient preferences.[2] A pilot study[73] reported the effects of use of a lower extremity night splint in patients with HIV disease and painful peripheral neuropathy. After 3 weeks of nightly use, splint wearers had significantly less pain and an improved sleep index score compared with a control group. The authors proposed that the improvements in sleep quality may prove beneficial breaking the vicious cycle of interrupted sleep and nocturnal pain, possibly enhancing the patient's quality of life.

Gale[74] reported favorable outcomes with microcurrent electrical stimulation in two cases, and Galantino et al.[72] reported improvement in functional activities and decreased muscle response latency after treatment with electroacupuncture. Randomized controlled trials on effectiveness of electrotherapeutic and other modalities in patients with HIV disease and DSP have not been published. A trial of various forms of electrical stimulation is recommended in an individual patient. If a clinically meaningful decrease in pain occurs in an individual patient after a particular form of stimulation, ongoing treatment with a home electrical stimulation unit should be considered. There is evidence in the literature that transcutaneous electrical stimulation or high-frequency muscle stimulation is effective in reducing pain in patients with diabetic peripheral neuropathy.[74-76] However, differences in pathophysiology of HIV-related peripheral neuropathy and diabetic peripheral neuropathy suggest caution should be used when applying results of outcomes studies performed on patients with diabetic peripheral neuropathy to patients with HIV-related neuropathy. Several studies have reported the effects of monochromatic infrared photoenergy (MIRE) therapy on patients with diabetic peripheral neuropathy. To date, the outcomes of these reports have provided conflicting evidence regarding the effectiveness of MIRE therapy on pain and sensitivity.[77] No published studies have reported on the effectiveness of MIRE therapy in patients with HIV-related peripheral neuropathy.

Pain Management Integrative Modalities: Acupuncture, Mind-Body Therapy, and Supplements

Use of complementary and alternative medicine (CAM) is prevalent among HIV-positive individuals despite the success of antiretroviral treatments and limited evidence of the safety and efficacy of CAM.[2,78,79] A systematic review of 40 studies of CAM use among HIV-positive people was conducted in 2008.[79] Findings confirmed that 60% of HIV-positive individuals report CAM use, and it is more common among individuals who are men who have sex with men, nonminority, better educated, and less impoverished. Other research found that former drug use, visits to a mental health professional, and a college education are factors associated with higher likelihood of CAM use.[78] In 2005, a systematic review of randomized clinical trials assessing the effectiveness of complementary therapies for HIV and HIV-related symptoms found 30 trials (between 1989 and 2003) that met predefined inclusion and exclusion criteria; most trials were small and of limited methodological rigor.[78,79]

The use of CAM is associated with longer disease duration and greater severity of HIV symptoms. HIV-positive users of CAM report that they use these modalities to prevent or alleviate HIV-related symptoms, reduce treatment side effects, and improve quality of life. Findings regarding the association between CAM use, psychosocial adjustment, and adherence to conventional HIV medications are mixed.[78,79] Although the reviewed studies are instrumental in describing the characteristics of HIV-positive CAM users, the literature lacks a conceptual framework to identify causal factors involved in the decision to use CAM or explain implications of CAM use for conventional HIV care.[79] Because of the long-term and often worsening symptoms of DSP, patients often seek use of CAM interventions to promote analgesia.

Acupuncture has been shown in many studies to be effective for reducing pain related to a variety of different medical conditions, as noted by the National Institutes of Health.[80] A clinical trial in the *Journal of the American Medical Association*[81] reporting use of acupuncture and amitriptyline in HIV-infected patients concluded that there was no effect for either acupuncture or amitriptyline on neuropathic pain compared with placebo. However, in a reanalysis of the data, acupuncture was effective in reducing attrition and mortality in this sample, especially when health status was taken into account, but results for pain relief were mixed.[82] In another study, the effect of acupuncture treatment comprising 5 weeks of 10 sessions of 30 to 45 minutes in a group setting on DSP found subjective pain and symptoms of DSP were reduced during the

period of individual acupuncture therapy delivered in a group setting.[83] When needles are unavailable, the use of electroacupuncture is another option for patients as they are instructed in the proper placement of electrodes over specific acupuncture points. In one pilot study, low-voltage noninvasive electroacupuncture was administered with skin electrodes over leg points BL60, ST36, K1, and LIV3 for 20 minutes every day for 30 days. Significant findings in the MOS-HIV 30-item quality-of-life instrument and H-reflex parameters were noted and support the use of low-voltage electroacupuncture to improve DSP.[84] Further clinical trials of acupuncture with improved methodological quality are needed to determine dose, duration, and mode of administration of acupoints for HIV DSP pain management.

When balance and strength impairments arise as a result of HIV-related neurological underpinning, the use of yoga and tai chi chuan may play a role in the rehabilitation process. Tai chi chuan has been shown to have an impact on function, quality of life, and psychosocial variables in individuals living in various stages of HIV/AIDS.[85-87] A review summarized research on the physical and psychological benefits of tai chi chuan and found improved balance and muscular strength as well as improved sleep and attentiveness and reduced anxiety.

Stress management may prove to be an effective way to reduce pain and increase quality of life in individuals with HIV/AIDS.[88] Mindfulness-based stress reduction (MBSR) for stress management in people living with HIV/AIDS is a behavioral intervention that practices insight-oriented (or mindfulness) meditation. Although research is limited, MBSR may be effective in the management of stress and anxiety for HIV-positive patients, as it has been with many other disease conditions.[89] Massage also has been shown to have similar benefits on the immune system as the MBSR approach. Massage may lower stress levels by reducing cortisol levels, which increases CD4 and CD8 cells and improves the general function of the immune system.[90]

A widening body of research indicates alternative supplements may be beneficial for HIV-related pain. Alpha lipoic acid, acetyl-L-carnitine, benfotiamine, methylcobalamin, and topical capsaicin are among the most well-researched alternative options for the treatment of DSP.[91] Other potential nutrient or botanical therapies include vitamin E, glutathione, folate, pyridoxine, biotin, *myo*-inositol, omega-3 and omega-6 fatty acids, L-arginine, L-glutamine, taurine, N-acetylcysteine, zinc, magnesium, chromium, and St. John's wort.[92,93] Although some CAM therapies have been shown to increase the quality of life of HIV-positive patients, other therapies have been shown to be detrimental.[94] Nutritional supplements and herbal remedies must be used with caution because some over-the-counter nutritional supplements may interact with drugs used in HAART. For example, St. John's wort, an herbal supplement used to improve mood, is known to interact adversely (owing to similar metabolic pathways) with certain protease inhibitors and nonnucleoside reverse transcriptase inhibitors that are commonly used in HAART. Patients should be advised to disclose and discuss use of any nutritional or herbal supplements with their infectious disease physician. Health care professionals need to be aware of the benefits and risks of herbal and nutritional supplements so that patients are properly informed and safety is ensured.

Decisions about using CAM in conjunction with HAART therapy are often poorly informed. Safety risks and potential drug interactions are frequently ignored because people who use HAART prefer to focus on the physical and mental benefits of using selected CAM therapies to promote their quality of life.[95] Researchers used a culture-centered approach to understand the experiences of people with treatment options for HIV-related peripheral neuropathy. Although participants reported that biomedical pills were an important context for understanding decision making regarding neuropathy treatment, they also expressed deep resentment and frustration with biomedically prescribed pills. Complaints about the pills worked to frame the holistic alternatives of acupuncture and massage therapy as better options for neuropathy and to establish a foundation for understanding how participants made particular health treatment decisions. As life expectancy increases, it is important for health professionals to be knowledgeable about the prevention, assessment, and treatment of HIV symptoms and treatment side effects of conventional and CAM treatments. Given the growing trend of using CAM by the general population, it is also important to understand the appropriate use of CAM for symptom management in HIV/AIDS care.

Other Types of Neuropathy Associated With HIV Disease

Less common forms of neuropathy occur in patients with HIV disease and are related to the stage of illness and the degree of immunodeficiency. Although DSP is still quite prevalent, the advent of effective HAART has led to a decline in many of these neuropathies.[95]

Autonomic Neuropathy

Autonomic dysfunction, involving sympathetic and parasympathetic nerve fibers, may be present in patients with HIV disease. Autonomic neuropathy is more likely in individuals with HIV/AIDS and may include symptoms such as hypotension, syncope, cardiac arrhythmias, anhidrosis, diarrhea, urinary dysfunction, and erectile dysfunction (in men).[10] The proposed etiology of autonomic neuropathy includes an autoimmune response or direct HIV infection of autonomic nervous system structures.[10] Medical management of the effects of autonomic neuropathy is often needed.

Inflammatory Demyelinating Neuropathies

Acute inflammatory demyelinating polyneuropathy (AIDP), a condition very similar to Guillain-Barré syndrome, may occur (albeit rarely) during the period of seroconversion and high CD4 counts (typically a few weeks after acute infection with HIV). This immune-mediated disorder may also occur in patients with advanced HIV/AIDS and advanced immunosuppression, especially when the opportunistic infection cytomegalovirus (CMV) is present.[3,10,38] AIDP, primarily affecting motor fibers, is associated with demyelination and axonal loss mediated by macrophages and lymphocytic infiltrates.[20] On EMG, demyelination and axon degeneration is evidenced by prolonged distal motor and F-wave latencies, reduced conduction velocity, partial conduction blocks, and other abnormalities[20] suggestive of a demyelinating neuropathy. Cerebrospinal fluid shows high protein content and mild mononuclear pleocytosis.[43] In HIV-positive patients with AIDP, cerebrospinal fluid lymphocytic pleocytosis is a common finding; this particular finding does not occur in HIV-negative individuals with AIDP.[20] Nerve biopsy shows segmental demyelination with onion bulb formations, macrophage activation, mononuclear cell infiltration of nerve fascicles, and endoneural edema.[5] Patients with AIDP typically present with a rapid onset of progressive weakness, especially in the lower extremities, and absent or diminished deep tendon reflexes. Sensory symptoms are minor. Weakness may progress to involve facial and respiratory muscles. Diagnosis is confirmed with nerve conduction studies, EMG, and lumbar puncture for detection of cerebrospinal fluid abnormalities. Medical interventions typically include intravenous immunoglobulin or plasmapheresis.[10] Corticosteroids are used with caution in patients with HIV disease because of their immunosuppressive effect. Recovery, which may be full or incomplete, typically occurs gradually over 1 to 2 years. Chronic demyelinating neuropathy shares many features with AIDP, with a more protracted onset (>8 weeks), periods of remission or relapse, and longer or incomplete recovery time.[20]

HIV-associated neuromuscular weakness syndrome, a clinically similar condition, includes other symptoms, such as nausea, abdominal distention, lipodystrophy, and hepatomegaly, and is associated with hyperlactatemia and lactic acidosis syndrome. This condition has been associated with treatment of HIV disease with NRTIs, which are thought to have a toxic effect on mitochondria.[5,10] This condition is thought to involve interplay between HIV-induced effects and drug toxicity.[3] In some cases, it can lead to severe morbidity or death.[3]

Mononeuropathies

Mononeuropathy involving one peripheral or cranial nerve (typically cranial nerve VII or V) or mononeuropathy multiplex (involving two or more peripheral or cranial nerves) is a rare complication in individuals with HIV disease that may occur in early stages of HIV disease.[10,38,43] Nerve involvement may be asymmetrical.[23] Mononeuropathies that occur in early stages of HIV disease are thought to be due to autoimmune mechanisms[10,23] or vasculitis of peripheral nerves.[5,20] Treatment may include corticosteroids, intravenous immunoglobulin, or plasmapheresis.[10,38] Neuropathies may occur around the time of seroconversion, when antibody production reaches measurable levels (typically a few weeks after acute infection), and may resolve spontaneously.[20,23] Signs and symptoms include sensory and motor impairments associated with the peripheral nerves involved. Electrophysiological studies show a multifocal pattern of reduction in evoked sensory and motor compound muscle action potential amplitudes,[5] suggesting axon degeneration. Severe cases may require treatment with corticosteroids, plasmapheresis, or intravenous immunoglobulin.[23] When mononeuropathies occur in patients with advanced disease, they may be related to CMV infection, varicella zoster, or other opportunistic infections, and medical management of the opportunistic infection is indicated.[3,10,23]

Neuropathy Associated With Infiltrative Lymphomatosis Syndrome

Infiltrative lymphomatosis syndrome is an uncommon systemic illness caused by hyperlymphomatosis of CD8 lymphocytes, with infiltration into visceral organs and epineurium and endoneurium of peripheral nerves.[5,20] It typically occurs in the early stages of HIV infection.[20] Peripheral sensorimotor neuropathies may result from infiltration of CD8 cells into axons and is associated with parotidomegaly, sicca syndrome, lymphadenopathy, and splenomegaly. Pain is typically multifocal and symmetrical,[5] although one third of patients have asymmetrical symptoms at onset.[1] Cranial nerve involvement may occur, typically in cranial nerve VII. Therapies include HAART and steroid therapy.[5,20]

Progressive Polyradiculopathy

Patients with advanced disease and CMV may present with progressive polyradiculopathy, a rare disorder affecting the lumbosacral nerve roots that causes a subacute onset of low back and lower extremity pain and paresthesias, lower extremity weakness, and cauda equine syndrome.[10,20] Low back pain and leg pain may precede sphincter and lower extremity weakness.[20] Rapid progression leads to flaccid paraplegia and, in some cases, involvement of the upper extremities.

Lumbar magnetic resonance imaging with contrast enhancement may reveal enhancement of lumbosacral nerve roots.[23] Electrophysiological studies show widespread denervation in paraspinal muscles and leg muscles.[5] Spinal fluid shows polymorphonuclear pleocytosis, elevated protein levels, and low glucose. This condition requires concurrent management of HIV and CMV. Prompt treatment of CMV with ganciclovir, foscarnet, or cidofovir often results in resolution of symptoms over several weeks.[5] Polyradiculopathies may also have other causes, such as syphilis, lymphomatous meningitis, herpesvirus, syphilis, cryptococcus, tuberculosis, or lymphoma.[20,23] Identification of these potential causes and appropriate treatment are indicated.

Neuropathies Related to Opportunistic Infections

Patients with HIV disease are at greater risk than the general population for herpes zoster (shingles) exacerbation, which typically causes pain and rash along the distribution of a dermatome, cranial nerve, or peripheral nerve. Although acute flares are often successfully managed with anti–varicella-zoster medication, some individuals may have incomplete resolution, and symptoms may persist as a postherpetic neuralgia, resulting in chronic and persisting symptoms.[10]

CASE STUDY

ML is a 48-year-old biomechanical engineer who learned he was HIV-positive 11 years ago. He had no HIV testing before that and does not know when he was initially infected. At the time he was diagnosed, his CD4 count was 575 cells/mm^3, and viral load was 8,000 copies/mL. ML was prescribed HAART 8 years ago and has been fully adherent with his medications since that time. At the time HAART was initiated, his CD4 count was 350 cells/mm^3, and his viral load was 12,000 copies/mL. Currently, his CD4 count is 650 cells/mm^3, and his viral load is undetectable (<40 copies/mL).

Since his diagnosis, ML has remained active. He currently runs 2 miles three times a week and takes an occasional yoga class. ML complains of a recent onset of intermittent numbness and burning-type pain in both feet, including all toes. His pain ranges from 2 cm to 5 cm on a 10-cm visual analog pain scale. Although often present at rest or at night, he reports that the pain in the plantar surfaces of his feet is worse after running. To help manage this pain, he takes NSAIDs after running. As a runner and biomechanical engineer, he has done some research on his own and is suspicious that his long-standing overpronation pattern may now be causing tarsal tunnel syndrome. He comes to the physical therapist for advice on management of his symptoms and to be evaluated for orthoses. Past medical history includes mild anxiety, which he manages with meditation and yoga.

Most recent laboratory values are CD4 count of 650 cells/mm^3 and viral load undetectable (<40 copies/mL). All other laboratory values are normal. ML's medications include HAART (Atripla) and over-the-counter NSAIDs as needed. ML lives with his wife and three children in a two-story home with several steps to enter the home. His wife and children have been tested for HIV and are negative. ML is independent in all activities of daily living and is working full-time as a biomedical engineer at a research university. His goals are to return to running pain-free and achieve relief of symptoms.

Systems review of ML shows the following:

Cardiovascular/pulmonary: Heart rate 76 beats/min, blood pressure 125/85 mm Hg, respiratory rate 14
Integumentary: Dry cracked skin along medial longitudinal arch
Musculoskeletal: Gross strength, range of motion (ROM), and symmetry within normal limits (WNL)
Neuromuscular: Transfers, gait, and gross motor function WNL; upper and lower quarter screening reveals slight decrease in light touch perception in all toes (nondermatomal distribution) and sluggish ankle jerk (1+) reflexes bilaterally
Communication, affect, learning: WNL
Tests and measures performed during examination show the following:
Posture and alignment (assessed in standing): Forward head with forward rounded shoulders, decreased lumbar lordosis, excessive bilateral calcaneal valgus and pes planus, mild hallux valgus bilaterally
Gait: Excessive pronation observed after weight acceptance and at midstance
ROM: WNL except for dorsiflexor passive ROM (with 0° knee), which is limited to 5° owing to heel cord tightness bilaterally
Manual muscle test: Upper extremity WNL; lower extremity WNL
Balance: 22 (out of 24) on Dynamic Gait Index
Sensation (additional testing performed because of deficits noted on lower quarter screening): 10g monofilament testing confirmed decreased light touch over all toes and decreased light touch sensation over dorsal and plantar surfaces of the feet; vibration sensation (128-Hz tuning fork) was diminished in the same areas
Proprioception: WNL
Special tests order showed the following:
Positive lower extremity neural tension test (straight leg raise with dorsiflexion): Provoked pain and paresthesias in the plantar surfaces of the feet
Positive (bilateral) Tinel test over tarsal tunnel: Reproduced paresthesias along medial arches

Palpation: No pain with passive extension of first metatarsophalangeal joint in standing; no tenderness along plantar fascia or at medial tubercle of calcaneus or elsewhere

Case Study Questions

1. What differential diagnoses need to be considered in this case?
   a. DSP alone
   b. Bilateral tarsal tunnel syndrome alone
   c. DSP and bilateral tarsal tunnel syndrome
   d. All of the above

2. Which of the following statements is most true regarding ML's prognosis if tarsal tunnel syndrome is diagnosed?
   a. The prognosis is poor because tarsal tunnel syndrome in individuals with HIV/AIDS is a progressive disease.
   b. Tarsal tunnel syndrome tends to be self-limiting and gets better without intervention.
   c. Antiretroviral drugs, in addition to their impact on immunosuppression, have a positive effect on neuropathy regardless of etiology.
   d. The prognosis is excellent with appropriate physical therapy.

3. Interventions for DSP include which of the following?
   a. Electrical stimulation
   b. Intrinsic muscle lengthening and strengthening
   c. Mobilization of mid-tarsal joints that exhibit decreased mobility
   d. All of the above

4. What would be appropriate topics for patient education at this time?
   a. ML needs to be informed that his symptoms may be due to two different problems (i.e., tarsal tunnel syndrome and DSP), and he should be educated regarding the nature and prognosis of these problems.
   b. ML should be taught to do frequent skin integrity checks, especially after running, and to change running shoes periodically.
   c. Discussion of self-management of DSP symptoms is needed.
   d. All of the above

5. Which of the following would be considered an inappropriate referral for ML?
   a. Referral for custom-made orthoses if taping and over-the-counter orthoses prove helpful but nonetheless inadequate
   b. Referral to an herbalist for a prescription for St. John's wort
   c. Referral to a neurologist or pain specialist
   d. Referral for EMG and nerve conduction velocity studies to confirm suspected diagnoses

References

1. Nicholas PK, Mauceri L, Slate Ciampa A, et al. Distal sensory polyneuropathy in the context of HIV/AIDS. *J Assoc Nurses AIDS Care.* 2007;18(4):32–40.

2. Baker WC. HIV-associated neuropathies. Not a necessary consequence of HIV infection. *Adv Nurse Pract.* 2003;11(11):83–86, 89–90.

3. Verma S, Micsa E, Estanislao L, Simpson D. Neuromuscular complications in HIV. *Curr Neurol Neurosci Rep.* 2004;4(1):62–67.

4. French MA. HIV/AIDS: immune reconstitution inflammatory syndrome: a reappraisal. *Clin Infect Dis.* 2009;48(1):101–107.

5. Ferrari S, Vento S, Monaco S, et al. Human immunodeficiency virus-associated peripheral neuropathies. *Mayo Clin Proc.* 2006;81(2):213–219.

6. Gonzalez-Duarte A, Cikurel, K, Simpson DM. Managing HIV peripheral neuropathy. *Curr HIV/AIDS Rep.* 2007;4(3):114–118.

7. Gonzalez-Duarte A, Robinson-Papp J, Simpson DM. Diagnosis and management of HIV-associated neuropathy. *Neurol Clin.* 2008;26(3):821–832.

8. Luciano CA, Pardo CA, McArthur JC. Recent developments in the HIV neuropathies. *Curr Opin Neurol.* 2003;16(3):403–409.

9. Dorsey SG, Morton PG. HIV peripheral neuropathy: pathophysiology and clinical implications. *AACN Clin Issues.* 2006;17(1):30–36.

10. Robinson-Papp J, Simpson DM. Neuromuscular complications of human immunodeficiency virus infection. *Phys Med Rehab Clin N Am.* 2008;19(1):81–96.

11. Simpson DM, Kitch D, Evans SR, et al. HIV neuropathy natural history cohort study: assessment measures and risk factors. *Neurology.* 2006;66(11):1679–1687.

12. Wulff EA, Wang AK, Simpson DM. HIV-associated peripheral neuropathy: epidemiology, pathophysiology and treatment. *Drugs.* 2000;59(6):1251–1260.

13. Ellis RJ, Rosario D, Clifford DB, et al. Continued high prevalence and adverse clinical impact of human immunodeficiency. *Arch Neurol.* 2010;67:552–558.

14. Fuller G, Jacobs J, Guiloff R. Nature and incidence of peripheral nerve syndromes in HIV infection. *J Neurol Neurosurg Psychiatry.* 1993;56:372–381.

15. Martin C, Pehrsson P, Osterberg A, Sonnerborg A, Hansson P. Pain in ambulatory HIV-infected patients with and without intravenous drug use. *Eur J Pain.* 1999;3:157–164.

16. Araujo AP, Nascimento OJ, Garcia OS. Distal sensory polyneuropathy in a cohort of HIV-infected children over five years of age. *Pediatrics.* 2000;106(3):E35.

17. Vance DE, Mugavero M, Willig J, Raper JL, Saag MS. Aging with HIV: a cross-sectional study of comorbidity prevalence and clinical characteristics across decades of life. *J Assoc Nurses AIDS Care.* 2011;22(1):17–25.

18. Nicholas PK, Kemppainen JK, Canaval GE, et al. Symptom management and self-care for peripheral neuropathy in HIV/AIDS. *AIDS Care.* 2007;19(2):179–189.

19. Ferrari LF, Levine JD. Alcohol consumption enhances antiretroviral painful peripheral neuropathy by mitochondrial mechanisms. *Eur J Neurosci.* 2010;32(5):811–818.

20. Hoke A, Cornblath DR. Peripheral neuropathies in human immunodeficiency virus infection. *Suppl Clin Neurophysiol.* 2004;57:195–210.

21. Scarsella A, Coodley G, Shalit P, et al. Stavudine-associated peripheral neuropathy in zidovudine-naive patients: effect of stavudine exposure and antiretroviral experience. *Adv Ther.* 2002;19(1):1–8.

22. Verma S, Estanislao L, Mintz L, Simpson D. Controlling neuropathic pain in HIV. *Curr HIV/AIDS Rep.* 2004;1(3):136–141.

23. Verma S, Estanislao L, Simpson D. HIV-associated neuropathic pain: epidemiology, pathophysiology and management. *CNS Drugs.* 2002;19(4):325–334.

24. de Freitas MR. Infectious neuropathy. *Curr Opin Neurol.* 2007;20(5):548–552.

25. Martin C, Solders G, Sonnerborg A, Hansson P. Painful and non-painful neuropathy in HIV-infected patients: an analysis of somatosensory nerve function. *Eur J Pain.* 2003;7(1):23–31.

26. Oh SB, Tran PB, Gillard SE, Hurley RW, Hammond DL, Miller RJ. Chemokines and glycoprotein120 produce pain hypersensitivity by directly exciting primary nociceptive neurons. *J Neurosci.* 2001;21(14):5027–5035.

27. Jones G, Zhu Y, Silva C, et al. Peripheral nerve-derived HIV-1 is predominantly CCR5-dependent and causes neuronal degeneration and neuroinflammation. *Virology.* 2005;334(2):178–193.

28. Acharjee S, Noorbakhsh F, Stemkowski PL, et al. HIV-1 viral protein R causes peripheral nervous system injury associated with in vivo neuropathic pain. *FASEB J.* 2010;24(11):4343–4353.

29. Simpson DM. Selected peripheral neuropathies associated with human immunodeficiency virus infection and antiretroviral therapy. *J Neurovirol.* 2002;8(Suppl 2):33–41.

30. Schifitto G, McDermott MP, McArthur JC, et al. Markers of immune activation and viral load in HIV-associated sensory neuropathy. *Neurology.* 2005;64(5):842–848.

31. Pardo CA, McArthur JC, Griffin JW. HIV neuropathy: insights in the pathology of HIV peripheral nerve disease. *J Peripher Nerv Syst.* 2001;6(1):21–27.

32. Lichtenstein KA, Armon C, Baron A, Moorman AC, Wood KC, Holmberg SD. Modification of the incidence of drug-associated symmetrical peripheral neuropathy by host and disease factors in the HIV outpatient study cohort. *Clin Infect Dis.* 2005;40(1):148–157.

33. Petratos S, Turnbull VJ, Papadopoulos R, Ayers M, Gonzales MF. Antibodies against peripheral myelin glycolipids in people with HIV infection. *Immunol Cell Biol.* 1998;76(6):535–541.

34. Moyle G. Mitochondrial toxicity: myths and facts. *J HIV Ther.* 2004;9(2):45–47.

35. McArthur JC, Brew BJ, Nath A. Neurological complications of HIV infection. *Lancet Neurol.* 2005;4(9):543–555.

36. Nagano I, Shapshak P, Yoshioka M, Xin K, Nakamura S, Bradley WG. Increased NADPH-diaphorase reactivity and cytokine expression in dorsal root ganglia in acquired immunodeficiency syndrome. *J Neurol Sci.* 1996;136(1–2):117–128.

37. Melzack R, Coderre TJ, Katz J, Vaccarino AL. Central neuroplasticity and pathological pain. *Ann N Y Acad Sci.* 2001;933:157–174.

38. Letendre S, McCutchan JA, Ellis RJ. Highlights of the 15th Conference on Retroviruses and Opportunistic Infections. Neurologic complications of HIV disease and their treatment. *Top HIV Med.* 2008;16(1):15–22.

39. Cherry CL, McArthur JC, Hoy JF, Wesselingh SL. Nucleoside analogues and neuropathy in the era of HAART. *J Clin Virol.* 2003;26(2):195–207.

40. Cherry CL, Wesselingh SL. Nucleoside analogues and HIV: the combined cost to mitochondria. *J Antimicrob Chemother.* 2003;51(5):1091–1093.

41. Hulgan T, Haas DW, Haines JL, et al. Mitochondrial haplogroups and peripheral neuropathy during antiretroviral therapy: an adult AIDS clinical trials group study. *AIDS.* 2005;19(13):1341–1349.

42. Simpson DM, Katzenstein D, Haidich B, et al. Plasma carnitine in HIV-associated neuropathy. *AIDS.* 2001;15(16): 2207–2208.

43. Moore RD, Wong WM, Keruly JC, McArthur JC. Incidence of neuropathy in HIV-infected patients on monotherapy versus those on combination therapy with didanosine, stavudine and hydroxyurea. *AIDS.* 2000;14(3):273–278.

44. Schifitto G, McDermott MP, McArthur JC, et al. Incidence of and risk factors for HIV-associated distal sensory polyneuropathy. *Neurology.* 2002;58(12):1764–1768.

45. Childs EA, Lyles RH, Selnes OA, et al. Plasma viral load and CD4 lymphocytes predict HIV-associated dementia and sensory neuropathy. *Neurology.* 1999;52(3):607–613.

46. Ances BM, Vaida F, Rosario D, et al. Role of metabolic syndrome components in HIV-associated sensory neuropathy. *AIDS.* 2009;23(17):2317–2322.

47. Banerjee S, McCutchan JA, Ances BM, et al. Hypertriglyceridemia in combination antiretroviral-treated HIV-positive individuals: potential impact on HIV sensory polyneuropathy. *AIDS.* 2006;25(2):F1–6.

48. Schifitto G, McDermott MP, McArthur JC, et al. Incidence of and risk factors associated for HIV-associated distal sensory polyneuropathy. *Neurology.* 2002;58:1764–1768.

49. Ellis RJ, Marquie-Beck J, Delaney P, et al. Human immunodeficiency virus protease inhibitors and risk for peripheral neuropathy. *Ann Neurol.* 2008;64(5):566–572.

50. Estanislao LB, Morgello S, Simpson DM. Peripheral neuropathies associated with HIV and hepatitis C co-infection: a review. *AIDS.* 2005;19(Suppl 3):S135–139.

51. Lopez OL, Becker JT, Dew MA, Caldararo R. Risk modifiers for peripheral sensory neuropathy in HIV infection/AIDS. *Eur J Neurol.* 2004;11(2):97–102.

52. Cettomai D, Kwasa J, Kendi C, et al. Utility of quantitative sensory testing and screening tools in identifying HIV-associated peripheral neuropathy in Western Kenya: pilot testing. *PLoS One.* 2010;5(12):e14256.

53. Cherry CL, Wesselingh SL, Lal L, McArthur JC. Evaluation of a clinical screening tool for HIV-associated sensory neuropathies. *Neurology.* 2005;65(11):1778–1781.

54. Ellis RJ, Evans SR, Clifford DB, et al. Clinical validation of the NeuroScreen. *J Neurovirol.* 2005;11(6):503–511.

55. Cornblath DR, Chaudhry V, Carter K, et al. Total neuropathy score: validation and reliability study. *Neurology.* 1999;53(8): 1660–1664.

56. Evans SR, Clifford DB, Kitch DW, et al. Simplification of the research diagnosis of HIV-associated sensory neuropathy. *HIV Clin Trials.* 2008;9(6):434–439.

57. Robinson-Papp J, Morgello S, Vaida F, et al. Association of self-reported painful symptoms with clinical and neurophysiologic signs in HIV-associated sensory neuropathy. *Pain.* 2010;151(3):732–736.

58. Herrmann DN, McDermott MP, Sowden JE, et al. Is skin biopsy a predictor of transition to symptomatic HIV neuropathy? A longitudinal study. *Neurology.* 2006;66(6): 857–861.

59. Zhou L, Kitch DW, Evans SR, et al. Correlates of epidermal nerve fiber densities in HIV-associated distal sensory polyneuropathy. *Neurology.* 2007;68(24):2113–2119.

60. Berger AR, Arezzo JC, Schaumburg HH, et al. 2′,3′-Dideoxycytidine (ddC) toxic neuropathy: a study of 52 patients. *Neurology.* 1999;43(2):358–362.

61. Hart AM, Wilson ADH, Montovani C, et al. Acetyl-l-carnitine: a pathogenesis based treatment for HIV-associated antiretroviral toxic neuropathy. *AIDS.* 2004;18(11): 1549–1560.

62. Breitbart W, Rosenfeld BD, Passik SD, McDonald MV, Thaler H, Portenoy RK. The undertreatment of pain in ambulatory AIDS patients. *Pain.* 1996;65(2–3):243–249.

63. Hahn K, Arendt G, Braun JS, et al. A placebo-controlled trial of gabapentin for painful HIV-associated sensory neuropathies. *J Neurol.* 2004;251(10):1260–1266.

64. Rosenstock J, Tuchman M, LaMoreaux L, Sharma U. Pregabalin for the treatment of painful diabetic peripheral neuropathy: a double-blind, placebo-controlled trial. *Pain.* 2004;110(3):628–638.

65. Simpson DM, McArthur JC, Olney R, et al. Lamotrigine for HIV-associated painful sensory neuropathies: a placebo-controlled trial. *Neurology.* 2003;60(9):1508–1514.

66. Lee K, Vivithanaporn P, Siemieniuk RA, et al. Clinical outcomes and immune benefits of anti-epileptic drug therapy in HIV/AIDS. *BMC Neurol.* 2010;10:44.

67. Simpson DM, Brown S, Tobias J. Controlled trial of high-concentration capsaicin patch for treatment of painful HIV neuropathy. *Neurology.* 2008;70(24):2305–2313.

68. Cherry CL, Affandi JS, Imran D, et al. Age and height predict neuropathy risk in patients with HIV prescribed stavudine. *Neurology.* 2010;73(4):315–320.

69. Abrams DI, Jay CA, Shade SB, et al. Cannabis in painful HIV-associated sensory neuropathy: a randomized placebo-controlled trial. *Neurology.* 2007;68(7):515–521.

70. Corless IB, Lindgren T, Holzemer W, et al. Marijuana effectiveness as an HIV self-care strategy. *Clin Nurs Res.* 2006;18(2):172–193.

71. Ellis RJ, Toperoff W, Vaida F, et al. Smoked medicinal cannabis for neuropathic pain in HIV: a randomized, crossover clinical trial. *Neuropsychopharmacology.* 2009;34(3): 672–680.

72. Galantino ML, Eke-Okoro ST, Findley TW, Condoluci D. Use of noninvasive electroacupuncture for the treatment of HIV-related peripheral neuropathy: a pilot study. *J Altern Complement Med.* 1999;5(2):135–142.

73. Littlewood RA, Vanable PA. Complementary and alternative medicine use among HIV-positive people: research synthesis and implications for HIV care. *AIDS Care.* 2008;20(8): 1002–1018.

74. Gale J. Physiotherapy intervention in two people with HIV or AIDS-related peripheral neuropathy. *Physiother Res Intl.* 2003;8(4):200–209.

75. Phillips KD, Skelton WD, Hand GA. Effect of acupuncture administered in a group setting on pain and subjective peripheral neuropathy in persons with human immunodeficiency virus disease. *J Altern Complement Med.* 2004;10(3):449–455.

76. Hamza MA, White PF, Craig WF, et al. Percutaneous electrical nerve stimulation: a novel analgesic therapy for diabetic neuropathic pain. *Diabetes Care.* 2000;23(3):365–370.

77. Harkless LB, DeLellis S, Carnegie DH, Burke TJ. Improved foot sensitivity and pain reduction in patients with peripheral neuropathy after treatment with monochromatic infrared photo energy-MIRE. *J Diabetes Complications.* 2006;20(2): 81–87.

78. Mill E, Wu P, Ernst E. Complementary therapies for the treatment of HIV: in search of the evidence. *Int J STD AIDS.* 2005;16(6):395–403.

79. Josephs JS, Fleishman JA, Gaist P, Gebo KA. Use of complementary and alternative medicines among a multistate, multisite cohort of people living with HIV/AIDS. *HIV Med.* 2007;8(5):300–305.

80. National Institutes of Health Concensus Conference. Acupuncture. *JAMA.*1998;280:1518–1524.

81. Shlay JC, Chaloner K, Max MB, et al. Acupuncture and amitriptyline for pain due to HIV-related peripheral neuropathy: a randomized controlled trial. *JAMA.* 1998; 280(18):1590–1595.

82. Shiflett SC, Schwartz GE. Statistical reanalysis of a randomized trial of acupuncture for pain reveals positive

effects as well as adverse treatment interactions on pain, attrition, and mortality. *Explore (NY).* 2010;6(4):246–55.

83. Shiflett SC, Schwartz GE. Effects of acupuncture in reducing attrition and mortality in HIV-infected men with peripheral neuropathy. *Explore (NY).* 2011;7(3):148–154.

84. Authier FJ, Gheradi RK. Peripheral neuropathies in HIV-infected patients in the era of HAART. *Brain Pathol.* 2003; 13(2):223–228.

85. Galatino ML, Shepard K, Krafft L, et al. The effect of group aerobic exercise and t'ai chi on functional outcomes and quality of life for persons living with aquired immunodeficiency syndrome. *J Altern Complement Med.* 2005;6:1085–1092.

86. Robins JL, McCain NL, Gray DP, Elswick RK, Walter JM, McDade E. Research on psychoneuroimmunology: tai chi as a stress management approach for individuals with HIV disease. *Appl Nurs Res.* 2006;19(1):2–9.

87. Field T. Tai Chi research review. *Complement Ther Clin Pract.* 2001;17(3):141–146.

88. Jam S, Imani A, Foroughi M, Alinaghi S, Koochak H, Mohraz M. The effects of mindfulness-bases stress reduction (MBSR) program in Iranian HIV/AIDS patients: a pilot study. *Acta Med Iran.* 2010;48(2):101–106.

89. Palmer R. Use of complementary therapies to treat patients with HIV/AIDS. *Nurs Stand.* 2008;22(50):35–41.

90. Head KA. Peripheral neuropathy: pathogenic mechanisms and alternative therapies. *Altern Med Rev.* 2006;11(4):294–329.

91. Cornblath DR, Hoke A. Recent advances in HIV neuropathy. *Curr Opin Neurol.* 2006;19(5):446–450.

92. Hasan S, Anwar M, Ahmadi K, Ahmed S, Choong C, See C. Reasons, perceived efficacy, and factors associated with complemenatary and alternative medicine use among Malaysian patients with HIV/AIDS. *J Altern Complement Med.* 2010;16(11):1171–1176.

93. Hoogbruin A. Complementary and alternative therapy (CAT) use and highly active antiretroviral therapy (HAART): current evidence in the literature, 2000–2009. *J Clin Nurs.* 2001;5(1):48–53.

94. Ho EY, Robles JS. Cultural resources for health participation: examining biomedicine, acupuncture, and massage therapy for HIV-related peripheral neuropathy. *Health Commun.* 2001; 26(2):135–146.

95. Cornblath DR, McArthur JC, Kennedy PG, Witte AS, Griffin JW. Inflammatory demyelinating peripheral neuropathies associated with human T-cell lymphotropic virus type III infection. *Ann Neurol.* 1997; 21(1):32–40.

GLOSSARY TERMS

A

Alcohol: Chronic alcohol ingestion is a common etiology of neuropathy (alcoholic polyneuropathy). The disorder is defined by a length-dependent axonal degeneration of motor and sensory neurons. Although the direct toxic effect of the alcohol on the nerve or the by-products of the metabolism of the alcohol are two potential etiologies, research has shown that vitamin deficiency as a complication of chronic alcohol ingestion plays a leading part in the development of the neuropathy.

Antiretroviral medications: The management of HIV/AIDS normally includes the use of multiple medications known as antiretroviral drugs in an attempt to control the infection. There are several classes of antiretroviral agents that act on different stages of the HIV life cycle. The use of multiple drugs that act on different viral targets is known as highly active antiretroviral therapy (HAART). HAART decreases the patient's total burden of HIV, maintains function of the immune system, and prevents the development of opportunistic infections that often lead to death. The National Institutes of Health (NIH) recommends offering antiretroviral treatment to all patients with HIV. Because of the complexity of selecting and following a regimen, the severity of the side effects, and the importance of compliance to prevent viral resistance, organizations such as the NIH emphasize the importance of involving patients in therapy choices and recommend analyzing the risks and the potential benefits to patients with low viral loads. Standard antiretroviral therapy (ART) consists of the combination of at least three antiretroviral (ARV) drugs for maximal suppression of HIV and to stop the progression of HIV disease. Huge reductions have been seen in rates of death and suffering when a potent ARV regimen is used, particularly in early stages of the disease. Expanded access to ART can also reduce HIV transmission at the population level, impact orphanhood, and preserve families.

Apoptosis: There are two methods of cellular death: necrosis and apoptosis. Necrosis occurs when a cell is damaged by an external force, such as a toxin, a medication, bodily injury, an infection, or an ischemic event such as a stroke. Necrosis results in an inflammatory cascade, which may cause additional local or systemic events. Apoptosis is often referred to as programmed cell death (PCD), and the process of apoptosis follows a controlled, predictable routine. When a cell is compelled to initiate the process of PCD, proteins called caspases go into action. Caspases break down the cellular components needed for survival, and they spur production of enzymes known as DNases, which destroy the DNA in the nucleus of the cell. An analogy is roadies breaking down the stage in an arena after a major band has been through town. The cell shrinks and sends out distress signals, which are answered by vacuum cleaners known as macrophages. The macrophages clean away the shrunken cells, leaving no trace, so these cells have no chance to cause the damage that necrotic cells do.

Arsenic: Arsenic is a metallic compound known for its use as a poison in homicide and suicide, but toxicity may also occur as a result of low-level exposure from various sources including the smelting of ores to the manufacture of integrated circuits. In some areas, arsenic is a groundwater contaminant. Symptoms are dose dependent and include gastrointestinal disturbances, arrhythmia, hypotension, cognitive changes, and peripheral neuropathy.

Assessment: An assessment is a plan of care that identifies the specific needs of the client and how those needs will be addressed by the health care system. The assessment is developed by a correlative process: the systematic review of all health-related data including the subjective history provided by the patient, previous medical records, laboratory tests, radiological tests, and physical assessment; discussion with consultants;

mutual goal setting by the health providers and the patient; and knowledge of the effectiveness of the proposed interventions. Interventions may range from preventive to therapeutic to palliative.

B

Balance: Balance is the ability to maintain the body's center of mass within the base of support with minimal sway. Sway is a horizontal movement of the center of gravity when a person is standing stationary. Maintaining balance requires coordinated input from the visual, somatosensory (kinesthetic/proprioceptive), and vestibular systems. Impairments of any of these systems results in decreased balance.

Behavior therapy: Behavior therapy is a broad term that refers to either psychosocial or behavior analytical intervention or a combination of the two therapies. In the broadest sense, the methods focus on just behaviors or behaviors in combination with thoughts and feelings. Behavior therapy consists of three disciplines: applied behavioral analysis, habit reversal training, and cognitive-behavior therapy. Applied behavioral analysis focuses on operant conditioning in the form of positive and negative reinforcement. Habit reversal training uses interventions to decrease habit-like behaviors. Cognitive-behavior therapy focuses on the thoughts and feelings behind mental health diagnoses with treatment plans in psychotherapy to remediate the issues.

Burner: A burner is also often referred to as a "stinger." A burner is a common nerve injury resulting from trauma to the neck and shoulder. Burners typically occur during a sporting competition. The injury is most often caused by traction or compression of the upper trunk of the brachial plexus or the fifth or sixth cervical nerve roots. Burners are typically transient, but they can cause prolonged weakness resulting in time loss from athletic participation. Also, they often recur. Treatment consists of restoring range of motion, improving strength, and providing protective equipment. Return to sports participation depends primarily on re-establishment of pain-free motion and full recovery of strength and functional status.

C

Capillary filtration coefficient: Urine formation results from glomerular filtration, tubular reabsorption, and tubular secretion. Rates at which different substances are excreted in urine represent the sum of three renal processes: (1) glomerular filtration, (2) reabsorption of substances from renal tubules into blood, and (3) secretion of substances from blood into renal tubules. This can be expressed mathematically as follows: Urinary excretion rate = filtration rate − reabsorption rate + secretion rate. Glomerular filtration rate (GFR) is determined by the sum of hydrostatic and colloid osmotic forces across the glomerular membrane, which gives the net filtration pressure and glomerular capillary filtration coefficient, K_{fc}. This can be expressed mathematically as follows: GFR = K_{fc} × net filtration pressure. Net filtration pressure is the sum of hydrostatic and colloid osmotic forces that either favor or oppose filtration across the glomerular capillaries.

Chronic kidney disease: Chronic kidney disease (CKD) is the progressive loss of kidney function over time. The primary function of the kidneys is to remove waste and excess water from the body. There may be no symptoms initially. The loss of function usually takes months or years to occur. It may be so slow that symptoms do not appear until kidney function is less than one tenth of normal. The final stage of CKD is called end-stage renal disease (ESRD). At this stage, the kidneys are no longer able to remove enough wastes and excess fluids from the body. The patient requires dialysis or a kidney transplant. CKD and ESRD affect more than 2 out of every 1,000 people in the United States. Diabetes mellitus and uncontrolled high blood pressure are the two most common causes of CKD. Many other diseases and conditions can damage the kidneys, including autoimmune disorders (e.g., systemic lupus erythematosus and scleroderma), congenital defects of the kidneys (e.g., polycystic kidney disease), toxic chemicals, glomerulonephritis, injury or trauma, renal calculi and infection, and ischemic kidney disease.

Classification of peripheral nerve injury: Classification of peripheral nerve injury assists in determining the severity, prognosis, and intervention strategy. Classification of nerve injury was described by Seddon in 1943 and by Sunderland in 1951. Generally, the lowest degree of nerve injury, in which the nerve remains intact, but there is a transient nerve conduction block, is called neurapraxia. The second degree of injury, in which the axon is damaged, but the surrounding connecting tissue remains intact, is called axonotmesis. The last degree of injury, in which both the axon and the connective tissue are damaged, is called neurotmesis.

Compression: Nerve compression, often called a trapped nerve or entrapment neuropathy, results from external compressive forces affecting a single nerve resulting in impairment of conduction of the afferent, efferent, and autonomic fibers. Nerve compression may result from trauma, congenital injury, abnormal development, overuse, repetitive strain, and disease.

Connective tissue disorders: Connective tissue disorders (often referred to as connective tissue diseases) results in injury to the target tissue. Connective tissue is any biological tissue that has an extensive extracellular matrix of supporting structures to facilitate function and protection. Some connective tissue disorders are heritable, whereas others are acquired. Most autoimmune diseases have a connective tissue component.

Contracture: A contracture is a permanent shortening of a contractile or noncontractile articular or nonarticular tissue. Contracture is usually in response to prolonged immobilization, disuse, hypertonic spasticity in a concentrated muscle area, congenital deformity, ischemia, or an inflammatory disease. When a contracture has matured, surgical release is often indicated. Physical therapy and occupational therapy interactions are very effective in the prevention of contracture.

Critical illness: Critical illness is the branch of medicine concerned with the diagnosis and management of life-threatening conditions requiring sophisticated and invasive monitoring. Examples include respiratory compromise requiring ventilator support, acute renal failure, and acute cardiac arrhythmia. Prolonged enforced bed rest often accompanies critical illness.

Critical illness myopathy: Critical illness myopathy (CIM) is a syndrome of widespread muscle weakness and neurological dysfunction that can develop in critically ill patients on prolonged bed rest. CIM is often distinguished largely on the basis of specialized electrophysiological testing or muscle and nerve biopsy, and its causes are unknown, although they are thought to be a possible neurological manifestation of systemic inflammatory response syndrome. Major risk factors include administration of intravenous corticosteroids and neuromuscular junction blocks. Previously a defined entity, CIM is now considered to be part of a larger diagnostic category referred to as critical illness myopathy/polyneuropathy.

Critical illness polyneuropathy: Previously a defined entity, critical illness polyneuropathy is now considered to be part of a larger diagnostic category referred to as critical illness myopathy/polyneuropathy.

D

Demyelination: Demyelination is a process resulting from a demyelinating disease. A demyelinating disease is any disease of the nervous system in which the myelin sheath of neurons is damaged. Demyelination impairs the conduction of signals in the affected nerves, causing impairment in sensation, motor control, autonomic regulation, cognition, or other functions depending on which nerves are involved. Demyelination describes the effect of the disease, rather than its cause; some demyelinating diseases are caused by genetics, some are caused by infectious agents, some are caused by autoimmune reactions, and some are caused by unknown factors.

Diabetes: Diabetes mellitus is a group of chronic metabolic diseases in which there are high levels of glucose in the blood as a result of the pancreas not supplying sufficient insulin or because cells do not respond to insulin that is produced. There are three main types of diabetes: gestational diabetes, type 1 diabetes mellitus, and type 2 diabetes mellitus. Untreated or undertreated diabetes can result in many complications, including diabetic ketoacidosis, nonketotic hyperosmolar coma, cardiovascular disease, chronic and acute kidney disease, retinopathy, stroke, and a spectrum of peripheral neuropathies.

Diagnostic testing: Diagnostic testing is a process of using valid and reliable procedures to confirm the presence of a disease, to rule out a disease, or to screen for a disease. The diagnostic journey is often begun with "screening" tests—tests that broadly evaluate for the presence of abnormalities but are typically not diagnostic. Screening tests are followed by specific tests and measures with a high sensitivity or specificity to rule in or rule out specific disease processes.

Disability and health: Persons with and without disability may be healthy and well. Disability is an umbrella term that includes impairments, activity limitations, and participation restriction. Impairment is a problem in body function or structure. An activity limitation is a difficulty encountered by an individual in executing a task or action. A participation restriction is a problem experienced by an individual in involvement in life situations and relationships. Disability is a complex phenomenon, reflecting an interaction between features of a person's body and features of the society in which the person lives. Health is the level of metabolic and functional efficiency of a living being; it is intrinsic to the organism.

Distal symmetrical polyneuropathy: Distal symmetrical polyneuropathy (DSP) is the most common form of peripheral neuropathy, a disorder of the peripheral nervous system affecting more than 20 million Americans. DSP is the most common type of peripheral neuropathy in people with HIV disease. It is characterized by paresthesia, motor neuropathy, and sensory neuropathy especially in the hands and feet.

Dynamic splint: A dynamic splint is any splint that incorporates springs, elastic bands, hydraulics, or other materials to produce a constant active force to counteract inherent resistance in a biological tissue.

E

Electrical stimulation: Electrical stimulation is the therapeutic use of electricity to decrease pain, improve range of motion, increase strength, improve coordination, normalize tone, assist with wound healing, and decrease edema. By varying the rate, amplitude, duration, waveform, and type of current, practitioners are able to elicit numerous physiological effects to improve healing.

Electromyography: Electromyography (EMG) is a technique for evaluating and recording the electrical activity produced by skeletal muscles during rest, minimal contraction, and maximal contraction. EMG is performed using an instrument called an electromyograph, which consists of recording electrodes, an amplifier, and an oscilloscope, to produce a record called an electromyogram. An electromyograph detects the electrical potential generated by muscle cells when these cells are electrically or neurologically activated. The signals can be analyzed to detect medical abnormalities, activation level, or recruitment order or to analyze the biomechanics of human or animal movement. Often EMG is used to describe the entire diagnostic process for nerve or muscle injury. Tests in addition to EMG include nerve conduction velocity tests and somatosensory tests. To avoid ambiguity, a better term to describe the diagnostic procedure is electroneurodiagnostic testing.

Endoneurium: The innermost layer of connective tissue in a peripheral nerve, forming an interstitial layer around each individual fiber outside the neurolemma, is the endoneurium. The matrix of tightly bound connective tissue also contains capillaries, mast cells, Schwann cells, and fibroblasts. The endoneurium appears to have two primary functions: to maintain the endoneurial space and fluid pressure—a homeostatic nerve fiber environment. A slightly positive pressure is maintained within the endoneurial tube. The collagen within the endoneurial tube is primarily longitudinal, evidence supporting the fact that the endoneurium assists with protecting the neuron from tensile challenges.

Epineurium: The epineurium, a loose connective tissue, is subdivided into internal and external components. The internal epineurium is the base collagenous tissue that physically separates the fascicles. It provides two basic functions: assisting the external epineurium in providing truncal protection from compressive forces and, more importantly, facilitation of gliding between the fascicles. As nerves stretch and rebound, fascicles glide within the base collagen matrix of the nerve trunk. There is a direct relationship between the diameter of the nerve and the volume of epineurium. There is also greater epineurium content in peripheral nerves as they cross joints and as they pass under or near fibrous bands, such as the flexor retinaculum at the wrist. The external epineurium surrounds the nerve trunk and provides protection from compressive and tensile forces.

Evaluation: The use of validated tests and measures with high sensitivity and specificity to rule in, rule out, or add to the differential diagnosis list begun during the clinical scripting process.

F

Fall prevention: Fall prevention modalities are evidence-based interventions that decrease fall risk. These include, but are not limited to, somatosensory rehabilitation, vestibular therapy, biomechanic/postural modification, visual acuity maximization, home modifications, strengthening, and education.

Fall prevention program: A fall prevention program uses evidence-based medicine and best practice designation to assist communities and individuals with reducing fall risk. Fall prevention programs range from individual consultations, assessments, and interventions to community-wide educational programs targeting specific cohorts at risk for falls.

Fall risk assessment: Fall risk assessment is the use of validated fall risk assessment tools to determine an individual's risk of falling. If the benchmark for fall risk is met, referral is made to a fall prevention program, and fall prevention modalities are prescribed.

Fibrosis: Fibrosis is the formation of excess fibrous connective tissue in an organ or tissue. Fibrosis is a hallmark event of the inflammation cascade. Initiated by trauma and regulated by cytokine concentration, excessive and aberrant tissue along with angiogenesis occurs at the site of injury. Fibrosis may occur intrinsic or extrinsic to the nerve. Intrinsic fibrosis may lead to adaptive shortening, and extrinsic fibrosis may lead to aberrant connections between the nerve and the adjacent structures.

F wave: When a motor nerve is stimulated and the electrical response of a muscle that it innervates is displayed on an oscilloscope, several responses can be observed. The initial response is the largest in amplitude and is termed the compound muscle action potential (CMAP). After the CMAP, several smaller responses are seen. These are called F waves. Action potentials in the motor nerve fibers that are caused by electrical stimulation travel in two directions. The action potentials that travel directly from the point of stimulation to the muscle elicit the CMAP. Some action potentials travel in the other direction on the nerve fibers, all the way to the motor neuron cell bodies in the spinal cord. These action potentials then travel back down to the nerve fibers to stimulate the muscles a second time, after a brief delay. F waves are called late responses because they are responses that occur later than the CMAP.

G

Gestational diabetes: Gestational diabetes is a condition in which a pregnant woman with no prior diagnosis of diabetes exhibits higher than expected concentrations of blood glucose. Gestational diabetes is a disease of the insulin receptors, most likely related to factors such as the presence of human placental lactogen that interferes with susceptible insulin receptors. Women with gestational diabetes have an increased risk of developing preeclampsia, delivery by cesarean section, delivering macrosomal infants, and developing type 2 diabetes.

Glomerular filtration rate: Glomerular filtration rate (GFR) is the volume of fluid filtered from the renal glomerular capillaries into Bowman's capsule per unit time. GFR is equal to the clearance rate when any solute is freely filtered and is neither reabsorbed nor secreted by the kidneys. The rate measured is the quantity of the substance in the urine that originated from a calculable volume of blood. Relating this principle to an equation, for the substance used, the product of urine concentration and urine flow equals the mass of substance excreted during the time that urine has been collected. This mass equals the mass filtered at the glomerulus because nothing is added or removed in the nephron. Dividing this mass by the plasma concentration gives the volume of plasma from which the mass must have originally come and the volume of plasma fluid that has entered Bowman's capsule within the aforementioned period of time. The GFR is typically recorded in units of volume per time (e.g., milliliters per minute [mL/min]). Several different techniques are used to calculate or estimate GFR (GFR or eGFR). The following formula applies to GFR calculation only when it is equal to the clearance rate: GFR = urine concentration × urine flow/ plasma concentration.

Guillain-Barré syndrome: Guillain-Barré syndrome is an acute polyneuropathy that affects the peripheral nervous system and spares the central nervous system. Hallmarks including ascending lower motor neuron paralysis with subtle sensory changes and pain more distal than proximal. Autonomic dysfunction is often present. The disease may be life-threatening especially if the respiratory muscles are compromised. Diagnosis is made by the clinical picture, cerebrospinal fluid analysis, and electroneurodiagnostic studies. The etiology is unknown, but the disorder is usually precipitated by a viral or bacterial illness. Treatment includes intravenous immunoglobulins and plasmapheresis, and the outcome is usually good.

H

Hemodialysis: The two main types of dialysis are hemodialysis and peritoneal dialysis. Dialysis removes wastes and excess water from the blood in different ways. Hemodialysis functions to remove wastes and water by circulating the blood outside the body through an external filter, called a dialyzer, that contains a semipermeable membrane. The blood flows in one direction, and the dialysate flows in the opposite direction. The countercurrent flow of the blood and dialysate maximizes the concentration gradient of solutes between the blood and dialysate, which helps to remove additional urea and creatinine from the blood. The concentrations of solutes (e.g., potassium, phosphorus, urea) are undesirably high in a patient with kidney disease but low or absent in the dialysis solution. Constant replacement of the dialysate ensures that the concentration of undesired solutes is kept low on this side of the membrane. The dialysis solution has levels of minerals such as potassium and calcium that are similar to their natural concentration in healthy blood. For another solute, bicarbonate, the dialysis solution level is set at a slightly higher level than in normal blood, to encourage diffusion of bicarbonate into the blood to act as a pH buffer to neutralize the metabolic acidosis that is often present. The levels of the components of dialysate are typically prescribed by a nephrologist according to the needs of the individual patient. In peritoneal dialysis, wastes and water are removed from the blood inside the body using the peritoneal membrane as a natural semipermeable membrane. Wastes and excess water move from the blood, across the peritoneal membrane, and into a dialysis solution called dialysate.

Hepatitis: Hepatitis refers to three disorders that affect the liver. Hepatitis A virus is found in the stool of persons with hepatitis A and is a short-lived infection. Most cases resolve within weeks or months, but some may have relapsing symptoms for up to 9 months. Patients rarely develop acute liver failure. Hepatitis A is spread by contact, often by putting something in the mouth that has been in contact with infected stool. Hepatitis A may also be spread by eating fruits or vegetables contaminated during handling, eating contaminated fish or

shellfish, or drinking contaminated water. Hepatitis B virus may result in an acute or chronic infection. Transmission of the virus is typically through sexual contact, sharing of needles for intravenous drug abuse with an infected person, tattooing, and sharing personal items such as toothbrushes with an infected person. Chronic hepatitis B can lead to liver damage. The hepatitis B vaccine is the best way to prevent infection. Hepatitis C infection is caused by hepatitis C virus (HCV). Virus transmission is similar to hepatitis B infection. Most persons with HCV have no symptoms. Long-term complications include cirrhosis and the need for a liver transplant. HCV infection is often associated with cryoglobulinemia. Peripheral neuropathy (PN) is a relatively common complication of cryoglobulinemia associated with HCV infection, and it is thought to be attributable to nerve ischemia. PN has been reported in only a few patients with HCV and cryoglobulinemia. The finding of HCV RNA in nerve biopsy specimens has suggested a possible direct role of HCV in the pathogenesis of PN.

Highly active antiretroviral therapy: Highly active antiretroviral therapy (HAART) is the name given to aggressive treatment regimens used to suppress HIV viral replication and the progression of HIV disease. The usual HAART regimen combines three or more different drugs, such as two nucleoside reverse transcriptase inhibitors (NRTIs) and a protease inhibitor, two NRTIs and a nonnucleoside reverse transcriptase inhibitor, or other such combinations. HAART regimens have been proven to reduce the amount of

active virus and in some cases can reduce the number of active virus until it is undetectable by current blood testing techniques.

Human immunodeficiency virus (HIV): HIV is a slowly replicating retrovirus that causes acquired immunodeficiency syndrome (AIDS). AIDS is a progressive failure of the immune system, allowing cancers and opportunistic infections to develop and thrive. HIV infection is spread through needle sharing and the transfer of blood or blood products, semen, pre-ejaculate, vaginal fluid, and breast milk.

Hypothesis-Oriented Algorithm for Clinicians (HOAC): Originally developed by Rothstein and Enternach (Rothstein JL, Enternach JL. The hypothesis-oriented algorithm for clinicians: a method for evaluation and treatment planning. *Phys Ther.* 1986;66:1388–1394), the HOAC is designed to aid practitioners in clinical decision making and patient management. The HOAC consists of two parts: a sequential guide to evaluation and treatment planning and a branching program used for re-evaluation and a systematic measure of intervention effectiveness. The HOAC requires the clinician to state a hypothesis list (differential diagnoses) and use diagnostic testing to rule in, rule out, or add to the hypothesis list.

I

Immobilization: Immobilization is the process of holding a joint or bone in place with a splint, cast, or brace. The purpose of immobilization is to prevent injury or to prevent movement to facilitate healing.

Infection: Infection is the invasion of body tissues of a host organism by disease-causing organisms such as bacteria, prions, viruses, viroids, parasites, and fungi. Many infectious organisms may lead to the complication of peripheral neuropathy.

Inflammation: Inflammation (from the Latin "to ignite or set afire") is part of the inflammatory cascade affecting vascularized tissues as a response to trauma, infection, illness, or repetitive injury. The cardinal signs of inflammation are pain, warmth, rubor, edema, and loss of function. When a tissue is traumatized, macrophages, monocytes, dendritic cells, histiocytes, Kupffer cells, and mastocytes release potent inflammatory mediators, which initiate the inflammatory cascade. These mediators facilitate vasodilation, angiogenesis, the laying down of fibrous tissue, and vascular permeability. They also mediate the release of bradykinin and other mediators that increase the sensitivity to pain.

Inflammatory demyelinating polyradiculopathy: Inflammatory demyelinating polyradiculopathy, also called chronic inflammatory demyelinating polyradiculopathy (CIDP), is a neurological disorder characterized by progressive weakness and impaired sensory function in the legs and arms. The disorder, which is sometimes called chronic relapsing polyneuropathy, is caused by damage to the myelin sheath (the fatty covering that wraps around and protects nerve fibers) of the peripheral nerves. Although it can occur at any age and in both genders, CIDP is more common in young adults and in men. It often manifests with tingling or numbness (beginning in the toes and fingers), weakness of the arms and legs, loss of deep tendon reflexes (areflexia),

fatigue, and abnormal sensations. CIDP is closely related to Guillain-Barré syndrome, and it is considered the chronic counterpart of that acute disease. Treatment for CIDP includes corticosteroids such as prednisone, which may be prescribed alone or in combination with immunosuppressant drugs. Plasmapheresis and intravenous immunoglobulin therapy are effective. The course of CIDP varies widely among individuals. Some may have a bout of CIDP followed by spontaneous recovery, whereas others may have many bouts with partial recovery in between relapses. The disease is a treatable cause of acquired neuropathy, and early initiation of treatment to prevent loss of nerve axons is recommended. However, some individuals are left with residual numbness or weakness.

Insulin: Insulin is produced by the beta cells of the pancreas and is the hormone responsible for regulating carbohydrate and fat metabolism and ultimately the concentration of glucose in the blood. When control of insulin fails, diabetes mellitus develops.

International Classification of Functioning: The International Classification of Functioning, Disability, and Health, known more commonly as ICF, is a classification of health and health-related domains. These domains are classified from body, individual, and societal perspectives by means of two lists: a list of body functions and structure and a list of domains of activity and participation. Because an individual's functioning and disability occur within a context, the ICF also includes a list of environmental factors. The ICF is the framework of the World Health Organization for measuring health and

disability at individual and population levels. The ICF was officially endorsed by all 191 WHO Member States in the Fifty-fourth World Health Assembly on May 22, 2001 (resolution WHA 54.21).

Intervention: When a valid diagnosis has been established, interventions (therapeutic modalities and treatments) determined by the evidence and clinical expertise are employed to remediate the impairment. The effectiveness of the intervention is determined by an outcome measure.

L

Laboratory testing: Laboratory testing is part of the diagnostic process to rule in, rule out, or add to the differential diagnosis list. Laboratory tests may be considered screening (nondiagnostic), such as complete blood count and sedimentation rate, or diagnostic, such as culture and sensitivity and enzyme immunoassay test for syphilis.

Lead: Lead toxicity is a leading cause of neuropathy in children but may occur in persons of all ages. Exposure is through ingestion and inhalation. The most common sources of toxicity are from paint in homes built between 1920 and 1970 and occupational settings such as battery manufacturers, auto radiator refurbishing, silver refining, and home demolition. Neuropathy is typically more motor than sensory and more distal than proximal. There may be associated cognitive loss, abdominal pain, headache, fatigue, and anemia.

Lower motor neuron: As a method of classification of nerve injury and nerve injury prognosis, motor nerves are considered upper or lower motor neurons. Lower motor neurons are typically the final neuron in the pathway from the motor cortex to the target muscle. Injury to the lower motor neuron results in flaccid paralysis, hypoactive deep tendon reflexes, and hypotonus. Examples of lower motor neuron disease include Guillain-Barré syndrome, polio, carpal tunnel syndrome, and L1 root lesion.

Lyme disease: Lyme disease is caused by a bite from the blacklegged tick, which infects the host with the bacterium *Borrelia burgdorferi*. The tick becomes infected by biting mice or deer that are infected with Lyme disease. The first reported case was in Old Lyme, Connecticut, in 1975. Stage I is where the infection is localized to the bite area. Symptoms are minimal but may include a "bull's-eye" expanding rash at the site of the tick bite. Stage II is called early disseminated Lyme disease, and symptoms may include chills, malaise, itching, articular and muscle pain, arrhythmia, and paralysis of the bulbar musculature. Stage III is called late disseminating Lyme disease, and symptoms include abnormal muscle synergies, dysarthria, motor neuropathy, and disseminated sensory neuropathy.

M

Macronutrient: Three primary macronutrients are defined as being the classes of chemical compounds consumed in the largest quantities by humans and that provide bulk energy. These are protein, fat, and carbohydrate. Carbohydrates include starches and simple and complex sugars. Proteins are foods that contain the standard amino acids. Fats include saturated fats, monounsaturated fats, polyunsaturated fats, and essential fatty acids. Failure to meet macronutrient needs may lead directly or indirectly to peripheral neuropathy.

Manual therapy: Manual therapy, also known as manipulative therapy, is a physical intervention used primarily to treat neurological and musculoskeletal impairments to remediate pain and disability. The scope of manual therapy is typically defined by the profession using the practice (for legal purposes) and by individual state practice acts.

Mercury: Peripheral neuropathy from mercury exposure commonly involves distal latency sensory slowing for short-term exposure and motor slowing for long-term exposure. Central nervous system effects are very common. Mercury toxicities, once quite common, are now mostly limited to industrial accidents. There continues to be concern related to mercury in dental amalgams and preservatives such as thimerosal.

Mesoneurium: The mesoneurium is one of the connective tissues supporting peripheral nerve trunks. It is classified as loose and areolar and is the entry portal for many of the arteries that supply the vasa nervorum, the highly anastomosing venous and arterial network within the nerve trunk. The function of the mesoneurium is not fully understood; however, the "slippery" surface of the mesoneurium limits frictional forces with longitudinal and side-to-side movement of the nerve trunk against local structures. There may also be substantial "sliding" motion between the mesoneurium and the external epineurium facilitating the extensibility characteristics of nerve. The mesoneurium may also provide limited protection from compressive and tensile forces affecting the nerve trunk.

Minerals: Minerals, also known as dietary minerals, are common chemical elements required by living organisms. There are seven major minerals: calcium, phosphorus, potassium, sulfur, sodium, chlorine, and magnesium. An additional group of minerals are known as "trace" minerals, and this list includes cobalt, copper, zinc, and iron. Mineral deficiency may lead directly or indirectly to peripheral neuropathy.

Modality: A modality is a therapeutic intervention. Modalities include medications, manual therapy, exercise, physical interventions such as ultrasound or electrical stimulation, teaching, counseling, and functional retraining.

Motor nerve conduction: The motor nerve conduction test is part of the overall nerve conduction study (NCS). The NCS is a test commonly used to evaluate the function, especially the ability of electrical conduction, of the motor and sensory nerves of the human body. Nerve conduction velocity (NCV) is a common measurement made during this test. NCV often is used to mean the actual test, but this may be misleading because velocity is only one measurement in the test menu. Motor NCS are performed by electrical stimulation of a peripheral nerve and recording from a muscle supplied by this nerve. The time it takes for the electrical impulse to travel from the stimulation to the recording site is measured. This value is called the latency and is measured in milliseconds (ms). The size of the response, called the amplitude, is also measured. Motor amplitudes are measured in millivolts (mV). By stimulating in two or more different locations along the same nerve, the NCV across different segments can be determined. Calculations are performed using the distance between the different stimulating electrodes and the difference in latencies.

N

Neurodynamic tests: Neurodynamic tests or testing refers to a group of physical maneuvers to assess for passive insufficiency and adaptive shortening of neural tissue. Neural tissue may be shortened by the inflammatory cascade as a result of trauma or infection, intraneural or extraneural scarring, and aberrant tissue connecting the neural tissue to adjacent structures. Examples include the median nerve tension test, straight leg raise test, and Kernig test.

Neurolysis: Neurolysis refers to the degradation of nerve tissue from injury or disease; the therapeutic destruction of neural tissue via chemicals, surgery, or radiofrequency ablation to block nerve pathways temporarily or permanently to relieve pain or spasticity; or the surgical removal of extraneural scarring or perineural adhesions tethering neural tissue to adjacent structures.

Neuroma: Neuromas can be differentiated into neoplastic and nonneoplastic neuromas. Neoplastic neuromas are tumors involving neural tissue affecting the neurons of the central and the peripheral nervous systems. Neoplastic neuromas may be benign or malignant. Nonneoplastic neuromas are typically the result of acute or chronic injury to a nerve. Many neuromas occur after a surgical intervention. The injured nerve fibers form an area of ineffective, random, and unregulated nerve regeneration. They are often palpable and painful. Nonneoplastic neuroma treatment ranges from conservative therapies to surgical excision.

Neuropathies: Neuropathies are a group of diseases and disorders that either directly or indirectly result in damage to a nerve. Peripheral neuropathy refers to damage outside the central nervous system; central neuropathy refers to damage within the central nervous system. Neuropathies may involve one nerve (mononeuropathy) or many nerves (polyneuropathy). Neuropathies may involve the sensory, autonomic, and motor nerves.

Neuropathy: Neuropathy is damage to one or more nerves as a result of trauma, illness, repetitive strain, or infection, which leads to motor, sensory, and autonomic dysfunction. There are hundreds and perhaps thousands of causes of neuropathy. Some disorders result in local neuropathy, and some result in patterned or systemic neuropathy.

Nitrous oxide: Nitrous oxide, used as an anesthesia, industrial additive, and recreational drug, was reported in 1978 as a potential source of peripheral neuropathy. Most neuropathies currently reported secondary to nitrous oxide abuse are related to recreational usage. As a recreational drug, nitrous oxide may cause analgesia, depersonalization, de-realization, dizziness, euphoria, and sound distortion. Similar to other N-methyl-D-aspartate antagonists, nitrous oxide has been demonstrated to produce neurotoxicity in the form of Olney's lesions. With chronic use, a subacute degeneration of the spinal cord, as described in classic vitamin B_{12} deficiency, occurs. The posterior white columns are involved with loss of position and vibratory sense, ataxia, and occasionally Lhermitte sign. Motor tract involvement may also occur with weakness,

spasticity, fecal and urinary incontinence, and clonus.

Nutrient: A nutrient is a chemical, molecule, or compound that an organism requires to live and grow or a substance used in an organism's metabolism that must be taken in from its environment. Nutrients are used to build and repair tissues and regulate body processes and are converted to specific compounds, which are used as energy. Methods for nutrient intake vary, with animals and protists consuming foods that are digested by an internal digestive system; most plants ingest nutrients directly from the soil through their roots or from the atmosphere. Organic nutrients include carbohydrates, fats, proteins, and vitamins. Inorganic chemical compounds, such as dietary minerals, water, and oxygen, may also be considered nutrients. A nutrient is said to be "essential" if it must be obtained from an external source, either because the organism cannot synthesize it or because the organism produces insufficient quantities. Nutrients needed in very small amounts are micronutrients, and nutrients that are needed in larger quantities are called macronutrients. The effects of nutrients are dose dependent, and shortages are called deficiencies. Deficiencies in nutrients may lead to disease, which may directly or indirectly result in neuropathy.

Nutritional deficiency: Nutritional deficiency results from a shortfall of the intake of, or the compounds that are manufactured into, essential nutrients. Nutritional deficiency may lead to disease, which may directly or indirectly result in peripheral neuropathy.

O

Operant therapy: Operant therapy uses the principles of

operant conditioning (punishment and reward) to change behavior. Operant conditioning is based on the premise that reinforced behaviors tend to continue and behaviors not reinforced tend gradually to end.

Overuse: High-force, low-repetition and low-force, high-repetition movements above the injury threshold of tissue result in overuse injuries. Overuse injury may affect nerve, muscle, tendon, enthesis, ligament, and paratendon areas.

P

Pain modulation: Most, if not all, ailments of the body cause pain. Pain is interpreted and perceived in the brain. Pain is modulated by physical modalities, medication, and counseling. Two primary classes of medications work on the brain: analgesics and anesthetics. The term analgesic refers to a drug that relieves pain without loss of consciousness. The term central anesthetic refers to a drug that depresses the central nervous system. Central anesthesia is characterized by the absence of all perception of sensory modalities, including loss of consciousness without loss of vital functions. Physical modalities that modulate the perception of pain include heat, cold, massage, electrical stimulation, ultrasound, and laser. Counseling indirectly affects pain through the reduction of anxiety and the use of behavioral modification.

Parasite: A parasite resides in close relationship with its host and causes the host harm. The parasite depends on the host for its life functions. Many parasitic infections may result in the complication of peripheral neuropathy. An example is the flagellate protozoan *Trypanosoma cruzi,* which is translated to humans by an insect vector and results in Chagas disease.

Paresthesia: Paresthesia is a subjective sensation of tickling, tingling, burning, pricking, formication, hot, cold, or numbness of a person's skin. Paresthesia is often described by the patient as a feeling of "pins and needles" or of a limb "falling asleep." The manifestations of paresthesia may be transient or chronic. Paresthesia may be benign, secondary to a minor neurapraxia lesion, or a symptom of a much more serious injury or illness.

Passive movement: Passive movement is the movement of a tissue or tissue structure that is not directly caused by muscle contraction. Tissues are often differentiated into contractile or noncontractile tissues. By definition, when a noncontractile tissue lengthens or shortens, it is passive movement. The lengthening or shortening may be caused by gravity or inertia or indirectly by associated muscle contraction. When a muscle contracts, this is termed active motion.

Perineurium: Each fascicle is surrounded by a layered sheath known as the perineurium. The perineurium has three primary functions: to protect the endoneurial tubes from normal articular movement patterns; to protect the endoneurial tube from external trauma; and to serve as a molecular diffusion barrier, keeping certain potentially neurotoxic compounds away from the perineurial and endoneurial environment via the blood-nerve barrier and the perineurial diffusion barrier.

Peripheral nerve: Peripheral nerves are neurons and the associated connective sheath that are located outside the central nervous system (brain and spinal cord). The peripheral nervous system includes nerves related to sensation, motor control, and autonomic regulation. In contrast to the central nervous system, the peripheral nerves are typically not protected by bone. Peripheral nerves may be injured from various sources, including trauma, overuse, medication, toxins, radiation, congenital deformity, and vitamin deficiency.

Peripheral neuropathy: Peripheral neuropathy is transient or permanent damage to an autonomic, sensory, or motor neuron outside the central nervous system. The injury may be primary (direct trauma to a nerve—e.g., median neuropathy associated with carpal tunnel syndrome) or secondary (as a complication of a disease process—e.g., diabetes mellitus). Peripheral neuropathy may affect one nerve (mononeuropathy) or many nerves (polyneuropathy).

Physical agent: Physical agents or physical agent modalities (PAMs) have been a component of interventional physical therapy for decades. PAMs traditionally include therapeutic ultrasound, electrical stimulation, short wave diathermy, and light. PAMs work by transmitting energy into tissues to stimulate them in ways that are not possible with patient exercise or manual therapy techniques. Original research and systemic reviews have provided a large paradigm shift in the effectiveness and indication of PAMs. Most often, PAMs are adjunctive to a comprehensive plan of therapy care. They may be particularly effective in the earlier stages of the treatment plan for numerous conditions, including reducing pain and edema, encouraging wound healing, and encouraging muscle contraction. PAMs allow therapists to treat symptoms and facilitate the introduction of other therapy interventions to achieve more rapid functional gains. The introduction of externally powered prostheses, orthoses, and exoskeletons not only for therapeutic exercise but also to improve and maintain function has added to the PAM menu of offerings.

Positive psychology: Positive psychology is a newer branch of psychology that is used to complement and not replace traditional areas of psychology. Positive psychologists attempt to find and nurture genius and talent, rather than merely treating mental illness.

Postural compensation: Postural compensation is one of the goals of balance rehabilitation for patients with visual, vestibular, or somatosensory loss. Patients are instructed how to use the remaining balance function, to develop compensatory mechanisms to use those balance functions, and to identify efficient and effective postural movement strategies.

Postural control: Postural control is the ability to sustain the necessary background posture to carry out a skilled task efficiently, such as walking, running, dressing, reading, or handwriting. The ability to stabilize the trunk and neck underlies the ability to develop efficient eye and hand movements.

R

Renal blood flow: Renal blood flow is the volume of blood delivered to the kidneys per unit time. In humans, the kidneys together receive approximately 22% of cardiac output, amounting to 1.1 L/min in a 70-kg man. Renal blood flow is closely related to renal plasma flow, which is the volume of blood plasma delivered to the kidneys per unit time.

Repetitive and overuse athletic movements: Repetitive and overuse athletic motions, also known as repetitive strain injuries or work-related musculoskeletal disorders, are either high-repetition/low-force movements or low-repetition/high-force movements. Either type has the potential of incurring tissue injury resulting in the inflammatory cascade with the hallmark local and systemic impact.

S

Safe position: With regard to hand positioning, the safe position is also known as the intrinsic plus position. The purpose of immobilizing in this position is to allow the hand to rest in this position without developing as much stiffness as would occur if the digits were positioned differently. In the intrinsic plus position, the metacarpophalangeal joints are flexed at 60° to 70°, the interphalangeal joints are fully extended, and the thumb is in the fist projection. The wrist is held in extension at 10° less than maximal.

Scalene muscle: The scalene muscles (from the Greek meaning "uneven") are a group of three pairs of muscles in the lateral neck: anterior, middle, and posterior scalene muscles. They originate on the transverse processes of C2–C7 and insert on the first and second ribs. The scalenes are innervated by the fourth through sixth spinal nerves. Together, they elevate the first and second ribs; ipsilaterally laterally flex the neck; contralaterally rotate the neck; and, acting bilaterally, flex the neck. Because of the intimate relationship with the subclavian vessels and brachial plexus, pathology related to the scalenes and their first rib insertion (scalene triangle) has been implicated in the development of neurogenic, venous, and arterial thoracic outlet syndrome.

Screening: The diagnostic process of ruling in, ruling out, or adding to the differential diagnosis list with the aim of determining the correct diagnosis often begins with screening tests. Screening tests are nondiagnostic for a particular disease but are capable of ruling in or out large classes of disease.

Sensory nerve conduction: The motor nerve conduction test is part of the overall nerve conduction study (NCS). The NCS is a test commonly used to evaluate the function, especially the ability of electrical conduction, of the motor and sensory nerves of the human body. Nerve conduction velocity (NCV) is a common measurement made during this test. NCV often is used to mean the actual test, but this may be misleading because velocity is only one measurement in the test menu. Sensory NCS are performed by electrically stimulating a peripheral nerve and recording from a purely sensory portion of the nerve, such as distally on a finger or toe. The recording electrode is the more proximal of the two electrodes. Similar to motor studies, sensory latencies are on the scale of milliseconds. Sensory amplitudes are much smaller than motor amplitudes, usually in the microvolt (μV) range. The sensory NCV is calculated based on the latency and the distance between the stimulating and recording electrodes.

Serial casting: Serial casting is a noninvasive procedure that helps children and adults improve specific joint range of motion to allow improved performance of daily activities. Serial casting is a process in which a well-padded cast is used to provide a mild extrinsic force to a restricted joint in a specific direction to improve range of motion. The cast is applied and removed on a frequent basis. Each cast gradually increases the range of motion in the affected joint.

Seronegative spondyloarthropathies: Also referred to seronegative spondyloarthritis, seronegative spondyloarthropathies are a group of related diseases that have an inflammatory component but are negative for rheumatoid factor. These diseases have a common spectrum of signs and symptoms including a relation to HLA-B27, an inflammatory axial/articular arthritis, oligoarthritis, a hereditary component, and enthesitis. Examples include psoriatic arthritis and Reiter syndrome.

Somatosensation: Somatosensation includes the components of the central and peripheral nervous systems that receive and interpret sensory information from organs in the joints, ligaments, muscles, and skin. This system processes information about the length, degree of stretch, tension, and contraction of muscles; pain; temperature; pressure; and joint position and provides real-time information related to joint position and muscle length during motion and at rest. Impairment of somatosensation may result in fall risk.

Static splint: A static splint is indicated to restrict active and passive range of motion of a joint to facilitate healing and prevent further injury. Materials used in the fabrication of static splints tend to be rigid and include steel, aluminum, high-density plastics, and plaster.

Subclavian vessels: The subclavian vessels consist of the subclavian artery and the subclavian vein. Because of the proximity to the first rib and scalene muscles, these vessels may be injured acutely or chronically secondary to trauma or cervical spine and glenohumeral overuse syndromes.

T

Tension: Tension neuropathy is the result of a longitudinal pulling force typically caused by aberrant, forceful, and excessive range of motion of an articular joint on a peripheral nerve. If the tensile forces are greater than the elastic ability of the nerve, deformation results leading to injury of the functional and connective tissue components of the peripheral nerve, resulting in loss of afferent, efferent, and autonomic nerve fiber conduction. Tension is the opposite of compression. Slackening is the reduction of tension.

Thallium: Thallium toxicity has been noted to produce dysesthesia, allodynia, distal muscle weakness, and sensory impairment. Pesticides and rodenticides were historically common sources of thallium poisoning, but these are no longer commonly used. Although industrial occupations may result in exposure to thallium, this is usually a low-level and chronic exposure. Consumption of contaminated food and water continues to be a common source of thallium exposure. The classic sign of thallium intoxication is alopecia.

Thoracic outlet syndrome: Thoracic outlet syndrome is a constellation of signs and symptoms related to an impingement of the brachial plexus, subclavian artery, or subclavian vein between the cervical spine intervertebral foramina and the insertion of the pectoralis minor on the humerus. Injury may be secondary to trauma, overuse, congenital abnormality, tumor, fracture, or maladaptive posture.

Three-point pressure: The controls incorporated in orthotic systems are based on three-point force systems that affect alignment by controlling two adjacent skeletal segments. The corrective force is located on the convex side of the curve at the joint addressed. Two counteractive forces are positioned on the opposite side above and below the corrective force. Increasing the distance of the counteractive forces from the corrective force increases the lever arms and the effectiveness. Based on the principle of pressure = total force/area of force application, the objective is to distribute the forces over a larger area to decrease the resultant pressures, which may result in skin breakdown. A well-fitting total contact orthosis that avoids bony prominences and uses an appropriate and effective three-point force system assists in achieving this objective.

V

Vasa nervorum: All peripheral nerves and the ganglia where the cell bodies of the autonomic nerves are located are surrounded by small-diameter blood vessels (arterioles and venules) known as vasa nervorum, which supply the blood necessary for the function of the neurons. All nerve trunks, from large ones such as the sciatic nerve to small ones such as the cavernous nerve, have their own vasa nervorum. The vasa nervorum of the peripheral nerve trunks can be divided into three groups: epineurial, perineurial, and endoneurial. Epineurial and perineurial blood vessels form a complex network known as the epineurial plexus. The epineurial plexus has prominent arteriovenous shunts, supplies the endoneurial vascular compartment, and is innervated by autonomic nerves such as sympathetic and peptidergic nerves. Injury to the vasa nervorum may result in ischemic (arterial) or compressive (venous) nerve fiber injury.

Vasculitic disorders: Vasculitic disorders, often referred to as the vasculitides, refer to a group of disorders that target the vascular system: lymph, arteries, and veins. A common variable of these disorders is the frequent association with common antibodies. Classification of disorders may be by etiology, location, or type or size of the blood vessel impacted. Examples include temporal arteritis, Behçet syndrome, and Buerger disease.

Vitamin: A vitamin is an organic compound required by an organism as a vital nutrient. Any required organic chemical compound (or related set of compounds) is called a vitamin when it cannot be synthesized in sufficient quantities by an organism and must be obtained from the diet or environment. The term is conditional on the circumstances and on the particular organism. For example, vitamin C is a vitamin for humans but not for most other animals. Vitamins are classified by their biological and chemical activity, not their structure. Each "vitamin" refers to a number of vitamer compounds that all show the biological activity associated with a particular vitamin. Such a set of chemicals is grouped under an alphabetized vitamin "generic descriptor" title.

W

Wallerian degeneration: Wallerian degeneration is a process that results when a nerve fiber sustains an axonotmetic or neurotmetic injury secondary to compression, tension, or disease. The axon separated from the neuron's cell body degenerates distal to the injury. A related process known as wallerian-like degeneration occurs in many neurodegenerative diseases, especially diseases in which axonal transport is impaired. Wallerian degeneration occurs after axonal injury in both the peripheral nervous system and the central nervous system. It occurs in the axon stump distal to a site of injury and usually begins within 24 to 36 hours of a lesion, but the process may take 3 weeks. Before degeneration, distal axon stumps tend to remain electrically excitable. After degeneration, the distal end of the portion of the nerve fiber proximal to the lesion sends out sprouts toward the intact connective tissue, and these sprouts are attracted by growth factors produced by Schwann cells in the tubes. If a sprout reaches the tube, it grows into it and advances about 1 mm per day, eventually reaching and reinnervating the target tissue.

Appendix: Case Study Answers

Chapter 1: The Anatomy and Physiology of the Peripheral Nerve

1. d. Nerve
2. a. Axillary
3. c. Axonotmesis
4. b. Teres minor
5. c. 2 months

Chapter 4: Peripheral Neuropathy and Vasculitic, Connective Tissue, and Seronegative Spondyloarthropathic Disorders

1. d. All of the above
2. c. Electroneuromyogram
3. a. A functional wrist splint placing the wrist in a neutral radial/ulnar deviation posture
4. d. All of the above
5. a. Rheumatoid vasculitis

Chapter 5: Environmental Toxic Neuropathies

1. a. Ingesting lead-based paint
2. d. Poorly healing wounds
3. a. Amy's mother may also have lead intoxication and may have passed the high level of lead to Amy while Amy was in utero.
4. d. All of the above
5. d. All of the above

Chapter 6: Critical Illness Polyneuropathy

1. d. Urinary tract infection
2. d. All of the above
3. a. Electrodiagnostic studies

4. d. All of the above
5. c. Skin breakdown

Chapter 7: Diabetes Mellitus and Peripheral Neuropathy

1. b. Monofilament testing
2. d. Hemoglobin A_{1c}
3. c. Inability to sweat
4. a. Painful paresthesias
5. d. Ankle

Chapter 8: Peripheral Neuropathy and Infection

1. b. Lyme disease
2. a. Erythema migrans
3. b. *Borrelia burgdorferi*
4. d. All of the above
5. a. Antimicrobials

Chapter 9: Peripheral Neuropathy Associated With Nutritional Deficiency

1. a. Beriberi
2. d. Skin rash
3. c. Peripheral edema and congestive heart failure
4. b. Guillain-Barré syndrome
5. a. Wernicke-Korsakoff Syndrome

Chapter 10: Peripheral Neuropathy and Chronic Kidney Disease

1. d. All of the above
2. c. Electroneuromyogram of both upper extremities
3. a. Lack of lower extremity symptoms

4. d. All of the above
5. d. All of the above

Chapter 11: Medication-Induced Neuropathy

1. a. Medication-induced neuropathy is a common side effect of pharmaceutical intervention, the symptoms may have a great impact on the quality of life of the patient, and effective treatment may be difficult to attain.
2. d. All of the above
3. b. Peripheral neurons
4. d. All of the above
5. a. A tactile sensory neuropathy involving the hands and feet

Chapter 12: Electroneurodiagnostic Assessment and Interpretation

1. d. All of the above
2. a. Wrist
3. d. All of the above
4. a. Neurapraxia, neurotmesis, axonotmesis
5. a. Myotonia

Chapter 13: Laboratory Investigation of Suspected Peripheral Neuropathy

1. d. The therapist cannot, with the current information presented, rule out diabetes as a cause of the falls.
2. a. Hemoglobin A_{1c}
3. d. Complete blood count
4. b. Urinalysis
5. d. 3 months

Chapter 14: The Examination: Evaluation of the Patient With Suspected Peripheral Neuropathy

1. b. Yes, because the patient could have two unrelated diagnoses
2. a. Paint removal
3. a. Loss of balance, sensory disturbances of the hand and feet, cognitive impairments
4. c. Serum lead levels
5. d. All of the above

Chapter 15: Overview of Rehabilitation Intervention for Peripheral Nerve Injury

1. d. Develop a trusting patient-therapist collaborative relationship
2. d. Inability to work secondary to gait instability
3. c. Eighth grade
4. a. Hypothesis-oriented algorithm for clinicians
5. b. Control inflammation

Chapter 16: Manual Therapy Techniques for Peripheral Nerve Injuries

1. a. Weakness of the ipsilateral digiti minimi muscle
2. b. Electroneuromyography
3. b. Lumbar thrust maneuver
4. d. All of the above
5. c. Neurodynamic treatment techniques

Chapter 17: The Role of Physical Agents in Peripheral Nerve Injury

1. "Unfortunately, the evidence of the effectiveness of electrical stimulation in human studies is poor. There are more effective interventions we should try."
2. a. TENS and amitriptyline are more effective than TENS alone.
3. b. A 2007 review of ES neither supports nor refutes the use of ES for the preservation of functional sarcomeres in denervated muscle.
4. c. Although there is considerable evidence of the effectiveness of US promoting nerve regeneration in a rat model, there is no quality evidence of the effectiveness in humans.
5. b. Based on rat models and cellular models, LLLT is a promising agent as an intervention for nerve injury.

Chapter 18: Orthotic Intervention for Peripheral Neuropathy

1. d. Elbow positioning
2. d. Both a and b
3. b. Figure-of-eight harness
4. d. All of the above
5. d. All of the above

Chapter 19: Counseling and Behavior Modification Techniques for Functional Loss and Chronic Pain

1. d. All of the above
2. a. Operant therapy is an approach designed to address the gross motor and cognitive/subjective responses to clinical pain.
3. d. All of the above
4. d. All of the above
5. b. The behavior of the family

Chapter 20: Guillain-Barré Syndrome

1. a. Areflexia and progressive weakness
2. b. Electroneuromyogram
3. c. Plasmapheresis and IVIG therapy
4. d. All of the above
5. a. Pain

Chapter 21: Peripheral Nerve Injury in the Athlete

1. c. Refer Bill for further testing with a tentative diagnosis of axillary nerve injury
2. d. Stop pitching and begin shoulder strengthening exercise
3. a. Venous thoracic outlet syndrome (Pagett-Schroetter syndrome)
4. d. All of the above
5. c. Biceps

Chapter 22: Effects of Peripheral Neuropathy on Posture and Balance

1. c. Severe
2. b. Afferent peripheral neuropathy
3. a. Expected destabilizations as a result of movement of the body limbs
4. d. All of the above
5. a. Increased lateral sway during quiet stance

Chapter 23: Brachial Plexopathies

1. a. Subclavian artery
2. b. First rib and transverse process
3. d. Shoulder impingement

4. b. Raynaud's phenomenon
5. b. A supraclavicular pulsatile mass

Chapter 24: Entrapment Neuropathy in the Forearm, Wrist, and Hand

1. a. Ulnar
2. c. Ulnar nerve impingement at the olecranon fossa
3. c. Abductor digiti minimi
4. d. All of the above
5. b. Electroneuromyogram

Chapter 25: Entrapment Neuropathies in the Foot and Ankle

1. b. Morton's neuroma
2. c. A positive Tinel sign between the second and third metatarsal heads
3. d. Electrical stimulation
4. d. All of the above
5. d. Women often wear high-heeled shoes

Chapter 26: Fall Risk and Fall Prevention Strategies for Individuals With Peripheral Neuropathy

1. c. BBS
2. d. Wheeled walker
3. b. Rigidity, no confusion, resting tremor
4. d. TheraBand for strengthening the anterior tibialis and the gastrocnemius/soleus in the seated position
5. d. The BBS alone cannot determine the cause of fall risk.

Chapter 27: Peripheral Neuropathies in Individuals With HIV Disease

1. d. All of the above
2. d. Excellent with appropriate physical therapy
3. d. All of the above
4. d. All of the above
5. b. Referral to an herbalist for a prescription for St. John's wort.

INDEX